KT-386-798

THE ELEMENTS OF
Nursing

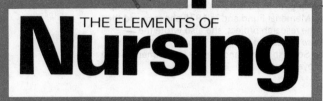

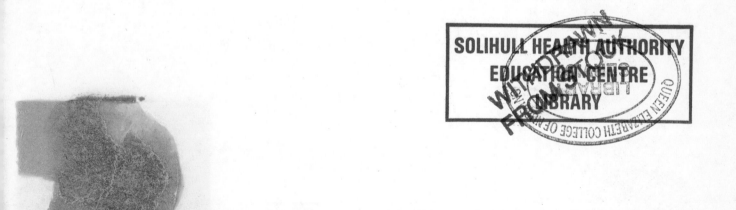

NANCY ROPER trained at the General Infirmary, Leeds, UK and later spent 15 years at the Cumberland Infirmary School of Nursing as Principal Tutor. In 1964 she became a self-employed writer. She is the editor of the *Churchill Livingstone Pocket Medical Dictionary*, *Churchill Livingstone Nurses Dictionary*, and *New American Pocket Medical Dictionary*; and the author of *Man's Anatomy, Physiology, Health and Environment* and *Principles of Nursing*. In 1970 she was awarded a fellowship from the Commonwealth Nurses' War Memorial Fund and in 1975 she received the MPhil degree for the thesis based on the research project; she also wrote the monograph *Clinical Experience in Nurse Education* (1976). From 1975–1978 she was Nursing Officer (Research) at the Scottish Home and Health Department. Since then she has continued as a self-employed author.

WINIFRED LOGAN is head of the Department of Health and Nursing Studies, Glasgow College of Technology, Scotland. She was Executive Director of the International Council of Nurses (ICN) from 1978–1980. She had already gained considerable knowledge and experience of nursing internationally, having worked or served as a consultant in Canada, the USA, Malaysia and Iraq. In 1971–1972 she acted as Chief Nursing Officer at the newly created Ministry of Health in Abu Dhabi. Prior to moving to the ICN she worked for 4 years at the Scottish Home and Health Department where she had responsibility for nursing education. She took to that post experience gained from a 12-year term of office, first as lecturer and latterly as senior lecturer, in the Department of Nursing Studies at the University of Edinburgh. She is an arts graduate of that university and did her basic nurse education at the Royal Infirmary of Edinburgh. She has served on various national committees associated with the General Nursing Council of Scotland, the Council for National Academic Awards, and the University Grants Committee.

ALISON TIERNEY is Director of the Nursing Research Unit in the Department of Nursing Studies at the University of Edinburgh, Scotland. From 1973–1980 she was a lecturer in the Department of Nursing Studies, a post which involved her in the development of the foundation nursing course for beginning students and in the clinical supervision of students at various stages of the integrated degree/nursing programme. She herself was one of the early graduates of that same programme. Her PhD degree was awarded for research undertaken in the field of mental handicap nursing while holding a Scottish Home and Health Department nursing research training fellowship (1971–1973). Dr Tierney is the editor of *Nurses and the Mentally Handicapped* (Wiley, 1983) and the author of a number of articles and chapters. She was a member of the course team which developed the Open University teaching package 'A systematic approach to nursing' (1984).

Nancy Roper, Winifred Logan and Alison Tierney are all gradutes of the University of Edinburgh. They came together in 1976 to work on the first edition of *The Elements of Nursing* which was published in 1980. Their second book *Learning to Use the Process of Nursing* was published in 1981. They edited a third book *Using a Model for Nursing* and it was published in 1983. In addition they have had published a number of journal articles concerned with the Roper, Logan and Tierney model for nursing, and bibliographical details are contained in Appendix 5, page 370.

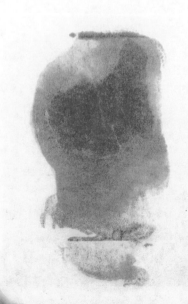

The authors can be contacted at their publisher's address:
Churchill Livingstone, 1–3 Baxter's Place, Leith Walk, Edinburgh, Scotland, EH1 3AF.
Telex 727511

THE ELEMENTS OF Nursing

NANCY ROPER
MPhil RGN RSCN RNT

WINIFRED W. LOGAN
MA DNS(Educ) RGN RNT

ALISON J. TIERNEY
BSc(Soc Sc-Nurs) PhD RGN

SECOND EDITION

Churchill Livingstone

EDINBURGH LONDON MELBOURNE AND NEW YORK 1985

CHURCHILL LIVINGSTONE
Medical Division of Longman Group UK Limited

Distributed in the United States of America by Churchill Livingstone Inc.,
1560 Broadway, New York, N.Y. 10036, and by associated companies,
branches and representatives throughout the world.

First edition 1980
Second edition 1985
  Reprinted 1986
  Reprinted 1987
  Reprinted 1988
  Reprinted twice 1989

ISBN 0-443-03028-6

British Library Cataloguing in Publication Data
Roper, Nancy
  The elements of nursing. — 2nd ed.
  1. Nursing
  I. Title   II. Logan, Winifred W.
  III. Tierney, Alison J.
  610.73   RT41

Library of Congress Cataloguing in Publication Data
'Roper, Nancy'
  The elements of nursing.
  Includes bibliographies and index.
  1. Nursing.   I. Logan, Winifred W.   II. Tierney, Alison J.   III. Title.
[DNLM: 1. Nursing Process. WY 100 R784e]
RT41.R724   1985   610.73   84-29342

Produced by Longman Singapore Publishers Pte Ltd.
Printed in Singapore.

Preface to the Second Edition

This second edition of *The Elements of Nursing* retains the format of the original text and, as before, is essentially for beginning nursing students. The fact that the first edition has been positively received, in particular because of its focus on a model for nursing (which incorporates the process of nursing), reassured us that there is still a need for an introductory text of this kind. However we wish to emphasise that this book is not intended as 'comprehensive'; the expectation is that it will be complemented by other nursing texts and literature from other disciplines such as human biology, psychology and sociology. Our extended use of references in this edition is intended to encourage students to read widely and, especially, to take account of research as a basis for nursing practice.

The contents of the book are basically as outlined in the preface of the first edition. Section 1, 'Nursing and health care', is still introductory but has been revised, updated and re-arranged.

In Section 2, the chapters on the 'Model of living' (Ch. 2) and the 'Model for nursing' (Ch. 6) have been rewritten for purposes of clarification and to incorporate refinements to the model which are the result of giving considerable further thought to our original ideas in the course of writing *Learning to Use the Process of Nursing* (1981), and of undertaking a project which is described in *Using a Model for Nursing* (1983). The middle chapters of Section 2—'Biological aspects of living' (Ch. 3), 'Developmental aspects of living' (Ch. 4) and 'Social aspects of living' (Ch. 5)—have been minimally revised and have been retained to provide beginning students with a brief overview of material which is relevant as a background to Section 3.

Section 3 consists of 12 chapters (Chs 7–18), one devoted to each of the 12 Activities of Living, the main focus of the model. All of these chapters have been substantially rewritten, obviously to update material but also to reflect the components of the model more clearly than in the first edition.

Section 4, consisting of one short chapter (Ch. 19), is new to this edition. One of the current major criticisms about nursing models is that although they may be of theoretical interest, there is difficulty in using them in the real world of nursing. This chapter therefore has been added to help readers to appreciate how the Roper/Logan/Tierney model can be applied in practice. To give some guidance for documentation, we discuss the proforma which developed out of the project of the third book *Using a Model for Nursing* (1983).

No one model can be perfect and no single text can possibly exhaust discussion of something as complex as a conceptual framework for nursing and its application to practice. We hope, however, that this new edition provides a clearer account of our model and a further analysis of those concepts which comprise the elements of nursing.

Edinburgh 1985   N.R. W.L. A.T.

Preface to the First Edition

It has been said and written scores of times that every woman makes a good nurse. I believe on the contrary, that the very elements of nursing are all but unknown.

FLORENCE NIGHTINGALE

We planned and wrote this book because of our conviction that the degree of complexity and specialisation of nursing today makes it more necessary than ever for the elements of nursing to be identified and understood. Today's nursing students right from the start of their education programme need to become familiar with those elements common to all branches of nursing and relevant to all patients.

Consequently we examined the core of knowledge required by nurses and we have presented it within a model for nursing which is based on a model of living. The model for nursing incorporates the process of nursing so that together they provide a conceptual framework for the book. It is hoped that this framework will assist learners to develop a way of thinking about nursing which will help them to provide effective and compassionate nursing for people of whatever age who have various problems and who are in different health care settings. In addition, as nursing experience is gained, this way of thinking should facilitate the acquisition of new and specialised knowledge.

In Section 1 the reader is encouraged to think about the meaning of health and illness and how a health care system develops within a country. Nursing's contribution to health care is examined and the section ends with a consideration of the educational preparation needed by today's nurses.

The two models—the model of living and the model for nursing—are described in Section 2. Both models focus on 12 Activities of Living (ALs): maintaining a safe environment; communicating; breathing; eating and drinking; eliminating; personal cleansing and dressing; controlling body temperature; mobilising; working and playing; expressing sexuality; sleeping; and dying. All Activities of Living have biological, developmental and social dimensions and so a chapter is devoted to each of these aspects of living within this section. Finally there is a discussion of the process of nursing, showing how this concept is used as a framework for the analysis of each of the Activities of Living.

This analysis of the 12 ALs makes up the 12 chapters in Section 3 of the book. In the first part of each chapter there is a description of the nature of the activity, the purpose of the activity, factors influencing the activity and body structure and function required for the activity. Guidelines are given on assessing an individual's performance of the activity. The second part of each chapter contains discussion of possible patients' problems associated with that AL. For example, among the problems discussed relating to the AL of eliminating are those arising from lack of privacy in the ward; dependence due to limited mobility or confinement to bed or psychological disturbance; urinary incontinence; urinary catheterisation; and anxiety associated with investigations of the urinary and defaecatory systems. Emphasis is placed on the problems as experienced by the patient, and related nursing activities are therefore presented as assisting the patient to solve, reduce or prevent problems which interfere with everyday living. Each chapter has a summary chart which shows how this problem-orientated approach is used in applying the process of nursing to the AL. Although a chapter has been devoted to each AL, in reality the activities are interrelated and it must be remembered that a problem with one can produce problems with any or all of the other ALs.

At the end of each chapter there are two lists, one of References and the other of Suggested Reading. Relevant research reports are included in both. Most of the listed articles and books contain references which will guide the reader who wishes to gain further information about a particular topic.

In the process of writing this book we were constantly clarifying and extending our thinking about nursing. All three of us feel that we now have a better understanding of the elements of nursing and a greater awareness of their complexity, which we hope we have conveyed to the readers of this book.

Edinburgh 1980
N.R. W.L. A.T.

Foreword to the First Edition

Professional practice is in constant need of review and refinement if it is to adapt to new demands and advances in knowledge. One of the most significant advances in nursing in recent years has been the move towards replacing ritualised and institutionalised approaches with those that are rationally planned and individualised.

The teaching of nursing in the past was often based on body systems, disease entities and procedures. The emphasis is now changing to one that concentrates on the essential nature of nursing action and the principles which underlie practice.

The authors of *The Elements of Nursing* have done a great deal to help us in this direction. They have given a model for nursing based on activities of living and incorporating the process of nursing. Components of the nursing function are analysed and guidelines are given for assessing the patient's functional abilities in each activity of living. A theoretical framework for assessment and nursing care evolves. The result is a unique amalgam of theory drawn from biological and behavioural sciences which should equip a nurse to function on a sound scientific basis.

The book begins with a quotation from Florence Nightingale:
'... the very elements of nursing are all but unknown.' The authors have accepted the professional challenge of those words and, 120 years later, they have done much to identify those elements of nursing which should help us towards rational, individualised nursing practice. I believe there is in their work a basis for innovation and improved quality of performance to which we all aspire.

January, 1980   McFarlane of Llandaff

Contents

Contents

SECTION **1**

Introduction

1

Nursing and health care

It has been said and written scores of times that every woman makes a good nurse. I believe on the contrary that the very elements of nursing are all but unknown.

Florence Nightingale (1859)

These words were written over a century ago but the profession is still refining its ideas about 'the elements' of nursing. This is not surprising. Nursing exists to serve society and as the conditions and needs of society have changed, practices have altered in response to the changes.

NURSING IN HEALTH AND ILLNESS

It must not be forgotten that sick people required and were given care long before nursing became an organised occupation; indeed, in the Western world until the end of the last century family members or domestic staff usually nursed the sick in their own homes and hospitals were used only for the pauper or the grossly mentally deranged. The family is the oldest and most used health care service in the world. Even now, in some countries, the family members are admitted to hospital with the patient, complete with bedding and cooking utensils while the 'trained' staff carry out specific treatments associated with the disease condition.

What is nursing?

Undoubtedly, however, during the last century nursing has been associated in the eyes of the public with care of the sick. And as nurses have become increasingly involved with the curative, technical treatments provided by medical staff they have come to occupy a strategic position. Nurses are the link between what are often stressful, complicated technical procedures associated with the disease condition and the maintenance of everyday bodily and mental functions which are so critical to the patient's comfort and so important to him as a person.

3

But nursing is not only associated with people who are ill.

Admittedly, looking back at the major professional developments in nursing in the Western world during the 20th century, it must be accepted that they have been associated mainly with the 'sickness' services. However knowledge about disease processes, developments in biological and social sciences, increasing sophistication in technology and a better-educated public have produced a new awareness about health care services in general, and there is increasing public interest in individual, family and community health. The hospital-based, disease-orientated health care system, and nursing within that system, is now being questioned. Nurses along with other health professionals are beginning to see the importance of putting increasing emphasis on maintaining health, preventing sickness, enhancing self-help and promoting maximum independence according to the individual person's capability. It is, therefore, difficult to define 'the elements' of nursing definitively when the needs and demands of society are in a state of flux and when the interface between health and illness is no longer so clearly defined. Before discussing nursing and the nurse's role in the health care team, it is useful to comment on changing concepts about health and illness.

If asked, most people would probably say that they are 'healthy' and that illness occurs only as brief isolated episodes in their lives. But what do they mean when they use these terms? Probably it is easier, first of all, to say something about illness. There is an abundant literature to indicate historical interest in conditions described as disease or illness.

What is illness?
From time immemorial, man has sought to explain illness, and his beliefs regarding cause have determined the role of the sick person, the role of the healer and the system of care provided. Primitive man attributed illness to evil spirits and sought to drive them out by practising witchcraft or assuaging their wrath by some sacrificial gift. Centuries later, the ancient civilisations — Egypt, Babylon, India, China, Greece, Rome — still thought of illness as a supernatural phenomenon. The healer might be a magician or a priest-physician or a god, and the care might be offered, for example, in a Greek temple of healing or a Roman military hospital.

With the advent of the Christian era, the sick received care from deaconesses; or from members, male and female, of religious orders; or during the Crusades, from members of the prestigious Order of the Knights Hospitallers of St John of Jerusalem; or under the feudal regime, from the lady of the manor. Care was given with Christian compassion and as illness was sometimes considered to be a just retribution for sinful word or deed, the care included concern for the soul as well as for relief of bodily distress.

In Europe, there was an historical watershed around 1500 and the long period of domination by the feudal system and by the Church was replaced by a great upsurge of new ideas, new discoveries and new inventions. It was during this post-Renaissance period that there were also great advances in man's knowledge about diseases and their treatment. The human body was studied in detail anatomically and physiologically, much of this investigation being made possible by the invention of the microscope.

From the evidence produced by historical researchers, it can be detected that down through the centuries there have been isolated attempts to use a scientific approach in determining the cause of disease but it was not till the 19th century that the caregiver moved away to any extent from magical techniques, religious practices and folk medicine. More reliance began to be placed on methods demanding systematic, objective, verifiable observations about the course of a disease and its treatment. And knowledge acquired was not considered to be static; there was the expectation that observations and conclusions would be constantly re-examined in an attempt to evolve more effective practices.

By the mid-19th century, the experiments of Pasteur were demonstrating the growth of microorganisms but when, in 1843, Holmes published a paper in the U.S.A. entitled, 'The Contagiousness of Puerperal Fever', the whole idea of infection was ridiculed by many learned contemporaries and continued to be so, even though objectively corroborated by Semmelweiss in Austria in 1867. This 'germ theory' however was given practical application by Lister in Scotland who started the use of substances called antiseptics, and subsequently used the 'aseptic method' which transformed the course of surgery. More sophisticated surgery became possible after Morton gave the first demonstration of the use of ether as an anaesthetic in Boston, Massachusetts, in 1846, and Simpson employed chloroform the next year in Edinburgh, Scotland. By the early 1900s, many of the microorganisms causing the commonly occurring infectious diseases had been isolated, thus providing a starting point for the development of specific agents, antibiotics, which could inhibit or kill specific pathogenic microorganisms in the human body and have contributed to the rapid growth of the pharmaceutical industry.

As more factual evidence became accepted, it was necessary to depart from single-cause theories of disease and from the idea of health and illness as disembodied states unrelated to the individual person. It is now realised that the health/illness status is determined not by one factor but by many factors, and in different combinations for any one individual according to heredity, environment, age, circumstance and culture.

Accordingly, it is no longer sufficient to concentrate only on the pathophysiological factors of disease. It is necessary to consider the social factors which contribute to the development of health problems including poverty and overcrowding; the cultural factors which determine individual lifestyles such as food preferences, and the symbolic significance of critical events such as birth, illness and death; the environmental factors including the effects of water and air pollution, poor sanitation and industrial hazards; the psychological factors including the manifestation of past experiences in present behaviour.

Age too is important. Two decades ago, according to world population statistics, the number of persons aged 60 years and over was 205 million. In the mid-1970s it was around 305 million and if current trends continue, it is expected to be 585 million by the year 2000. Most older people are generally healthy, both physically and mentally, but their social problems can be considerable. Especially in industrialised countries, they include loneliness, isolation, boredom, change in social role, reduced income because of enforced retirement and loss of contacts. These social, economic, vocational and psychological problems are as important as physical disability in creating difficulties in life for the older person.

Knowledge about these many variables can influence the care provided for the individual and also affect the level of health within social groups and indeed, in the general population of a country. And they affect attitudes to health, and public expectations about the meaning of health.

What is health?

Perhaps the people of the ancient world were much more aware of maintaining health than we are now. In Ancient Greece, there is little doubt that the pursuit of excellence, encapsulated in the Platonic ideal, required a sound mind in a sound body; both contributing to the good of the soul. In Plato's *The Republic* it is declared that:

... in a well-run society each man ... has no time to spend his life being ill and undergoing cures ... there's nothing worse than this fussiness about one's health ... it is tiresome in the home, as well as in the army or in any civilian office.

Perhaps a 'good' state of health was possible in the heyday of the Greek city state. Some time later, Galen (130-201 AD) the celebrated physician, accepted that health in the abstract was an ideal state to which no one attained, yet he found difficulty regarding as unhealthy, all who did not function perfectly. He therefore was prepared to overlook small ailments and to consider health as a state of reasonable functioning and freedom from pain:

... that state in which we do not suffer pain and are not impeded in the activities of life, we call health; and if anyone wishes to call it by any other name, he will accomplish nothing more by this than those who call life perpetual suffering.

Quoting Galen, Brockington (1958) commented that perhaps little can be added — health is not an absolute quantity but a concept which is continually changing with the acquisition of knowledge and with changing cultural expectations. If, however, the dividing line between health and disease is placed just this side of death, said Brockington, then all life represents some measure of health; and within this concept 'not only does the absence of disease not exhaust the possibilities of health, but health and disease co-exist.' Brockington maintains that this stance allows us to consider 'positive health' and that it was within this framework that the World Health Organization (Appendix 1) defined health in its constitution as 'a state of complete physical, mental and social well-being, and not merely the absence of disease or infirmity'. (WHO, 1946).

When WHO defined health in this way however it was genuinely believed that there was a clear distinction between health and ill-health. For example in the early 1940s when Lord Beveridge, the well-known British economist was helping to plan the National Health Service in the U.K., it was assumed that there was a strictly limited quantity of illness which, if treated, would be reduced; indeed the planners expected that the annual cost of the health service would decrease as treatment reduced the incidence of illness, and people were transferred from the 'ill' category to the 'healthy' category (OHE, 1971). With the advantage of hindsight, this interpretation of health is too simplistic and in recent years, it has become accepted by most people that there is no such clear-cut distinction between health and ill-health.

In the first place, in strictly scientific terms, it is not possible to demonstrate a cut-off point between an individual's healthy state and diseased state, says the OHE monograph (1971). For a range of biochemical and physical observations which can be made on the individual, there is a continuous distribution curve for the population as a whole, for example for haemoglobin levels or blood pressure readings. The distribution of measurements ranges smoothly from those for the obviously healthy to those for the obviously diseased; and there is a substantial overlap area in the middle where one cannot objectively draw definite conclusions from the measurements. In fact it is probable that for many measurements the optimum varies from person to person so that correcting an abnormality by treatment and bringing the measurement to some average value, would be unnecessary.

In any case, it is a purely subjective judgement on the part of the individual whether he is feeling well or feeling unwell, and this to some extent is dependent on prevailing attitudes. For example in the U.K., disabilities which were tolerated as inevitable in the 1930s are now thought to justify treatment. Formerly, for example, deafness, lack of teeth and failing sight were accepted as part of the ageing process whereas now, corrective treatment is the expectation and often considered as a right. Also sophisticated procedures such as renal dialysis and transplant surgery offer the possibility of treatment to people who, even 10 years ago, were resigned to an incurable afflication and an early demise.

Nowadays too, life styles have changed the public's concepts of health and illness. Gross obesity, alcoholism, drug abuse, excessive stress are regarded as conditions which can be treated. Previously they would have been considered an individual responsibility or a family concern or perhaps the domain of the clergy. They are now considered to be the responsibility of the health service.

In essence, health can be defined only in relation to the individual and his expectations, and in relation to his optimum level of functioning in everyday living. A growing number of writers and practitioners now consider that the health status of the individual is dependent on his ability to adapt to, and cope with the challenges he meets throughout life. In fact, they go so far as to say that someone who feels well and lives in a way which he finds socially and economically satisfactory may be considered 'healthy' even though he may have a disease or significant disability such as a physical or mental handicap. On the other hand, someone with no detectable evidence of physical illness may be judged 'unhealthy' because he feels unwell. It is relatively easy to identify an individual's 'maladaptive' behaviours. It requires a much more subtle understanding of human reactions to detect 'adaptive' behaviours/coping mechanisms and to evaluate whether or not they should be supported and maintained.

Although in industrialised countries, the individual has come to be so dependent on the state and in particular, on the health services provided — and all countries in Europe, for example, have some form of health service — it is fascinating to note a resurgence of interest in self-determination in relation to matters of health. In an article on the subject of self-care, Levin (1981) explains that health professionals are having to be educated to reconsider ordinary people as self-providers of health and health care. Self-care is a term that is used increasingly to denote health care activities which include health caring services of the family, extended family, friends, lay volunteer groups, mutual and self-help groups, religious organisations, and in some instances, a whole neighbourhood. Although most published statistics about self-care are confined to the industrialised nations, self-care is the dominant form for most of the world's rural people in developing countries.

Several factors have been suggested as sources of our increasing awareness of self-care and its potential, and have been the subject of various WHO symposia. Levin (1981) summarises them:

- in the industrialised nations, the massive shift in disease patterns during the last 50 years to almost a

trebling of the incidence of chronic diseases when lay caring is a partnership with professional resources
- an erosion of professional mystique; and the public's awareness of rights and of options
- the public's awareness of alternative health care strategies
- a change in public attitudes to disease prevention and health promotion involving personal lifestyle and collective action
- the public's awareness of the economic implications of health care.

Levin ends his discussions claiming that this is an exciting period in the transition of health planning from a professional/industrial to a social model and concludes: 'we shall need a new conceptual vocabulary free of the we/they dichotomy'.

These concepts of health and illness have, inevitably, had an effect on the evolution of health care systems throughout the world.

NURSING AND HEALTH CARE SYSTEMS

Many health care systems have evolved in a fragmented way in response to local demand. Others are planned at national level and an attempt is made, although not always successfully, to provide services which are accessible to the whole population, even in remote areas. There are many variations between these two extremes and to a large extent they reflect the economic status of the country — its financial capacity to provide services — and the stated goals of the health care system.

Financing a health care system

It is becoming increasingly important that, no matter how rudimentary, each country's health care system, while essentially a service, should also provide value for money. In the post-Second World War era of growth, expansion and prosperity, the rhetoric of health care in industrialised countries seemed to assume that society had a duty to provide all the health care from which each of its members could conceivably benefit. Of course such a goal is beyond the reach of even the most wealthy nations, mainly because of lack of means to meet such an open-ended commitment. As a result, some form of rationing exists for almost everyone, either by ability to pay or by queueing for a share of a limited service to which everyone has access — what Godber (1982) succinctly described as 'the most for the most and not everything for the few'. Obviously, the priorities vary in different countries according to circumstances and it is only by having an adequate data base that planned priorities can be selected. Once identified, they have to be provided within a fixed financial envelope.

Money necessary for the economic viability of a country is obtained from a variety of sources, some of which are hidden assets, but every citizen is aware of various forms of taxes which are levied: it may be a percentage of personal income, tax on certain luxury goods, a flat rate tax on all goods, or a local levy of 'rates' based on the size and location of the house of each citizen. Whatever the source, a country's financial income is finite and the government in power must arrange priorities accordingly, allocating shares to health, welfare, social security, education, housing, law and order, roads and transport, defence and external affairs, nationalised industries, economic development and so on. And no matter how desirable it may seem for the health care system to respond to influences in its environment, it can only be done within the constraints of financial allocation.

It is customary to compare the costs of various services within a country and express them as percentages of the gross national product (GNP) or the gross domestic product (GDP). Sometimes, however, the cost of one service (for example health care) in various countries is compared, and although published statistics take no account of the different health structures that exist in different countries, the figures give a useful rough guide of comparative costs. The following figures provided by the Office of Health Economics for 1982, give some indication of the amount of GNP spent in a sample of countries:

Country	% GNP spent on health
Australia	7.6
Denmark	7.5
Eire	8.5
Finland	6.8
France	8.1
Germany (West)	8.8
Holland	8.7
Japan	5.7
Norway	7.1
Sweden	9.6
Switzerland	6.8
U.K.	5.3
U.S.A.	9.9

These figures do not distinguish between private expenditure on health and public expenditure; nor do they give any indication of the extent of the services provided by public expenditure. For example in all European countries there is some form of nationalised health system covering most services whereas in the U.S.A., only people over 65 years of age and the very impoverished have a service paid from public sector finance. So the figures are useful but should be interpreted with caution.

It is useful also to note the proportion of the health budget spent on nursing personnel. In the U.K.,* for

* Throughout the text mainly U.K. statistics are quoted; nurses from elsewhere will need to refer to the relevant sources in their own countries for the equivalent statistics.

example, three-quarters of the health budget is expended on staff and as over half of the National Health Service staff is on the nursing establishment, nursing manpower is a critical component in terms of numbers and cost. As a professional group, nurses are in great demand to carry out direct nursing, to teach, to administer and more recently, to carry out research in nursing. The health care system could not function adequately without nursing personnel.

Of course, the slice of the national budget apportioned to the health care system, and the allocation of monies within the system are related to the stated goals.

Goals of a health care system

During this century in industrialised countries the tendency has been to provide increasingly specialised services which, at vast expense, have focused on ever more elaborate techniques for diagnosing disease, and on providing hospitals to house the expensive equipment and the people being cured. This method of providing care has been described as a 'disease-based, hospital-based, medical-based' model of health care. For some time it has been under criticism because it has reached only a small proportion of the population. Nevertheless, a great deal of excellent work has been done using this model, bringing relief to many sufferers. The knowledge gained has been used not only to cure disease but also to control the environment and prevent disease. However, even some of the most affluent countries have come to realise the great disparity between the high cost of care in these systems and the low health benefits.

In many of these countries it is now recognised that greater emphasis should be given to community-based health care. And with this in mind, the attention of health professionals has been directed more to the desirability of maintaining and promoting health rather than concentrating so much on the individual's isolated episodes of illness which are treated in hospital.

With this change in emphasis, there is a trend to shift some of the finance from hospital to community services; from heavy concentration on physical aspects to social, behavioural and economic aspects of care; from the paternal dictates of health staff to a situation where the patient is playing a more active role in the decisions regarding his own care.

In many of the developing countries, the conventional Western pattern of health services has been emulated and in practice this has meant the construction of hospitals with emphasis on the treatment of the minority who are hospitalised. A study carried out by the Executive Board of the World Health Organization in 1973 found 'widespread dissatisfaction' by populations with their health services which, by and large, were found to be concentrated on urban areas to the neglect of rural areas where about 80% of the world's population live. Even in urban areas, it was said, health services scarcely touched the under-privileged groups such as children of the urban poor and shanty-town dwellers. Obviously a more appropriate pattern of health care provision was needed in the developing countries, even more than in the countries of the industrial world.

A system referred to as Primary Health Care (PHC) was presented in a WHO/UNICEF* Report (1978) which, it claimed, is equally valid for all countries. Irrespective of the level of economic development in a country, it is desirable to provide services which are relevant to the needs of the whole population. This means that services must be easily accessible to individuals/families in the community, by means available to them, and at a cost which that community and country can afford. PHC services which reflect the economic conditions and social values of the community will, therefore, vary from country to country but, says the Report, should include:

promotion of proper nutrition and an adequate supply of safe water; basic sanitation; maternal and child care, including family planning; immunisation against the major infectious diseases; prevention and control of local endemic diseases; education concerning prevailing health problems and the methods of preventing and controlling them; appropriate treatment for common diseases and injuries.

PHC is presented as a practical approach to achieving an acceptable level of health throughout the world and 'for developing countries it is a burning necessity'.

The Report suggests that for many developing countries, the most realistic way of reaching the total population with essential health care would be to employ community health workers who can be trained in a short period of time to perform specific tasks. In many instances, it would be desirable for such people to come from the community and indeed, be chosen by the local inhabitants. Assistance can be sought too, it is suggested, from traditional medical practitioners and birth attendants who are found in many societies and often have high social standing in the locality, with the capacity to exert considerable influence. These indigenous practitioners could provide effective assistance in organising efforts to improve the health of their community. For advice on complex health problems, however, the community worker should be able to turn to more highly trained staff in health centres or hospitals where it is possible to have the support of a formal health care system.

But whereas conventional health systems have concentrated on authority which descends from the top downwards, in PHC the accent is on the community and its self-reliance. Whereas the conventional health systems have concentrated on health in isolation, the PHC approach puts it in the context of the total human environment and involves not only the health sector but all related sectors of national and community development, in particular agriculture, animal husbandry, food, industry, education, public works, communications and so on. It demands the co-ordinated action of all these sectors at government and at local level.

This PHC approach on an international scale offers a tremendous challenge to nurses who, in most health care systems, are already strategically placed to teach the public about self-care and to teach, supervise and assist primary health workers and indigenous practitioners. Indeed, in many countries, nurses are already functioning in this manner but the contribution they make to community health has not always been sufficiently recognised at government level, and in some instances, has not been given effective support.

To help to co-ordinate the efforts of nurses in its member organisations, the International Council of Nurses (ICN) (Appendix 2) made a statement on nursing's contribution to PHC; it was presented by ICN's representative at the WHO/UNICEF Conference on PHC held in Alma Ata in 1978. The following year, at its meeting of the Council of National Representatives in Kenya, the ICN members discussed PHC and produced guidelines for its 1 million members around the world in *The Role of Nursing in Primary Health Care*. This thrust has been followed up at subsequent ICN international meetings; at local/area workshops; and at the World Health Assembly in 1983 when the 'Role of nursing/midwifery personnel in the strategy of "Health for All"' was outlined as a Resolution of the World Health Assembly.

The PHC approach offers great promise for the future. But to look forward with vision, it is sometimes wise to glance backward, not to be bound by history, nor to blame our predecessors, but to reflect on and learn from the past. For example there is a great deal to be learned by looking at the development of the nurse's role in the health care system of an industrialised country such as the U.K.

The nursing team in a health care system — in the hospital

In the U.K. during and since the Second World War, many new categories of health workers have been introduced in the health care services. In a hospital ward during the early 1940s the nursing personnel would probably have consisted of a ward sister/charge nurse, one or two registered nurses, several students preparing to be registered nurses and perhaps an orderly in a male surgical unit. But the scene changed. In 1943 the category of enrolled nurse was introduced along with pupil nurses preparing to be enrolled nurses; then in the 1950s, nursing auxiliaries, many without educational preparation were recognised as members of the health care team, as also were nursing cadets, although the latter did have an educational component built into their employment.

* UNICEF — United Nations Children's Fund.

Around the same time, working conditions for all nursing personnel began to improve, resulting in shorter hours of duty and longer holidays. With fewer man-hours available per staff member and the resulting shortage of staff, it was not surprising that part-time staff came to be employed. By so doing, the number of communication links required to keep all staff informed about changes in patients' nursing plans was greatly increased. Therefore, not only were there changes in the numbers of nursing staff in a hospital but also changes in the number of categories of staff, some of whom had very little training. In this more complex management setting, different methods of organising nursing evolved. There are three main methods (Fig. 1.1):

1. *Task assignment or job assignment.* Several decades ago, when carrying out scientific experiments in industrial settings, it was found that 'division of labour' was an economical method of production, and the method became popular in the commercial world. Using this idea in a nursing context means that the care of the patient is fragmented into a series of jobs and these are assigned to different members of staff with different levels of ability, thus creating a hierarchy of people and a hierarchy of jobs. One nurse can do the same procedure for many patients and with constant repetition becomes very quick. Personal hygiene activities, which sometimes involve relatively lengthy nurse/patient contact time rank low on the scale of activities to be performed, in some people's estimation, so the most junior staff are allocated to these tasks. On the other hand, the most competent staff, the registered nurses, are allocated tasks which involve less patient/nurse contact. Indeed, often the tasks involve or-

ganisation and co-ordination of work and personnel, and are not performed in the presence of the patient at all. In the U.S.A., during the 1950s, this phenomenon was referred to as 'the RN flight from the bedside'.

In some wards where this task assignment method is used, it has to be admitted that the patient almost becomes subordinated to the system, a rigid system, and it is difficult for the person performing one nursing task to see it in relation to the total care of the patient as a person. It must be remembered, however, that many patients have survived this method of providing nursing; even today it is the one most commonly used in hospitals in the U.K.

2. *Patient allocation.* In this method, all nursing for one patient during any one period of duty is carried out by one nurse. It may be carried out on a 1:1 nurse: patient ratio but more commonly one nurse is responsible for several patients. Unless there is some personality clash, the patient usually finds this a very reassuring relationship and the nurse, given entire responsibility for a set number of patients, usually finds such an assignment professionally satisfying.

A variation on the theme is *primary nursing.* The primary nurse holds 24-hour, 7-days-a-week responsibility for planning care, although only actually giving care during the hours on duty. When off duty, nursing is carried out by an 'associate' nurse, who follows the nursing plan developed by the primary nurse. This type of organisation is designed to provide continuity and individual attention; and responsibility and accountability are established for each patient (Pearson, 1983).

3. *Team nursing.* This method involves allocating some

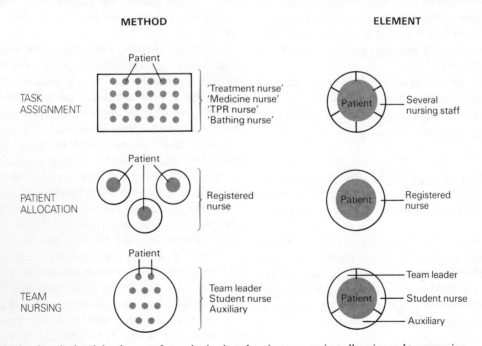

Fig. 1.1 The organisational method and the element of organisation in task assignment, patient allocation and team nursing

members of the nursing staff (the team) to be responsible for a group of patients and on any one ward there can be two or three teams. This is not simply a registered nurse in charge of a task assignment arrangement in miniature. The registered nurse gives total nursing to some of the patients in her group and supervises the work of other members of the team (student nurses or auxiliaries) nursing other patients in the group. All members of any one team have a particular interest in all patients in that group so for the staff it is possible to know in detail about the nursing plan for each patient.

The organisational method called 'team nursing' was devised primarily to provide non-professional nursing personnel with more supervision from the registered nurse so that, with her help, they would give planned nursing rather than perform isolated functional tasks for the patients. But 'team nursing' also emphasises the position of the registered nurse as a 'team leader' and provides the staff nurse with a meaningful role. For the patient too, it is desirable. Each patient has fewer nursing staff contacts to make in any one day than in the job assignment method.

An important feature of this method is the daily conference held by the 'team leader', when observations can be made, assessments can be discussed, problems identified, solutions suggested, goals revised and all team members can learn to participate in planning and evaluating nursing; and at the same time it is an excellent teaching/learning opportunity.

The team idea is not new. Any good ward sister/charge nurse encourages group action, group interest, group response to leadership — in fact, a team spirit. Of course, assigning a registered nurse, a student and an auxiliary to work in a ward team does not necessarily constitute a team. Unless each member is united in the common purpose of nursing a group of patients and has respect for the leader, there is no team.

This alternative to the traditional task assignment method of nursing does not change the purpose of the endeavour, it merely changes the method by which it is achieved.

These then are the principles of the three main organisational methods but there are several variations on each, and the method adopted must be chosen to suit local conditions.

Currently, there are some interesting developments. In the hospital setting, for example, particularly in specialised areas, the nurse clinician or clinical specialist as she is called, is being accepted in a nurse consultant rôle and instead of being attached to one ward unit, she usually is peripatetic, giving advice about specialised nursing wherever a patient may require it.

The nursing team in a health care system — in the community

By the beginning of the 20th century, efforts were in progress in the U.K., as indeed in many parts of Europe, to promote community care in the form of preventive and health promotion services. To a large extent this was provided by the nursing team made up of *district nurses*, *community midwives* and *health visitors*. They visited the homes and were close to the people in the community. In some areas these services were highly successful but were not universally available throughout the country. With the coming of a state health service in 1948, there was a more even distribution of personnel but by that time hospital services had mushroomed, had become highly sophisticated, and were receiving much of the finance and most of the prestige. In the structure of the reorganised National Health Service (1974) there was an attempt to regain more emphasis on the community services and to make provision for more effective links between hospital and community in order to provide an 'integrated' health service and this emphasis is ostensibly reflected in the 1982 re-structure.

The district nurse. In the community services, as in the hospital services, various categories of nursing staff are also used. The district nursing sister visiting the sick at home includes in her team, for example, enrolled nurses, bath attendants and 'night sitters'. Never more so than now, district nurses are in demand because the recently inaugurated, integrated health service in the U.K. is placing a new emphasis on providing health care in the home rather than in a hospital setting. This is exemplified by 'early discharge' schemes, and '5-day wards' which necessitate referral from hospital to community services and involves the expertise of the district nurses.

A current practice in the district nursing service is the employment of 'specialist' nurses. One example is the registered general nurse with a specialist training helping all the patients in a prescribed area who have a stoma (p. 200). Another example is the community psychiatric nurse (CPN) who cares for mentally ill patients following discharge from hospital and in many instances, gives preventive nursing which makes admission to hospital unnecessary. There are now established courses to prepare nurses to function with this level of expertise.

But the district nurse is not only concerned with the sick. She plays an important role in preventive care and health education, and because she visits the home for some specific and obvious reason, the patient and family are likely to be receptive to advice from her about physical, emotional, financial and social problems. It is the imaginative co-ordination of nursing, medical and rehabilitative services and their interpretation to the patient which is the hallmark of the effective district nurse.

In more remote areas of the country, the practice of district nursing is sometimes combined with midwifery and health visiting. The additional qualifications are, of course, necessary for this 'triple-duty nurse' who has the challenging responsibility of combining so many aspects of nursing for a whole community.

The community midwife. In the U.K., most babies are delivered in hospital, but there are still some areas where midwives are employed in the community. Indeed currently there are some pressure groups which are advocating that childbirth should be demedicalised and that more women should be delivered in their own homes. Where home deliveries are planned, the community midwife is responsible and she also cares for the mother during confinement in the few hospital units where general practitioners deliver their patients. The community midwife may see expectant mothers in their homes or in general practitioners' surgeries or in local health centres. She is involved in teaching parentcraft to expectant mothers and fathers. Following delivery, and especially in the areas where there is a hospital policy for 'early discharge', the community midwife cares for the newly delivered mother and the baby at home, until the health visitor takes over surveillance as an integral part of her statutory responsibility for the pre-school child. The midwife and health visitor may collaborate in providing family planning advice where this is appropriate.

The health visitor. As a registered nurse with a special postbasic preparation, the health visitor is pre-eminently concerned with the promotion of health and the prevention of disease. She provides this service to individuals and social groups, and the work has five main aspects:

- the prevention of mental, physical and emotional ill health or the alleviation of its consequences
- early detection of ill-health and the surveillance of high risk groups
- recognition and identification of need and the mobilisation of appropriate services where necessary
- health teaching
- provision of care such as support during periods of stress; advice and guidance in cases of illness; care and management of children

A health visitor's workload covers the age continuum from childhood to old age. Most of the work is concerned with care of children although the former emphasis on routine visiting of children under 5 years is changing in favour of establishing priorities so that selective family visiting based on need is now more common. 'At risk' families can thus be accorded additional, more concentrated attention. Even in a family where there are no small children, the support of the health visitor is valuable when a family member has a long-term or terminal disease; or when one of the family is physically or mentally handicapped; or following bereavement; and so on. Elderly people, too, may need help to maintain a valued degree of independence and the health visitor can mobilise appropriate community resources to this end.

During the last few years there have been interesting developments in community nursing services in the U.K. Health visitors, district midwives, district nurses and their teams have tended to become 'attached' to general practitioner practices, and carry out duties in relation to clients on a practice list rather than, as formerly, to a population in a defined geographical area. Also, with the increasing emphasis on community aspects of mental health, the use of community psychiatric nurses has become increasingly popular. In most instances, they have been used to follow up patients who have been discharged from psychiatric hospitals and their work has reduced the number of hospital readmissions, but more and more they are using their expertise in the prevention of mental breakdown. These developments serve to emphasise the importance of the multiprofessional health care team.

The health team in a health care system

In the U.K. at the beginning of the century there were only two groups of care workers associated with the provision of direct services to the patient, namely the nurse and the doctor. Even within the sophisticated structure of the present health care system, nurses and doctors are still the two professional groups who work together most frequently. The doctor is concerned with identifying the medical diagnosis of the patient's problems. He prescribes treatment to alleviate or cure the condition and in this, the nurse may assist the doctor with some of the procedures — this relationship is sometimes referred to as the *dependent* role of the nurse.

When assisting with the care, treatment or rehabilitation of the patient, the nurse may have an *interdependent* role with the doctor and with other members of the health care team such as the physiotherapist, who is expert in assisting with physical mobility, or the dietitian, expert in diet therapy.

But in most of the caring, comforting role associated with the patient's activities of everyday living, the nurse is acting as an *independent* practitioner and helping the patient to become as self-sufficient as his disability or dysfunction will permit, or helping him to remain well, or helping him to face death with dignity.

So the nurse has an independent role and also an interdependent collaborative role as one member of the health team: nurses, doctors, physiotherapists, occupational therapists, speech therapists, dietitians, social workers, employment officers, housing personnel and so on (Fig. 1.2). Traditionally the doctor has been seen as the decision-maker in relation to health care but with the introduction of the team concept in the provision of care,

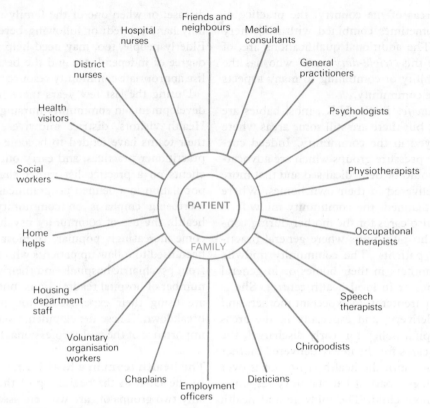

Fig. 1.2 Some members of the health team who assist the patient and family

it is recognised that there are occasions when other members of the team take the initiative, or indeed when the patient may take the initiative.

It is beginning to be accepted that of all the members of the health team, the nurse is usually in most constant contact with the patient. Especially in the community, the nurse is in a strategic position to identify changing patient/family needs, to assess the home environment and to initiate the use of community support services, both professional and voluntary. Particularly in the care plan for patients with long-term illness, some professionals consider that the nurse has a role as leader of the health team, undertaking a co-ordinating and integrating function. In fact in two WHO Reports (1976, 1977) it was suggested at international level, and is now accepted by many that under such circumstances the nurse is acting as an independent professional practitioner who calls in the expertise of other health team members when appropriate.

As well as contributing to direct patient care, nurses are increasingly appointed to posts within the management and planning structure of the health system. Nurses are also involved in teaching and research and are part of the health policy-making structure at local and national level, so the opportunity for nursing input is provided at critical points within the system. These are examples of the team concept being reflected in a health care system's structure.

The nurse's ability to function as an independent practitioner, as a member of a nursing team, and as a member of an interdependent professional team requires an educational preparation that includes a range of knowledge and skills from the biological and social sciences insofar as they relate to nursing knowledge, skills and attitudes. The educational programme is of the utmost importance.

Nursing education in a health care system

Florence Nightingale was one of the first people to appreciate the need to provide a planned teaching programme for nurses. After the Crimean War, a grateful nation had provided her with an endowment fund which she used to establish the first school of nursing at St Thomas' Hospital, London, in 1860 and enabled it to be financially independent. In her inimitable way she wrote:

An uneducated man who practises physic is justly called a quack, perhaps an imposter. Why are not uneducated nurses called quacks or imposters? . . . till the last 10–20 years, people in England thought that every woman was a nurse by instinct.

Nightingale, 1859

But she also recognised that proficiency could not be attained without adequate experience in the practical situation and her *Notes on Nursing* leave no doubt about her emphasis on careful and accurate observation of the patient. Education and service were equally important aspects of the nurse's preparation.

Following in her precepts, other hospital schools of nursing were created in various parts of the U.K. and indeed overseas. Consequently, when the First World War was declared in 1914, a considerable number of British nurses had been trained and could meet the demands for skilled nursing required by service and civilian personnel. Again, as in the Crimea, a war had highlighted the inestimable contribution made by nurses, mostly women, so the nation in recognition prepared to accord them opportunities for political, social and economic emancipation. One of the significant results for nursing was the passing of the first Nurses Act in 1919 which among other things set minimum standards for entry to the profession and by so doing, was a form of protection to the public. The General Nursing Councils (since 1983, the United Kingdom Central Council for Nursing, Midwifery and Health Visiting) were created to implement the Act, and they set up the machinery for curriculum development, for final examinations and for maintaining a national register of nurses. This was a significant event because a form of statutory registration has become the hallmark of professional status for nurses, doctors and the paramedical groups who are part of the health care team. Actually, in some countries such as those of the European Economic Community (EEC) there is automatic reciprocity of registration for registered general nurses and midwives (Appendix 3).

Meantime, the International Council of Nurses (see Appendix 2) had been founded in 1899 and the first President, Mrs Ethel Bedford-Fenwick, a Britisher, when speaking at the Congress in 1902, advocated university education for nurses. A few years later, in 1909, the first degree/basic nursing programme in the world was started at the University of Minnesota, in the U.S.A. In Europe, however, it was not till 1960 that an integrated degree/nursing programme was created at the University of Edinburgh.

The type of programme and the type of educational establishment used for nursing education varies from country to country. In some, for example Canada and the U.S.A., the theoretical education of nurses is now to a large extent sited in establishments of general education and there is usually a department of nursing within the establishment. In others, most though not all nurse education is carried out in monotechnic schools of nursing; that is, all students in the educational establishment are preparing to be nurses.

As would be expected, the availability of educational preparation affects the quality of the nursing service provided, which in turn has an effect on the public image of the nurse. In some countries, much of the nursing is provided by personnel who have minimal formal preparation or none at all and in these circumstances, the 'nurse'

in the eyes of the public, is accorded a relatively low social status. In others, a carefully planned theoretical and practical preparation is demanded before the nurse is given the legal right to practise, and nurses hold senior, well-paid clinical, managerial and teaching posts in the health care system. It is not surprising that in these circumstances, the nurse has a good public image.

The accorded status colours the nurse's view of her professional responsibilities, and her position vis-à-vis medical and paramedical staff. Although it may seem alien to many nurses, there are still parts of the world where nursing services are administered by non-nurses or where nurses have little say in the planning and execution of health care. However, there is a growing acceptance among health professionals of a team approach to patient care and in some countries, students from the various health professions share the same preparation for selected parts of the educational programme. To function effectively as a qualified nurse in such a complex, rapidly changing, demanding role requires scientific knowledge and intellectual skills as well as concern for people and manual dexterity.

But what should be the content of the educational programme? What is nursing? Is it only a 'mix' of other established sciences or are there some elements which are peculiar to nursing? Is it helpful to postulate a conceptual framework for nursing which assists the student to identify relationships between the different elements, yet which is also sufficiently flexible to incorporate future change?

A CONCEPTUAL FRAMEWORK FOR NURSING

In the mid-19th century Florence Nightingale deplored the fact that nursing was then considered to be 'little more than the administration of medicines and the application of poultices'. It is curious that even today many people consider nursing to be simply a series of tasks carried out by the nurse. Undoubtedly, observable tasks are a very important aspect of nursing but this restrictive interpretation does not take account of the thinking processes which are involved before, during and after any observable task. Nor does it take into account the knowledge and attitudes which must be acquired to accompany the dextrous performance of a nursing activity which is only a part of a deliberate plan of nursing.

Throughout the world, various authors have attempted to find a definition of nursing which puts emphasis on why activities are performed rather than limiting attention to what is done — the observable tasks — and the following definition by Virginia Henderson is one of the most frequently quoted:

Nursing is primarily assisting the individual (sick or well) in the performance of those activities contributing to health, or its recovery (or to a peaceful death) that he would perform unaided if he had the necessary strength, will or knowledge. It is likewise the unique contribution of nursing to help the individual to be independent of such assistance as soon as possible.

Henderson, 1960

Henderson enlarged on this theme, recognising that many nursing activities were simple until their application to the particular demands of a patient made them complex. She implied that there are thinking, decision-making and action elements in nursing activities; that the physical situation in which the activity is performed can increase its complexity; and that a management expertise is needed to co-ordinate all the elements. In recent years, in literature on both sides of the Atlantic, attempts have been made to elaborate on these thinking/decision-making/action elements in the nurse-patient interaction and, by dint of common usage, the term 'nursing process' has come to be used to illustrate this integration of the intellectual activities and the observable skills which the nurse performs.

The process of nursing

The use of the term 'nursing process' and discussion of the concept began to be popular in North America during the 1960s, and writers such as King (1971), Orem (1980) and Roy (1981), who have been developing conceptual frameworks related to nursing over the last two decades, were using the nursing process approach. The term was not used in the U.K. literature until the 1970s and when first introduced met with considerable resistance. However it gained remarkably rapid recognition and in 1977 the professional registering body, the General Nursing Council (England and Wales) decreed that 'the nursing care of patients should be studied and practised in the sequence of the nursing process'. Its use in Europe was given enormous impetus when the Regional Office of the World Health Organization decided to use the nursing process as an integral part of its Medium Term Programme for Nursing/Midwifery for Europe in order to identify nursing aspects of health needs within populations (Farmer, 1983). Eleven countries within the WHO European Region are collaborating in this multinational study which commenced in 1983 and WHO has established focal centres in interested countries:

- Collaborating Centres. These must be adequate in terms of academic and technical resources and a nurse in employed — the Research Programme Manager — to develop the research designs for use in the study.
- Participating Centres. In Type 1 participating centres nurses use the nursing process approach and are directly involved in the WHO project. In Type 2 participating centres, groups of nurses who are interested in the development and improvement of nurs-

ing are brought together, but although perhaps engaged in research, are not directly involved in the WHO project. The Research Programme Manager co-ordinates the activities of the Participating and Collaborating Centres.

It is an ambitious programme and will do much to stimulate research into nursing in Europe. Throughout all the discussions about the nursing process since the 1960s, a number of terms have been used for the various phases, but for the project WHO has decided to use *assessment*, *planning*, *implementation* and *evaluation* to describe the cycle of events in the nursing process.

The process itself is not new in nursing; the 'good nurse' has always used it. Often, however, she did not analyse what she was doing. Nor did she verbalise the stages of the process or commit them to paper, probably because, until recently, the stages had not been identified so specifically as a composite of intellectual and observable skills. And students learning to be nurses have found it difficult to appreciate the often rapidly executed mental activity which determines the experienced nurse's actions, because the qualified nurse has not explained the intellectual aspect of the process to the onlooking learner.

Of course, the four phases of the process are simply a logical mode of thinking, and it is not peculiar to nursing. Assessing, planning, implementing and evaluating could be applied equally in education, in sociology, in psychology and so on. What makes it peculiar to nursing is its application within a nursing context and this is explained in more detail in Chapter 6. The process on its own is *in vacuo*. It has to be used in the context of a conceptual framework.

Especially within the last two decades, various models have been suggested as a conceptual framework for nursing.

Models for nursing

Models are useful in any discipline. They provide a visual representation of the discipline's theoretical framework, indicating relationships between various components. Models should not be set in marble however; indeed they should be constructed in the knowledge that essentially, they indicate growing points for further thinking about the discipline. And as new, scientifically acceptable theories are proposed to explain observed practice, the model may be modified, or improved, or indeed discarded.

A model could be described as an overall image made up of ideas and concepts. In relation to a patient/client for example, a collection of several fragmented 'raw' observations is not a nursing assessment. Observations are made within a set of concepts which help the practitioner to simplify and organise them into a manageable form. So a model could be useful for nurse practitioners, nurse educators, nurse managers and nurse researchers.

In practice terms, a model can provide a framework for what the nurse does and how she does it; in education, it can provide a framework which organises the knowledge, skills and approach necessary for learning about practice; in management, it can outline the common goals to be achieved; in research, a model can provide guidance about what should be studied to extend nursing knowledge and improve practice.

Discussion about models is topical. In recent years a number of writers created and presented models which they have found useful in their own thinking about the discipline of nursing. It is interesting to consider the various models and in the following examples, the authors have incorporated the nursing process approach.

Dorothea Orem, for example, first wrote about her concepts of nursing in 1959 and her central ideas were self-care, and maintaining the patient's quality of life in a state of equilibrium. Orem assumes that man has an innate ability to be self-caring and when unable to do this (a self-care deficit) nursing compensates by means of the nursing system. In this model, the nurse only becomes involved when the patient's ability to apply therapeutic care fails, and equilibrium is lost. Orem developed this theme in 1971 and more recently in *Nursing: Concepts of Practice* (1980). Man is still the focus of her model and she maintains 'it is a nurse's mastery of key organising concepts that influences his or her selection and use of knowledge in a wide range of nursing situations'. Nursing, she declares, has as its special concern 'the individual's need for self-care action and the provision and management of it on a continuous basis in order to sustain life and health, recover from disease or injury, and cope with their effects'. When self-care is not maintained, illness, disease or death will occur. So the nurse must determine the need, design the system, plan the implementation, control the system of self-care; the goal being the patient's optimal level of self-care.

Another frequently quoted model was developed by King. She views man as the centre of three general systems: the social system or society; the interpersonal system or groups; the personal system or individual. In 1968 she identified five concepts for organising knowledge which would be used in nursing practice and in 1973 reduced them to four: social systems, interpersonal relationships, perceptions, and health. According to King, man is seen as functioning in *social systems* through *interpersonal relationships* in terms of his *perceptions* which influence his life and *health*. Nursing is described as 'a process of action, reaction, interaction and transaction whereby nurses assist people of any age and socio-economic group to meet their basic needs in performing activities of daily living, and to cope with health and illness at some particular point in their life-cycle' (1971).

The Roy systems model (1981) is also frequently quoted. Her focus is man and his position on a health-illness continuum which is influenced by his ability to adapt to stimuli; focal, contextual and residual. The goal of nursing is to promote patient adaptation to stimuli in one or more of four adaptive modes outlined under: physiological needs; self-concept; role function; and interdependence. Man is seen as a biopsychosocial being who is in constant interaction with his internal and external environments and nursing assists man towards health by promoting and supporting his adaptive powers. Although the Roy adaptation model was developed at the individual level, the 'client' of nursing may be a person, a family, a group, a community, or a society.

Of course, over 30 years ago, Henderson was writing about man as a whole, complete and independent being and she described 14 basic activities. In her view the goal of nursing was to substitute for what the patient lacks in physical strength, will or knowledge to make him complete, whole or independent. At that time, she was talking about the nature of nursing rather than using the term 'model' and she greatly influenced current and subsequent thinking, partly because of her related monograph *Basic Principles of Nursing Care* written for the International Council of Nurses, and translated into over 20 languages.

The model described and used in this book — the Roper/Logan/Tierney model for nursing — was to some extent influenced by Virginia Henderson's concept of nursing. As explained in Chapter 6 our model is based on a model of living (Ch. 2) which focuses on Activities of Living. In conjunction with the process of nursing, the model makes it possible for the elements of nursing to be identified, and for nursing activities to be planned, implemented and evaluated after assessing the patient/client and identifying actual and potential problems. For creators of models, their construction can be an exciting, intellectual exercise. The reader, however, should only adopt the model if it is usable. This book is written particularly to help student readers to learn about nursing; the model offers a framework which gives cohesion to activities which must often appear to the novice to be strangely disparate and unconnected.

Section 2 describes the Roper/Logan/Tierney model of living and the model for nursing.

REFERENCES

Brockington F 1958 World health. Penguin, Harmondsworth
Farmer E 1983 Planned change in nursing. Nursing Times Occasional Paper 29 (9) April 20: 41–44
Godber Sir G 1982 Striking the balance: therapy, prevention and social support. World Health Forum 3 (3): 258–275
Henderson V 1960 Basic principles of nursing care. International Council of Nurses, Geneva, p 3
King I 1971 Toward a theory of nursing. Wiley, New York
Levin L 1981 Self-care in health: potentials and pitfalls. World Health Forum 2 (2): 177–184

Nightingale F 1974 Notes on nursing. Blackie, London (original 1859) p 6 and p 3

Office of Health Economics 1971 Prospects in health. OHE, London

Orem D 1980 Nursing: concepts of practice. McGraw Hill, New York

Pearson A 1983 Primary nursing. Nursing Times 79 (40) October 5: 37–38

Roy C, Roberts S 1981 Theory construction in nursing: an adaptation model. Prentice Hall, New Jersey

World Health Organization 1976 Report on two working groups. The definition of parameters of efficiency in primary care. WHO, Copenhagen

World Health Organization/UNICEF 1978 Primary health care. WHO, Geneva, p 7

ADDITIONAL READING

Aggleton P, Chalmers H 1984 Models and theories. (First of a series.) Nursing Times 80 (36) September 5: 24–28

Expert Committee on the Education and Training of Nurse Teachers and Managers 1984 Primary health care. WHO, Copenhagen (Information Sheet)

Holmes P 1984 Holistic nursing: Acupuncture (First in a series) 80 (16) April 4: 28–30

Inglis B, West R 1983 The alternative health guide. Michael Joseph, London

Knobs D 1983 Nursing in primary health care. International Nursing Review 30 (5) September/October: 141–145

Mahler H 1981 The meaning of 'health for all by the Year 2000'. World Health Forum 1 (1): 5–22

World Health Organization 1983 Clinical practice of nursing: identification, development and evaluation. WHO, Copenhagen

World Health Organization 1983 Collaborating Centre Network for Nursing in Europe. WHO, Copenhagen

A model for nursing based on a model of living

2

Model of living

The background to the model for nursing which is utilised in this book has already been referred to in the preceding chapter and, for reasons briefly explained, it is based on a *model of living*. This chapter provides an outline of the model of living, and an account of the model for nursing is presented in the last chapter (Ch. 6) of this section of the book.

To encapsulate all of the complexities of 'living' in a model which is simple enough to be meaningful is, of course, impossible! The model of living presented here is only an attempt to identify the main features of a highly complex phenomenon, and to indicate relationships between the various components of the model. The model of living is made up of five components and these are labelled as follows:

- Activities of Living (ALs)
- Lifespan
- Dependence/independence continuum
- Factors influencing the ALs
- Individuality in living

These components are now described in turn, following which the model of living is presented as a whole by means of a diagrammatic representation.

ACTIVITIES OF LIVING
(ALs)

A model of living obviously must offer a way of describing what 'living' entails. If asked to describe what everyday living involves, probably most people — irrespective of their age and circumstances — would mention activities such as eating and drinking, working and playing, and sleeping. If prompted they would agree that breathing, communicating and eliminating are also activities which are an integral part of living, even if at times they may be hardly aware of performing them. All of these activities, and others — such as maintaining a safe environment and personal cleansing and dressing — collectively contribute to the complex process of living. They are the *activities of living*.

It is this concept which is used as the focus of the model of living; and a set of Activities of Living (ALs), 12 in number (Fig. 2.1), makes up the main component of the model.

ACTIVITIES OF LIVING

Maintaining a safe environment
Communicating
Breathing
Eating & drinking
Eliminating
Personal cleansing & dressing
Controlling body temperature
Mobilising
Working & playing
Expressing sexuality
Sleeping
Dying

Fig. 2.1 Activities of Living

The term 'Activity of Living' (AL) is used as an all-embracing one. *Each* 'Activity' has many dimensions; indeed it could be thought of as an overall activity composed of a number of particular activities, rather as a compound is made up of a number of elements. The more one analyses the Activities of Living the more one realises just how complex each one of them is. Compounding this complexity is the fact that they are so closely related. For example, communicating is related to many of the other ALs: just imagine eating and drinking, working and playing, and expressing sexuality without communicating! And breathing is essential for all of the ALs. So only for the purpose of description can they be separated, and here only a brief description of each AL is necessary by way of introduction.

Maintaining a safe environment

In order to stay alive and carry out any of the other activities of living, it is imperative that actions are taken to maintain a safe environment. In fact, each day, many activities are carried out with this purpose although, because they are such a routine part of everyday living, they are performed almost without conscious effort. For example, steps are taken to prevent accidents in the home by guarding fires, keeping poisonous substances in a safe place and carpets in good condition. Everyday, too, pre-

cautions are taken to prevent accidents when travelling and while working and playing. Maintaining a safe environment on the roads and in the workplace is not only a shared responsibility of individuals but also, through action and legislation, of the government. Some people, in addition to ensuring their own personal safety, engage in activities — such as campaigning for nuclear disarmament or action to prevent pollution of the environment — which they consider will help to ensure for future generations an environment which is as safe as possible.

Communicating

Human beings are essentially social beings and a major part of living involves communicating with other people in one way or another. Communicating not only involves the use of verbal language as in talking and writing, but also the non-verbal transmission of information by facial expression and body gesture. Communication of this type also provides the vehicle for transmission of emotions: long before a baby has acquired verbal skills, feelings such as pleasure and displeasure can be communicated to others. Communication through touch is equally subtle although less frequently used except in intimate personal relationships and here, as in verbal language, there are distinct cultural differences.

By its very nature, the activity of communicating permeates the whole area of interpersonal interaction and human relationships which are such a fundamental and important dimension of living.

Breathing

The very first activity of a newborn baby is breathing. The ability to do this is vital since by this action the cells of the body will receive from the air, oxygen which was previously supplied from the mother's blood. But, thereafter, breathing becomes an effortless activity and people are not consciously aware of performing it until some abnormal circumstance forces it to their attention. Oxygen is absolutely essential for all body cells; there is irreversible damage to the brain cells when they are deprived of it, even for a few minutes. Consequently all other Activities of Living — and life itself — are entirely dependent on breathing.

Eating and drinking

A baby is born with the ability to suck and swallow so that nourishment can be obtained without which survival and growth are impossible. Human life cannot be sustained without eating and drinking so this activity, like breathing, is absolutely essential. Eating and drinking is also a time-consuming activity since apart from the time spent eating meals, food itself has to be procured and prepared. The way meals are taken, and the food and drink selected, reflect the influence of sociocultural factors on this AL. For most people, eating and drinking are pleasurable activities but the fact that great numbers of people in the world die daily from starvation serves as a reminder of the essential nature of this Activity of Living.

Eliminating

We have chosen to describe urinary elimination and faecal elimination together because, although two distinct body systems are involved, there is no good reason to separate them in the context of an Activities of Living framework. The essential nature of this AL is such that in infancy elimination occurs as a reflex response to the collection of urine in the bladder and faeces in the bowel. The acquisition of voluntary control over elimination and independence in this AL are important milestones of development in the early years of life.

Eliminating, like eating and drinking, is a necessary and integral activity of everyday life. However, interestingly, whereas eating and drinking and many other ALs are performed in the company of others, eliminating is regarded as a highly private activity. Throughout the world people are socialised into eliminating in private and this contributes to many strongly held attitudes and taboos which are associated with this Activity of Living.

Personal cleansing and dressing

Cleanliness and good grooming are commended in most cultures, whatever the particular standards and norms. Apart from taking pride in their appearance, people have a social responsibility to ensure cleanliness of body and clothing. The term 'personal cleansing' was deliberately chosen in preference to 'washing' because in addition to handwashing, body washing and bathing, the activities of perineal hygiene and care of the hair, nails, teeth and mouth are also carried out. In relation to dressing it is interesting to appreciate that clothing not only fulfils the function of protection of the body but also reflects important aspects of culture and tradition; has sexual associations; and is a medium of non-verbal communication.

Controlling body temperature

Unlike cold-blooded animals whose body temperature is subject to the temperature of the external environment, man is able to maintain the body temperature at a constant level irrespective of the degree of heat or cold in the surrounding environment. The heat-regulating system is not fully sensitive at birth but, once its function is established, the temperature of the human body is maintained within a fairly narrow range. This is essential for many of the body's biological processes and also ensures personal comfort in continually varying, sometimes dramatically changing, environmental temperatures. Human tissue cannot survive very long when subjected to extremes of heat or cold; trauma and even death can occur from either heatstroke or hypothermia.

Although body temperature is essentially self-regulating, people have to perform certain deliberate activities to avoid the hazards and discomforts of heat or cold. Therefore activities such as adjusting the temperature and ventilation of the surroundings; varying the amount and type of clothing and regulating the amount of physical activity are all carried out with the objective of helping to control body temperature.

Mobilising

Although a rather clumsy word 'mobilising' seemed more explicit than 'moving' to describe the capacity for movement which is one of the essential and highly valued human activities. The devastating effects — physical, psychological and social — of any serious long-term limitation on movement bear witness to this fact.

The AL of mobilising includes the movement produced by groups of large muscles, enabling people to stand, sit, walk and run as well as groups of smaller muscles producing movements such as those involved in facial expressions, hand gesticulations and mannerisms.

The relationship of mobilising to other ALs should be readily apparent: behaviour associated with the activities of breathing, eating and drinking, eliminating, working and playing and so on, all involve movement and, even in sleeping, the body systems continue their ceaseless activity.

Working and playing

When not sleeping most people are either working or playing. Indeed play has been described as the child's work. Usually for most adults working provides an income from which, after essential costs are met, leisure activities are financed. The activities of working and playing can have very different meanings for different individuals. The old adage 'one man's work is another man's play' illustrates this well; for example, one person might earn an income by growing flowers and vegetables whereas, for another, this might be a hobby.

For most people, the sense of belonging to work and leisure groups, the satisfactions from challenge and achievement, and the prevention of boredom, are all important aspects of this AL. Both working and playing can be seen to have positive and negative effects on personal health and well-being. Because both involve physical and mental activity, each can contribute positively to physical and mental health. Conversely, enforced lack of working (as in unemployment or retirement) or insufficient playing may contribute to physical or mental ill-health.

Expressing sexuality

So important is the subject of 'sex' in life today that it cannot be ignored ... but how were we to describe this as an Activity of Living? The specific activity which tends to be directly associated with sex is sexual intercourse. Of course this is an important component of adult relationships — and essential for the continuation of the human race — but there are also many other ways in which human sexuality is expressed.

An individual's sex is determined at conception and throughout the lifespan sexuality is an important dimension of personality and behaviour. Femininity and masculinity are reflected not only in physical appearance and strength but also in style of dress; in many forms of verbal and non-verbal communication; in family and social roles and relationships; and in choices relating to work and play.

Sleeping

It may seem strange to describe sleeping as an 'activity' until it is realised that body processes do not stop being active during sleep. All living organisms have periods of activity alternating with periods of sleep. In human beings this is a 24-hour rhythm of sleeping and waking. Babies spend the major part of the time asleep and even adults spend up to one-third of their entire lives sleeping and so, in terms of time alone, this is an important AL. It is an essential one too; growth and repair of cells take place during sleep and sleep enables people to relax from, and be refreshed to cope with, the stresses and demands of everyday living. Without adequate sleep people suffer discomfort and distress, and a variety of ill-effects result from accrued sleep deprivation.

Dying

The inclusion of 'dying' in our list of ALs has been questioned: for example, it has been pointed out that it seems illogical without also including 'being born'. Death is what marks the end of life just as the event of birth marks its beginning. However, the concern is not solely with the event of death, but rather with the process of dying. It could be said that the process of living is a fatal one and certainly, in the process of dying, all the Activities of Living are affected and eventually cease with death. In describing 'living' it seems essential to acknowledge that death is the only really certain thing in life. The whole of a person's life is lived in the light of the inevitability of death, for some people overshadowing living and for others giving positive meaning to life. And of course people do not live only in anticipation of their own eventual death, but also in the knowledge that loved ones will die. It has been said that 'grief is the cost of commitment' in our lives. Grieving is the activity, inextricably linked with dying, through which a bereaved person comes to terms with the death of a loved one and finds the courage to begin living fully once more.

Even from such a brief description of the 12 ALs, it is clear that conceptualising 'living' as an amalgam of 'ac-

tivities' is a helpful way of beginning to think simply yet constructively about the complex process of living. All of the ALs are important, although obviously some have greater priority than others; the AL of breathing is of prime importance. The order in which the ALs are listed does not reflect an order of priority because, according to circumstances, the priorities change. Also, as previously mentioned, although the 12 ALs are described separately, they are very closely related to each other. Indeed, although the ALs are presented as one component of the model, they should not be thought of in isolation since they are affected by the other components and these too are closely related to each other. However, in their own right, each of the components contribute another dimension of 'living', as the following discussion will show.

LIFESPAN

It is easy to appreciate why a lifespan is included as one component of the model of living. 'Living' is concerned with the whole of a person's life and each person has a *lifespan*, from conception to death.

The lifespan is represented in the diagram of the model by a line, arrowed to indicate the direction of movement along it from conception to death (Fig. 2.2).

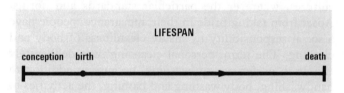

Fig. 2.2 The lifespan

As a person moves along the lifespan there is continuous change and every aspect of living is influenced by the process of physical, intellectual, emotional and social development which occurs throughout life. An account of these developmental aspects of living is provided in Chapter 4. There the concept of the lifespan, which is very simply represented in the model and only briefly mentioned here, is developed in more detail. The lifespan is broken down into a series of 'stages' — prenatal, infancy, childhood, adolescence, adulthood, old age — and these are discussed one by one.

DEPENDENCE/INDEPENDENCE CONTINUUM

This component of the model is closely related to the lifespan and to the ALs. It is included to acknowledge that there are stages of the lifespan when a person cannot yet (or for various reasons, can no longer) perform certain activities of living independently. Each person could be said to have a *dependence/independence continuum* for each AL. As shown below (Fig. 2.3A), the term 'total dependence' and 'total independence' are used to describe the poles of the continuum and the arrows indicate that movement can take place in either direction according to circumstances.

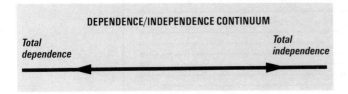

Fig. 2.3A Dependence/independence continuum

To emphasise that the dependence/independence continuum relates to each of the ALs — for on its own the concept is too global to be meaningful — the continuum appears in the diagrammatic representation of the model of living alongside each of the 12 activities (Fig. 2.3B).

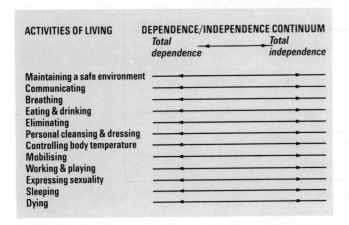

Fig. 2.3B Dependence/independence continuum related to the ALs

A person's position could be plotted on each continuum (at either pole or somewhere between) to provide an impression of the degree of dependence/independence in respect of the 12 Activities of Living. If repeated at intervals of time, any obvious change in direction of movement along the continua would become apparent.

Comparing the dependence/independence status of people at different stages of the lifespan illustrates the close links between these two components of the model. Newborn babies are dependent upon others for help with almost every Activity of Living. From this state of almost total dependence, each child according to his capacity can be visualised as gradually moving along the continuum towards the independent pole for each AL. At 5 years old the picture might look like Figure 2.3C: independence has been acquired in the ALs of breathing, eliminating, controlling body temperature, mobilising and sleeping, whereas the child is far from independent in the ALs of communicating and maintaining a safe environment, for example. However, by the time the child is 10 years old, a greater degree of independence has developed and the picture could look like Figure 2.3D. Often in the declining years there is some loss of the complete independence attained, and Figure 2.3E could apply to an infirm elderly person.

The pattern which has been outlined of links between dependence/independence in the ALs and stage on the lifespan is, of course, only the norm and there are always exceptions to even the most general of rules. By no means everyone has the capacity or opportunity to achieve or retain independence in all of the Activities of Living. Not all children are born with the potential for 'total independence', whether as a result of severe physical or mental handicap or both. In such circumstances, progress during infancy and childhood cannot be measured against normal developmental milestones and the goal is maximum

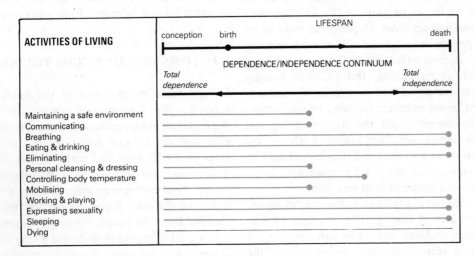

Fig. 2.3C Dependence/independence at 5 years old

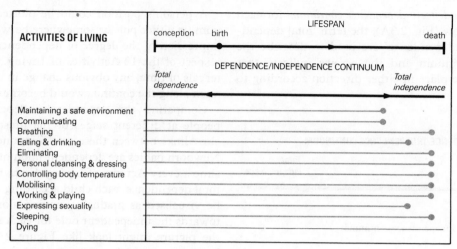

Fig. 2.3D Dependence/independence at 10 years old

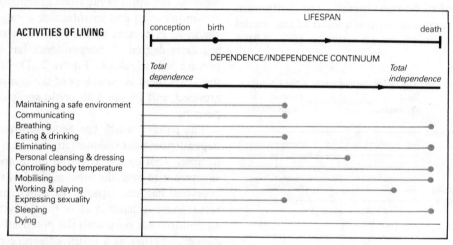

Fig. 2.3E Dependence/independence in declining years

independence in the ALs according to the capacity of the individual child.

Even in adulthood, there are circumstances which can result in dependence in one or more of the ALs: obvious examples are illness and accident. Dependence may be on help from other people or on special aids and equipment: for example, a wheelchair which provides 'aided independence' for the AL of mobilising. Indeed, even healthy able-bodied adults are dependent on others and on aids for their so-called 'independence' in many of the Activities of Living: for example, for the AL of eating and drinking there is dependence on people such as the farmer, fisherman, factory worker and shopkeeper and on various types of equipment which aid preparation, cooking, serving and consumption of food and drink.

There is, therefore, no absolute statement of 'independence' in the Activities of Living. The concepts of 'dependence' and 'independence' are really only meaningful when considered as relative to one another, hence the reason for presenting these ideas in the model of living

by means of a dependence/independence *continuum*. Change in dependence/independence status for one AL can, because the ALs are so closely related, cause change in status for one or more of the other activities.

FACTORS INFLUENCING THE ALs

So far, three components of the model have been described — the Activities of Living, the lifespan, and the dependence/independence continuum. However although everyone carries out Activities of Living (at whatever stage of the lifespan and with varying degres of independence) each individual does so differently. To a large extent these differences arise because a variety of factors influence the way a person carries out ALs, and these 'factors' form the fourth component of the model.

It would be possible to devise a long list of the different factors: for example, physical, intellectual, emotional, social, cultural, ethical, spiritual, political, economic and legal factors. However, one of the purposes of the model is to achieve succinctness and ease of recall, so the *factors influencing the ALs* are described in five main groups (Fig. 2.4).

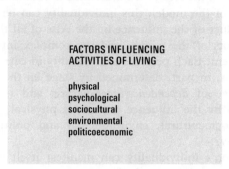

FACTORS INFLUENCING ACTIVITIES OF LIVING

physical
psychological
sociocultural
environmental
politicoeconomic

Fig. 2.4 Factors influencing the ALs

The factors are deliberately focused on the Activities of Living. It would be possible to focus them on the individual as a total entity discussing in general terms the effects of the five groups of factors on lifestyle, but this is too global. In preference, discussing them as they influence each of the 12 ALs highlights the individuality in living.

In discussing the first three components of the model, the fact that they are closely related has been emphasised. This is also true in relation to this component and, indeed, the five groups of factors are so closely related that it is only for purposes of description that they can be separated. Perhaps the simplest way to explain what the five 'factors' which influence the ALs entail, and to illustrate how they are related, is by means of an example. The AL of eating and drinking provides a good example because it is an activity with which everyone is familiar and which is clearly influenced by physical, psychological, sociocultural, environmental and politicoeconomic factors.

Eating and drinking are essentially *physical* activities. A functional hand (or substitute) is necessary for food and drink to be conveyed to the mouth. Although not so immediately obvious, physical body structures are required to chew and swallow, and then for food and fluid to be conveyed to the stomach and small intestine. There, by the process of digestion, nutrients and water are absorbed into the blood and lymph circulating in the body for utilisation by the cells. And, of course, in order to procure food and drink in the first instance, the individual must have the physical capacity to shop, prepare and cook food and, in some instances, to grow the food, or farm or fish.

However, there are also intellectual and emotional aspects to eating and drinking — the *psychological* factors. A certain level of intelligence is required: for example, to cope with infant feeding; or for planning a diet during pregnancy; or to meet the nutritional requirements of various members of a family. It requires numeracy for careful calculation to manage the budget for family food shopping. Emotional factors also influence this AL. Great pleasure can be obtained not only in preparing food and presenting meals, but also in the consumption of food and drink. Entertaining people to a meal is a mark of friendship in most cultures, and in some instances a meal is a form of celebration to mark a special occasion. However, eating and drinking are not only associated with pleasurable psychological states. If a person is unhappy or anxious there may be reduced appetite, perhaps resulting in loss of weight; or conversely, overindulgence in food or drink resulting in obesity or alcohol dependence.

While both psychological and physical factors influence body weight and shape, to some extent so too do *sociocultural* factors. In some cultures, a curvaceous figure is regarded as desirable and is an outward sign of wealth and abundance. However, elsewhere a slender body is the desirable image and the popularity of slimming diets in the Western world is a tribute to the power of the advertiser's persuasion in this respect. Religion is subsumed in sociocultural factors and in various ways it can have a very powerful influence on the AL of eating and drinking. What a person eats, when it is eaten and how it is prepared is often dictated by religious regulations: for example, orthodox Jews consider every meal a religious rite and eat specially prepared Kosher food; Muslims will not eat pork and during the month of Ramadan they fast during daylight hours; Buddhists and Hindus adhere strictly to a vegetarian diet.

Environmental factors certainly influence the AL of eating and drinking. Geographical position, soil fertility, climate and rainfall influence the type of food which can be grown locally and the availability of meat, poultry and fish; and fuel supplies will affect cooking and the capacity for certain types of food preservation and storage. In many parts of the world, something so basic as water is difficult to find and when available may not be safe to drink because of contamination, often by sewage. Accessibility and distribution of food and water in the local environment certainly contribute to the ease of eating and drinking and two-thirds of the world's population are entirely dependent on the local environment for food and drink.

Because ensuring an adequate supply of food and drink for any nation is a responsibility of government, and because food and drink are commodities with a price, the AL of eating and drinking is influenced by *politicoeconomic* factors. In a number of developing countries people die daily as a result of starvation and the lack of drinking water because of drought. In contrast, countries of the Western world are faced with problems of affluence — namely obesity and alcohol-related disease. Of course, even in these so-called developed, wealthy countries there are some people who are unable to afford a diet which is nutritionally adequate. It is a political decision whether or not a government provides assistance for these groups, those most in need usually being the very young and the very old.

This example has illustrated, albeit briefly, the variety of ways in which physical, psychological, sociocultural, environmental and politicoeconomic factors can influence an Activity of Living. A more detailed discussion of this component of the model for each of the 12 ALs is provided in later chapters (Chs 7–18) of the book. In more general terms, some background knowledge which is relevant to an understanding of these 'factors' is contained in Chapters 3, 4 and 5 which are concerned with biological, developmental and social aspects of living.

INDIVIDUALITY IN LIVING

The model of living attempts to provide a simple conceptualisation of the complex process of 'living'. However, the concern of the model is with living as it is experienced by each individual and this fifth and final component —

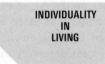

INDIVIDUALITY
IN
LIVING

Fig. 2.5 Individuality in living

individuality in living — serves to emphasise this point.

The Activities of Living were selected as the main component of the model and, although every person carries out all of the ALs, each individual does so differently. In terms of the model, this individuality can be seen to be a product of the influence on the ALs of all the other components of the model, and the complex interaction among them. Each person's individuality in carrying out the ALs is, in part, determined by stage on the *lifespan* and degree of *dependence/independence*; and is further fashioned by the influence of various physical, psychological, sociocultural, environmental and politicoeconomic *factors*.

A person's individuality can manifest itself in many different ways, for example in:

- *how* a person carries out the AL
- *how often* the person carries out the AL
- *where* the person carries out the AL
- *when* the person carries out the AL
- *why* the person carries out the AL in a particular way
- what the person *knows* about the AL
- what the person *believes* about the AL
- the *attitude* the person has to the AL

The idea that this component of the model — individuality in living — is a product of the other components, is conveyed in the way it is depicted in the diagram of the model of living (Fig. 2.6)

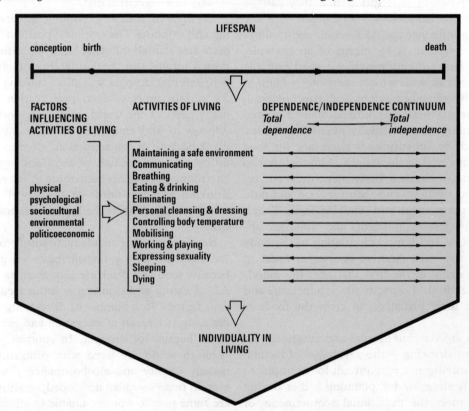

Fig. 2.6 Diagram of the model of living

THE MODEL OF LIVING

The model of living was described in the introduction to this chapter as comprising five components and these have now been outlined one by one. A diagrammatic representation of the whole model made up of its five components is shown in Figure 2.6:

- Activities of Living(ALs)
- Lifespan
- Dependence/independence continuum
- Factors influencing the ALs
- Individuality in living

Remember that the diagram of a model is merely an aide-memoire and, indeed, has little meaning without explanation. Although each of the five components was described separately, the fact that they are closely related was emphasised and the relationships are portrayed in the diagram both by position and the addition of arrows. In other words, the whole model is more than simply the sum of its parts.

Before the model for nursing which is based on this model of living is presented (in Ch. 6), some further discussion of the complex process of living is provided in the form of three chapters which, in turn, focus on biological, developmental and social aspects of living.

3

Biological aspects of living

Throughout life every person can be placed at a particular point on the lifespan. Yet how does each person's life begin? What does living mean in a biological context? What does sharing the environment with many millions of microorganisms mean in a health context? What sort of body defence mechanisms does man possess for safely interacting with his environment? What is the value of pain as a warning of danger in the environment or of disease affecting his body?

To begin to answer these questions a brief account of the biology of cells, including some of the disease-producing ones will be given. There will be an overview of the human body and its defence mechanisms, followed by a discussion of pain as a protective mechanism, which when it has served this purpose needs to be controlled by diverse means.

THE LIVING CELL

Animals and plants have in common the fact that they are composed of living cells, the number being different according to their complexity. The cell then can be thought of as the basic unit of life. This idea is called the 'cell theory' but it is more a statement of fact than a theory; nevertheless it now ranks with Darwin's theory of evolution as one of the foundations of modern biology. So what is a cell?

Cell structure
A cell is the smallest collection of matter about which it can meaningfully be said 'this is alive'. Most cells are infinitesimal in size and cannot be seen by the naked eye. However, the invention of microscopes and the development of laboratory techniques have permitted observation of their structure and behaviour. Cells are described as having four identifiable components: nucleus, nuclear membrane, cytoplasm and cell membrane (Fig. 3.1).

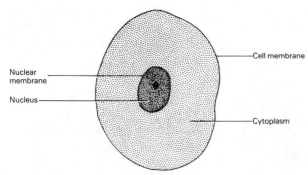

Fig. 3.1 A cell

Nucleus. This is a complex jelly-like mass which carries the chemical instructions or genes that are found in long chains called chromosomes. Its position within a cell can vary. The main constituents of genes and therefore of chromosomes are the highly specialised deoxyribonucleic acids (DNA) which are needed for the maintenance of cells and reproduction. The chemical instructions for production of enzymes pass into the cytoplasm to complicated structures which secrete the enzymes (Fig. 3.2). The nucleus therefore acts as an enzyme-controller.

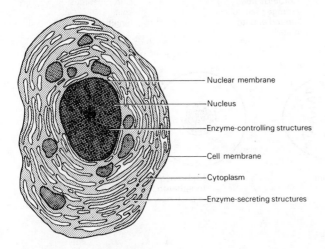

Fig. 3.2 Structures within a cell

Nuclear membrane. The boundary of the nucleus is provided by this 'elastic' membrane through which water passes easily; substances suspended or dissolved in the water can be held up on either side of the membrane in varying amounts depending on, for example, their concentration and the size of their molecule. The nucleus is on the inside and cytoplasm on the outside of the nuclear membrane.

Cytoplasm. This is a sticky watery substance containing proteins, fats, carbohydrates, minerals and vitamins. Within it are complex enzyme-secreting structures. The enzymes are secreted in response to information from the genes; they facilitate the many chemical processes occurring in the cytoplasm. Usually an enzyme is concerned

with only one particular chemical reaction so several specific enzymes may be involved in any one biological function such as growth, respiration, nutrition, elimination or reproduction.

Cell membrane. Enclosing the cytoplasm is the cell membrane which is as complex in structure and function as the nuclear membrane and regulates which substances pass into and out of the cytoplasm.

Intracellular activity

There is constant intense chemical activity going on within cells; the complex food molecules ingested from the environment are broken down into a simpler form and simple ones are then built into the exact complex molecules needed by the cell. The building process is called *synthesis* and the sum total of these activities is called *metabolism.* Oxygen is essential for these processes and it is obtained from the environment via the cell membrane. The products of metabolism — carbon dioxide and other waste materials — have to be excreted, again via the cell membrane. The movement of substances in both directions between the cell and its environment is by diffusion and osmosis. *Diffusion* is the process whereby gases and liquids of different densities, when in contact, intermingle until the density is equal throughout. *Osmosis* occurs when two liquids of different densities are separated by a semipermeable membrane which allows some components of a solution to pass through and holds back others. The diffusible components will tend to flow from the less concentrated solution into the more concentrated solution. Osmosis, then, is the selective flow of diffusible components.

Movement of cells

A unicellular organism, for example the amoeba, moves by pushing out part of its cell membrane in response to a stimulus from the environment provided by something like a food particle (Fig. 3.3). The contents of the cell then flow into the pushed-out part. The projecting part of the cell encloses the food particle and digests, absorbs and assimilates (metabolises) it, a process called *phagocytosis.*

In cells other than the amoeba this movement is called amoeboid action. In the human body white blood cells can move from their containing vessel, enter the tissues and engulf pathogenic microorganisms, thus acting as a protection agaist infection. Also some of the cells lining the blood vessels in the liver, spleen and bone marrow are phagocytic, that is they ingest and therefore remove unwanted particles of solid matter, ranging from microorganisms to worn-out red blood cells (corpuscles).

Division of cells: mitosis

Unicellular organisms are asexual and they perpetuate their species by dividing into two, in preparation for

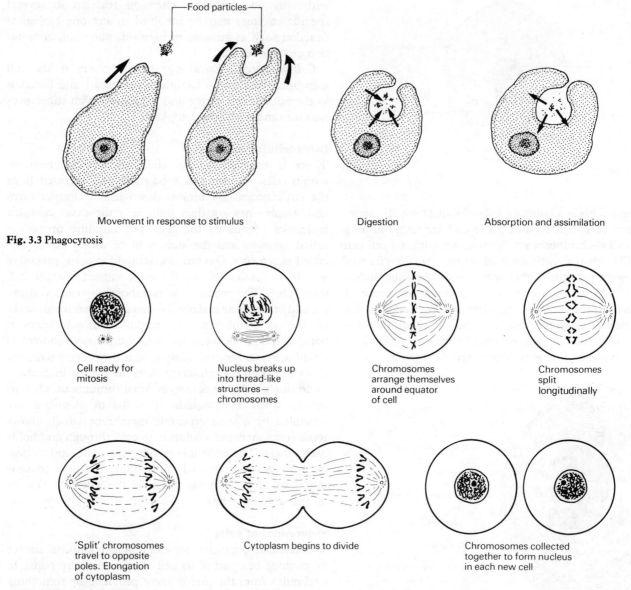

Food particles

Movement in response to stimulus   Digestion   Absorption and assimilation

Fig. 3.3 Phagocytosis

Cell ready for
mitosis

Nucleus breaks up
into thread-like
structures—
chromosomes

Chromosomes
arrange themselves
around equator
of cell

Chromosomes
split
longitudinally

'Split' chromosomes
travel to opposite
poles. Elongation
of cytoplasm

Cytoplasm begins to divide

Chromosomes collected
together to form nucleus
in each new cell

Fig. 3.4 Mitosis

which each chromosome is duplicated. The chromosomes with their sets of genes are then distributed in exact replication to each new cell (Fig. 3.4). Thus the unicellular organism is capable of reproducing itself precisely, generation after generation. Microorganisms are unicellular and sometimes they take only 20 minutes to reproduce themselves; if the organism is disease-producing (pathogenic), illness can result very quickly.

Disease-producing cells: pathogens

There are elaborate classification systems with complex nomenclature for pathogenic microorganisms. Their general appearance, behaviour and modes of reproduction vary considerably but collectively there are three main groups: bacteria, fungi and viruses.

Bacteria

These are small cells about one micron in transverse diameter, a size difficult to imagine but something like three hundred of the smaller ones could fit across the diameter of a pin's head! They are larger than viruses and smaller than fungi and are classified according to their shape; some are spherical, others look like rods and yet others resemble spirals (Fig. 3.5).

Spherical cells include the cocci which are further differentiated according to their arrangement. When they appear in clusters they are called staphylococci; when they appear in pairs they are diplococci and when in chains they are streptococci. Other terminology indicates the disease which they produce, for example pneumococci cause respiratory infection and gonococci cause gonorrhoea.

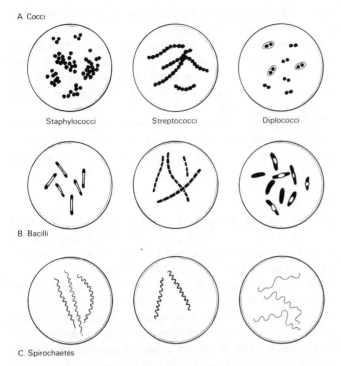

A. Cocci

Staphylococci   Streptococci   Diplococci

B. Bacilli

C. Spirochaetes

Fig. 3.5 Bacteria

Specific rod-shaped cells are capable of producing for example tuberculosis, anthrax, tetanus, gas-gangrene and botulism. Bacillus is the designation used for all these pathogens.

The spiral-shaped cells resembling a corkscrew are called spirochaetes. One spirochaete causes syphilis; another carried by rats causes a severe and often fatal type of jaundice.

Fungi
Though still microscopic, fungi are larger than viruses and bacteria. One type of fungus causes an infection called thrush which more commonly occurs in the mouth but can occur on other moist surfaces of the body, such as the vagina. Another fungus causes ringworm and yet another is responsible for athlete's foot.

Viruses
Viruses are the smallest microorganisms and can only be seen through a highly sophisticated electron microscope. They differ from other microorganisms in that they can only reproduce within living tissue. Pathogenic viruses cause many of the so-called 'infectious diseases' including the common cold. The study of viruses (virology) is still in its early stages.

The important thing to remember about the biology of all these pathogens is that, in the one cell, intense chemical activity is constantly going on. For this they require nourishment, warmth and moisture and many flourish away from the light. With these requirements each one

can divide into two exact replicas, sometimes in as short a time as 20 minutes.

THE LIVING BODY

In a biological context man is a highly complex organisation of many millions of cells. Nevertheles, human life begins as a single living cell even though the child has two parents, so how is this accomplished?

Cells of the body
Each human cell is characterised by *46 chromosomes* and each cell reproduces by mitosis (p. 29) as in unicellular organisms. However the reproductive cells — sperms in the male and ova in the female — reproduce by a special reduction division known as *meiosis* whereby only 23 chromosomes are contributed by each parent in the gamete cells (Fig. 3.6). Whichever male gamete cell is fertilised by whichever female gamete cell, the resulting fertilised cell will have 46 chromosomes.

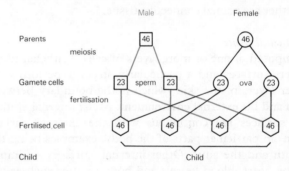

Fig. 3.6 Meiosis

Two of the 46 chromosomes in each cell are *sex chromosomes*, known as X and Y in the male; X and X in the female. The 46 chromosomes in each cell can therefore be written as $44+X+Y$ for the male and $44+X+X$ for the female. In the process of meiosis only one sex chromosome can be contributed by each parent. Hence, if the father's X chromosome pairs with the mother's X chromosome the offspring will have $X+X$ chromosomes and so will be female (Fig. 3.7). If the father's Y chromo-

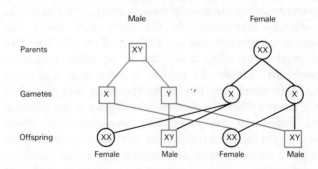

Fig. 3.7 Determination of sex by meiosis

some pairs with the mother's X chromosome the off-spring will have X + Y chromosomes and will be male. The sex of the offspring is therefore determined by the father's gamete.

It is striking that the highly complex, multicellular human being has a unicellular origin. A few days after fertilisation of the ovum, a cluster of cells develops as a result of cell division by mitosis, and the functional properties of the cells begin to change. Gradually there is differentiation and specialisation of cells into various tissues, a tissue being an aggregation of similar cells. These changes enable the complex interactions that take place between man and his environment.

Body tissues

There are numerous types of tissues in the human body and each plays a special role in body functioning. The tissues which are mainly protective are called epithelial tissue; those which produce movement are called muscular tissue; those which transmit information from one part of the body to another are known as nervous tissue; and those which hold the different structures of the body together are named connective tissue.

Epithelial tissue

Composed of one or more layers of cells, epithelial tissue covers surfaces and a particularly strong type forms the outer layers of the skin, which is the boundary between man and his external environment. Moist internal epithelial surfaces are continuous with the external surface (skin) in particular parts of the body, examples being the mouth and the anus. Other internal 'surfaces' — linings of the heart, blood vessels and body cavities such as the cranium, thorax and abdomen — have no connection with the outside but, being 'surfaces', they too are composed of epithelial tissue.

The functions of epithelial tissue are a consequence of their positions; being 'surfaces' they are subject to wear and tear and therefore in this sense they are protective. Epithelial cells are constantly dying and being replaced; the skin, for example, is constantly being shed and renewed.

In some areas of the body, epithelial tissue has special characteristics. In the digestive tract, it secretes a sticky substance called mucus and consequently is referred to as a mucous membrane. In the respiratory tract, this mucous membrane has on its surface small, hair-like structures, the cilia, hence the name ciliated mucous membrane. These cilia help to enmesh dust and other materials which are foreign to the body and therefore they act as a filter. To facilitate the organs in the thoracic and abdominal cavities gliding smoothly, the lining membranes secrete a thin watery substance — serum — so they are called serous membranes. Epithelial tissue is found in joint cavities producing a clear thick liquid which lubricates the joints; the name is synovial fluid and the tissue is synovial membrane.

Epithelial tissue also controls the passage of substances into and out of the body: the stomach and intestines absorb nutrients; urine is excreted by epithelial cells in the kidneys; and oxygen enters the body through the epithelial lining of the lungs.

It is important to note that all sensory stimuli enter the body via epithelial tissue since it is an important constituent of sensory organs such as the nose, eye, ear and skin.

Muscular tissue

The one-celled amoeba is capable of undifferentiated movement, but the quick, cleverly co-ordinated movement found in humans is possible only because of muscle tissue, of which there are three main types:

Skeletal voluntary muscle covers the bony skeleton. Movement of skeletal muscle is generally initiated by sensory stimuli conveyed to it by nerves; the muscle response is rapid — it contracts and relaxes quickly in readiness for new stimuli. The word voluntary is applied to skeletal muscle because it is controlled voluntarily.

Smooth involuntary muscle is not under voluntary control, and unlike skeletal muscle tissue it is relatively slow to contract. It is found, for example, in the walls of blood vessels and of structures in the alimentary and respiratory tracts, and in the uterus and urinary bladder.

Cardiac muscle is exclusive to the heart and is not controlled voluntarily. Usually muscle tissue will contract only when stimulated by a nerve, but cardiac muscle is unique in that it has the property of automatic rhythmical contraction, independent of nerve stimulation.

Nervous tissue

Nerve cells vary considerably in size and shape (Fig. 3.8). The nerve cell has a central body with its nucleus, but the cytoplasm is drawn out into one or more processes of varying length, termed nerve fibres. The cell bodies form the grey matter of the central nervous system and are

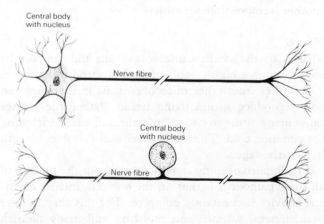

Central body with nucleus

Nerve fibre

Central body with nucleus

Nerve fibre

Fig. 3.8 Nerve cells

found mainly on the periphery of the brain and at the centre of the spinal cord.

The long fibres form the white matter of the central nervous system and are found deep within brain tissue, at the periphery of the spinal cord and as spinal nerves extending a considerable distance from the cell body.

All the complexities of behaviour and conscious thought are dependent on the fundamental activity of the nerve cell: the capacity to transmit electrical impulses to other cells. Though their function is the same — to transmit impulses — nerves are usually classified into two main groups:

Sensory afferent nerves transmit impulses from the periphery of the body to the spinal cord and then to the brain for interpretation.

Motor efferent nerves convey impulses from the brain to the spinal cord and hence to muscle, stimulating movement.

Connective tissue

The term connective tissue includes several different types of tissue formation involved in carrying out a wide variety of functions. There are two broad functional classes:

Supportive connective tissue makes up the hard supporting skeleton which forms a framework for the body; it is protective to delicate organs and permits mobility. This skeleton is made up of cartilage and bone. Cartilage has a certain degree of resilience but bone, in contrast, is a rigid non-elastic tissue. It is composed of a strong protein matrix into which salts such as calcium and phosphorus are deposited, not only to make it hard and able to bear weight and strain, but also to act as a store from which they can be released to the blood as necessary. 'Hard bone' forms the surface layer of all bones; 'spongy' or cancellous bone is found inside the hard bone and the spaces in it are usually filled with red bone marrow. The large marrow cavity in the long bones is filled with yellow bone marrow.

Binding connective tissue such as is found in tendons and ligaments is required because physical activity makes certain structural demands on the human frame. Tendons bind muscles to bones and are subjected to constant stress when the muscle contracts and the bone moves. Ligaments which envelope bones at joints are elastic and resilient.

A type of connective tissue also binds nerve fibres together and binds organs together in a loose yet powerful manner, keeping them in position yet allowing movement. This type of tissue provides a base in which the innumerable blood vessels and nerves are embedded.

Adipose tissue is another form of connective tissue and consists of cells filled with fat globules. Fatty or adipose tissue is found binding and supporting organs, such as the eyes and the kidneys, as well as under the skin, where it also helps to preserve body heat and give the body a smooth continuous profile.

In summary, epithelial, muscle, nerve and connective tissue are examples of different kinds of body tissue; they illustrate the way in which the cells of the body are differentiated in order to allow for the specialisation of function needed for the variety of complex activities going on within the human body.

Organs and systems of the body

To form any particular *organ* such as the heart and the brain, several types of tissue are grouped together. Organs function interdependently and those which work together for a similar purpose comprise a *system*. The various systems of the human body interact in an organised way to allow the body to perform its various activities of living. Only a brief overview of each system is given here, relating it to the appropriate Activity of Living (AL). In Section 3 a chapter is devoted to each AL and in it, the body structure and function required for the AL is briefly described.

The respiratory system with its AL of breathing is essential for all other Activities of Living. Oxygen is absorbed from the air in the lungs into the blood flowing nearby, whereas waste products pass from the blood to the air.

The cardiovascular system is essential for all other Activities of Living in a similar way, since all cells in the body must receive oxygen and nutrients and get rid of their waste. This is accomplished by the blood flowing in vessels — arteries, veins and capillaries — carefully controlled by the pumping action of the heart. The constant circulation of blood, especially through organs of high chemical activity with consequent heat production, distributes heat throughout the body and in this way assists in the control of body temperature.

Because the functions of the respiratory and cardiovascular systems are so interdependent they are sometimes considered as one system: *the cardiopulmonary system* and the AL associated with it is breathing.

The lymphatic system affects all the ALs indirectly yet cannot be closely related with any one of them. It comprises lymphatic glands and lymphatic vessels into which the fluid part of blood which has exuded from the blood vessels, bathed the cells, and failed to re-enter the blood vessels, is collected, filtered and returned to the blood. Because of its filtering function, this system performs a preventive activity.

The nervous system, composed of the brain and spinal cord together with nerves which supply all the body tissues, deals with the rapid conduction of stimuli. These are in the form of electrical impulses which generate intellectual, emotional and muscular activity, consequently the nervous system is primarily related to the AL of communicating which involves both verbal and non-verbal communication.

The sensory system is made up of the five senses which interpret touch, sight, sound, taste and smell; it plays a large part in the ALs of maintaining a safe environment and communicating. As its name implies the sensory system is entirely dependent on the nervous system for effective functioning.

The endocrine system is composed of several glands situated in various parts of the body. The glands secrete hormones — chemicals — which circulate in the blood and control the functions of many cells and tissues, particularly the transmission of nerve impulses across the junction of nerve fibres, so that the term 'neurochemical transmission' is used to describe such activity within the nervous system. Therefore the AL to which the endocrine system is appropriately related is communicating.

The digestive system is closely associated with the AL of eating and drinking. After food is ingested it must be digested because the body cells cannot be nourished until the food is broken down into its constituent molecules. As a result of this process of metabolism, energy is available for all the other ALs. The function of the lower part of the digestive tract, the large bowel, is formation and elimination of faeces. For this reason the term *defaecatory system* is sometimes used for this portion of the digestive tract, and this term relates it to the AL of eliminating.

The urinary system functions to balance the body's fluid and electrolyte levels. The kidneys maintain the constancy of the body fluids by producing urine which is excreted from the body. The urinary system is consequently associated with the AL of eliminating.

The musculoskeletal system, comprising the muscles, bones and joints, produces co-ordinated movement in conjunction with the nervous system, thus facilitating the AL of mobilising.

The reproductive system consists of the organs for perpetuation of the human species and they are necessarily different in the male and the female. The sex hormones play a very significant role in the development and functioning of the reproductive system, an essential feature of the AL of expressing sexuality. In the male, the penis is part of the reproductive system and it is also part of the urinary system.

Body fluids

The human body is made up of approximately 60% water. Of this, 66% is within cells and the other 34% is outside the cells. Many substances are dissolved in this water giving the different body fluids particular characteristics as described below.

Cellular fluid. This is present not only inside the cells of the body but also between them; the fluid inside the cells is called *intracellular*, while the fluid outside the cell, separating the cell from a nearby blood capillary (Fig. 3.9),

is called *extracellular* or tissue fluid. Both these fluids contain oxygen, proteins, fats and carbohydrates, together with vitamins and also minerals, mainly sodium, potassium, iron, calcium, phosphorus, magnesium, chloride, sulphur and iodine. All these substances are suspended or dissolved in water, as are several waste products from cellular metabolism. The substances are present in varying densities in the intracellular and extracellular fluids and the nearby blood throughout each moment of the day. Consequently diffusion and osmosis are constantly going on in order to maintain an equilibrium — a condition known as homeostasis.

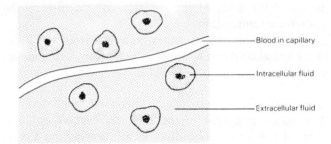

Fig. 3.9 Cellular fluid

Mucous fluid. Thick and sticky, this fluid is secreted by glands in mucous membranes which line the cavities and passages that communicate with the exterior of the body. It has a protective and lubricating function.

Serous fluid. In contrast, this fluid resembles water and is present as a fine film between two layers of serous membrane surrounding an organ so that the organ can carry out its function without friction, as the fluid permits gliding. The serous membrane round the heart secretes pericardial fluid; that round the lungs secretes pleural fluid while the membrane surrounding the abdominal organs secretes peritoneal fluid. Cerebrospinal fluid (CSF) not only surrounds the brain and spinal cord but is also present in a central canal within the cord and in several hollow spaces (ventricles) in the brain. It therefore forms a 'water cushion' and acts as a shock absorber protecting the delicate nervous tissue.

Synovial fluid. This is a clear thick fluid which lubricates all freely movable joints in the body. It is protective in that it prevents friction on movement.

Digestive juices. As the name implies, several juices manufactured in the body are poured into the digestive tract. They contain enzymes which break down the complex molecules in food into simpler substances that can be absorbed from the tract.

Bile. A greenish, bitter-tasting fluid, bile is produced in the liver cells and stored in the gall bladder. Although bile does not contain an enzyme it plays an important part in emulsifying fats and colouring and deodorising faeces.

BODY DEFENCE MECHANISMS

Although there are many agents in the environment which can cause injury or disease, the body has several mechanisms for combating the adverse conditions that are an inevitable part of living. For instance, the body has many reserve capacities which ensure that vital functions can continue even when an organ is injured or diseased: there is more lung tissue than is normally required, there is reserve liver tissue, there are two kidneys, eyes and ears. Apart from this 'over-provision' there are other mechanisms.

Defence mechanisms against injury/disease

Physical barriers and secretions
The skeleton acts as a physical barrier and is protective; the hard bony skull protects the brain; the vertebral column protects the spinal cord; and the ribs protect the lungs and heart. The intact skin acts as a barrier to many potentially harmful agents. The filtering function of lymphatic tissue enables the tonsils and adenoids to trap pathogens. The cilia in the respiratory tract hasten the exit from the body of possibly harmful foreign material. By reflex action — a mechanism of the nervous system — the threatened hand is instantly withdrawn and the threatened eye closed. The eye is further protected by the constant secretion of tears.

The inflammatory process
Inflammation is another defence mechanism and is a reaction of living tissue to infection, injury and irritants. Regardless of the cause, the reaction is similar. A substance, histamine, is produced by injured cells; it causes capillaries in the area to dilate thus bringing greatly increased amounts of blood to the site of injury. If this occurs on or close to the skin, it can be observed as redness and it feels warm to the touch. As well as dilating, the capillaries become more permeable and allow fluid to escape into the tissues, which produces swelling. In many instances, this swelling is enough to produce pressure on sensory nerves causing pain; to minimise the pain, the patient keeps the part as still as possible. The cardinal features of inflammation are therefore redness, heat, swelling, pain and loss of function. But these features are protective since they usually induce rest and aid healing. Furthermore inflammation is frequently accompanied by fever and an increased temperature is unfavourable to survival of some microorganisms.

The process of tissue repair
As inflammation subsides and damaged tissue cells are cleared away in the blood, repair begins in one of two ways:

- *repair by first intention* occurs when there is replacement by cells identical to those which were damaged. The best example is a surgical incision, which is sutured and heals without complication of infection. Only a small amount of new tissue is required to fill the gap.
- *repair by second intention* occurs when a lot of tissue has been lost and the wound edges cannot be approximated; a mass of new tissue is required to fill the gap. First, the damaged tissues are sealed with tissue fluid and blood, which clots. Then blood vessels invade the clot and connective tissue cells from the blood enter the clot and form fibroblasts. At this stage the healing area is reddish in appearance and is referred to as granulation tissue. The fibroblasts are then converted to fibres which, when they contract, draw the wound edges together. As the process proceeds many blood vessels become nipped and the scar tissue changes in colour from red to white.

The healing process is completed when epithelium grows in from the edge and covers the granulation tissue. If, however, too much granulation tissue is produced and it protrudes above the surface, epithelium will not grow over it until it has been decreased by application of a cauterising agent, then healing can take place. The skin and the tissue in the digestive tract heal quite rapidly; bone takes longer and the cells of the brain and spinal cord, once damaged, cannot be replaced.

The rate of healing is influenced by several factors:

- *degree of injury* is pertinent; the repair process takes longer when extensive areas of tissue have been damaged
- *nutritional state* of the tissues is important; substances such as protein and vitamin C are essential for rapid healing. Protein is needed for the formation of new tissue and vitamin C for the maturation of fibrous tissue
- *blood circulation*, particularly any occlusion of blood flow, delays healing by depriving the cells of nutrients and oxygen, so vital to tissue repair
- *age* can affect the rate of healing which is usually more rapid in younger than in older people. This is partly due to the decreased circulatory effectiveness in the elderly
- *infection* inevitably delays wound healing because the pathogenic microorganisms destroy tissue

The process of immunity
Immunity is another type of defence mechanism usually arising in response to an infection. The basic response to infection is inflammation; another response is related to immunity. The body reacts to the entry of any foreign materials (antigens) by developing substances called im-

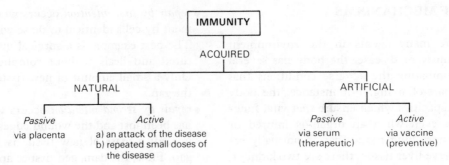

Fig. 3.10 Types of immunity

mune bodies. Immune bodies which destroy microorganisms are called antibodies and those which destroy toxins produced by microorganisms are called antitoxins. For purposes of description, the process of immunity can be classified into four main types (Fig. 3.10).

Natural passive immunity. Antibodies and antitoxins circulating in the pregnant woman's blood are passed via the placenta to the fetus. This inherited, natural, passive (the baby has not produced it) immunity to, for example, measles and whooping cough usually lasts only for a few months after birth. Thereafter, the baby is vulnerable to such infections and this is borne in mind when organising immunisation programmes for the child.

Natural active immunity. This type of immunity can be naturally acquired in two ways both of which involve the production of antibodies:

- By having an attack of the infectious disease the body is stimulated to produce appropriate antibodies not only to assist recovery but also to provide a sufficient quantity to remain in the blood for a longer period, sometimes throughout life, for example after an attack of rubella
- By being exposed to repeated small doses of the infecting agent. The amount is insufficient to cause the classical signs and symptoms of the disease but is sufficient to stimulate the body to produce antibodies which remain in the blood throughout life. Most adults have developed an immunity to tuberculosis in this manner

Artificially initiated active immunity. This is produced by injecting a small dose of the antigen into the body and allowing time for the person to produce antibodies himself, which then remain in the body for a variable time. It may be short-term, for example as a protection against influenza, or almost life-long, for example against diphtheria. The antigen can be a modified toxin called toxoid and it stimulates the body to make antitoxins.

Artificially initiated passive immunity. This is produced by injecting ready-made antibodies (usually developed in the blood of another human or in a horse serum and suitably treated for injection purposes). This technique is only used when a person is dangerously ill and his own blood would not have time to develop the antibodies. It can be life-saving.

The phenomenon of shock
The body responds to both physical and emotional trauma by a phenomenon known as shock. When it occurs, the body defences immediately try to compensate.

Basically shock is a state of circulatory failure. The average adult body contains about 6 litres of blood and if all the innumerable blood vessels were widely open simultaneously, there would be insufficient blood to fill them. The body functions with this relatively small volume of blood by controlling the muscle tissue in the walls of the small arteries (arterioles), thereby narrowing (vasoconstricting) or widening (vasodilating) the lumen. The control is very exact and normally it is a state of vasoconstriction. However, when the control is disturbed and the lumen of many arterioles are simultaneously vasodilated, the volume of blood is insufficient to maintain effective circulation and there is some degree of shock.

In shock, the body defences immediately try to compensate by permitting the vessels supplying blood to vital organs such as the brain, heart and kidneys to continue to do so, while the supply to muscles, skin and intestines is severely restricted. In a severe form of shock, the body temperature falls; the blood pressure falls; the pulse increases; the person complains of feeling cold; the skin is grey, cold and moist; and there is generalised prostration. If the cause of shock is treated satisfactorily, these adverse changes will be reversed but if not, the blood pressure falls further and death will ensue.

The most common causes of shock are the inhibition of vasoconstriction due to:

- loss of blood, as in haemorrhage
- loss of plasma, as in severe burns
- loss of electrolytes, as in continued vomiting and/or diarrhoea, and heat exhaustion
- alteration in permeability of blood vessel walls, as in injured tissue
- severe pain
- severe fright, as when hearing bad news or seeing horrifying sights

When there is, for example, loss of blood or plasma (sometimes called oligaemic shock) the reason for circulatory failure is more readily understood and expected because there is actual loss of circulatory volume. But in instances of severe pain or severe fright there is no loss of fluid; shock (sometimes called neurogenic shock) is due to reduced vasoconstriction. It is just as important to expect and recognise the body's warning signals of neurogenic shock so that it can be effectively treated.

All of these mechanisms — the inflammatory process, the process of tissue repair, the process of immunity and the phenomenon of shock — are body defence mechanisms against injury and disease. But there are other mechanisms to control man's internal environment.

Physiological homeostasis

The composition of all of the body fluids has to be kept within a narrow range of normal throughout every minute of each 24-hour day. The constantly occurring processes of osmosis and diffusion help to accomplish this. There are also elaborate feedback mechanisms whereby the secretion of enzymes and hormones further regulate the composition of man's internal environment.

After a meal there is a temporary storage of glucose by the action of the hormone insulin secreted by the pancreas, a part of the endocrine system. During the period between meals glucose is gradually released back into the blood to maintain its glucose content within the narrow range of normal. When fasting for any reason, the body can synthesise glucose from protein and fat, such is the essential nature of homeostasis.

After drinking large quantities of fluid, a hormone secreted in the brain influences the kidneys to filter out more water in the urine. Excretion of very dilute urine is almost as rapid as absorption of fluid from the intestine so that there is no drastic fluctuation in the body's fluid and electrolyte levels.

The blood is normally slightly alkaline, yet exercise produces acid bodies. The buffering mechanisms of the blood deal with some of these, while the rate and depth of breathing increases in order to get rid of the acid carbon dioxide permitting the blood to remain in its slightly alkaline state. This is an example of circulatory and respiratory adaptation.

Exercise raises the body temperature, as do many other internal activities such as all the ongoing chemical reactions as well as external factors like a high environmental temperature. Sweating is a physiological cooling mechanism that attempts to return the temperature of the body to normal.

These are a few examples stated briefly to illustrate the importance for living of physiological homeostasis.

Mechanisms for coping with stress

It is also essential for living that man is able to maintain a 'psychological equilibrium' and to achieve this he develops mechanisms for coping with stress.

Although the word 'stress' is a familiar one, there is much confusion about its definition. Some writers (Woolstone, 1978) seek an analogy in engineering and point out that the words 'stress', 'strain', 'tension' and 'pressure' are used when the load becomes too great and a breaking point is reached; it is the point where the strain is so great that metal ceases to bend and it snaps. Hans Selye, who pioneered the stress concept in the 1950s, concluded that stress was the wear and tear on the body in response to stressful agents. These he called 'stressors' and said that they could be physical, physiological, psychological or sociocultural.

The physical, chemical and nerve-initiated regulatory activities to achieve physiological homeostasis have been mentioned. The microorganisms causing inflammation and infection and the antigens producing immunity are also stressors. Added to these are psychosocial stressors which can be associated with life crises and which often cause feelings of fear and anxiety. Life crises can be developmental in nature: weaning, toilet training and puberty are examples that characterise all people's lives. Others are the periods of inevitable stress and anxiety surrounding incidents like changing school, job or house; getting married or divorced; child bearing, and death of loved ones.

The stress reactions in the body from fear and anxiety are similar. The word fear is used when there is a specific cause for the reaction, such as fearing that one will not arrive in time to catch the train connection. But psychologists point out that fear motivates all the activities carried out every day to prevent for example fire and accident. Anxiety, on the other hand, has a vague, generalised and not easily identifiable cause, indeed psychiatrists use the term 'free-floating anxiety.' Again psychologists point out that anxiety is a motivator, in that people are anxious to finish a job in the specified time and so on.

'Fight or flight' mechanism

For survival, man is capable of an extreme response to perceived danger — an immediate stressor. Activated by the autonomic nervous system, additional hormones are instantly secreted. They increase the heart rate, raise the blood pressure, increase the flow of blood to muscles, and increase the rate and depth of respiration. To effect this extra activity, the blood supply to the skin and mucous membranes is diminished so that there is paleness of skin, dryness of mouth and slowed digestion. In these ways the body is physiologically prepared for 'fight or flight'.

For most of the time most people's reaction to fear is much less intense. Physiologically the body reacts to anxiety in a similar way, but frequently the reaction is of much longer duration. Anxiety can be troublesome and most people can be helped to overcome its effects by learning simple relaxation techniques. Currently there is great interest in helping tense people to relax and lower their blood pressure and pulse rate by constant visual technological monitoring of these functions called biofeedback.

As the feeling of anxiety is so unpleasant, everyone, sometimes consciously but mostly subconsciously, attempts to avoid it. To do so, everyone indulges in an enormous diversity of coping mechanisms in an attempt to reduce stressful anxiety to a tolerable level. These mental mechanisms result in observable behaviour and are important aspects of living.

Mental mechanisms

Compensation is mainly a constructive defence mechanism for coping with stress arising in one sphere of living. For example a person who suffers anxiety because of real or imagined deficiency in say domestic activities may become highly competent in another sphere, for instance the academic field.

Conversion can occur when living becomes intolerably stressful. An example might be a writer not meeting deadlines losing the movement in his hand. This is not deliberate, it is the result of the unconscious mental mechanism of conversion. It is important to understand that the loss of movement is not due to paralysis; for paralysis there has to be a deficit in the nervous system.

A commonly used mechanism is that of *denial*. If the anxiety is about a feeling like hating Mr X, the hatred, being consciously unacceptable, is subconsciously denied. Should the anxiety be about a forthcoming event like fairly imminent death, the event being consciously unacceptable is subconsciously denied, commonly a part of the dying process (p. 335).

Most people use the mechanism of *displacement*. For example, a conscious feeling of anger in reaction to what one's employer said can be followed by 'angry' banging of the typewriter and this behaviour can be observed by an onlooker. A version of this mechanism is called 'scapegoating' in which the displacement is to a person, always the same person — the scapegoat.

Most people at times use the coping mechanism of *fantasy*, otherwise known as daydreaming. It brings temporary escape from pressing anxiety-producing problems. If indulged in to excess it ceases to be a means of coping and becomes a problem.

To help sustain oneself in, for instance, becoming the sort of person one wants to become, many people use the coping mechanism of *identification*. They model their behaviour on a person or persons who are seen to have the desired qualities.

When people are aware that they have unacceptable feelings or attitudes to others, they sometimes cope by projecting their feelings to others. *Projection* is not a conscious coping mechanism; people often criticise faults in others, unaware that these are deficiencies in their own make-up.

Probably the most commonly used coping mechanism in stressful situations is *rationalisation*. It consists of providing socially acceptable reasons for one's behaviour. Sometimes this mechanism is employed deliberately, at other times it functions at a subconscious level.

In periods of stress some people cope by regressing to behaviour which was acceptable at a previous stage of development. Again when over-indulged in, *regression* can paradoxically create problems for the person, mostly in human relationships. Many people indulge in this coping behaviour when they are ill.

When things like unpleasant memories or impending unpleasant tasks are causing stress, the coping mechanism of *repression* removes them from memory. *Suppression* is a lesser version of repression in that the suppressed material can be recalled.

Sublimation is a mechanism by which some people cope with the energy from what — to them — are unacceptable urges by transferring the energy to a socially acceptable activity. For example the energy from the sex drive is channelled into career development.

A very commonly used defence mechanism to keep the level of anxiety within tolerable limits is that of *withdrawal*. Most people respond at times by removing themselves from the anxiety-producing stimulus.

These, then, are some of the mental mechanisms used in coping with stress and anxiety which, if not kept to a tolerable level, will adversely affect all activities of living and may indeed cause physical or mental illness.

PAIN: A PROTECTIVE MECHANISM

Pain is yet another biological aspect of living. Of all the signs and symptoms of illness, it is probably the most common. Pain is disagreeable; in some instances it is described as unbearable, yet nevertheless it is a protective mechanism; it is a warning signal. It is the body's response to any one of a large number of stressors, ranging from microorganisms to trauma.

The phenomenon of pain

There are many different kinds of pain: headache, earache and toothache, to name some of the most common. They are particular kinds of pain, which can vary in intensity from a mildly uncomfortable feeling to one of absolute misery.

Most people who know what it feels like to be in pain regard it as an unpleasant sensation and something to be avoided if at all possible. But, equally, the value of pain cannot be disregarded; pain is a protective mechanism because it warns that something harmful is happening to the body.

People bereft of the ability to feel pain are therefore constantly in danger of accidentally being burned, bruised or cut, and of failing to recognise the onset of disease. At the opposite pole are people who experience pain even in the absence of any apparently painful stimulus. These two extremes are part of the phenomenon of pain.

The physiology of pain

Pain is manifested by the nervous system and research carried out over the past 20 years has greatly increased our understanding of the phenomenon. At the site of pain certain chemicals are released; they sensitise the nerve endings and help transmit the impulse to the spinal cord, from where it is relayed to the thalamus resulting in consciousness of the pain, then on to the cerebral cortex where the type, intensity and location of the pain are recognised. However, the painful stimulus can be so intense that the impulse is not transmitted to the brain and an immediate response is initiated by a reflex action, which is processed in the spinal cord. The classic example of this is the reflex withdrawal of the hand on touching something very hot, such as a baking tin straight from the oven.

For a long time it was thought that painful stimuli were received by special pain receptors in the tissue and transmitted along special pain pathways to a pain centre in the brain. However, this theory, called the *specificity theory*, does not account for the complexities of pain perception. A more acceptable explanation was provided by *pattern theory* which assumes that the pathways in the central nervous system are not narrowly specific but deal with patterns of impulses, pain therefore being transmitted along pathways which convey other sensations too.

One of the widely accepted theories of pain is the *gate theory* put forward by Melzack & Wall (1965). The human body cannot possibly cope with all the sensory input which could occur and the central nervous system must have the ability to exert control over the input of sensations. This is the idea underlying gate theory.

As the name suggests, gate theory proposes the idea that there is a mechanism at spinal cord level which acts as a gate. It can decrease or increase the number and intensity of pain signals which reach the brain from the peripheral sensory receptors. Also, impulses from the higher centres of the brain (for example, anxiety or suggestion) can descend and modulate the ascending pain impulses. The gate-control theory helps to explain some of the strange features of the pain experienced, such as why the amount of pain perceived does not necessarily correlate with the intensity of the painful stimulus and why the emotional status of the person appears to influence the process of pain perception.

In fact the role of the brain itself in suppressing pain sensations is now accepted as an area of knowledge crucial to understand. In 1975 at the University of Aberdeen, Scotland, Hughes & Kosterlitz (Medicine, 1984) discovered a powerful pain-blocking chemical which they called endorphin, present naturally in the human brain and spinal cord. Since then several such substances (endorphins) have been identified, as well as some non-opiates (enkephalins) which are produced in the body and they all have a complicated part in closing the gate to pain. These discoveries add a new and important dimension to understanding the physiology of pain.

Perception of pain

This aspect of the pain experience is one of the most fascinating. It concerns the individual's interpretation of the meaning of the signals received in the brain — his perception of the pain.

Individuals vary in their perception of pain. Two people can be given an injection and one may find that it really hurts while the other may hardly feel it. Pain perception also varies in the same individual under different circumstances; for example, although the injection felt sore the first time, it is possible for another to be given when it would be experienced as virtually pain-free.

Cultural factors, too, are recognised as influencing the way people grow up to perceive and react to pain. In Western societies childbirth is generally considered to be a very painful experience, whereas in other parts of the world women appear to experience little pain in labour. Members of some tribes in India and Africa engage in ritualistic ceremonies involving piercing of the lips and cheeks with needles and stakes: they do not appear to experience pain and the resulting wounds heal quickly.

Past experience of pain is another important factor and children are influenced by the attitudes of their parents to pain. Some mothers make a great fuss about even a fairly minor injury whereas others reserve attention for more severe pain; as a result the children concerned will adopt different ways of responding to pain.

The influence of suggestion on the intensity of pain is increasingly being recognised. For example the 'placebo effect' is well-known: placebo drugs (often, innocuous confections of sugar) can relieve a person's pain simply because of the implicit suggestion that 'drugs make pain better' (Alagaratnam, 1981).

It is often said that these variations in the perception of pain are the result of people's different 'pain thresholds' — some people having a low threshold and feeling only slightly painful stimuli, and others having a high threshold and being immune to everything except the most intensely painful stimuli. In fact, all people have the same 'sensation threshold' (that is, the point at which sensation of any kind is experienced): it is the *'pain perception threshold'* — the point at which the sensation of pain is experienced — which varies between individuals.

Of course, the ability to perceive pain requires a fully

functioning nervous system and any damage to the sensory nerve endings, sensory tracts in the spinal cord or the involved areas of the cerebral cortex of the brain will interfere with pain perception. For example, there may be no perception of pain affecting the lower limbs in a person paralysed from the waist down. Sometimes, on the other hand, there is an increased sensitivity to pain and this often occurs in neuritis, an inflammatory condition affecting nerve tissue. Level of consciousness is also relevant; as the level lowers, the pain perception threshold is correspondingly depressed.

Reaction to pain
Most people will have among their friends or acquaintances at least one person who could be described as a stoic because of his ability to suffer pain in silence, and another who fits the description of a coward because of fear of pain and inability to control the misery and annoyance brought on by it. Like the perception of pain, the reaction to pain is highly individual. Despite these individual differences, there are physiological manifestations of pain which can be observed in all people: the pulse becomes more rapid, blood pressure rises, breathing quickens, skeletal muscle tenses and the skin may become pale and sweaty. Anorexia, nausea, restlessness, irritability and insomnia may also occur.

Again, like the perception of pain, the way an individual reacts to pain is largely determined by upbringing, personality and sociocultural factors. Cultural differences are very distinct; 'keeping a stiff upper lip' is the British reaction, whereas people of Latin origin characteristically express their feelings by crying and groaning aloud.

The reaction to chronic pain is different from that to acute pain; it is often less easily recognised and is sometimes extremely complex, causing personality changes and psychological disturbance. Over time, pain makes people anxious and depressed or irritable and aggressive. The tiredness caused by pain lessens the person's ability to control and tolerate the continuous pain. Often when the chronic pain is associated with a malignant disease the person's reaction is to concentrate his whole attention on this pain and everything else is ignored, but Carus-Wilson et al (1983) give an account of the successful control of chronic pain in a young woman.

Types of pain
Pain manifests itself in different ways according to the location, cause, intensity and duration. There is no one definition, but it is possible to categorise pain into various types.

Superficial pain describes that which is felt in the superficial body structures, that is, the skin and subcutaneous tissue. As a rule, the individual is able to locate the pain fairly accurately. Often there is an obvious cause such as heat, pressure or mechanical trauma.

Deep pain, in contrast, describes that associated with the deeper structures of the body, such as muscles and joints. This is often less easy to locate exactly and is usually of a duller nature which may be described as 'aching' or 'gnawing'. Frequently it is long-lasting and of considerable intensity.

Visceral pain arises from pain in an organ of the body. Very often its character is highly specific to the particular organ involved and to the cause, which is usually a disease process. For example, angina is a heart pain caused by a reduction in oxygenated blood reaching the myocardium (the muscle layer of the heart). Characteristically the pain of angina is a central chest pain, often described as a 'tightness', which may radiate to the neck, shoulders and arms, more commonly the left arm.

Neuralgic pain arises from damage to the peripheral nerves of the body. This may be from infection, inflammation or poor circulation. An example is shingles, a condition in which a virus produces very painful inflammation along specific sensory nerves.

Referred pain is an interesting type in that it is felt in a place other than the diseased or damaged tissue. For example, heart disease is often accompanied by shoulder pain and disease of the gall-bladder may result in a pain which feels as if it originates in the right epigastrium and radiates to the angle of the scapula. The patterns of referred pain are so consistent from individual to individual that often a medical diagnosis can be made on the basis of the patient's description of it.

Phantom limb pain is an intriguing type; it has long been known that, following amputation of a limb, pain is experienced in the lost limb. The pain is actualy felt in specific parts, such as the toe, and is usually described as a tingling or 'pins-and-needles' sensation. This syndrome may continue for months or even years although fortunately it usually does disappear eventually. Sometimes other regions of the body become involved as trigger areas so that touching these can produce pain in the phantom limb. It is also known that people who suffered prolonged pain in the affected limb prior to amputation are more likely to develop phantom limb pain.

Psychogenic pain is the term used to describe the experience of pain in the absence of any apparent painful stimulus. It is increasingly being recognised that psychological factors can cause pain which is as troublesome as that resulting from mechanical trauma or physical disease. Psychogenic pain is not 'imaginery'; to the person experiencing it, it is real.

Assessment of a person's pain
Because pain is a subjective experience and such a complex phenomenon it is not easy to assess. Obtaining the person's own description of the pain and observing the individual's reaction to it are the two main methods of assessment.

The location of the pain is one of the first facts to ascertain. The person may be able to point to or describe the gross area involved, such as in the arm. He may need help to locate it more specifically.

The temporal pattern of the pain may be important in diagnosis, for example, whether stomach pain occurs before, during or after a meal. The time of the onset of the pain, the duration and the time at which it gets worse or less or better can be established from questioning.

The intensity of pain must be assessed as the patient's own perception and is not necessarily reflected by the pain reaction. An effective way of finding out how intense the patient's pain is, and how the intensity varies, is to use a 'painometer'. This is not a scientific intrument but simply a continuum drawn on a card (Fig. 3.11) which the person is shown and asked to point to the appropriate rating. This method is more informative than spontaneous verbal statements such as 'I can't bear it' or 'It's terrible'. There is another illustration of a painometer, side by side with a pain chart, in BNDU News Letter (1984).

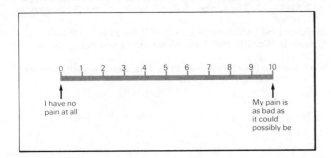

Fig. 3.11 A 'painometer'

The reaction to pain, if observed carefully, may provide important information particularly when the person has difficulty in communicating verbally or has a depressed level of consciousness. Pallor, rapid breathing, a raised blood pressure and excessive sweating may accompany intense pain. Facial gestures such as screwing up the face or gritting the teeth are common reactions to pain. Body posture may also be relevant; for instance with stomach pain the person often curls up whereas with chest pain he may want to lean forward or lie on the affected side. Crying and groaning may occur and if the pain is intermittent and very intense, the person may shout aloud or shriek.

The character of the pain is the way it is described. Some of the ways in which pain can be described have already been mentioned; 'aching', 'gnawing', 'tightness', 'tingling' are a few of the words commonly used. Some others are 'stabbing', 'burning', 'twisting' and 'shooting'. Sometimes the description is a comprehensive statement of the pain being experienced; for example, the patient may say 'I have a sharp pain in my chest when I breathe

in' or 'I have a burning pain when I pass water' or 'I get cramp-like stomach pains with my periods'.

Factors precipitating the pain are important elements for identification in assessment. Pain is often related to everyday activities of living such as eating and drinking, eliminating, breathing, working and playing, to name a few. Whether pain is associated with mobility or whether it occurs even at rest is of crucial importance. Environmental factors such as noise, and psychological factors such as anxiety or fear may also precipitate pain. The person may describe without difficulty what precipitates his pain: 'The pain in my chest comes on when I get short of breath, for instance after climbing a flight of stairs'.

Past experience of pain is relevant in assessment because it may affect subsequent pain experiences. Discussion can also provide information about measures which have been effective in alleviating pain, or it may indicate sources of anxiety which could be reduced by adequate understanding of what to expect, for instance regarding an operation, and so prevent pain in the postoperative period.

Measures which relieve the pain aim at preventing the stimuli from getting through the gate by competition from other sensations. Consequently rubbing or slapping an injured part can reduce the pain. Transcutaneous electrical nerve stimulation is another 'competitive' measure; electrodes are attached to the skin over a painful area and a mild current is generated to compete with the pain stimuli (Allan 1981). Acupuncture (Chung & Dickenson 1981) and biofeedback (Broome & Khorshidian, 1982) also come into this category. At another level, any sensory distraction or diversion such as change of position, application of heat or cold, and relaxation techniques will provide competition of stimuli and will reduce the pain signals.

Controlling pain

The relief of pain and suffering is one of the most important objectives of health care. The search for new and more effective techniques of pain control goes on year by year. Anything which seems promising is investigated with hope and, at various times, different methods seem to be in vogue. For all people suffering chronic pain it is essential to devise a pain control plan and to accomplish this multidisciplinary pain control clinics have been established in several countries (Latham, 1983). These clinics offer diverse methods of pain control which can be summarised under three headings — physical, psychological and pharmacological:

physical	{	change of position
methods		applications of heat/cold
of	{	massage and vibration
pain		electrical stimulation techniques
control	{	neurosurgical techniques
		acupuncture

psychological methods of pain control	communicating
	sensory distraction and diversion
	music therapy
	relaxation techniques
	desensitisation
	hypnosis
	biofeedback

pharmocological methods of pain control	analgesics (local and general)
	drugs to treat the cause of the pain
	tranquillisers to reduce anxiety
	anaesthetic blocking agents (for example, epidural anaesthesia)
	inhalations (for example, Entonox)

As it is essential for nurses to increase and use their understanding of pain, there is further discussion in the chapter on communicating (p. 133) of pain which is not specific to any other AL. When pain is causing a problem with a particular AL, for example, mobilising, it is discussed in the second part of the appropriate AL chapter 'Patients' problems and related nursing activities'.

Summarising this chapter on the biological aspects of living — it started with a brief account of the biology of cells including pathogens. An overview of the human body was given together with its defence mechanisms — physical barriers and secretions, the inflammatory process, the process of immunity, the phenomenon of shock, physiological homeostasis and mechanisms for coping with stress. It looked at pain as a protective mechanism, which when it has served that purpose needs to be controlled by diverse means. The chapter provides students with information which will be useful when they read about the biological factors influencing each of the 12 ALs in Chapters 7 to 18 and it leads to the next chapter in which the developmental aspects of living are considered.

REFERENCES

Alagaratnam W J 1981 Pain and the nature of the placebo effect. Nursing Times 77 (43) October 28: 1883–1884

Allan D 1981 The use of transcutaneous nerve stimulation in patients with severe pain. Nursing Times 77 (40) September 30: 1721–1722

BNDU News Letter 1984 Nurses and pain. Nursing Times 80 (19) May 9: 58

Broome A K, Khorshidian C E 1982 Psychological treatments of chronic pain. Nursing Times 78 (31) August 4: 1305–1306

Carus-Wilson E, Griffin C, Banks A J 1983 Controlling chronic pain. Nursing Times 79 (17) April 27: 51–53

Chung S, Dickenson A 1981 The last piece in the puzzle. Nursing Mirror 152 (6) February 5: 40–41

Latham J 1983 1. The pain relief team. Nursing Times 79 (17) April 27: 54–57. 2. The nervous system. Nursing Times 79 (18) May 4: 57, 59–60

Medicine 1984 Unlocking pain's secret. Time 24 June 11: 40–47

Melzack R, Wall P D 1965 Pain mechanisms: a new theory. Science 150: 971

Woolstone A S 1978 Stress — a call for a humane approach. Nursing Times 74 (14) April 6: 599–600

4

Developmental aspects of living

Looking at even the smallest newborn baby it seems impossible that a human being starts off as one tiny cell, as small as the point of a pin. But, as described in the previous chapter, this is the case. How does the fertilised egg cell grow into a human being? Having lived in the protective environment of its mother's uterus, how can the newborn baby survive in the external environment? What happens during the first few years of life to transform the helpless infant into an active and curious child? How does adolescence prepare a person for adult life? What are the responsibilities of adulthood? What are the difficulties and rewards of old age? These are some of the questions which are answered in the following description of developmental aspects of living.

The chapter is divided into sections, each dealing with one stage of the lifespan. In the diagram of the model of living (Fig. 2.6) the lifespan component was simply represented by a line, arrowed to indicate the direction of the person's movement along it from conception to death. This line forms the basis of Figure 4.1 and added to it are the various distinct *stages of the lifespan*, with approximate ages alongside.

Of course, all people do not live through all of the stages of the lifespan: some die before birth or at birth and some otherwise healthy people die prematurely, for example as a result of accidents, disease, natural disasters or war. So although each individual has a lifespan from conception to death, its length is not predetermined. Collection of statistics, usually at national level, allows life expectancy to be predicted according to the average age of death. In most countries of the Western world, the majority of people have a lifespan of 65 years or more. This description of the lifespan and its stages is based on that norm, but it needs to be remembered that the average lifespan is much shorter in some of the developing countries of the world.

In discussion of the lifespan component of the model of living, it was said that as a person moves along the

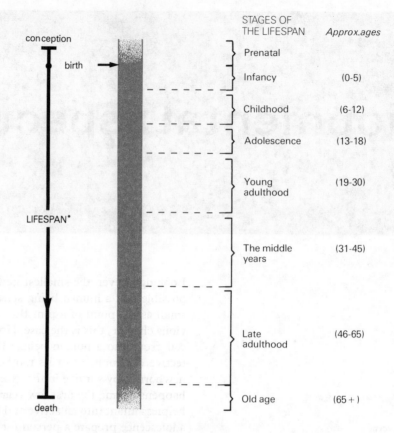

conception

birth

LIFESPAN*

death

*see **Model of Living** (Chapter 2)

STAGES OF THE LIFESPAN	*Approx.ages*
Prenatal	
Infancy	(0-5)
Childhood	(6-12)
Adolescence	(13-18)
Young adulthood	(19-30)
The middle years	(31-45)
Late adulthood	(46-65)
Old age	(65 +)

Fig. 4.1 Stages of the Lifespan

lifespan there is continuous change. Every aspect of living, and all of the activities of living, are influenced by the process of development which occurs throughout life. This process of development is complex and has many dimensions. This account of developmental aspects of living discusses these dimensions in terms of 'physical', 'intellectual', 'emotional' and 'social' development for each of the stages of the lifespan, beginning with the prenatal stage.

PRENATAL DEVELOPMENT (conception-birth)

The unborn child, although a living being, is a person no one knows. Not even the parents know what their child will look like, what kind of an individual it will turn out to be. However, taking conception rather than birth as the start of the lifespan is useful. For one thing it reminds us that the process of living begins before birth itself. For another, it draws attention to the important fact that many aspects of a person's individuality are shaped, some even absolutely determined, in the prenatal stage of the lifespan.

It is interesting to reflect that until very recently, knowledge of this stage of the lifespan was largely based on information from animal research or from examination of the human fetus from pregnancies which for one reason or other terminated early. Now, since the advent of advanced technology such as ultrasonography and in utero photography, it has become possible to observe, photograph, listen to and monitor in minute detail the hitherto almost unknown world of prenatal life. Even the very beginnings of human existence are now better understood as a result of these advances in science. Human life begins as a single living cell, a fertilised ovum. Within a few days of conception the fertilised ovum implants in the wall of the uterus, which gives it shelter and protection. As early as 3–4 weeks the embryo has a body shape with a head, trunk and tail and, in rudimentary form, a nervous system with a brain and spinal cord. At 8 weeks, the embryonic stage complete, the fetus is connected by the umbilical cord to the placenta which keeps the fetus supplied with oxygen and nutrients from the mother's blood. At the same time, carbon dioxide and other waste products are excreted via the placenta. This important organ also functions as a defence mechanism against certain pathogenic microorganisms and noxious substances. The liquor amnii, fluid surrounding the fetus, acts like a protective 'shock absorber' and also keeps constant the surrounding temperature. The liquor and the fetus are enclosed in a double layer of membranes, the amnion and chorion.

At 12 weeks the fetus weighs only about 57 g (2 oz) and is roughly 9 cm (3½ inches) long. By this time the fetus is beginning to look human; the face and head resemble the characteristic profile of a baby, the lips open and close and the head turns. Arms and legs constantly move and sucking and grasping reflexes occur frequently. The ears begin to function as early as the fourth month; the eyes open during the seventh.

From the fourth to the ninth month of pregnancy the fetus gains in weight and size. At term, its weight is about 3 kg (7 lb) and its length 50 cm (20 inches).

Ideally, the baby should be born at full term, which is between the 38th and 42nd week of pregnancy: if much earlier than this the baby may be of low birth weight, and any later he is likely to be deprived of oxygen and nourishment because the placenta begins to deteriorate. Labour is the process by which the fetus, placenta and membranes are expelled from the uterus through the birth canal (the vagina). The onset of labour is triggered off by a combination of physiological factors. For the mother, the signs of labour are the onset of contractions, 'the show' (a mucous vaginal loss) and rupturing of the membranes.

In the first stage of labour uterine contractions cause the cervix of the uterus to open to allow the baby to pass out into the vagina. The second stage of labour involves the actual delivery of the baby and, for the first time, the mother sees the human being which has grown inside her throughout the months of pregnancy. During the third and final stage of labour the placenta and membranes are expelled from the uterus. However, just before this, the umbilical cord is cut: the prenatal stage of development is complete and the baby is separated from the mother and ready to begin to live as a unique human being.

DEVELOPMENT IN INFANCY (0–5 years)

The first weeks

Having lived in the warm and protective environment of the uterus, the newborn infant must quickly adapt to very different circumstances. At first, the most fundamental needs are for oxygen, nourishment, rest, warmth and human contact. Taking a breath of air is the very first activity of living to be performed after birth. Sometimes the newborn baby is put straight to the breast to suckle; within a few hours regular feeding is established. Nourishment is provided by the milk and equally important, feeding times provide the ideal opportunity for the mother to cuddle and be close to her baby, thus establishing the bonding relationship. This also occurs while changing and bathing the baby; keeping the skin clean and dry is essential very frequently because eliminating

happens reflexly to ensure that the body's waste products are removed. Keeping the baby dry is also important in preventing loss of body heat because temperature regulation is unstable in the newborn and there is always the risk of hypothermia (an abnormal decrease in body temperature; p. 241). Much of the care which the baby needs in the first weeks of life simply ensures that basic biological needs are met and that infection and injury are prevented. Most of the time, when not feeding or being cuddled and admired, being changed or crying, the newborn baby sleeps.

It is not long, however, before the baby begins to be more awake and becomes interested in his environment, learning about it through the senses which, although not yet acute, do function. Very soon the baby will watch his mother intently as she talks to him, then begin to follow moving images and later to look around. Suddenly too the baby begins to become more active and, given freedom, will kick his legs and wave his arms about. This is quickly followed by two developments which turn the helpless newborn infant into a very responsive human being: he begins to experiment with vocalisations and he smiles.

Physical development during infancy

Height and weight. During the first year of life the infant increases in length by over a third and the weight almost triples. As the limbs and trunk lengthen, the head begins to look more in proportion to the body. By the age of 2, the average child is round about 90 cm (3 ft) tall and 13 kg (27 lb) in weight. The most rapid growth after that is in the legs, until by 5 years the average child is getting on for 100 cm (40 ins) tall.

As the body grows, so too do the internal organs, such as the heart, lungs and kidneys, in order to cope with the increasing demands made on them. Very important to all of this growth is good nourishment but, of course, it is equally necessary to prevent obesity (p. 167). During these years of rapid growth adequate sleep is imperative (p. 317).

Mothers, and those involved in child health, use height and weight as measures of healthy growth and, although children do develop at different rates, failure to thrive is often a warning sign of malnutrition, disease or sometimes emotional difficulty.

Independent mobilising is one of the most obvious acquisitions during infancy; the first random movements of the newborn baby are followed by a sequence of development which involves sitting, crawling, walking, managing stairs, jumping, running, hopping and skipping. The 5-year-old is agile and speedy on his feet and, as a result of increasing manual dexterity, he becomes competent at a range of manipulative skills.

Independence in some of the ALs results from gaining mobility and dexterity. The ability to feed independently is one of the first milestones and then, from the second year onwards voluntary control over elimination is gained (p. 187) and the skills for personal cleansing and dressing are perfected. These achievements do not just happen of course; the child needs to be taught and encouraged and he also requires a certain level of intellectual functioning.

Intellectual development during infancy

In very general terms 'cognition' is about knowledge and knowing; the term 'cognitive development' is often used to refer to the process of acquiring intellectual skills — such as thinking, reasoning and problem-solving — which are as essential for survival as physical abilities. There are two main processes involved in cognitive activities: perception and conceptualisation.

Perception is the process by which a person obtains information about himself and the surrounding environment. Through the senses, even the newborn baby perceives many stimuli such as pressure, pain, warmth, cold, taste, sound, changes in light intensity and various visual images. The response to many of these stimuli is simply a reflex action: for example, the baby will blink in bright sunlight or withdraw his hand from something hot. In general, the infant's responses basically are either ones of pleasure (smiling and gurgling) or displeasure (frowning and crying) and highly differentiated responding is not possible until the cerebral cortex and conceptual processes begin to develop.

Conceptualisation, the process of concept formation, is an intellectual activity which facilitates thinking, reasoning, remembering, problem-solving, and so on. It would be extremely difficult to do these things if the brain did not have the ability to interpret, organise and store the huge amount of information it receives. Concepts allow sense to be made of the complexities of the environment and they help in the identification of components of the environment. One of the first concepts which infants master is one called 'the object concept'; initially, the distinction is made between 'me' and 'not me'; later, there is differentiation between objects; and then, there is distinction between 'objects in sight' and 'objects out of sight'.

Jean Piaget's theories of cognitive development are among the best known. He maintains that, like all biological organisms, human beings have a characteristic internal organisation which is responsible for their unique mode of intellecual functioning. According to Piaget, there are three main stages in cognitive development.

The *sensori-motor* stage lasts from birth to 2 years and involves development from a reflex level of behaviour to a state in which adjustments to the environment are well organised functionally and do not depend on verbal communication.

The second stage is from 2 to 7 years and is called the *preoperational* stage. It is concerned with preparations for formal thought and the capacity to symbolise and conceptualise. At this stage, although the child can distinguish himself from objects and others, he cannot conceive of any way of experiencing events other than his own. So preoperational thinking is largely intuitive.

The development of formal thinking enables the child to go beyond his own experiences and this development is accomplished in the third stage of cognitive development — the stage of *concrete and formal operations* that lasts from 7 to 16 years. During the first of these, that of 'concrete operations', the child's thought becomes less egocentric and more systematic. After about age 12, the child begins to cope with 'formal operations' in which concrete systems are extended to include ideas of the interdependence of variables and so he becomes able to cope with quite complex problem-solving tasks.

With the emergence of formal thought, the process of cognitive development is complete, although throughout the rest of childhood and adulthood increasingly complex conceptualisation, abstract reasoning and problem-solving are gradually learned.

It is clear that the acquisition of language is crucial to satisfactory cognitive development in the first years of life. The infant whose mother continually talks to him, sings and tells stories, will become attuned to sounds quickly and so he will try to imitate these. Learning to talk is one of the amazing achievements of the early years and this and other forms of communicating (Ch. 8) enable the child to relate to the people in his environment. The formation of relationships is important to social and emotional developments which occur at all stages of the life-span.

Emotional development during infancy

The need for love is one of the most obvious needs of young children. From a stable and close relationship in infancy the child can grow with self-confidence and a feeling of security.

Feedback from others enables the child to develop a self-concept; if this is to be of self-acceptance and self-approval then he must have the acceptance and approval of parents and friends. Much of a child's behaviour is concerned with seeking acceptance and approval; children love to please and, in turn, to be praised and loved.

Smiling is one of the first ways an infant has of responding in a positive way to adult attention and love. On the other hand, his crying is likely to make his mother annoyed, less able to love him and in extreme cases perhaps even to drive her to physically harm him.

The mother–infant relationship is founded on love and grows in mutual affection. Whether deprivation of love, by separation of a child from his mother or due to some other cause, can have lasting consequences has been the subject of considerable debate. The concept of 'maternal deprivation' attracted great interest when John Bowlby

(1953) published the results of a study he undertook for WHO on the needs of homeless children. His evidence supported the generally held view that children deprived of a normal home life may suffer from mental ill-health and may grow up to become parents incapable themselves of giving a child the experience of a warm, intimate and loving relationship.

Although he later modified his stance, there is no doubt that Bowlby's concern encouraged those responsible for child health and care to pay more attention to the emotional needs of children. Nurses of sick children now realise the importance of comfort and contact and how essential it is that parents can visit and even actually stay with the child, even though it may be less easy for the nurses to have a routine and order in their day's work.

However, as Rutter (1972) points out, there has been some misunderstanding of the concept of maternal deprivation. The stress on the need for a continuous and intimate relationship has been taken to imply that the mother (or mother substitute) alone must provide care without interruption all day, every day. There is no evidence to show that this is necessary or, indeed, the most desirable option.

The development of personality is one of the outcomes of emotional development. The psychoanalytic theory of *Sigmund Freud* is a theory of personality development as well as an explanation of psychosexual development. Personality is viewed as the outcome of reciprocally urging and checking forces and central to psychoanalysis, is the assumption that sexuality is the most basic human drive. However, in infancy, and at various stages of development, certain erogenous zones of the body assume particular importance as sources of pleasure. In the first year and a half of life, the obvious source of satisfaction is the mouth and Freud names this stage of psychosexual development the 'oral stage'. The second stage (18 months–3 years) is the 'anal stage' and the third (3–5 years) is the 'phallic stage'. During the phallic stage the child discovers that the genital area can be a source of pleasure. At the same time, boys tend to show a marked emotional attachment to their mother (called the Oedipus complex) and girls to their father (the Electra complex).

Freudian theory considers the first 5 years of life to be the most important in the development of personality. Also, it states that certain experiences which occur at critical periods may have an adverse effect on later development. Such ideas, for example that a punitive approach to toilet training will result in fixation at the anal stage, are largely unfounded and, in fact, there is very little scientific evidence to support much of the psychoanalytic theory attributed to Freud.

Erik Erikson's theory of personality development is also well known but it emphasises the social rather than psychosexual dimension of development. Erikson suggests that there are eight stages of development during life, each stage involving particular extremes of attitude which must be resolved.

In his analysis, the task of the first stage — the stage of infancy — is the resolution of the 'trust versus mistrust' dichotomy. The infant is said to develop both basic trust and mistrust attitudes and must find a way to strike a balance between these two inherently conflicting attitudes in order to develop emotional stability and satisfactory relationships with others.

Social development during infancy

The family is the first and most important social institution for a child. Indeed for the first year or so of life the home and parents constitute the infant's social world: it is not until going to nursery and later to school that others feature significantly in a child's social network.

Even children living with their natural parents as a family are not guaranteed an ideal upbringing. For instance, those of large families can suffer because a lot of the parents' time is spent on activities to keep the members adequately fed, clean and clothed so that there is relatively little time for talking and playing with the children.

Social roles — those of child, brother or sister, grandchild, playmate and schoolchild — are gradually acquired during social development in infancy. Initially whether a baby is male or female is hardly discernible but, in no time at all, boys and girls become socialised into different roles. Play provides the opportunity for experimentation with role-playing so that the child learns what social expectations and conventions accompany which relationships. Playing at 'houses' allows children to enact their role in the home and imitate parental roles; playing with toys teaches the child the importance of respect for belongings and the rules governing cooperation and competition; pretending to be doctors or nurses, shopkeepers or policemen promotes insight into adult occupational roles and social structures and reflects the child's growing sexual self-image and interests and aspirations; and picture books, stories and television further extend his understanding of the society in which he lives.

DEVELOPMENT IN CHILDHOOD (6–12 years)

Physical development in childhood

The rate and amount of growth are much less dramatic than in the preceding 5 years. Between the ages of 5 and 8, the body weight and height increase at a fairly constant rate with only slight changes in body build. Individual variations in size become more apparent as do physical differences between the sexes later in childhood. Developments in the child's motor skills are closely related to two specific attributes: speed and strength. Co-operative games, an important feature of social interaction in this age group, demand a high degree of speed, strength, agility, coordination and precision.

People who say about a child 'He's only playing' do not realise the importance of play. As described later in Chapter 15, play is as important to children as work is to adults. Through play the child learns about the complexities of his environment and the people in it; control is gained over physical skills and feelings; and through the fantasies of child's play, there is temporary escape from the frustrations and demands of the real world and immeasurable satisfaction from being, for once, the 'king of the castle' or the 'angry father' or the 'Lady of the Lamp' instead of just a small, unimportant child.

Play can also be purposefully directed along these lines. For example, a child can be helped to anticipate the experience of hospitalisation if, through play, he learns that nurses and doctors are kind even though sometimes they do things — like giving an injection — which hurt.

Intellectual development in childhood

In most societies with a formal education system, the child now attends school full-time where he learns the complex skills of reading, writing, spelling and counting. According to Piaget's theory, this is the period of 'concrete and formal operations'. Verbal language skills are further developed with an increased vocabulary and fluency of speech. Some children learn more quickly than others and differences between children become evident in terms of their rate of intellectual development and level of ability. Sometimes 'intelligence tests' are used to measure such differences. 'Intelligence' is simply an indicator of how an individual uses cognitive processes for adaptive purposes. Although the potential to be highly intelligent or otherwise may be influenced by hereditary factors, much more important are the opportunities for learning afforded to a child by his school and family.

Emotional development in childhood

The child who is developing physically and intellectually in accordance with advancing age is likely to gain self-confidence and to enjoy the satisfaction of his own achievements.

As the child learns to be more specific in his expression of positive and negative emotions, he also learns to misuse these responses in being devious and mischievous. He begins to learn the effects of manipulation of his own behaviour on others. Social interactions with his parents, siblings, peers and school teachers become more complex and subtle. The child still relies on others for encouragement and praise and, although increasingly self-reliant, still needs comforting and protection from sources of fear and anxiety. The school-age child may suffer from loneliness or from feeling unloved in his family or unpopular at school.

An important dimension of the child's concept of self at this stage is his or her increasing awareness of self as male or female. Early sex-related behaviour patterns tend to be strengthened and the child often models himself on the parent of the same sex. Parents remain very significant to the child and continue to influence his social behaviour, emotional development, self-concept, interests, and keenness to learn at school. In addition, they shape his gradual acquisition of social mores, norms and moral standards. Although a young child still misses his parents if separated from them, he can cope with a temporary separation because he is able to conceptualise time and to understand reasoning and promises.

Social development in childhood

Social development has an important new dimension in that it becomes less family-dominated than in infancy. The child's peers provide opportunities for co-operation and competition and he usually associates with a number of different groups — school friends, cubs or Brownies, Sunday school, and neighbours — each group providing social relationships of various strengths and types. The loss of a close friend, for example if the family moves to another district, can be a very distressing event for a child.

From time to time, most children do experience unhappiness and anxiety; childhood is not without its problems, however trivial they may seem to adults. Apart from transient difficulties some children, because of personal, family or social circumstances, may not have a happy childhood. Among these are children of large low-income families and those who have to live apart from their parents, or with one parent only because of marital breakdown. In addition, children with physical or mental handicap are particularly vulnerable to stress and anxiety.

However, most children are protected during these early years from the responsibilities and obligations of adulthood; learning to assume a greater degree of independence and to make decisions of consequence are important tasks of the next stage in the process of development.

DEVELOPMENT DURING ADOLESCENCE (13–18 years)

The time period of adolescence — which means 'passing from childhood to maturity' — is less easy to define in terms of age because it varies between individuals and to a large extent is culturally defined. In Western societies, the end of adolescence is usually arbitrarily determined by the school-leaving or voting age. In some developing countries, entry into adulthood is achieved much earlier, being defined as the time when sexual maturity is reached. Because becoming an adult is such a significant step in life, the event is marked in some cultures by a social ceremony — a *rite de passage* which stresses the change of social status and the new responsibilities.

Physical development in adolescence

Growth in adolescence is dominated by the development of sexual maturity, the onset being called puberty. In the female, the first signs of approaching puberty are the enlargement of the breasts and the growth of pubic hair. This can occur at any time from the age of 8, but usually happens around the age of 12. At the same time the shape of the body undergoes change. The hips widen and fat deposits are laid down to give the characteristic female body outline. The abdominal organs enlarge, particularly those of the reproductive system. The onset of menstruation (the menarche) completes sexual maturity; the average age for this in the U.K. is about 13 years. The menstrual cycle is discussed further in Chapter 16.

Boys tend to reach puberty a little later than girls. From the age of 12 or so, the body size and strength of muscles increase greatly and the amount of body fat decreases. Physiological changes accompany these overt physical ones — the blood pressure rises, heart rate falls, blood volume increases and respiratory efficiency improves. The overall effect is a substantial gain in strength and physical ability. The age at which these changes take place varies between boys; delayed puberty can be a source of extreme distress and at this age, boys are often very self-conscious about their body sometimes feeling particularly embarrassed when in the company of females.

The growth of the male sex organs and the appearance of secondary sex characteristics (body and facial hair and deepening of the voice) complete the development of sexual maturity in the male. Although boys are capable of erection of the penis before puberty, the ability to ejaculate semen and the production of active spermatozoa are developments of puberty itself.

Intellectual development in adolescence

Intellectual development continues through formal education and the pursuit of personal interests. At school, through academic studies, the adolescent can achieve a refined level of logical thought, conceptual ability and creativity. Scholastic attainment shows an even more marked differentiation between individuals, some choosing to take advanced examinations and others failing to reach an acceptable standard of literacy and numeracy. The decision regarding what job or career to take up becomes an important issue in late adolescence.

Emotional development in adolescence

Emotional development during the teens is very closely linked to the physical changes of puberty. Although cap-

able of the adult function of sexual reproduction, adolescents are without the emotional maturity needed for adult relationships and this causes one of the conflicts inherent in adolescence. Relationships with parents undergo change and the adolescent begins to assert his individuality and desire for independence by resisting adult authority and advice. An awareness of his own sexuality may make the adolescent feel uncomfortable about the intimacy of the parent–child relationship. As a result, he may become secretive and detached.

Adolescence is often a period of emotional turmoil and insecurity caused by the conflict between need and desire for independence and need to hang on to a child-like dependence on others. The adolescent often displays swings of mood and experiences confused emotions. He can be both happy and miserable, selfish and idealistic, submissive and rebellious, full of energy one moment and lazy and lethargic the next.

Social development in adolescence

Social development is rapid and involves an expansion of the network of social relationships and a diversification of social activities (Fig. 5.2).

The acquisition of sexual maturity results in an increasingly marked differentiation in the social roles of males and females. Boys tend to reinforce their masculinity and channel their physical energies by grouping together and engaging in sports or other male activities. Many boys experience homosexual attractions and, though a natural feature of development, this can cause feelings of guilt and confusion. Girls tend to become concerned with their appearance and femininity, and their associations with each other are often competitive rather than cooperative and friendly.

Later in adolescence heterosexual attachments become more common and, although often transient, can be intense and traumatic. Often they involve varying degrees of sexual experimentation and sometimes pairings established in adolescence may develop into full sexual relationships. There is then the risk of unwanted pregnancy. Despite the wider availability of contraceptives today (p. 299) illegitimacy is still a problem of contemporary society.

The problems of cigarette smoking, drug dependence and alcoholism (pp. 143, 288 and 177), with all their attendant health hazards, often grow from habits established in the teenage years. Parents who realise the long-term dangers of adolescent experimentation may try to overprotect their child rather than encourage freedom within a framework of guidance. But this may not be helpful, because society expects the adult to assume responsibility: unless responsibility is given, the adolescent cannot learn to exercise it.

DEVELOPMENT IN EARLY ADULTHOOD (19–30 years)

Physical development in early adulthood

Physical changes are minimal during this stage of the lifespan. It is a time of stability when full physical maturity has been reached and before the process of ageing begins. The young adult male is at his peak of physical fitness. The young adult female has major physical adaptation to make only in respect of pregnancy, if this occurs. In industrialised societies the incidence of morbidity and mortality is very low compared with other age groups, and so most young adults can expect to be unthreatened by major illness.

Intellectual development in early adulthood

Intellectual development continues to take place throughout adult life, although in a less formalised and more personal way than during the school years. In all aspects of living, the adult uses his intellectual skills and cognitive processes. Some people so inclined choose jobs which demand a high level of intellectual ability. The choice of, and establishment in, an occupation is one of the major tasks of young adulthood. The significance of the AL of working is discussed fully in Chapter 15.

The choice of occupation is influenced by factors such as family background, educational qualifications, interests and motivations and employment opportunities. Although the income level of a job is a basic consideration, for most people job satisfaction is also important and influences choice. People who find their job tedious or unsuitable can be under considerable stress, as are those unable to obtain a job. Some jobs involve working under unpleasant or dangerous conditions; others are known to create mental stress or predispose the individual to ill-health. The type of employment, then, considerably influences an individual's life-style, economic status, social standing and health. Choosing and starting a job is therefore an important and demanding task for the young adult.

Emotional development in early adulthood

In the early years of adulthood emotional development concerns adjustment to independent adult life and centres on the formation of adult relationships. Erikson describes the conflict of this stage of development as that between 'intimacy and solidarity' and 'isolation'.

Of the relationships developed in this period, the central one in a society based on the nuclear family is the marriage relationship—a long-term, reciprocal, total relationship with an adult of the opposite sex. The sexual component of this relationship is discussed in Chapter 16. Whether or not the non-reproductive functions of sex are important depends to a large extent on sociocultural factors which affect the marriage relationship. In Western societies there is considerable emphasis on marriage as a romantic relationship giving security and companionship. In other cultures, marriage is seen more as a vehicle for child-rearing and commercial enterprise.

Although still an important social relationship, marriage has undergone considerable change in recent times. Premarital and extramarital sexual relationships are more common and divorce much more frequent. Husband and wife roles are tending to become less stereotyped with a greater sharing of economic, domestic and parental responsibilities. While these changes may bring greater flexibility and personal freedom in marriage they also carry stresses and difficulties for the young adult.

The birth of the first child is a most important event for young parents and it completes the 'formation' phase of the family life cycle (Table 5.1). Becoming a parent demands major adaptation in role and function and requires a readjustment of the emotional relationship between husband and wife. Often parenthood, especially motherhood, is rather idealised by the media and so people may not be emotionally prepared to face the demands made on emotions, energy, time and money. The constraints on every aspect of living may be adversely affected. Preparation for parenthood is assuming greater importance in prenatal care these days.

Although the monogamous, heterosexual relationship of marriage is for many the central relationship in adulthood, there are other kinds of relationships in which emotional satisfaction may be gained. A minority of adult males and females remain unmarried by the age of 30, by chance or choice. They may or may not choose to form a long-term heterosexual relationship or to engage in short-term relationships. Others may form homosexual relationships. Some may continue to live in their parental home or be required to devote their attention to ageing parents or relatives. Still others may set up 'one-parent' families or live communally within a group. These are but a few of the life-styles which adults choose to adopt and within which emotional relationships are established and emotional satisfaction gained.

Social development in young adulthood

For the young adult this takes place within the context of his job and network of relationships. These provide opportunities for him to fulfil a variety of social roles — workmate, husband, father — and to enter into a number of different social systems. Leisure pursuits provide another means of social integration. The individual may also begin to influence the society in which he lives and, through politics or other activities, he can become an agent of social change.

DEVELOPMENT IN THE MIDDLE YEARS
(30–45 years)

For most adults in the fourth decade of life, the major tasks of career establishment and family formation are well underway and the related family, social and occupational roles have emerged with some degree of stability and permanence. As a result, this phase of life is a relatively settled one and can be one of the most productive and satisfying periods.

But equally, just because of its settled nature, it can be a crisis period for some because of the apparent lack of challenge, change and external pressure. As they pass through their 30s, some adults experience a sense of disillusionment, boredom or frustration. The previous challenges of the new job may subside into an onerous routine; the excitement of establishing a home may give way to irritation at its continual need for redecorating and the cost of its upkeep; the satisfactions of rearing young children may be forgotten as the trials of adolescence begin to develop; their own parents may be ageing and beginning to make demands upon them; the marital relationship may have lost some of its novelty; the wife may be facing the demands of coping with a family and a job or may be fearing a return to work after an absence; and the reality of problems of society at large may impinge on the adult and depress him. Married couples may envy the apparent freedom of their unmarried counterparts' life-style, while the bachelor or spinster may begin to feel the burden of loneliness.

DEVELOPMENT IN LATE ADULTHOOD
(46–65 years)

Physical and intellectual changes in late adulthood

The forties are often described as the years of 'middle age'. It is a good description because at this time the balance between physical growth and physical degeneration begins to alter and finally settles on the side of degeneration.

Physically, the effects of ageing become quite noticeable, particularly on the face and in the skin. Men experience quite a rapid decline in physical strength, agility and speed of movement. The significant physical change for women is the menopause, the process whereby menstruation ceases marking the end of female fertility (see p. 299). Due to the effects of the hormonal changes involved, many physical discomforts can be experienced and this 'change of life' is frequently tiresome and tiring for women.

In the face of declining physical fitness, many men find the demands of their job more tiring. Men and women in professional jobs may be reaching the height of their careers which although satisfying, may involve excessive stress. Sometimes the acuity of senses and intellectual skills may deteriorate and it becomes difficult to concentrate and retain information. In contrast, people in manual or unskilled occupations may by this stage have little interest or challenge left in their job and suffer from boredom and apathy or extreme physical tiredness. In either case, working may dominate life and there may be little time or energy left for playing.

Emotional and social changes in late adulthood

When grown-up children leave home (the 'contraction' phase of the family life cycle — Table 5.1), the middle-aged parents are freed of their arduous parental responsibilities. For some, this will seem a tremendous loss and the experience of the menopause for a woman is often worsened by her regret at the loss of her role and function as mother. For others, the freedom will bring relief and enjoyment and the vicarious parental experiences gained from being grandparents are often more than just a substitute.

Both sexes are apt to be less flexible at this age, less able to cope with major upheavals such as changing jobs or moving house. Stability of routine tends to be favoured, even though this in itself may result in a sense of boredom. Stability in marriage is reflected in the dramatic reduction in the divorce rate within this age group. Many couples begin to appreciate the close companionship which marriage provides, although some experience marital problems associated with the loss of parental roles and a declining interest in the sexual aspect of the relationship.

A major event which occurs towards or at the end of this stage of the lifespan is retirement from work. Preparation for a healthy and satisfying retirement is now regarded as extremely important (p. 276).

Although people of this age group still have a long expectancy of life ahead, loss of a spouse by death is not uncommon and widowhood demands an enormous change of lifestyle with the bleak prospect of having to embark alone on the final stage of the lifespan.

DEVELOPMENT IN OLD AGE (65 years +)

Although the average lifespan in countries of the Western world has increased over the last century to around 70 years, the maximum attainable length of life has not increased significantly throughout history. It is still extremely rare for people to survive to the age of 100 years or more. The significant fact is that more people are living longer and as a result the proportion of elderly people in the population has increased. We now live in an ageing society.

It is one of the most significant demographic changes of this century (and of Western societies in particular) that the elderly make up, at least temporarily, a larger proportion of the total population than ever before. It is in the 75 years and over age group that the current increase is greatest. This has important implications for health and social services because members of this age group are likely to succumb to various problems which affect health and independence and are unlikely to have relatives to look after them.

For nurses and others involved with the elderly, an understanding of developments of old age is essential. It should of course be remembered that many people who are over 65 are not really 'old' in the way that word tends to imply. However, there is a definite and irreversible acceleration in the biological ageing process and, sooner or later, its effects begin to be noticeable.

Physical changes in old age

Ageing involves the gradual physical deterioration of the body; all living organisms undergo some kind of degenerative process. The most obvious signs of ageing in humans are changes in the extracellular matrix. The tissues appear to 'dry out' and as a result the skin loses its elasticity and turgidity, the walls of the blood vessels deteriorate in quality, joints stiffen, muscle mass and strength reduce, and all the organs of the body function less efficiently and are less able to tolerate the demands made upon them. The body becomes increasingly less efficient as a biological organism.

The result is that old people may experience problems with various Activities of Living; for example, there may be difficulty in breathing on exertion, loss of appetite or discomforts associated with digestion in relation to the ALs of eating and drinking. Also, mobility may become impaired or restricted and the AL of eliminating may be affected by incontinence of urine or chronic constipation.

As the body becomes increasingly less efficient, illness occurs more readily than in youth and some pathological changes are very closely associated with advancing age and biological degeneration. Narrowing of the arterial blood vessels (atherosclerosis), high blood pressure (hypertension), disease of the joints (such as arthritis) and malignant tumours (cancer) all have a high incidence among the elderly. Another problem likely to arise among the elderly who live alone is malnutrition.

Defects of sight and hearing are also common. A common cause of death in old age is a stroke, properly called a cerebral vascular accident (CVA). This can cause speech difficulties (the problem of aphasia is discussed on p. 129) or perceptual disorder and usually results in upper and lower limb defects (p. 266).

Irrespective of the disease process involved, health problems in old age may often lessen the elderly person's capacity to be independent in the Activities of Living.

Intellectual changes in old age

The total number of cells in the human body decreases during the ageing process and the effects are most noticeable in respect of the brain cells. There is a gradual decline in intellectual functioning. The old person eventually begins to suffer from loss of memory and slowness in thinking and becomes less able to concentrate. The acuity of the senses also reduces: eyesight weakens, hearing becomes impaired, and the senses of touch and smell may be less acute. Overall, intellectual functioning becomes increasingly less efficient.

Again, this degeneration can result in problems with activities of living. The elderly are particularly prone to difficulties in communicating because the senses are less acute. Maintaining a safe environment in the home may become difficult when memory fails. As opportunities for working and playing become less, boredom or loneliness may result. Maintaining sensory and intellectual stimulation is an important responsibility of all who care for the elderly.

Social aspects of old age

It is remarkable that, in spite of the problems associated with ageing, the majority of elderly people do manage to remain in their own homes. In the U.K. for example, only a very small minority of the elderly population has to be looked after in institutions. However, as the numbers of very old people increase it will become more and more important for disability and dependence to be prevented if institutional care is to be kept to a minimum.

As a social group, the elderly are vulnerable to many social difficulties including poverty, poor housing, and social isolation. In a society which emphasises youth and independence the rewards are not rich for those who have contributed to it a lifetime of work and a new generation of children. In contrast, other cultures such as in China regard the elderly as a group worthy of respect, and special care and honour are bestowed upon them.

Emotional aspects of old age

The way society views old age inevitably affects the way in which the elderly see themselves. If society does not value and respect its senior members and emphasise the positive aspects of ageing rather than all the negative ones it is not surprising that many old people experience a loss of self-respect and a sense of worthlessness. Erikson, in his theory of individual development (p. 47), described the task of old age as reconciling the conflict between 'integrity' and 'despair'.

This conflict is related to the prospect of approaching death which, inevitably, is something every old person thinks about. Dying (Ch. 18) is the final act of living and reaching acceptance of impending death involves major emotional adjustment. On top of this, there are many adaptations to be made in coping with the physical effects of the process of ageing and in adapting to declining intellectual ability.

As opportunities for social integration become fewer, and as friends and family die, the elderly may have to rely increasingly on the company of younger people who inevitably have their own interests and may have difficulty in appreciating the feelings and needs of members of an older generation. Tremendous patience and empathy are needed to understand and tolerate the slower pace of life in old age, the lability of emotions of the elderly and their fierce resistance to help which they may interpret as charity. Often the old person finds that the pace and outlook of modern society does not suit him and he prefers to live in the past, reminiscing about the 'good old days' and criticising the ways of the present. Some old people may refuse to accept the inevitability of death and, feeling unfulfilled, may become depressed and even angry about their old age. Others will appreciate the experience which life has given them and, accepting old age and death as natural, will move towards the end of their life with confidence and dignity.

This chapter has provided an overview of developmental aspects of living — a resumé of the physical, intellectual, emotional and social developments in the various stages of the lifespan, from conception through to death. It is clear that every aspect of living and specifically, all of the Activities of Living, are influenced by this complex and continuous process of development which occurs throughout the lifespan. Later in the book (Chs 7–18) the specific effects of the lifespan on each of the 12 Activities of Living are described. Prior to that (Ch. 6) there is discussion in general terms to show how an understanding of developmental aspects of living is relevant in the context of nursing.

REFERENCES

Bowlby J 1953 Child care and the growth of love. Pelican, Harmondsworth
Rutter M 1972 Maternal deprivation reassessed. Penguin, Harmondsworth

5

Social aspects of living

It is clear from the preceding discussion that, like physical, intellectual and emotional development, socialisation is a lifelong process. How does an understanding of a person's social background help to explain his attitudes and behaviour? In what ways does the kind of community a person lives in affect the style and quality of his life? What circumstances alter a person's role and status in society and how does status affect interpersonal relationships? Why are relationships among kin so important and why does the social institution of the family survive as the basic unit of society? These are some of the questions examined in this chapter which looks at some *social* aspects of living.

LIVING IN SOCIETY

Society, culture, community

It is usually only in adulthood that a person becomes regarded as a fully fledged member of *society*, the social environment within which living takes place. Indeed, with rights such as the right to vote, an adult has an opportunity to change the society of which he is a member, so he has a degree of control over it as well as being influenced by it.

However, during childhood and adolescence, individuals develop under the influence of the society into which they are born: they undergo a process of *socialisation*. It is as a result of this process that individuals of a particular society share in common certain values and beliefs, and function harmoniously within its organisation.

Within every society there is some kind of organisation of people into groups and of activities into institutions. The social organisation may be simple, as in a nomadic tribe in which members belong to a family group and work is divided into 'men's work' and 'women's work'; or it may involve a highly elaborate network of groups and specialised structures, as in technologically advanced countries.

Whatever the basic structure of society each individual becomes socialised into it and accustomed to the set of sanctions, sentiments and values which characterise its way of life and make it unique.

Culture is the word used in sociology to refer to the way of life of a particular society and cultural differences exist in even the most basic of everyday living activities. Such cultural idiosyncrasies are highlighted for each AL in Section 3.

Different systems of health care throughout the world show that culture influences the way societies deal with health and illness. Deep-rooted cultural beliefs and traditions affect an individual's behaviour when ill — for example, responses to pain vary according to ethnic origin. Also cultural factors influence the way people treat others who are ill so that some types of handicap and certain diseases carry a degree of stigma in some societies. The mentally handicapped may be shunned or feared even today because of the legacy of the view once held that idiocy was inflicted on people as punishment for their sins. Sociocultural factors are therefore important in understanding an individual's health behaviour and his response to illness and hospitalisation.

As well as belonging to a society and sharing its culture, every person is a member of a *community*. The term is most often used to describe a locality with a sub-culture of its own and even a small town can have several communities, such as the industrial estate and the housing scheme. The kind of community a person lives in greatly affects the quality of his life; even his personal safety is to a large extent dependent on the maintenance of safety in the community at large, for example in its schools and transport systems.

Housing

For most people *a house* provides a reference point within a community and it is the pivot around which life is lived. But some housing factors — poor amenities, high-rise flats and overcrowding — can predispose to health problems and interfere with growth and development.

Poor amenities. In old, often dilapidated property in urban areas, lack of a piped water supply, a hot water system and a fixed bath pose many health problems. Every drop of water for personal washing and laundering of clothes has to be heated on a stove. If the toilet is out of doors, there is the additional problem of carrying out the preventive activity of hand washing after elimination. These inner city slums are often the result of urban change as new towns and industries are moved to the outskirts of the city, the inner areas are deprived of their communities of workers. Only the poor, the elderly and the handicapped remain and the vacant dilapidated dwellings are occupied by low-income groups such as new immigrants and large working-class families.

In these poor amenity areas children can become emotionally disturbed and they may act out their resentment and disillusion by indulging in vandalism and petty thieving. This is likely to happen after they go to school where they are exposed to the reality of comparison and realise that they are different from the predominantly middle-class teachers and other more affluent children.

High-rise flats. In many countries vertical building was hailed as the solution to slum clearance since hundreds of families could be housed on one building site, land being an expensive item in the provision of houses. Far from being a solution, it has brought in its wake social problems that are as vexing as those created by the overflowing slums. Long cold concrete corridors; every front door exactly the same; 20 floors up and the lift only working half the time; two lifts for 400 people and each lift carrying only eight people — these can be the harsh facts about life in a multistorey flat.

Social isolation in multistorey flats can be severe resulting in statements such as 'The whole family could be dead and nobody would know a thing about it' and 'As soon as you shut the door you are cut off from the rest of the world'. Mothers with infants have pram problems and they are afraid to allow the older children to play out of doors because of the difficulty of keeping an eye on them. Some local authorities have a rule that families with young children should not be housed above the fourth floor, but in reality this is difficult to observe: such children, as well as their mothers, can be socially deprived.

Overcrowding. Some children have to share a bedroom with siblings while others share their parents' bedroom. There are other households where all members sleep in the living room. Bed-sharing is also frequent and it can be a cause of disturbed sleep, bed-wetting, sexual precocity, cross infection and infestation. These patterns prevent each child from having space to call his own in which he can keep his personal and 'private' possessions, an important part of developing a self-concept.

The constraint of lack of privacy affects all members of the family in their development of a concept of body privacy — the females in relation to personal cleansing necessary during menstruation and the parents in relation to sexualising activities. Clearly, the social circumstances of an individual's community, and in particular his home, exert a considerable influence on his lifestyle and his health status.

Role and status

The concept of *role* is helpful in describing the part an individual plays in society. There are many different social roles and each carries very specific expectations and makes specific demands on the individual. From birth, a male baby may occupy the roles of son, brother and grandson and these differ from the daughter, sister and granddaughter roles of a female baby. These are examples of 'ascribed' roles, i.e. those allocated to people at birth according to their sex and existing kinship network. Others are 'achieved' as a result of personal choice and endeavour, for example occupational roles.

Even such fundamental roles as man or woman and child or parent have to be learnt. One of the important functions of the family is the socialisation of children, the process whereby they are taught and learn about the characteristics, expectations and responsibilities attached to the whole range of social roles.

Each person has his or her own repertoire of different roles and Figure 5.1 illustrates one individual's role set. At any time, there is a central role being played (in this case, that of 'wife') and a number of peripheral roles. According to the circumstances, any role can become the central one. Although each role has distinct characteristics, most are closely interrelated and interdependent. Sometimes the role of 'mother' and 'nurse' may be almost indistinguishable but at other times, they may clash; for example, there are many conflicts inherent in a woman's dual role as 'mother' and 'worker' (in this case, as a nurse).

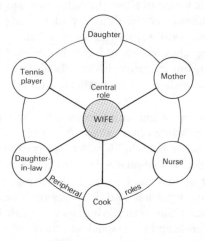

Fig. 5.1 An individual's role set

Of particular interest to those involved in the delivery of health care is what happens to an individual's role and status when he becomes ill. Talcott Parsons, a sociologist, described this phenomenon in what he termed the '*sick role*' (Parsons, 1966). He pointed out that most societies exempt a sick person from some of his usual obligations and responsibilities as long as he fulfils a corresponding obligation to seek medical care and co-operate in the process of getting well. In many parts of the world there is in fact legislation to ensure that the sick are given special entitlements; for example, there are government schemes which provide the employee with sickness leave along with protection from financial hardship caused by loss of earnings (p. 278).

However, as other writers have pointed out, there are many social implications of illness not considered in Parsons' analysis. It does not acknowledge the subjectivity involved in defining 'health' and 'illness' or take account of the fact that some sick people will never get 'well' and others may not wish to co-operate in attempts to restore them to health. It is probably more helpful to view the role transition from 'well' to 'sick' as a gradual process (except in cases of acute illness) during which the individual's role and status undergo modification. Sometimes, if the term 'sick role' is interpreted in a broad way, the term 'patient role' is preferred when referring to people actually receiving health care (Anderson, 1973).

Assuming the role of 'patient' involves many role changes: for example, a young mother is expected to receive rather than give care; the managing director usually responsible for many employees becomes the responsibility of others; and the lawyer and the miner are treated as equals despite occupying quite different social positions in real life.

In general, in any society there are differences in the degree of *status* attached to particular roles and in the importance attributed to ascribed as compared to achieved roles. In some parts of the world the roles of women are less valued than those of men whereas in others they are still delineated into 'child-rearing' and 'wage-earning' roles respectively, but are nevertheless regarded with equal importance. Some societies afford very special privileges and advantages to some occupational roles; for instance, traditionally in Europe and North America doctors and lawyers obtain high salaries and have considerable political power and high social prestige.

Relationships and groups

The expectations society attaches to various roles are displayed in patterns of social interaction and interpersonal *relationships*. For example, the doctor's high social status is reflected in the way patients tend to behave subserviently to him, submitting to his authority and accepting his advice unquestioningly. Such behaviour also serves to reinforce the traditional assymetrical doctor–patient relationship. In fact, throughout the whole health care system there is an elaborate set of expectations and rules about the kinds of interaction considered to be appropriate between members of different health care professions and between professionals and patients.

Each individual has his own unique network of relationships. Initially, this emerges from the kinship network into which the person is born and it comprises relationships with members of the nuclear family and the extended family. Later, as the child interacts with people outside the family, the network grows to include relationships with peers and friends, neighbours and members of various social groups. Figure 5.2 shows the type of network of social relationships which an adolescent may have. Further extension of the network occurs in adulthood from relationships arising from marriage, childbearing and an occupation. An example of an adult's network of social relationships is shown in Figure 5.3. During adult life, a person's network continually changes and expands; in old age there is a gradual retraction in the number and variety of social relationships.

An individual does not interact only with another individual. Co-operation plays an important role in a complex society and to this end a great deal of social interaction takes place within *social groups*. An individual begins life as a member of the most generic social group, his family. Thereafter, he spends his entire life joining and leaving various groups which exist in society to serve a multitude of functions: social, occupational, recreational, educational, political and religious. The family and peer groups, and groups associated with working and playing, are among the most significant. Absence from these, as happens during a period of hospitalisation, may cause loneliness or boredom. Other groups, for instance religious and political organisations, may be very important for some people but less so for others. However, in general, membership of groups is extremely important for the fulfilment of love and belonging needs and the development and enhancement of self-esteem. Those individuals not strongly integrated with social groups may suffer from social isolation and become lonely and depressed, even sometimes suicidal.

Social structures and institutions

While social groups provide an important framework for the interaction of individuals, society itself must have some kind of overall structure to ensure that basic needs are met. The existence of a health care system shows that

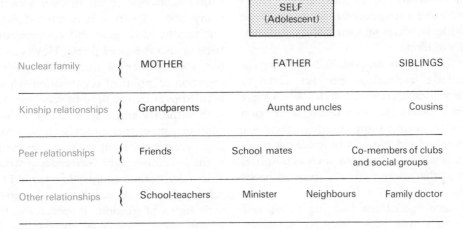

Fig. 5.2 Adolescent's network of social relationships

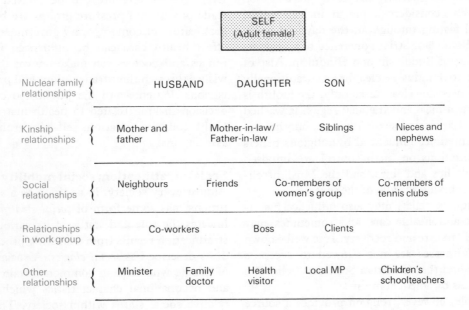

Fig. 5.3 An adult's network of social relationships

the society recognises the need to maintain health, for example. All societies therefore have certain *social structures*. Some of the basic structures or institutions are:

- the family: to ensure replacement of population
- education: to socialise the new population, train members to fulfil tasks, and transmit culture
- religion: to maintain a sense of purpose and morality
- economics: to ensure the production and distribution of goods, services and money
- health: to maintain the health of the population
- government: to preserve law and order

If the basic needs of society are to be met the existence and continuation of these social institutions are essential. In a complex industrialised society this requires a high degree of organisation, a large workforce and expenditure of a great deal of public money.

For each individual the family is, at least initially, probably the most influential of the institutions. However, the others too exert a tremendous influence on the behaviour of individuals, shaping their habits and attitudes in all activities of living.

The influence of religion on individual behaviour for example is particularly fascinating, religious doctrines often dictating a very circumscribed lifestyle. When there is religious unity in a society the culture and the religion are almost inseparable; within some countries there are many ethnic sub-cultures and so many religions are practised. This is a fact of which institutions such as hospitals must take account so that every patient's spiritual needs may be appreciated.

Many religions have regulations affecting eating and drinking habits which will affect nursing activities. Orthodox Jews, for instance, consider every meal a religious rite and must eat specially prepared 'kosher' food at all times. Muslims consider the pig an unclean animal and observe total fasting throughout the daylight hours in the month of Ramadan. Strict adherence to a vegetarian diet is a feature of Buddhism and Hinduism. Also of great importance to Hindus is cleanliness; traditionally the right hand is used for clean tasks only, the mouth is rinsed out after each meal and the anal region is washed after defaecation. Expressing sexuality is yet another activity of living sometimes influenced by religious beliefs and customs: limitations on birth control are imposed upon Roman Catholics and Jews, and the Muslim religion prohibits free mixing socially of the sexes.

A person's religious beliefs may also influence his attitudes to health and health care and sometimes may present an obstacle to care and recovery. It is well-known that Jehovah's Witnesses are not allowed to accept a blood transfusion and that Christian Scientists believe in the healing of illness by spiritual means.

For many people, however, religion provides a source of hope and comfort during illness. Sometimes, as in the Roman Catholic church, special sacraments may be offered to the sick and the dying. Baptism, thought by some to be necessary for a person's salvation, is carried out for any infant in danger of death or for a stillborn child (or fetus). The Sacrament of the Anointing of the Sick (formerly known as Extreme Unction or Last Rites) is often performed for a Roman Catholic during illness to aid healing and give moral strength or as a preparation for death. In general, for the dying and the bereaved religion often assumes a role of great importance, and this subject is returned to in Chapter 18. In fact religion, as a social institution, plays a key role in determining attitudes and customs on matters of life and death in nearly every existing society, regardless of whether the members actively practise the religion.

The relevance of government as a social institution, too, is of great importance in the growth and development of a society and in its organisation, as well as in the preservation of law and order. In some societies, for example in many parts of Africa, it is often difficult to separate the institutions of religion and government: the chief of the tribe is also the chief priest. However, in the more complex societies of that continent there is increasing differentiation of political organisation whereby the kingdom is ruled over by the head of state and others are endowed with authority and responsibility for judicial, legislative, administrative and military functions of government. Even greater differentiation and specialisation is inherent in the governments of Western industrialised societies.

In a democratic country like the United Kingdom, citizens can exert their influence on government through their rights of freedom of speech and the vote. In such a system each member of society who is motivated and politically aware can act as an agent of social change. Even greater pressure can be exerted collectively, and trade unions and pressure groups are becoming an integral feature of contemporary government. Policies which affect health care can be influenced in this way, and nurses and doctors can make known their opinions and wishes through their trade unions and professional organisations. Patients and the public too can participate in decision making related to health matters through local health councils or various self-help groups and consumer associations.

Social stratification; social mobility

Almost every society, in addition to a set of social institutions, has some form of *social stratification* which delineates the role and status of its various groups. Social stratification results from a layering process which creates units described as *social classes*. A social class is a group of people who have in common certain social, economic and occupational characteristics which determine their relative social status within society. There are different systems of class used throughout the world. In industrialised countries, the class system is often based on occupational grouping and in the U.K. the Registrar General's Social Class Scale is used to categorise social class according to occupation (p. 278). In general, people tend to think of three social classes — 'upper', 'middle' and 'working' class — and to attribute to each a stereotyped set of characteristics.

The concept of social class is useful in order to understand the variations in lifestyle of different social groups. For example, it is known that methods of child-rearing and the value placed on education vary between social classes. Power and status in society are also related to social class, those of the higher classes usually having greater political power and social influence.

There is also an important correlation between social class and health status. Infant mortality tends to be higher in the lower social classes, a baby born into a working-class home being more likely to have a lower birth weight and more likely to die in the first week of life. In general there are differences in the types of illnesses that affect members of high and low social classes. For example, statistics show that heart disease is more prevalent among professional people and respiratory conditions are more common among working-class groups.

There is also an apparent correlation between social class and response to illness. The best possible use of health services tends to be made by members of the higher social classes; others often fail to take advantage of provisions such as child health or family planning clinics. Added to this is the advantage which professional people gain from their ability to interpret symptoms of illness and to know which ones should have immediate medical attention. For example, a number of studies have shown that the symptoms of blood in the urine (haematuria) and a lump in the breast are usually considered to merit medical attention by members of higher social classes whereas those of lower classes often fail to appreciate their significance.

The movement of individuals or social groups from one stratum of society to another is known as *social mobility*. In a system of social class based on occupation, individuals are able to 'better' their social status by obtaining a more skilled and remunerative job and so achieve 'upward' social mobility. Sometimes, as happens if unemployment is high, an individual may be forced to accept a lower social status. Either way, even if the person's lifestyle remains virtually the same, social mobility results in a change of 'class consciousness' — his own and other people's.

In some societies there is no opportunity at all for social mobility, for instance within the Indian caste system. Although less rigid than it once was, there are five major castes, based on occupation, and a person is born into a caste. There is no mobility across caste lines even as a result of marriage or a change in occupation. In addition, the caste system places limitations upon interpersonal interaction and involves many legal and religious restrictions.

Whether or not there is the opportunity for social mobility later in life, the social class of a child is determined at birth according to the father's social position. In this and many other matters, it is the social institution of the family which determines and shapes an individual's personal process of socialisation.

LIVING IN THE FAMILY

The family as a social institution
It was pointed out at the very beginning of Chapter 1 that the family is the oldest and most used health care service in the world. Even where there exists a comprehensive health care system the family remains an important adjunct to care, looking after its members during illness and infirmity and providing support during hospitalisation when this is necessary. Depending on the degree of organisation of the social structure in different societies, the family also fulfils or assists with the tasks of other institutions: in various ways the family is an educational establishment, an economic unit and a focus for the preservation of morality and law and order.

Responsible for the primary socialisation of children, the family shapes an individual's habits and attitudes in all activities of living. It is so important that the family can be considered as the basic unit of society and through procreation it ensures that the population is replaced and that society itself continues to exist.

Throughout the world there are numerous different patterns of family structure and lifestyle. Even within one nation, there are many variations between families according to social class and whether or not the community is a rural or urban one, for example. However, when studying the family as a social phenomenon, two broad categories are usually identified: the extended family and the nuclear family.

The extended family
The extended family comprises several generations of a family living together as one domestic group. The group may be entirely self-sufficient and, through division of labour, carry out all the functions necessary for the survival and satisfaction of all its members. Division of function is possible because there are so many adults and, while some women will be responsible for care of the children, others will do the cooking and cleaning. This kind of family structure was common before industrialisation and still exists as the norm in some developing countries. This includes the father, mother and their children; the other wives of the father and their children; and the father's brothers and their wives and children.

All members live in huts in close proximity and all the children regard each other as brothers and sisters.

The extended family is in many ways a very stable and satisfactory kind of social institution. The position of the elderly is usually secure because there are sufficient younger people available to look after them and take over domestic and occupational roles. Although there is inevitable grief, the effect of the death of a parent on a child is likely to be less traumatic in an extended family where others are readily available to take over the parental function.

Sometimes in the U.K. the term extended family is used to refer to a modification of the structure in which a family of father, mother and children live in one house with grandparents, aunts, uncles and cousins living nearby (Fig. 5.4 illustrates the structure of an extended family). However, in this and other industrialised countries, the nuclear family is the most common form of communal living.

This increased mobility further decreases opportunities for mutual help among kinship groups and lessens the influence of one generation on another. Lacking close bonds with their families of origin, the husband and wife are more dependent on each other than in the extended family and children have to find company in peer groups outside the kinship network. The trends towards a higher divorce rate and a greater number of working mothers are other sources of strain for the nuclear family and, of course, illness and unemployment cause considerable difficulties for this small and unsupported domestic unit.

Like all social institutions, the family is not a static structure but one which changes as society develops. In addition, any one nuclear family undergoes a series of changes, and Table 5.1 shows how it can be described as having different phases according to the events which typically occur within its lifetime.

The phases of the family life-cycle of course have relevance for each member of the family. An individual

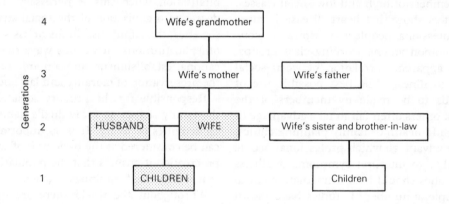

Fig. 5.4 An extended family

The nuclear family
The nuclear family comprises not more than two generations living together (see Fig. 5.5) — the father and mother and their children. Usually they do not live very close to near relatives such as grandparents or siblings and contact between the nuclear family and relations is often infrequent. This type of family structure developed following industrialisation which encouraged workers to move to urban centres of employment, and often nowadays families move several times during the working life of the parents.

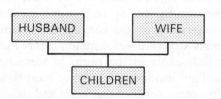

Fig. 5.5 The nuclear family

passes through the different phases at different stages of his lifespan and various dimensions of this intricate interrelationship of family circumstances and age are highlighted in Chapter 4.

Table 5.1 Basic model of a nuclear family life-cycle.

Phase of family life-cycle	Events characterising beginning	Events characterising end
Formation	Marriage	Birth of first child
Extension	Birth of first child	Birth of last child
Completed extension	Birth of last child	First child leaves home
Contraction	First child leaves home	Last child leaves home
Completed contraction	Last child leaves home	Death of first spouse
Dissolution	First spouse dies	Death of survivor

Source: World Health Organization.

Other types of 'family'

In conventional sociological analysis of the family, other types of 'family' are increasingly becoming recognised in addition to the two ideal types of extended and nuclear. For example, in industrialised countries where divorce is becoming more common, there are more 'one-parent' families; and with the trend for adolescents to leave home after finishing school education, hostels, university halls of residence and shared flats have become established forms of communal living for many young people.

The reasons why some children have to live apart from their natural parents — in residential care, hospitals or temporary foster homes — range from gross emotional inadequacy of the parents to profound mental or physical handicap of the child. Adults, too, because of chronic physical or psychiatric illness, may have to leave their families to live in an institution. A small proportion of the elderly population is cared for in old people's homes or geriatric hospitals.

Some of these other types of 'family' do provide a reasonable substitute for the natural family; however others unfortunately seem to predispose individuals to a variety of emotional, social and health problems.

One-parent families. Nowadays a considerable number of children in industrialised countries are brought up by one parent only, usually the mother, because of marital breakdown. Life for the child consists of day nursery or school, and, in the evening, exposure to an already tired parent perhaps preoccupied with domestic chores and financial difficulties. The effects on physical, emotional, social and intellectual development of children who grow up in one-parent families are as yet little understood. However, because these families are likely to suffer financial hardship, the child may well be deprived of a comfortable way of life, good nutrition and opportunities to develop certain leisure interests. It does appear that children of divorced parents are more likely than others to show disturbed behaviour and experience emotional difficulties.

Substitute families. Fostering has always been a way of providing a substitute family and is practised almost universally, in animal kingdoms as well as human societies. If a foster-child experiences stable and continuous family care and parental love then he is probably better off than a child living with natural parents but in an impoverished or discordant atmosphere.

Permanent adoption is generally considered a much more satisfactory solution for a child, at almost any age, who lacks a normal home life. But because most societies lay great emphasis on the importance of the 'blood tie' adopted children often feel, or are made to feel, disadvantaged and this may be all the more so in the case of those adopted into a family of different ethnic origin and skin colour.

Residential care. Many children 'in care' could be described as suffering from multiple deprivation; they are often illegitimate, or born prematurely or of low birth weight, and so begin life at a disadvantage. Often the reasons for a child being taken into care include problems of the parents, such as dependence on alcohol or criminality. The child may have lived his life in a large family within a poor community and with little opportunity to develop intellectually or emotionally. From such a background the child enters residential care which itself may not allow for a normal process of socialisation. Deprived of stable loving relationships the child in care may fail to learn how to trust and how to love.

Short-term care, as often happens during a mother's hospital confinement, is not usually harmful although young children are distressed when moved to an unfamiliar environment. Long-term care is now generally regarded as most unsatisfactory and when it is unavoidable every attempt is made to provide at least one 'parental' relationship (with a housemother or father), thus providing some sort of substitute for the absence of a family.

Institutional care. The need for this type of care is negligible in non-industrialised societies where the extended family assumes responsibility for looking after the sick, the handicapped and the elderly. In contrast, the health care systems of industrialised countries increasingly must provide institutions for long-term care in addition to hospitals designed to deal with short-term admissions.

Life in an institution such as a hospital for the mentally handicapped or a psychiatric or geriatric hospital — especially if it is old and large and cut off from the local community — is most abnormal for a member of a society whose basic social unit is the nuclear family. The adverse effects of 'institutionalisation' were first noticed in long-term psychiatric wards. At first it was thought that the patients' tendency to become totally apathetic, withdrawn and dependent was a result of psychiatric illness itself. Then it was realised that this behaviour was actually the effect of the patients' resignation to the unchallenging and unchanging institutional environment. This syndrome has been described as 'institutional neurosis' (Barton, 1966).

Now that this problem is recognised, members of the health care team lay great emphasis on helping patients in long-term care to be as independent as possible. Doing this utilises the concept of each individual having a dependence/independence continuum for each AL as described in the models of living and nursing (p. 22 and p. 69). Recently the concept of the 'therapeutic community' has been introduced into psychiatric care. This means that the hospital is made to operate as far as possible like a normal community; it is equipped with a shop and hairdressing salon, for example, and patients are expected to fulfil working and leisure roles and to participate in decision-making and community life. As a result, the risk of institutional neurosis is considered to be decreased and there is greater potential to restore health and improve social skills.

Taken a step further, this idea has led some hospitals to experiment with 'family living units', a system designed to replace institutional life altogether. Homes are provided (either actually in the community or by modifying the hospital environment) and these are occupied by small groups of patients with nurses acting as houseparents — in fact, a system exactly modelled upon the oldest and most basic social institution of all, the family.

Chapters 3, 4 and 5 provide a general outline of some major issues concerned with biological, developmental and social aspects of living. They give some substance to the model of living and are related to the factors which influence the Activities of Living. In general terms, the biological aspects are relevant to physical factors; devel-

opmental aspects to both physical and psychological factors; and social aspects to sociocultural, environmental and politicoeconomic factors. At risk of repetition, it has to be said that in the real life situation, these aspects and factors are not separate entities; they are related and interacting. It is only for purposes of description that they are dealt with separately.

The description of the model of living along with the content of these three chapters provide the framework for discussion of the model for nursing.

REFERENCES

Anderson E 1973 The role of the nurse. The study of nursing care project reports. Royal College of Nursing, London
Barton R 1966 Institutional neurosis. Wright, Bristol
Parsons T 1966 On becoming a patient. In: Folta J R, Deck E (eds) A sociological framework for patient care. Wiley, New York

6

Model for nursing

There is now much more general acceptance of the need for nursing to loosen its attachment to the 'disease' model, which has been in the ascendancy in many countries in the world throughout this century. In part this move reflects that nurses, along with others involved in health care, have become increasingly aware that people's health and the illnesses from which they suffer are inextricably linked with their lifestyle and the activities of living. In view of this, there are good reasons for offering as relevant to contemporary nursing, a *model for nursing* which is based on a *model of living*.

After all, most people require nursing only episodically during their lifetime and our rationale for linking 'nursing' with 'living' was the idea that this would encourage nurses to aim for minimal disruption of a person's established lifestyle while being nursed — to base individualised nursing on individuality in living.

Although based on concepts such as individuality, normality and healthy living, the model should not be seen as ignoring the concept of disease, or the interdependence of nurses and doctors, for both are fundamentally important to patient care (Mitchell, 1983; Tierney, 1983). However, the purpose of the model for nursing is to provide a framework for nurses to plan individualised nursing of those activities which are nurse-initiated and related to the patient's ALs. Of course a nursing plan also includes activities which are derived from the medical prescription, and from that of other members of the health care team. The carrying out of these delegated activities is an important function of the nurse. However, the model is essentially concerned with the nurse-initiated aspects of nursing. This is an important point to appreciate in relation to the model for nursing and, indeed, to the whole of this book.

A model for nursing which is based on a model of living may seem to be a rather broad and somewhat simple view of nursing. In fact, this is deliberate on both counts. While acknowledging the importance and necessity of specialisation within nursing, we believe that, underlying this, there is — and should be — a consensus among nurses as to the beliefs, goals and practices which are common to nursing, whatever the particular setting or circumstances, disease condition or patient/client group involved. Certainly for nurse learners we consider it essential that they are helped to see some connecting thread or theme to provide continuity and cohesiveness in the practice they observe and carry out in various settings, and in the various components of their theoretical instruction. This model for nursing is, we believe, sufficiently broad and flexible to be used as a framework for the process of nursing in any area of professional practice, and as a means of appreciating the underlying unity of the various branches of the profession.

And, certainly, the model is simple — as simple as the model of living on which it is based. This is not to suggest that either 'living' or 'nursing' are simple processes because, of course, they are not. However, we believe that to be useful, a model should be simple and in the case of nursing, directly relevant and applicable to practice. There is no necessity for a model to exhaust every aspect of the subject and, indeed if its presentation is excessively complicated by detail, its application to practice is unlikely to be readily apparent, however interesting and academically respectable it may be. This model is deliberately uncomplicated: it is offered as an overall framework to assist learners to develop a way of thinking about nurs-

ing in general terms, which then can be utilised in practice as a means of developing individualised nursing.

THE MODEL FOR NURSING

The diagrammatic representation of the model for nursing (Fig. 6.1) is, as will be immediately apparent, based on the diagram of the model of living (Fig. 2.6). Indeed it is exactly the same with one exception: '*individualising nursing*' takes the place of 'individuality in living'. The other four components – the *Activities of Living*, the *lifespan*, the *dependence/independence continuum* and the *factors influencing the ALs* — are all transferred directly from the model of living to the model for nursing.

The way of thinking about 'living' generated by the model of living will now be transferred to nursing in the following discussion of each of the five components of the model for nursing. Only an outline is provided in this chapter because the next section of the book comprises 12 chapters (Chs 7–18), one devoted to each of the ALs, in which detailed discussion of the five components of the model is presented in the context of nursing.

ACTIVITIES OF LIVING (ALs)

As in the model of living, the Activities of Living (Fig. 6.2) are considered as the main component of the model for nursing.

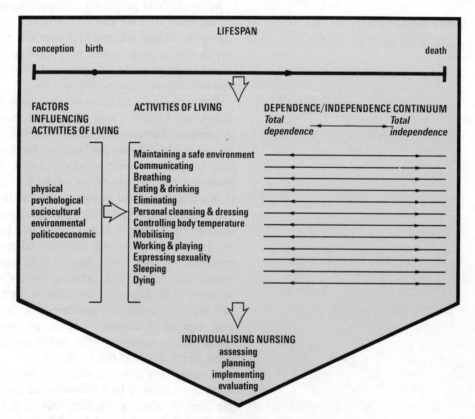

Fig. 6.1   Diagram of the model for nursing

ACTIVITIES OF LIVING

Maintaining a safe environment
Communicating
Breathing
Eating & drinking
Eliminating
Personal cleansing & dressing
Controlling body temperature
Mobilising
Working & playing
Expressing sexuality
Sleeping
Dying

Fig. 6.2   Activities of Living

The ALs are the focus of the model because they are central to the underlying view of nursing. *Nursing is viewed as helping patients to prevent, solve, alleviate or cope with problems with the Activities of Living.* Implicit in that statement is recognition of the fact that patients' problems with the ALs may be *actual* or *potential* and, therefore, that nursing not only responds to existing problems but is also concerned with preventing problems, whenever possible. The kinds of problems which patients may experience with the ALs are many and varied and they result from a variety of causes and circumstances. Some problems result simply from the *change of environment and routine* which is an inevitable consequence of admission to hospital; others occur when illness or disability causes a *change in usual habit or mode of carrying out an AL*; others are a consequence of *change in dependence/ independence status*; and another category of problems is *discomforts associated with the ALs.* These groups of patients' problems and related nursing activities associated with each of the 12 ALs are identified and discussed in the chapters which make up Section 3 of the book, each opening with an analysis of the AL in the context of healthy living. So far, only a brief outline of each of the ALs has been provided in discussion of that component in the context of the model of living (pp. 20–22). Rather than focus here on the 12 activities individually, the remainder of this section offers some comments on the ALs collectively.

Use of the concept of ALs
There is, of course, nothing highly original about using the concept of activities of living within a nursing model. Virginia Henderson's definition of nursing was quoted in the introductory chapter (p. 13) and the kinds of *activities* she was writing about (14 in number) are activities of living, although that particular term was not used. More recently, however, the term has become a familiar one in nursing and for that reason it is pertinent to make a few

comments about how we came to use the concept of ALs as we did, for the purposes of our model.

We deliberately chose to use the concept of activities of living in preference to 'basic human needs', a concept which has been widely used in nursing, based on Maslow's analysis of human needs. He categorised needs and then arranged them in order of priority, creating a 'hierarchy'. The hierarchy is frequently illustrated in the form of a pyramid — the physiological needs at the bottom; safety and security needs next, followed by needs for love and belonging, and self-esteem needs; and, at the top, the need for self-actualisation — inferring that those in the lowest category need to be at least minimally fulfilled before motivation is established to seek fulfillment of needs in the next category, and so on to the top. To some extent, this thinking is relevant to the concept of activities of living but, unlike needs, ALs have an advantage for a nursing model in that they are observable and can be explicitly described, and, in some instances, objectively measured.

The terms we chose to name the ALs also merit comment. Although anxious to avoid jargon, finding suitable names for some of the activities was difficult. The names of the 12 ALs were chosen in an attempt to be consistent in emphasising their active nature (therefore, 'eliminat- *ing*' rather than 'elimination') and their comprehensiveness (for example, though 'washing and dressing' is the more common term, we decided on 'personal cleansing and dressing' because it is all-embracing of the various activities subsumed within that AL). As a consequence, some of the names may seem rather strange at first but we believe that familiarity with the 12 ALs should result in acceptability of our deliberately and carefully chosen terms.

The set of 12 ALs is unique to our model. Many of the activities are contained in other lists, for example Virginia Henderson's. But, in addition, our list contains some activities (such as 'expressing sexuality') which have not always been included alongside the more obvious activities (such as 'eating and drinking') despite the fact that they are integral to the process of living and, therefore, relevant in the context of nursing.

Complexity and relatedness of the ALs
The fact that each AL is highly complex because it subsumes a variety of activities was a point mentioned in discussion of the AL component of the model of living (p. 20). The point is worth reiterating here because it explains why, in the context of nursing, there is such diversity in the patients' problems and related nursing activities associated with each of the 12 ALs. This will become apparent from discussion of nursing and the ALs in Section 3 of the book (Chs 7–18).

The relatedness of the 12 ALs was also commented on (p. 20) and this too is an important consideration in the context of nursing. In the course of obtaining information (by assessment) about any one AL, the nurse is likely to find out a great deal about other closely related ALs. For example, discussion of eating and drinking habits leads naturally to description of eliminating habits. A problem with one AL may well cause problems with one or more of the others: for example, mobilising difficulties are likely to cause problems with other ALs, such as 'personal cleansing and dressing' and 'working and playing'.

Priorities among the ALs

Although every AL is important in the process of living, some are more vital than others. The AL of breathing must be considered as of prime importance because it is essential for all the other ALs and, indeed, for life itself. The notion of priorities among the ALs was briefly mentioned in discussion of the model of living (p. 22) and in the context of nursing is an extremely important consideration.

With the exception of the AL of breathing, there is no fixed order of priority among the ALs because depending on the prevailing circumstances and individual choice, priorities among the ALs alter. Although eating and drinking are activities which are usually carried out regularly at fixed times there are occasions when other activities, such as working and playing, are afforded a higher priority. On the whole, however, those activities which are vital to survival and safety take precedence over others and, in nursing, this principle certainly applies in circumstances of acute illness and any condition which is considered to be life-threatening. Therefore, although the 12 ALs all have relevance to nursing, not all of them are necessarily relevant to all patients or to any one patient all of the time. Although it takes up much time in ordinary life, the AL of working and playing will assume a low priority during a period of critical illness. For a patient who has suffered a myocardial infarction, the AL of expressing sexuality may only seem important again when the person is recovering and, looking ahead, may wish information about whether and when it will be safe to resume sexual relations again. However, for a woman having a mastectomy many aspects of that same AL may assume great importance, both pre- and post-operatively and in the long-term too. What is important is for nurses to be aware that different circumstances create different priorities and, therefore, to apply common sense and professional judgement in making decisions about the relevance and relative priorities of the ALs.

LIFESPAN

The reason for including a lifespan as one component of the model of living has previously been explained (p. 22)

and, in Chapter 4, the main features of development in the various stages of the lifespan were described. In the model for nursing, the lifespan (Fig. 6.3) serves as a reminder that nursing is concerned with people of all ages: that an individual may require nursing at any stage of the lifespan, from conception to death.

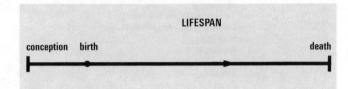

Fig. 6.3   The lifespan

So relevant is the concept of the lifespan to nursing that some branches of the profession, and some professional qualifications, are linked specifically to certain stages of the lifespan: for example, midwives are concerned with the prenatal stage, birth and the immediate postnatal period; paediatric nurses and health visitors with the stages of infancy and childhood; and geriatric nursing is the speciality concerned with old age. Their special knowledge and understanding of the processes of normal growth and development in a particular stage of the lifespan enables them to monitor development and to detect any delay or deviation from the parameters of 'normal'.

Taking account of a patient's age — the fact which identifies the stage of the lifespan involved — has always been recognised as important in nursing. It influences all phases of the process of nursing — assessing, planning, implementing and evaluating — and is an important consideration in individualising nursing.

The following brief comments on each of the main stages of the lifespan help to illustrate the relevance of this component of the model for nursing.

Prenatal stage (conception–birth)

Midwives, and in some instances other nurses such as health visitors, work in close collaboration with obstetricians and others to provide what is referred to as 'prenatal care'. A detailed knowledge of growth and development in the prenatal stage of the lifespan (briefly outlined on p. 44) is utilised to monitor fetal growth, allowing for early detection of problems which can occur in pregnancy and for appropriate treatment to be initiated.

Another important nursing function in prenatal care is health education: for example, teaching expectant mothers about the dangers of smoking, taking alcohol and drugs and the importance of a balanced diet, exercise and adequate rest. There is knowledge about all the Activities of Living which can be imparted so that the parents-to-be can adapt their lifestyle during the pregnancy with the aim of maximising the mother's health and that of the baby.

Attending a woman in labour is universally the role of the midwife, the word meaning 'with woman'. The great advances in obstetric care which have taken place in this century have markedly reduced both maternal and fetal mortality, and birth is now safer than ever before. It is the event of birth which marks the end of the prenatal stage of the lifespan and the midwife shares with the parents this profoundly important experience. By cutting the umbilical cord, the midwife separates the newborn baby from the mother to begin existence as an independent human being. It is interesting to reflect that almost every person is literally brought into the world by a member of the nursing profession.

Infancy (0–5 years)

The first moments of life after birth are crucial and, here too, the midwife plays a vital role. She ensures, for example, that the AL of breathing is satisfactorily established; that there is immediate opportunity for communication between mother and baby; that the baby is dried and kept warm to prevent problems with the AL of controlling body temperature; and so essential to life is the AL of eating and drinking, that the midwife may encourage the mother to suckle her baby at the breast very soon after the birth. Helping the mother to learn to feed and care for her baby is a major concern of postnatal nursing, for after all the baby is totally dependent on the mother in respect of almost all the Activities of Living.

Throughout the first year of life, even the most healthy of babies remain vulnerable to the hazards of infection and injury and susceptible to a variety of problems with the ALs, for example, hypothermia, malnutrition and dehydration. In all countries with a developed health care system, child health services are afforded a high priority and nursing makes an important contribution to efforts aimed at achieving ever lower rates of infant mortality and morbidity.

There are of course some babies and young children who, for a variety of reasons, require nursing in a neonatal unit or children's hospital. Their nursing care is provided by specially trained nurses who, in addition to knowing about treatment of disease, require an in-depth understanding of the normal processes of development in the early years of the lifespan. This is essential for nursing care to be tailored to the very different needs and abilities of children of different ages; and to prevent the experience of hospitalisation from adversely affecting the child. There is now widespread acceptance of the need to avoid the adverse effects of separation and for this reason parents are encouraged to visit freely (p. 284) and take an active part in nursing their baby or young child.

Some children have the misfortune to suffer from a chronic illness or a fatal disease or a condition which results in long-term physical and/or mental handicap. Frequent readmission to hospital and, in some cases, long-term hospitalisation or community nursing support may be necessary. In such cases nurses play a very significant part in the child's early years of the lifespan.

Childhood (6–12 years)

Childhood tends to be a period of relatively good health for the majority, with death an unusual occurrence. In the Western world the single most important cause of death in this age group is accidents (p. 84).

Serious illness is rare too. Apart from transient illness, such as respiratory infections or the infectious diseases of childhood, the majority of children have little need for medical treatment or nursing care. The exceptions are those children with a chronic illness or long-term physical or mental handicap. For nurses involved in their care, whether in hospital or the community, one of the important considerations is to provide nursing in such a way that there is minimal interference with normal development in this stage of the lifespan, such as progress at school; involvement in family life and friendships; and increasing independence in all of the Activities of Living.

However, even 'well' children come into contact with nursing through the school health service. Like health visitors with the younger age group, school nurses are primarily concerned with the monitoring of growth and development, and the early identification of problems: for example, defects of hearing and sight, speech difficulties, dental caries, malnutrition, obesity, inadequate hygiene, poor posture, foot malformation, urinary incontinence or infection, and conditions underlying excessive fatigue or anxiety. In some cases, the nurse may provide treatment but equally important is her ability to refer the child and parents to the appropriate source of help.

Many of the problems mentioned can be considered essentially as potential problems of childhood and prevention through health education is another important aspect of the work of school nurses. Increasingly, health education is viewed as more than simply information giving, and through discussion, debate and experimentation, children are being encouraged to appraise their personal health practices and to develop positive health values at an early age.

Adolescence (13–18 years)

In describing development during this state of the lifespan (p. 48) it was noted that adolescence is dominated by puberty. Sex education in school and at home during the years of childhood helps to prepare the adolescent to anticipate and cope with the physical and emotional changes which are associated with puberty.

Many of the problems which can arise in adolescence are related to physical and psychological aspects of sexual development. Some adolescents experience severe emotional or psychological problems, such as depression or anxiety, which require psychiatric treatment; some require treatment for drug dependence (p. 289); some may benefit from psychosexual counselling; some need treatment of sexually transmitted disease. Many adolescents use family planning centres for advice about contraception and selection of contraceptives; and girls who do become pregnant may seek an abortion or require obstetric care. Thus it can be seen that a variety of nurses come into contact with adolescents — psychiatric nurses, nurse counsellors, school nurses, nurses who work in genitourinary clinics, and those in family planning services, gynaecology and midwifery.

For all of these nurses, an understanding of adolescence is essential. They are unlikely to deal effectively and sympathetically with an adolescent's problems, whatever they may be, in the absence of an appreciation of the emotional turbulence of this stage of the lifespan and of other features, such as a teenager's changing relationship with parents, the pressures of school and worries about future employment.

Appreciating these difficulties and remembering that adolescence is a period of transition, with fluctuation between the desire for adult independence and regression to child-like dependence, is certainly essential for nurses involved with adolescents who require hospital or home care, whether short- or long-term. Adolescence is, like childhood, a stage of the lifespan when illness is uncommon. For those affected that fact must make illness or incapacity harder to accept when it occurs; for example, an adolescent who becomes physically disabled following an accident or an adolescent with diabetes mellitus.

Even short-term hospital care of an adolescent presents the nurses with a considerable challenge. On the one hand there may be the desire to be talked to and treated as an adult but, on the other hand, the circumstances may well precipitate some regression to child-like behaviour. This may be manifest in signs of fear and anxiety, or in a desire for parental closeness; or perhaps in a reluctance to accept responsibility for self-care and independent decision-making.

The swings of mood common in adolescence may make for difficulties in the nurse-patient relationship and ambivalent feelings towards authority may be projected on to nurses and doctors. Self-consciousness about physical development and relationships with members of the opposite (or same) sex may cause the adolescent patient to experience considerable embarrassment in some physically intimate nursing activities; for example, those related to the ALs of personal cleansing and dressing, and eliminating.

The nursing of adolescents, whatever the circumstances, requires sensitivity and knowledge of 'normal' development in this stage of the lifespan.

Adulthood (18-65 years)

In discussion of development during the lifespan in Chapter 4, adulthood was described as comprising three stages — young adulthood (19–30 years), the middle years (31–45) and late adulthood (46–65 years). Here, all three stages are discussed together.

It is easy to appreciate the necessity of adapting nursing to the very specific needs and abilities of children of different ages. Adults of different ages do have special requirements too but, because of their independence in the Activities of Living and their ability to communicate their needs and desires, there is not the same need to adapt nursing so specifically to age as there is with children. It is also the case that the parameters of 'normal' are very much wider in adulthood, resulting in much greater diversity in lifestyle, abilities and attitudes than among children of a certain age. Appreciating the diversity though is helpful because it warns against making assumptions, pointing to the need to collect relevant information about each adult patient as an individual.

However, remembering what was described about the three stages of adulthood in Chapter 4, there are two dominant areas of concern for all adults, namely, work and family life. Both are directly affected by illness and hospitalisation and, therefore, individualised nursing must take account of the adult patient's work and family circumstances. In some instances these circumstances may be directly related to the patient's need for nursing: for example, a patient who has suffered an accident at work or, in relation to family life, nursing services which are concerned with family planning, pregnancy and childbirth, and parenthood.

Therefore, work and family life not only bring adults into direct contact with nursing but are directly affected, often disrupted, by illness and hospitalisation. There are, too, direct links between work and family life and health and ill-health.

Early adulthood was described as a stage of relative stability, with both physical fitness and intellectual ability at their peak. Apart from those young adults who are continuing to cope with a life-long physical or mental handicap, serious ill-health is uncommon and the death rate is low. The more common conditions include bronchitis, peptic ulceration, gall bladder disease, alcoholism, back injury and psychiatric illness, particularly depression. With advancing age into the middle years of life, ill-health becomes more common. There is a sharp increase in the death rate in late adulthood with three conditions responsible — heart disease, cancer and stroke.

Knowing the causes of morbidity and mortality in the various stages of adulthood gives some idea of the reasons why adults come into contact with the health care system, and with nurses. But there is a more important reason: if the causes of ill-health are understood, then appropriate preventive measures can be directed at people of a particular age. Many of the diseases of adulthood are, to some extent at least, preventable. It might seem trite to point it out, but it is true that much ill-health and injury would be avoided if adults did not smoke cigarettes, drank less alcohol, avoided becoming obese, took more frequent and more vigorous exercise, and learned to avoid or cope more effectively with stress. Health education is one means of encouraging adults to adopt a more healthy lifestyle, and there are many ways in which nurses can contribute to this effort.

Old age (65 years +)

Nowadays many more people are living longer. Elderly people now make up a larger proportion of the total population than ever before and, with proportionately fewer younger people available to look after them, the needs of the elderly are now a matter of considerable concern to many groups, not least to nursing. It has already been pointed out (p. 52) that the majority of people in this last stage of the lifespan do manage to remain in their own homes, often totally independent, though sometimes in need of assistance with some of the Activities of Living. The reasons for decreasing independence in the ALs were outlined in Chapter 4 in terms of a gradual decline in old age of physical and intellectual function, and the effects of ageing on health.

The fact that ill-health is more common in this stage of the lifespan than in any other is reflected in the numbers of elderly patients in the wards of general hospitals. To some nurses this comes as something of a surprise and it certainly would seem to contradict the belief that old people are the concern only of the specialist geriatric services. All nurses, (with certain obvious exceptions such as paediatric nurses) nowadays require extensive knowledge of the process of ageing; a sympathetic understanding of the needs of old people; and a positive attitude towards their care and rehabilitation. Individualised nursing is as necessary for an old person as for a child or a young adult — even more so it might be argued, for there is a longer established individuality in living!

When physical or mental disability is such that an elderly person can no longer stay at home, or cope within a community care setting, placement in a 'continuing care unit' may be the only solution. In such a setting, the primary aim is to help the person to maintain what independence there still is in the Activities of Living and, of course, to provide an atmosphere and environment which is like 'home' as far as is humanly possible. Long-stay geriatric wards have not enjoyed a good reputation on the whole and, while inadequate conditions are certainly to blame, staff attitudes probably contributed to the unnecessary routinisation and institutionalisation which prevailed. The emphasis nowadays on individualised nursing, through the process of nursing method (which is incorporated in this model) offers a way of en-abling long-stay patients in a geriatric unit to continue their individuality in living.

The inevitable preoccupation of old people with death was mentioned in discussion of this stage of the lifespan in Chapter 4 and this is something which should always be borne in mind by nurses who are involved with the elderly. In Western society most people die in old age and skilled and sensitive nursing may help a person to come to the very end of the lifespan, to the event of death, in comfort and with the greatest possible dignity.

In this overview of the relationship between stages of the lifespan and nursing, various activities of living have been mentioned. The specific effects of the lifespan on each of the 12 ALs are described in Chapters 7–18; and from that it will be apparent how a patient's age is a relevant consideration in all phases of the process of nursing. Therefore, the lifespan component of the model for nursing is closely related to the AL component, as it is to the dependence/independence continuum which will now be discussed.

DEPENDENCE/INDEPENDENCE CONTINUUM

The reason for including the dependence/independence continuum in the model of living was described (p. 22). The concept of dependence/independence has been widely utilised in nursing and, as a component of the model for nursing, is related directly to the 12 Activities of Living (Fig. 6.4).

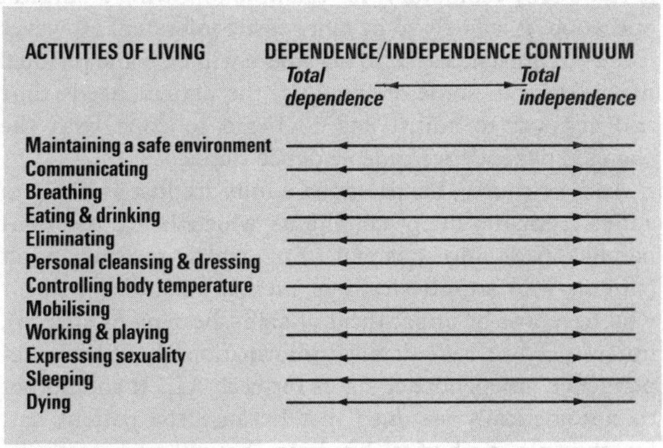

Fig. 6.4 Dependence/independence continuum related to the ALs

There is also a close link between this component of the model and the lifespan. Nursing care for newborn babies acknowledges their total dependence in respect of almost every Activity of Living whereas children's nursing must take account of the fact that the early years of the lifespan are associated with increasing independence in the ALs. Some children do not have the capacity to acquire this independence, to the same extent or at the 'normal' rate, either due to physical or mental handicap. Where nurses are involved in care of such children, whether at home or in an institutional setting, the objective is an individualised programme for the acquisition of maximum independence for each AL. For any child, an episode of illness or injury as a result of accident will not only affect the level of independence already achieved in the ALs but may also require a stay in hospital. Young children are very easily upset by any change in environment or alteration to their daily routine. For example, a child who has recently achieved independence in certain personal cleansing activities, or who is able to dress without help, is likely to be confused if the nurse washes or dresses him. A child may be very distressed if expected by the nurses to exercise a degree of independence in the ALs which has not yet been acquired: for example, being given a knife and fork with which to eat when he is still spoonfeeding; or being expected to use the WC when still at the stage of using a potty; or being given a game to play with or books to read which are beyond his level of comprehension. It is obvious that nurses require to have detailed information about what each child can and cannot do independently in relation to each AL so that the nursing plan is tailored to the individual child, as well as to the circumstances of his illness or injury.

For the majority of people, independence is a central feature of adulthood. When for any reason there is enforced dependence, for example as a result of illness or injury, many people find this hard to cope with. If the period of dependence in relation to any or all of the ALs is to be only temporary, for example following a surgical operation, it is likely to be more easily tolerated. However if the circumstances mean that there will be some residual dependence in some of the ALs, the patient needs time and support to adjust and to begin to cope with the changed dependence/independence status.

And, of course, handicapped adults are just as likely to suffer from the many conditions which bring the non-handicapped into hospital. So, when nursing adult patients who are physically or mentally handicapped (or who have loss or impairment of sight, hearing or speech), nurses need to have detailed information about their dependence/independence status for each AL. It should not be automatically assumed that because the patient has, for example, a physical handicap, he will necessarily be dependent on the nurse. However, he may well require to continue to use the coping mechanisms, aids or equipment which have enabled him to remain independent in the ALs outwith the hospital, and nurses should ensure that this is made possible and that relevant information is provided on the patient's nursing plan.

Even for the most able people, independence in the ALs is generally acquired over a long period of time. In old age the loss of independence can be equally gradual and it is seldom for all of the ALs. The AL of mobilising is often one of the first affected and because movement is required to perform many other activities, this may result in loss of independence in some of the other ALs. The elderly patient may be reluctant to bath and careful questioning may elicit that it is due to fear of falling. Difficulties with personal cleansing and dressing activities may in fact be due to problems with mobilising. There are now many gadgets available to help elderly people with such difficulties and provision of these may permit a patient to retain independence, albeit 'aided' independence in these activities. It is worth repeating a point made in the context of the model of living that old age does not necessarily bring about loss of independence, and there is seldom dependence for all ALs. An important skill in nursing is developing professional judgement in relation to patients' abilities and never depriving a patient, however old, of independence in those ALs for which he is capable. There is, of course, a fine line between this and misjudgement in demanding independence when a patient is incapable of so being.

It is, equally, a skill in nursing to know when a patient is in a state of dependence, or should be helped to accept that this is necessary. Although the emphasis in nursing is generally on encouraging patients to achieve or regain maximum independence in the ALs, there are circumstances (for example, unconsciousness or severe illness) when patients are totally dependent on nurses. There are other circumstances when, although the patient may desire to be independent, this is not in his best interests. At certain times (for example, immediately postoperatively), in certain illnesses (for example, severe respiratory conditions) and for other reasons (for example, immobilisation in traction), it is important for the patient to move as little as possible and for energy to be conserved. Such patients may need to be helped to accept that their dependence is necessary and their distress is likely to be lessened if nurses carry out activities on their behalf in a willing manner and in a way which does not offend the patient's dignity and self-esteem.

Therefore, sometimes nurses help patients towards independence in the ALs and, at other times help them to accept dependence. The dependence/independence continuum in the model for nursing, as in the model of living, is arrowed to indicate that movement can take place along it in either direction — an important dimension of the concept of dependence/independence in the context of nursing. A very important aspect of nursing is assessing a patient's level of independence in all of the Activities of Living and judging in which direction, and by what amount, he should be assisted to move along the dependence/independence continuum; what nursing assistance he needs to achieve the goals set; and how progress in relation to these goals will be evaluated.

This discussion of the dependence/independence continuum as one component of the model has been presented in general terms. In later chapters of the book (Chs 7–18) the concept is discussed more specifically in relation to each of the 12 ALs. In each case there is a section which identifies causes of change in patients' dependence/independence status, and some of the related nursing activities.

FACTORS INFLUENCING THE ALs

In introducing this component in the model of living (p. 24) the reason for its inclusion was given as the need to explain why there are many individual differences in the way the ALs are carried out. As described there, the various 'factors' which influence the ALs were categorised into five main groups and in the model for nursing this component is similarly presented (Fig. 6.5).

**FACTORS INFLUENCING
ACTIVITIES OF LIVING**

physical
psychological
sociocultural
environmental
politicoeconomic

Fig. 6.5 Factors influencing the ALs

A brief outline of some of the knowledge which provides a background understanding of these five groups of factors has been provided in Chapter 3 ('Biological aspects of living'), Chapter 4 ('Developmental aspects of living') and Chapter 5 ('Social aspects of living'). More is said later in the book (Chs 7–18) about ways in which physical, psychological, sociocultural, environmental and politicoeconomic factors influence the 12 Activities of Living. Therefore, at this point, all that is presented is by way of illustrating how thinking about this component of the model in the context of 'living' is transferred to the context of 'nursing'.

INDIVIDUALISING NURSING

Individualised nursing can be accomplished by use of a systematic approach to patient care known as the process of nursing. This comprises four phases — assessing, planning, implementing and evaluating — and it is illustrated in Figure 6.6. These four phases are more usually referred to as the 'nursing process' but the process is not unique to nursing; it is used by many disciplines. We prefer the term the 'process of nursing'. It is neither a

INDIVIDUALISING NURSING

assessing
planning
implementing
evaluating

Fig. 6.6 Individualising nursing

'model' nor a 'philosophy' as is sometimes written but simply a method and it needs to be used with an explicit nursing model. This is the rationale for incorporating the process of nursing into our model for nursing (Fig. 6.1).

Comparing Figure 6.1: Model for nursing, with Figure 2.6: Model of living (p. 26) it will be readily apparent that 'Individualising nursing' is developed from its equivalent component 'Individuality in living'. In both illustrations the arrows make it clear that this fifth component takes account of the interaction of the others. We have already stated the rationale for using the model of living as a base for nursing (p. 63) and here we repeat our belief that the patient's individuality in living should be borne in mind throughout all four phases of the process of nursing.

When introducing the process of nursing to hospital wards, the proposed change means moving away from expecting newly admitted patients to fit into the nursing routine, to organising work in a sufficiently flexible way to take account of the individuality of patients. Furthermore newly admitted patients are likely to have an increased level of anxiety as Wilson-Barnett (1978) discovered, and this may make it less easy for them to cope with change. In the case of long-term patients the result of an inflexible daily routine may be boredom and institutionalisation, characterised by apathy, dependence and a lack of personal responsibility. Individualised nursing could help to prevent this.

Throughout all four phases of the process the patient should wherever possible be an active participant: for example, making decisions about continuing to carry out some activities such as eating and drinking, and perhaps agreeing to undertake some new activities such as deep breathing and foot exercises to prevent complications like pneumonia and deep vein thrombosis. Of course participation may not be possible in the case of a child, a confused or an unconscious person. In these instances family members or significant others are usually willing to participate in giving information and helping with decisions and possibly carrying out some of the activities, as is usually the case when patients are nursed in their own homes.

Patient participation demands a somewhat radical approach to nursing by both patients and nurses. To take patients first — in the past the majority accepted what happened to them while they were in the health care service, apparently on the grounds that the doctor/nurse knew best. With the social changes which have occurred in the last few decades, particularly the influence of the mass media, more and more patients are knowledgeable about what is happening to them; they have acquired part of the medical vocabulary and are capable of, and indeed many expect to have the opportunity to ask questions and discuss their health problems with nurses. What they may be less aware of is how they can help achieve specific goals by for example charting their fluid intake and output, or collecting a midstream specimen of urine. Nurses need to be able to give clear instructions about such activities and ascertain the patient's understanding so that responsibility for the task can be accepted. However there are still a large number of people who are not sufficiently assertive to ask for the information which would help to make them feel less anxious and more comfortable, and part of nursing is learning to identify and help such patients whether they are attending a clinic, are at home or in hospital.

The idea of patient participation has had repercussions in nursing too. For example the acceptance of any responsibility by the patient must be clearly stated on the nursing plan so that any nurse will know exactly what the patient has agreed to do, and will be able to supervise and give support. In some instances it may be easier and quicker for the nurse to carry out the task but it might not be in the best interests of the patient, examples being a person relearning dressing skills, or a person learning to take medicines so that when independence is achieved there can be discharge from hospital to home. Some of the skills required by the nurse to cope with the change to patient participation are described by Faulkner (1981).

To take account of these changes nursing is gradually moving away from task/job assignment — a method whereby routinised tasks are carried out by one nurse for all patients — to a system of patient allocation (p. 9) and using the process of nursing to achieve individualised nursing.

Although the process is described as comprising four phases, this is merely for the purpose of description and discussion. The implication in describing four phases is that they are carried out sequentially but in reality all four phases are ongoing. It is important for nurses to realise this from the outset so that knowledge and thinking will not be rigid and compartmentalised. Before any further discussion of general aspects of the process of nursing, a description will be given of each of the phases.

Assessing
The world 'assessment' has been adopted for the first phase of the process of nursing by the majority of nurses including those who organised the 'nursing process project' in Europe, which was carried out under the auspices of the World Health Organization; it is described by Farmer & Ashworth (1981). However we think that over-use of the word assessment encourages the idea that it is a once-only activity and we prefer greater use of 'assessing' to encourage recognition of the ongoing nature of the activity. There is some dubiety about what assessment includes, so it is necessary to clarify our use of the word; it includes:

- collecting information from/about the patient
- reviewing the collected information
- identifying the patient's problems
- identifying priority of problems

The information will be gained by observing, interviewing, examining, measuring and testing as appropriate: that gained at the initial assessment forms a base-line against which any further information can be compared. It is likely that as rapport with the patient is established, more information will be forthcoming and when relevant will be recorded. There is discussion about such documentation in Section 4 (p. 347).

The primary source of such information is the patient when capable of cooperating, but secondary sources such as previous health records can be used, and this can make the nurse's initial interview with the patient more relaxed: in conversation the patient can be given the opportunity to verify the information. Another secondary source will probably be family members and sometimes it is customary to record the names of those who have given information. This source is especially important in the case of children, disoriented, unconscious or severely mentally ill or handicapped patients and in such circumstances there may have to be more than usual reliance on previous records.

Information volunteered by the patient is classified as subjective, whereas nurses are taught to develop the skill of recording any information collected by observing, in as objective a way as possible. This involves describing exactly what is seen or heard without any interpretation, inference or opinion. For example, a patient may have a mask-like face, be very still when sitting for long periods and eat little at each mealtime: these are descriptive observations and should be reported as such and not as 'patient seems depressed'. Crow, in Kratz (1979), discusses subjective and objective information in more detail.

In a further attempt to provide objective information especially when assessing and evaluating there are a few data collecting instruments, and their use is described in the appropriate chapters. There is the Norton scale for identifying patients at risk of developing pressure sores

(p. 72) and the Glasgow coma scale (p. 326) which measures the level of consciousness. These two scales give a numerical index as base-line data and re-use of the instruments will reveal whether there is improvement or deterioration. On the other hand, pain is a subjective experience, nevertheless a measuring instrument — a painometer (p. 41) — can be used at time intervals to show whether that particular patient's pain is increasing or decreasing. Nurses are increasingly using established rating instruments for detecting and monitoring extreme anxiety and depression. Although the patient gives subjective information on these self-recording instruments, they have been researched and tested so that a number can be attached to the degree of anxiety being experienced. Reusing such instruments will obviously reveal whether the anxiety is increasing or decreasing.

At every meeting of two people, each makes observations about the other, and this is no less true when a nurse meets a patient for the first time. Attention will therefore be paid not only to appearance but also to what is said, how it is said, facial expression and body gesture. The first meeting may be during admission (whether as an emergency or from the waiting list), or at home, or at a health centre. In hospital, it may well be that after the greeting and establishing the patient's identity, he is accompanied to the bed which he will occupy, introduced to nearby patients and shown the toilet and bathroom facilities. The rationale for this is that it gives the patient time to settle and become composed before the nurse returns at a suitable time to carry out the 'initial assessment'. However the patient may be so ill that only members of staff introduce themselves as they carry out essential treatment. Assessing as part of individualising nursing should ideally be carried out as early as possible in the patient's stay. In reality it is often not possible to collect extensive information within a few hours of admission, and McFarlane & Castledine (1982) illustrate a 'first stage history format' which they say 'provides enough information for the nurses to start looking after the patient', then it is followed as soon as possible by using a more detailed second stage format. There are however some subjects about which information must be collected early. Any bleeding or injury would of course be assessed immediately; information about pressure sores or any bruises is essential; it is customary to record the temperature, pulse and respiration, blood pressure and the result of testing a specimen of urine. It is also necessary for the staff to know of any sensitivities, allergies and any medicines which are currently being taken.

Many wards now provide specific stationery on which the information from assessment is written. Beginning nurses may be confused by the various names which are used for it — nursing assessment form, patient assessment form, nursing Kardex, nursing history and patient profile. Whatever the name and format, the objective is to record two different sorts of information: one we call the patient's biographical and health data, and the other is about the effect the current health problem and related medical treatment, if any, is having on the individual's ability to carry out the Activities of Living. We designed suitable proforma for recording these two different sorts of data and they are illustrated in Figure 19.2, pages one and two: the following discussion is based on them.

Biographical and health data
The patient's biographical and health details include such obvious items as name, sex, age; next of kin and the usual place of residence. This list is deceptively simple! Take the name; the custom in Western countries is to use the surname of the family, or in the case of a married woman, the husband's family name, but this is not so in all cultures and nurses may need to seek expert help so that the 'correct' surname is recorded. Likewise it used to be customary to talk about 'Christian' names but with changing social mores the word 'Forenames' is now widely used. In addition to the forename/s which appear on the birth certificate, another one or more can be given at a later religious ceremony and this may give further differentiation if there is more than one patient with the same surname. Increasingly nurses are directed to ask patients what form of address they prefer as some people use a name other than the one on the birth certificate, and use of the familiar one can help them to retain a sense of personal identity.

A word needs to be said about 'next of kin' and relationship to the patient. The rationale for this information is that the hospital needs to know who to contact should there be any deterioration of the patient's health status. A person separated from a spouse is still legally in a husband/wife relationship but may not wish that person to be contacted. Again as social mores are changing, nurses have to remember that a couple who are cohabiting may prefer that partner to be contacted.

It is becoming more common to record the type of living accommodation — information which is particularly relevant to community nurses on relief duty when visiting patients in their own homes, and indeed for hospital nurses participating in a multidisciplinary rehabilitation programme, so that they know for instance whether the patient will need to climb stairs at home. Increasing mobility of the population may mean that a patient's near relatives are abroad or otherwise not available for constant visiting, and the immediate significant others may be neighbours or a home-help. It is usual to record any support services being used such as meals-on-wheels or visiting by the community psychiatric nurse as on discharge, arrangements for their resumption may have to be made.

Occupation is a useful piece of information. From a health point of view it may have contributed to the need for admission, for example an employee in an asbestos factory who has breathing problems. Or in some instances the reason for admission may be incompatible with return to former employment, for example when an accident causes paraplegia. Religion too may be important because there are people whose religious beliefs will have to be catered for while they are ill such as the saying of special prayers or taking part in a special ceremony for the sick. The recording of major life events may sometimes be relevant. Nurse learners may not realise that illness can follow a life crisis such as change of school/work/house/ marital status and so on, and this is the reason for its inclusion.

It is useful too to know the patient's and the family's perception of the patient's current health problem. Asking the patient about the reason for admission/referral can give an indication of the patient's level of understanding or it can reveal a lack of knowledge, perhaps that an 'operation' is scheduled, when in fact it is an investigation. It is usual to record the address and telephone number of the patient's own doctor and consultant. Some proforma direct the admitting nurse's thoughts to 'plans for discharge' and this in fact alerts nurses to their role as health teachers.

This outline gives an idea of the sort of information which might be collected at the initial assessment. It gives an individual account not only of the 'patient' but of the people who are important to him. These biographical and health data are unlikely to change and will be useful and should be available to all nursing staff whether the patient's stay is long or short.

Assessing ALs

Attention will now be paid to the second part of assessment information which concerns the effect that the current health problem and related medical treatment, if any, are having on the patient's Activities of Living. Use of the ALs for assessment is central to our model for nursing. Those who will nurse the patient need to know about his previous mode of living; whether or not there are any problems or discomforts associated with any AL; if so, whether these have been experienced previously and if this is the case, how they have been coped with. The following provides only an introduction to assessing the ALs because each AL is developed more comprehensively in its particular chapter in Section 3. Also in Roper, Logan & Tierney (1981) examples are given of the sort of questions that a nurse might bear in mind when assessing a patient.

Assessing ability to maintain a safe environment is of particular importance if the patient is physically or mentally handicapped. The nurse needs to know whether or not he appreciates the dangers in the environment and knows how to prevent accidents. Assessing the level of safety in the home is an important responsibility of the nurse who visits, in their homes, elderly people or families with young children.

Assessing communicating skills is necessary in order to discover the patient's level of communication and this is important whether in the home, health centre or hospital. It is very important for nurses who have an extensive vocabulary to remember that not all patients do. Communicating is a two-way process; it is tempting to some nurses to use their 'medical' vocabulary without discovering what meaning, if any, these words have for the patient; it is especially important to remember this if deliberate teaching/learning is required. The nurse should observe whether the patient is reticent or forthcoming at talking about his home and his health problems. It is sometimes possible to discern from his conversation whether he is gregarious by nature or more fond of his own company. It may be necessary to gather specific information about one of the sensory organs if the nurse suspects a deficiency or dysfunction which is affecting the patient's AL of communicating.

Assessment of breathing may involve counting the number of respirations per minute. For the majority of patients, however, it is simply a case of the nurse noting whether there is an apparent breathing difficulty. Subsequently, the nurse may notice that the patient has a morning cough with sputum. This observation may offer an opportunity to discover whether or not he smokes and if so how much. The nurse should attempt to discover his perception of the multiple ill-effects of smoking and whether or not he would welcome help with giving up the habit. More detailed assessment of breathing is necessary when a patient is unconscious, still under the effects of an anaesthetic or suffering from a disease affecting the cardiopulmonary system.

Assessing eating and drinking routines is relatively easy because most people enjoy talking about this AL. When nursing underweight and overweight patients it is especially important to talk with them about what they eat, as well as when and how much. Nurses will need information about how handicapped people have managed this activity. When the patient complains of discomfort associated with eating or drinking, more specific assessment will be required.

Assessing a patient's eliminating habits is a nursing function even though admission to the health care system may not have been associated with bowel or urinary dysfunction. But there may well be a persistent problem with, for example, constipation and this may be elicited from the assessment. Many people find it embarrassing to talk about elimination and the nurse needs to broach the topic with sensitivity and phrase the questions carefully to avoid embarrassment yet elicit information.

Initial *assessment of personal cleansing habits and dressing* is possible by observing the result of these activities; ill-cared for clothes may be an indication of financial hardship or a lack of self-esteem which can characterise exhaustion or mental illness. The nurse may discover unhygienic practices for example related to cleaning teeth or lack of handwashing after visiting the toilet. With this knowledge she can plan to include relevant teaching in her nursing.

Assessing control of body temperature is carried out by using measuring equipment, usually a thermometer. Regular measurement/assessment of this AL may become necessary if the patient is suffering from pyrexia or hypothermia. There are other ways of assessing this AL — observation may reveal flushing of the skin, excessive perspiration, the presence of goose flesh, shivering, and excessively hot or cold hands and/or feet.

When assessing mobilising, initially it may only be necessary to observe that the patient does not appear to have any problems. But close observation might reveal for example stiffness of the joints on rising after sleep, a common occurrence for the older person. People who have persistent back pain often adopt a posture to minimise low back movement and it gives a characteristic gait which nurses learn to recognise. They also have a characteristic way of getting out of bed. Other mobilising problems are usually self-evident and nurses need to know how the patient copes with them.

Assessing working and playing routines is an essential part of an initial assessment. By the way that the patient talks about these activities, the nurse will gather which parts he finds challenging and which are boring. The physical conditions at the patient's place of work may have contributed to the accident or illness which has necessitated admission to hospital. On the other hand, difficulty in social relationships because of personality problems or mental illness may have contributed to admission.

Assessing the AL of expressing sexuality involves observing how people express their gender in a general way for example in mode of dress, use of cosmetics and so on. Specific assessment is not usually necessary or appropriate unless the patient's problems or potential problems are somehow associated with sex and reproduction; most people find it embarrassing to talk with strangers about this private AL. However, the observant nurse will perceive cues which are expressions of sexuality or indicators of anxieties or ignorance about expressing sexuality. With sensitivity the nurse can create an atmosphere in which patients feel able to discuss sex-related problems and when these are raised, a detailed assessment may become necessary.

Assessing sleeping routines at an early stage is important so that nurses have information on which to base nursing activities aimed at promoting sleep. Patients are not usually admitted to hospital because of a sleep problem as such, but adequate sleep is important for progress towards recovery, whatever the reason for admission.

Assessing the needs of the dying is a very important role of the nurse in hospital and in the community. Constant sensitivity and acute observation are necessary to recognise whether or not the patient wants to talk about the many aspects associated with death, dying and bereavement.

Assessing is not a once-only activity and it is likely that additional data will be collected as the nurses have further opportunity to observe patients and talk with them and there is discussion in Section 4 (p. 355) of where this additional data should be documented. Acknowledging that assessing is an ongoing activity, the data may need to be recorded frequently as in a one-to-one relationship with a very ill patient, or they may only need to be recorded intermittently, such as weekly for longstay patients, unless of course there is any sudden/gross change which will be recorded immediately. However, in life-threatening emergency situations, of course only minimal data can be collected before the patient is transferred to the operating theatre or before resuscitation techniques are implemented. Assessing therefore is not a rigid routine carried out at a particular time; it is an ongoing activity as nurses are constantly observing; the idea of assessing helps nurses to focus their attention not on nursing procedures but on patients and their problems and potential problems.

Assessing is just as applicable to patients who are in the health care system for surveillance or maintenance of health as for those who are in for investigation and/or treatment. The examples given for use in the model of living (Figs 2.2, 2.3 and 2.4), whereby a child's increasing independence and an older person's decreasing independence are plotted along the continua, are relevant here. Some nurses think that the identification of patients' problems is not applicable to health maintenance, but in healthy living the aim is to avoid potential problems becoming actual ones and the problems which endanger health may be sociocultural, environmental or economic, rather than physical.

Health authorities in various countries are using the *problem-oriented approach to the recording of patient data*. This has provided a change of focus in records away from the disease and towards the patient and his problems. The problem of a man with bronchitis, for instance, is not bronchitis as such but his breathlessness, lassitude, restricted mobility, and these items will appear in the problem-oriented record. This type of record can be used by nurses only, or it can be used by other or all members of the multidisciplinary health team, each 'problem' being recorded on its own sheet and each member of the health care team entering day-to-day information.

It cannot be too strongly stressed that the objective in collecting information about the ALs is to discover:

- previous routines
- what the patient can do for himself

- what the patient cannot do for himself
- problems ⎫
- discomforts ⎭ previous coping mechanisms

Identification of problems
Another activity included in 'assessing' is identification of the patient's problems and deciding which are amenable to nursing intervention. It is helpful to couch the problems in the patient's words, after all, that is how they are being experienced. Most of the ALs are familiar to the patients, who are all too aware of any *actual* problems with them, such as having no appetite for food. This problem can be verified by observing/measuring the amount of food eaten but the patient's statement of the usual amount eaten has to be accepted: any further deterioration of appetite will be observed as less food eaten. Patients may have a priority among their actual problems and one that springs readily to mind is pain: many patients do not eat until the pain has been relieved; and personal hygiene is often of secondary importance to relief of pain.

It is the concept of *potential* problems which highlights the aspects of nursing which are concerned with promotion of health; for example the majority of hospital patients have a potential problem of boredom which interferes with self-esteem, and lack of self-esteem is not conducive to health.

The idea of potential problems also emphasises the preventive aspects of nursing — preventing conditions which sometimes are referred to as 'complications'. Patients are also aware of some potential problems such as dental caries if attention is not paid to diet and mouth hygiene, so it is important for nurses to ensure that there is no disruption of patients' previous routines, unless of course they are found to be unsatisfactory.

It has to be remembered that there can be a nurse-perceived problem of which the patient is not aware; an example might be infestation with head lice. It must be noted so that it can be treated, otherwise lice may be transmitted to other people in the immediate environment. Equally the patient can have a problem of which the nurse is not aware, such as having overheard a worrying conversation and assuming it is about him.

A clear statement of the patient's problems, as ascertained from the nursing assessment, is increasingly being referred to as a nursing diagnosis. In an article entitled 'Can nurses diagnose?' Marks-Maran (1983) says that the garage mechanic tells her that he has 'diagnosed' what is wrong with her car; he is not afraid of the word 'diagnosis'. The development of nursing diagnoses is still in its infancy but we believe that they should be descriptions of the problems which patients experience with ALs, whereas the medical diagnosis is usually concerned with pathological changes. Returning to Marks-Maran's article, she states that a patient with one medical diagnosis may have several nursing diagnoses.

The advantage in using the AL framework for assessing is that it can provide information about all of the patient's 'living', as well as particulars about the style of carrying out each AL, and the type of problem being experienced with one or more of them. For the few ALs which are presenting problems, the nursing plan will start with a statement of the goals — more will be said about this later. To return to the unproblematic ALs, for example it might be sleeping, information on the assessment form could be: retires at 21.00 hours, wakens refreshed at 06.00 hours, double bed, two pillows, downie. This will be useful information throughout the patient's stay and should be available to a nurse beginning a spell of duty.

This outline of the first phase of the process of nursing gives an idea of the sort of information that might be collected at an initial assessment. It gives an individual account not only of the 'patient' but of the people who are important to him. It shows how patient participation wherever possible enhances the identification of problems, which when clearly stated are a nursing diagnosis.

Priority of problems
Life-threatening problems which result in an emergency admission to hospital will obviously be attended to before collecting information about the other ALs. Such problems can concern most of the ALs. More is said about this in Section 4 (p. 353). In the case of non-emergency admissions to any part of the health service, the priority will be decided in collaboration with the patient and may be with the family. The patient's priority may not be the same as the nurse's, but his priority is likely to contribute to his motivation to co-operate in the carrying out of the interventions to achieve the set goals.

Planning
The second phase of the process of nursing is planning — the objective of the plan being *to prevent* the identified potential problems from becoming actual ones; *to solve* actual problems; where possible *to alleviate* those which cannot be solved; and *to help the patient cope with* those problems which cannot be alleviated or solved. To achieve this a goal has to be set for each actual and potential problem in collaboration with the patient whenever possible and may be with the family, so that goals are not imposed on the patient. Instead of the word 'goals' some nurses prefer the phrase 'patient outcomes'; it is a matter of preference.

Goal setting
It may seem trite to say that goals should be realistic but a frail 75-year-old person is hardly likely to want to walk 3 miles; although this may well be realistic for a younger patient. Goals should be achievable within a patient's in-

dividual limits otherwise there is the danger of disheartenment. Whenever possible goals should be observable, measurable and capable of being tested as these provide objective data. Obviously all of these adjectives will not apply to each goal but they should be borne in mind when setting goals. Most writers agree to the idea of long- and short-term goals. The idea of adding a date by which the goal will be achieved may be particularly relevant to short-term goals when they can be graded gradually and precisely, for example 'will walk × metres by 21 July'; 'will walk × + 1 metres by 22. July' and so on. The positive feedback of achievement will give encouragement and provide motivation for further effort. In the case of long-term goals, even with patient participation, there is an element of 'guesswork' about pre-dating goals. However, if the patient/family understands this, and at the same time are willing to co-operate in achieving the goal by the set time, no harm should result because the goal was set in good faith and with agreement of all concerned.

To give a few more examples of goal setting — should the patient's problem be a coated dry mouth, the goal would be a clean moist mouth which is observable. If the problem is associated with pyrexia, the goal would be a return to that patient's usual body temperature which is measurable. When the problem is itching on passing sugar-containing urine then the goal would be freedom from itching on passing sugar-free urine and this can be confirmed by testing the urine.

Setting goals is the first activity in the planning phase of the process of nursing, and the last activity is evaluating which is dependent on the goal statement. To reach a destination when travelling, the destination must have been stated in advance, and this is no less true of goal setting and evaluating in nursing.

Nursing plans

Before nursing plans can be written, account has to be taken of existing resources which in a nursing context may be equipment, personnel and physical environment: available support services may have to be considered when a patient is being nursed at home. Possible alternative nursing interventions may be determined by the availability of resources. Decisions have to be made about such things as, for instance, should the patient use a commode at the bedside independently or walk 15 steps to the toilet assisted by two nurses? Walking would perhaps best meet the patient's mobility needs but it necessitates the availability of two nurses at the required time.

Having considered the resources, the next step is to make decisions about what the nurse and possibly the patient agree to do to achieve the goals related to each of the patient's problems with ALs. For those activities which the patient agrees to do, the associated nursing activity is supervision. *A plan* is then made of all the necessary nursing activities stated in sufficient detail so that any other nurse, on reading it, would be aware of, and carry out, the planned nursing. There is no argument against this being essential since no one nurse can be on duty throughout the 24 hours.

Some nursing interventions will be derived from the medical prescription, obvious examples being: giving medicines and dressing wounds. We have devised a Nursing Plan on which to record the nursing interventions derived from problems with ALs separately from those derived from medical/other prescription (pages three and four, Fig. 19.2) and use of this plan is discussed in Section 4 (p. 354).

The nursing plan is not a static thing and will require revision. For instance when evaluation reveals that a goal has not been achieved for a particular patient's problem, there may have to be a change in the nursing intervention which will then be recorded in the nursing plan.

Social changes such as decreased working hours, and an increase in both annual leave and use of part-time staff, have made it essential for nurses to develop the skill of communicating by writing adequate nursing plans. If such social trends continue, it may well be that the nursing plan will assume even greater importance as a means of communication between nurses. And furthermore, assessing a patient and writing a nursing plan helps the nurse to know the patient which aids the establishment of a satisfactory nurse/patient relationship, the unique basis of the nursing contribution to a patient's health care.

Summarising the planning phase of the process — it involves writing a nursing plan which contains the following information: stated goals for each problem; a date on which the goals are expected to be achieved; the nursing interventions to achieve the goals, and where relevant any activities which the patient has agreed to do to achieve the goals. The objective of the nursing plan is to provide the information to facilitate individualised nursing.

Implementing the nursing plan

Implementing the plan is the third phase of the process of nursing. Traditionally nursing has been associated with 'doing', so nurses have less difficulty in understanding the necessity for this phase. However it is being increasingly recognised that nurses need to make explicit the thinking which must precede the nursing intervention, be part of the procedure, and accompany any necessary observations after the nursing intervention.

Some nursing activities may well be derived from the information on the patient assessment form, for example, making sure that the patient is supplied with a vegetarian diet whatever type of meal service is provided in the hospital (p. 171). This need not be recorded on the nursing plan because the patient does not have a 'problem' with the AL of eating and drinking but merely has a diet preference, a fact which the nurse discovered in the assessing phase of the process.

During implementation a nurse will require to use an amalgam of skills of which the following are brief examples merely to alert the beginning nurse to the complexities of nursing:

observing patients for any change in their condition or in their non-verbal behaviour

listening not only to what patients say but how they say it

talking with patients in such a way as to convey that what they are experiencing is important to the nurse

phrasing sentences so that they convey the intended meaning — being supportive, encouraging, empathic, assuring, reassuring, non-judgemental and so on

phrasing questions so that generally they are open-ended, that is, cannot be answered by just a 'yes' or 'no'

timing conversation with patients so that it can be unhurried; and timing the sequence of tasks so that a patient is not being disturbed frequently

enabling patients to be as independent as their condition allows, yet to be dependent when this is in their best interests

facilitating 'aided independence' when appropriate by procuring the necessary equipment

teaching patients who are re-learning basic skills such as dressing, walking, speaking; some patients have to be taught to give injections or care for a colostomy; and some patients require advice about the resumption of sexual intercourse after gynaecological operations or a myocardial infarction

preparing patients for a variety of operations, investigations and discharge

measuring such things as body temperature, blood pressure, fluid intake and output

testing urine

counting, for example, the frequency of the pulse or the episodes of incontinence

administering such diverse items as medicines, suppositories, enemas, oxygen and injections

carrying out aseptic technique while dressing surgical wounds, catheterising and so on

preparing equipment for the doctor to carry out procedures such as lumbar puncture

managing the work environment so that it is uncluttered and as safe as possible

liaising not only with other nurses, but also with other staff so that the patients will benefit

This is by no means an exhaustive list and it is merely intended to demonstrate the wide variety of activities which comprise nursing.

A day-to-day record must be made of the nursing interventions, when they were carried out, and by whom, together with any relevant information; for example, the patient may have experienced nausea while his wound dressing was being changed. More is said about documentation of the implementing phase of the process of individualising nursing in Section 4 (p. 355).

Summarising the implementing phase of the process — it has traditionally been perceived as the 'doing' part of nursing but with a backward glance at the list of examples of required skills, it will be realised that many are not 'observable' physical skills. The thinking before, during and after an activity is the difference between a routine task and nursing. Readers will learn more about the non-physical skills when they attend the psychology course in their programme.

It has been shown that some nursing activities are derived from information on the patient assessment form; they do not derive from a problem with an AL and do not need to be written on the nursing plan.

Other nursing interventions are derived from the patient's problems with one or more ALs; they are carried out to achieve the set goals. Yet other nursing interventions derive from medical prescription and they are designed to deal with the cause of the problem. And there may be nursing interventions which arise from liaising with paramedical staff — supervising particular exercises perhaps of the limbs or of the muscles required for speech.

Evaluating the nursing plan

It is difficult to justify the prescribed nursing interventions if it cannot be demonstrated that they benefit the recipient in some way, hence the fourth phase in the process of nursing. However a particular criticism of treatises on 'the nursing process' is that the evaluating phase receives only scant attention. In some ways this is understandable as evaluating can only be as good as the goals set; and the goal setting depends on the identification of actual and potential problems; the quality of identification relies on the review of the assessment data; and this is dependent on the data base being accurate and comprehensive.

Each phase of the process of nursing is equally important and each is interdependent. But how can evaluating be described? Put in simple terms it is determining whether or not the set goals have been or are being achieved, and the set goals are the criteria used in evaluation.

The skills which can be used in assessing can also be used in evaluating — observing, interviewing, examining, testing and measuring. Whereas they are used in assessing to provide baseline data, in evaluating they are used to discover whether or not the set goals are being or have been achieved: in other words evaluating involves comparison against an objective.

Goal achievement in effect cancels the nursing intervention. However it may be necessary to ask the question 'Was the goal set too low?' A reconsideration of the original goal setting might answer this question. But after goal achievement (that is resolution of the problem) it may become a potential problem, pressure sores being a classic example.

In the absence of complete goal achievement the nurse might ask:

● is it partially achieved and is more information needed from a further full assessment?
● is the problem unchanged/static and should the nursing intervention be changed in order to achieve the goal?
● is there a worsening of the problem and should the goal and the planned nursing intervention be restated?
● was the goal incorrectly stated?

There are times however when no change is good! In the case of a potential problem of developing deep vein thrombosis the goal might be stated as 'calf measurement remains unchanged; temperature of calf skin remains unchanged; no pain in calf' — so no change in these measurements would mean goal achievement. If evaluation reveals that the potential problem has become an actual one then there will have to be collection of extra assessment data, setting of a different goal to be achieved by a different nursing intervention. Solving of this actual problem may render it a potential problem!

Of course, sometimes evaluating is carried out immediately after the nursing intervention, an example being comparison of temperature pulse and respiration with the previous recording. Some nursing interventions as well as needing immediate evaluation, involve use of the nurse's knowledge of 'normal' as the criterion, for example, the result of an enema.

Earlier, in discussion of the assessing phase of the process, measuring scales (p. 72) were mentioned as a means of providing base-line data. The subsequent goal setting would indicate the direction in which movement on the scale was anticipated. Re-use of the instruments in the evaluating phase would reveal whether or not the goal has been achieved.

All of the foregoing description of evaluating rests on the assumption that the goal was achieved solely by the nursing intervention and in many instances this may not be so. Nurses need to recognise and acknowledge the contribution from other health workers in a multidisciplinary team.

From this albeit brief survey of the fourth phase of the process of nursing it can be seen that it has many facets and it is entirely dependent on the other three phases — assessing, planning and implementing.

In this chapter it has been shown how the model for nursing is developed from the model of living which was discussed in Chapter 2. The 12 ALs are the main component of the model for nursing and they are influenced by others — the lifespan, the dependence/independence continuum and the factors influencing ALs: physical, psychological, sociocultural, environmental and politicoeconomic factors. All of these components interact and have to be considered when describing the component, individualising nursing, which is accomplished by assessing, planning, implementing and evaluating, activities which are conventionally called the process of nursing. And we end the chapter by reiterating that the process is only a logical method which we consider has to be used with a model for nursing to give it meaning.

REFERENCES

Castledine G 1982 The patient's progress. Nursing Mirror 155 (16) October 20: 41
Crow J 1979 Assessments. In: Kratz C (ed) The nursing process. Bailliere Tindall, London, p 45–48
Farmer E, Ashworth P 1981 Who does what in Europe. Nursing Mirror 152 (7) February 12: 37–38
Faulkner A 1981 Aye, there's the rub. Nursing Times 77 (12) February 19: 332–336
Marks-Maran D 1983 Can nurses diagnose? Nursing Times 79 (4) January 26: 68–69
McFarlane J, Castledine G 1982 A guide to the practice of nursing using the process of nursing. Mosby, St Louis, ch. 4
Mitchell J R A 1984 Is nursing any business of doctors? A simple guide to the 'nursing process'. Nursing Times 80 (19) May 9: 28–32 (reprinted from British Medical Journal)
Roper N, Logan W, Tierney A 1981 Learning to use the process of nursing. Churchill Livingstone, Edinburgh, p 1–5
Tierney A J 1984 Defending the process. Nursing Times 80 (20) May 16: 38–41
Wilson-Barnett J 1978 Factors influencing patients' emotional reaction to hospitalisation. Journal of Advanced Nursing May 3: 221–229

Nursing and the activities of living

7

Maintaining a safe environment

The activity of maintaining a safe environment

It is imperative that all people attend to the maintenance of a safe environment in which to carry out their Activities of Living. Every day in fact from the time they waken until they go to bed, people are engaged in carrying out many activities with the specific purpose of maintaining a safe environment, whether at home or at work or at play or travelling. In order to maintain health, both personal and public, much energy has to be directed at maintaining an environment which is as safe as possible for people to live in and for future generations to inherit.

THE NATURE OF MAINTAINING A SAFE ENVIRONMENT

Throughout history man has been concerned with controlling the external environment or adapting to its vagaries. To an amazing degree man has conquered the dangers inherent in the physical environment and has devised methods of protecting his family, his dwelling, his crops and his livestock. Most humans no longer live in constant threat of danger, although there are powerful natural forces such as earthquakes, floods and drought which man is impotent to control. The fact that this is the case is illustrated by events in recent history, such as the devastating forest fires in South Australia in 1983 and the continuing drought in parts of the African continent which has taken the lives and livelihood of countless people. It should not be forgotten either that in this so-called era of peace, there are wars going on in many parts of the world which means that some people are living in an unsafe environment and in constant danger.

Even under normal circumstances, however, people throughout the world are still exposed to a variety of environmental hazards which jeopardise their safety, health, happiness and, indeed, survival. Increasingly too, in this age of technological and scientific advancement, there are yet new hazards to be contended with — such as the risks associated with radiation, chemical waste, drugs and modern war weaponry — and these, in contrast to natural forces, have been created by man himself.

There are many dimensions to the AL of maintaining a safe environment and, obviously, not all can be discussed in this chapter. Many different kinds of activities contribute to maintaining a safe environment and, because most are essentially *preventive* in nature, the remainder of this section considers the following topics:

- preventing accidents
- preventing fire
- preventing infection
- preventing pollution

Preventing accidents

Accidents can occur anywhere and at any time. Frequently, though not always, they are avoidable. Preventing accidents — in the home, at work, at play and while travelling — can and should be everyone's concern, both for their own personal safety and that of others. The human suffering which results from an accident can be severe and can result in some form of life-long disablement or disfigurement for the victim, not forgetting the stress and guilt which is borne by the person who may have had some responsibility for the accident occurring.

In recent years the problem of accidents and accident prevention has come very much to the fore because the huge scale of the problem is now recognised. In Europe, accidents are now the third most important cause of death, and yet fatalities represent only the tip of the iceberg. *Accidents in childhood* are of particular concern. Although by no means in a poor position on the world league table, in the U.K. *accidents account for 30%* of fatalities among preschool children. Again, fatalities represent only a small fraction of accidents and, even though by no means all injuries sustained require medical treatment, many hundreds of thousands of children do receive treatment each year on account of accidents. Data collected on 128 000 cases admitted to hospital in 1977 showed that nearly 11% were the result of road accidents and more than 20% occurred in home. Of the road accidents, 86% involved children between the ages of 5 and 14 years (boys outnumbering girls 2 to 1). Conversely, 63% of home accidents were to children aged 1–4 years (boy: girl ratio at 1.5:1): and the major causes were poisoning (29%), intracranial injury (27%), and burns

(14%) (OHE, 1981). These statistics show that, for children, accidents in the home and accidents on the roads are of particular concern and more is said on these subjects later.

Specific issues aside, what is now generally realised is that unless something is done to reduce accidents, other measures taken for the good of a nation's health are being undermined. Health care professionals have a vital role to play in accident prevention, though the problem needs to be tackled by multidisciplinary effort, organised at national and international levels. Health education is an important aspect of prevention but that is unlikely to be effective in the absence of increased safety measures and legislation. Individual effort is also vital. Accident prevention cannot be viewed only in terms of the elimination of hazards. The potential for accidents will always exist, and so each individual must become skilled at maintaining safety in the face of hazards inherent in the environment. Some of the ways in which this can be achieved are described in the discussion which follows of preventing accidents *in the home; at work; at play; and while travelling.*

Preventing accidents in the home

Most people probably think of their home as a 'safe' place but, in reality, the average home is potentially a very dangerous environment. Even in countries where housing standards have improved immeasurably, and the promotion of safety in the home has been of long-standing concern, the problem of accidents is one of some magnitude. As has already been mentioned, young children are particularly at risk and they must rely on adults to protect them from the dangers in their home environment.

In 1982 in the U.K., the Royal Society for the Prevention of Accidents marked its golden jubilee with a major publicity compaign to draw the public's attention to hazards in the home, and make them more aware of the simple measures which can be taken to prevent accidents. The Society emphasised the magnitude of the problem by pointing out that there are 6000 deaths and 1 million injuries in British homes each year, a situation which affects one family in four and costs the nation £45 million a year to treat home accident cases in hospital.

What then are some of the hazards in the home environment which can cause accidents? Some different groups of hazards are described below, along with related preventive measures.

There are *fire* hazards. Open fires are increasingly less common in homes today but, where they do exist, the crawling child and toddler need to be protected. A large safety guard securely fixed to the wall will prevent a child coming into contact with a fire, and children's neightwear should be flame resistant. Much modern household furniture is a fire hazard, and burning cigarette ends in lounge suites or beds can cause serious fires.

There are *electrical* hazards. No matter how new and safe the wiring is in a home, there is always the danger of injury and electrocution. Faulty electrical appliances should be repaired by an electrician and even simple procedures, such as fixing a new plug or renewing a light bulb, can be hazardous if a mistake is made. In any home where there is a young child, socket guards should be fitted to prevent a finger or pencil being poked into the dangerous socket.

There are *chemical* hazards. Poisoning comes high on the list of accident causes, especially to children, and all toxic substances should be kept labelled and carefully stored in a safe place, preferably a specific cupboard in the kitchen, bathroom, garage or garden shed. Wherever they are kept, they should be out of reach of children and, where appropriate, under lock and key. The increasing use of child-proof containers for medicines is helpful, but vigilance is still necessary. It is unwise to keep medications in a handbag which could be lost or might be explored by a child, with disastrous results. Apart from medicines, there are many other potentially dangerous chemicals, solid or liquid, which may be in any ordinary home: for example, substances for cleaning and decorating, and killing weeds and rodents. One particularly toxic cleaner found in the kitchen is dish-washer powder. One should not forget other commonly used substances, such as bleach and hair dye or nail polish and perfumes, which may well be left out in the bathroom or bedroom.

There are *thermal* hazards. If tapwater is very hot, it can easily scald sensitive skin and one precaution is to run the cold water into the bath before the hot. Hot liquids, whether in a kettle or pot on the cooker, or in cups on the table or in the hand, should always be dealt with carefully and especially when there are young children about because even an apparently small volume of liquid can cause severe burning. Use of a cooker guard, not using a tablecloth and not holding a cup of hot liquid while holding or feeding a baby are precautions to be recommended. Other hazards in the kitchen include the hot cooker and hot baking utensils, and protecting the hands with heat-resistant gloves will help to avoid burns.

There are hazards associated with *sharp equipment*. In the home, there are scissors, pins and needles used for sewing; razor blades in the bathroom; sharp knives and, possibly, a food processor with sharp blades in the kitchen; nails and other sharp instruments in the toolbox; and shears and other tools in the garden shed. All need to be used and stored with forethought and care, especially in the interests of children.

There are hazards associated with *house design*. Houses vary structurally and can be more or less dangerous for the inhabitants. Safety should be considered in relation to positioning of lighting in the house and access areas, particularly where there are steps or stairs. Provision of a stair guard, and secure door and window locks, are sensible precautions with children. For elderly people, grab rails at strategic places (including the bathroom/toilet) and use of a non-slip bath mat are devices likely to prevent accidents from occurring. Similarly, use of non-slip polish and non-skid pads under rugs, and prompt repair or replacement of frayed carpets, will help to keep the floor trip-free. Glass is another danger and modern house design tends to favour large areas of glazing — glass doors and full length glass panels, either fixed or sliding — to allow for maximum natural lighting. The cost of safety glazing has deterred its use in private dwellings. However, one inexpensive precaution is to apply self-adhesive warning stickers on the glass at eye level: for example, on a patio door which someone might inadvertently walk or run into while their attention is fixed on the garden beyond.

Whatever precautions are taken to minimise the hazards mentioned, accidents still can and do happen. At the risk of repetition, it is worth mentioning again that children (especially those of preschool age) are particularly vulnerable to home accidents, the major ones being poisoning, head injury and burns. For infants under 1-year of age, the majority of fatal accidents are caused by choking on food or by suffocation. When constant adult surveillance cannot be assured, young children can at least be protected by being put in a playpen or securely fastened in a bouncing cradle (placed on the floor), highchair or pram. However, physical restraint is not a solution to accident prevention and, indeed, excessive over protection will only deny a child the opportunity to explore and learn about the environment. All children have to develop a concept of safety and an ability to cope with the hazards which exist in that environment. Parents and, depending on the circumstances, grand-parents and childminders too, have a vital role to play in preventing accidents in the home. Because they go into homes, health visitors have a unique opportunity to assess levels of safety and to offer appropriate guidance and help to parents. However, to accomplish this, nurses need to be well informed about the subject of home accidents. Articles by Moore, Ray and Ahamed are collected together, along with a fact sheet, in an issue of 'Community Outlook' (1982) which is devoted to the subject of home accidents and clearly shows that there are many ways in which the nursing profession can contribute to their prevention. But others, too, must accept their share of responsibility for safety in the home. They include house designers and manufacturers, especially those concerned with the production of child safety equipment; children's furniture and toys; and household products, especially commonly used chemicals and other potentially dangerous substances and articles.

Apart from children, the other group most vulnerable to accidents in the home are those at the other end of the lifespan, the elderly. Falls are of particular concern.

There is a high mortality associated with old people who lie undetected for a long time, both related to the injury sustained and to complications; such as hypothermia, dehydration, bronchopneumonia and breakdown of pressure areas (Wild et al, 1981). Fear of this happening may cause old people to be admitted to residential homes though, as Wild (1983) shows, falls are by no means uncommon in that setting either; they are most likely to occur among those who have suffered previous falls indoors and have impaired gait and balance. Broadly speaking, falls in the elderly can usually be attributed to either medical or environmental causes and prevention must tackle both aspects. The fact that many simple preventive measures are possible is well illustrated in an article by Mitchell (1984) and these range from encouraging elderly people to wear well-fitting shoes rather than slippers, to the use of alarm systems, and the involvement of neighbours and regular callers to an old person's house. Again, as in childhood accidents, prevention of accidents in the home to the elderly requires a variety of approaches. Everything possible needs to be tried if, as the numbers of elderly people increase by the year, the sought-after goal of independent life at home in the community is to be achieved.

Preventing accidents at work
Even when at work the AL of maintaining a safe environment cannot be forgotten. Wherever people gather together there is a danger of fire from smoking. But in some industries it is the major hazard and workers have to agree to be searched on entry; matches, lighters and cigarettes are not allowed on the work site. Education and training of the workers so that they are aware of the particular hazards are of paramount importance.

What has already been said about thermal hazards can also apply at work. Where automatic stoking equipment is not in use, furnace workers wear heat-resistant clothing, especially gloves; and also goggles to protect eyes from glare and sparks. This also applies where substances like molten steel, lead, glass and tar are poured. In some climates, outdoor workers have to be trained to take protective measures against brilliant sunshine.

At the other end of the scale, there are industries where excessive cold is used, refrigeration in the fishing industry being one example, and cold storage rooms in the catering industry another. Workers need to understand how quickly human tissue freezes, and the necessary precautions to prevent its occurrence. Workers who can be exposed to excessively cold weather conditions have not only to know about survival measures during over-exposure, but be able and willing to carry them out.

Workers in the pharmaceutical industry and in laboratories obviously have to be knowledgeable and skilled to avoid the many chemical hazards that can threaten the safety of their environment. When the chemicals could damage the skin or the eyes, adequate protection is essential. Careful use of fragile glassware minimises injury from broken glass. Very strict measures for preventing infection are also necessary in those laboratories where workers handle infected material.

Where workers make sharp equipment, or use machines with cutting edges and moving parts, use of adequate guarding is essential to maintain safety in their environment. Wherever possible automatic safety factors are built into the machines, for instance by making them unworkable unless the guards are in place. If this is not the case, it is imperative that workers build safety factors into their work pattern from the beginning.

Some groups of health care workers are subject to certain types of injury and accident. For example, back injury is common among nurses and there is growing concern about the need to instruct nurses in proper lifting techniques (p. 248) and to encourage them to use mechanical lifting devices as much as possible. Exposure to radiation is another area of concern, affecting radiologists, doctors, dentists and nurses who are involved in the use of X-ray procedures and care of patients undergoing treatment with radioactive substances. Female staff of childbearing age, particularly women who are known to be pregnant, require special protection from radiation hazards. Finch (1983a) reviews how the codes of practice which apply to radiotherapy and X-ray procedures affect nurses.

So important is the subject of a safe work environment that most countries have legislation requiring protective practices at all places of employment. Standards are set for ventilation, heating, lighting, hygiene, safety features of tools and equipment, fire precautions, first aid facilities and provision is made for occupational health services. In the U.K., the Health and Safety at Work Act 1974 is an important piece of legislation in this respect. It imposes statutory obligations on employers to set down and implement policy to safeguard the health and safety of their employees. However, the employees also have responsibilities and are required both to exercise reasonable care, and to co-operate with their employers' health and safety policies. Clarke (1982) and Finch (1983b) discuss this aspect of the Act in relation to nurses.

At international level, the International Labour Organization (ILO) and the World Health Organization (WHO) collaborate to produce various recommendations which seek to establish worldwide standards of safety with the purpose of preventing avoidable accidents at work.

Preventing accidents at play
It seems paradoxical that man must attend to the AL of maintaining a safe environment even during leisure activities. But for those who choose arduous out-door recreations like climbing and ski-ing this is particularly so. A necessary motto is 'Be prepared' by wearing suitable at-

tire, paying attention to the weather and the forecast, and by having extra rations and a heat-reflective sheet for keeping warm in an adverse environment.

Those who pursue water-related sports should learn to respect natural events like tides and floods. For safety they should co-operate when local authorities display signs, warning that the seashore is dangerous. Becoming a competent swimmer is obviously sensible and for those who sail in boats a knowledge of seamanship is essential.

Even at festive times like Christmas, extra safety precautions need to be taken with Christmas trees, fairy lights and decorations. Extra precautions are necessary on other occasions when bonfires and fireworks form part of the festivities. An increasing number of countries are moving towards a policy of prohibiting the sale of fireworks to the public and having organised displays operated by experts.

In spite of knowledge about precautions, injuries from accidents during sport and leisure activities are commonplace and account for a significant proportion of emergency admission to hospitals. This may reflect the fact that people today have more leisure and money to spend on such pursuits than in the past. Certainly sports such as motor-cycling, hang-gliding, ski-ing, skating, yachting, diving and squash have become popular among a broad cross-section of the community. All of these, some more than others, carry the risk of injury from accident and even the safety of some long-standing sports — notably boxing — has become a focus of attention. It is not only players of a sport who risk injury, but in some cases the spectators too, and for example the problem of 'football hooliganism' has become a matter of concern in the U.K. In an attempt to prevent violence and injury, steps have been taken to combat drunkenness at football matches and to improve crowd control. Of course even in a well-controlled crowd there are bound to be accidents when many thousands of spectators are gathered together, and Sadler (1983) describes the medical problems which commonly occur and how they are managed on such a large scale, with particular reference to the nurse's role.

In the main, sporting accidents affect young adults because involvement is more competitive, and dangerous sport is a pastime of that age group. However, accidents do happen to school-age children in the course of play, and consistent with the activities of this age group, they suffer fewer accidents in the home (compared with pre-school age children) but more accidents outdoors and in the school playground. The results of a study undertaken in Cardiff (Wales, U.K.) of 10 000 school children injured by accident are reported by Maddocks (1981). In the 5-9 year age group, 15% of injuries happened in school and 24% out of doors (compared with 23% at home); and for 10-15-year-olds, 29% occurred in school and 26% out of doors (compared with 11% at home). The comment is made that the proportion of accidents in school

is high, considering the relatively small part of total time spent there. It is also relevant to note that 55% of school injuries occur in the playground. Here again in this context, as in the home, preventing accidents needs to balance the necessity of supervision and restriction in the interests of safety, against the need for children to enjoy themselves and to develop a sense of personal responsibility for their own safety.

Preventing accidents while travelling
Every person has a responsibility for maintaining safety while travelling. Laws and regulations can lay down safety standards but individuals have to comply with those standards. Ignorance is no plea in law, so people have to be taught about safety while travelling, and have to be encouraged to develop a positive attitude and strict self-discipline in relation to prevention of accidents.

This is said to be the 'age of travel'. Certainly this century has seen incredible advances in the speed of travel, both inter-city and international, and in the distances people travel — indeed as far as the moon. Holidays and business trips abroad are now commonplace occurrences and an elaborate network of international communication ensures the safety of travellers by land, sea and air. There are also carefully planned strategies to cope with emergencies and the victims of major travel accidents, wherever they may occur in the world.

At national level, the major concern is with preventing accidents on the roads. Safe road surfaces, adequate street lighting and sign posting, compulsory driving tests, road use regulations, compulsory speed limits and minimum mechanical safety standards for vehicles are all examples of measures taken by national governments to maintain a safe environment on the roads and to prevent accidents. In addition, many governments have extended legislation to other areas, for example, laws which permit police to use a breathalyser test to detect and detain drivers who have been drinking in excess of the alcohol limit.

In an increasing number of countries, use of seat belts in cars is now obligatory. Even in the short time since the introduction of seat belt legislation in January 1983 in the U.K., there has been a demonstrable reduction (of approximately 25%) in the number of deaths and serious injuries (e.g. internal chest injuries and fractured skulls) among front seat car occupants. Pressure groups are now campaigning for the law to be extended to cover back seat passengers too, principally with the safety of children in mind but also to protect front seat occupants who can be injured in a crash if an unrestrained person in the back is thrown forward. It is interesting to see how a law has so rapidly effected a dramatic and important change in people's behaviour concerning safety while travelling where even aggressive publicity campaigns apparently failed to make the necessary impact.

In an article on road accidents, Smith (1981) argues

that we must change our fatalistic attitude to road accidents. He provides an interesting and revealing analysis of the statistics. The number of people killed or seriously injured on British roads during the 1970s exceeded 750 000, and in one year alone (1979) there were 6352 deaths and over 80 544 serious injuries and 247 617 minor injuries. Smith suggests that these figures, though alarming, fail to reveal the true impact of road accidents as a cause of death, pointing out not only that they share first place with cancer as the number one killer of the under 40s, but also that they steal many more years of life expectancy because road accident victims tend to be younger than those who die from cancer. Smith argues also that there are serious moral questions involved when one appreciates that, apart from the risks to car drivers, passengers and motorcyclists themselves, the *pedestrian* casualty figures are alarming. He points out that safety campaigns aimed solely at the pedestrian are not sufficient in view of the fact that a substantial proportion of pedestrians are run down and killed or injured, not on the road but on the pavement. Smith concludes his articles, saying:

We must escape from the fatalistic attitude to road accidents which has clouded our thinking for so long, and realise that death and injury on the present scale are no more an inevitable consequence of mortality in a technological society than is cholera or bubonic plague an inevitable consequence of living together in cities.

Preventing fire

Any activity which aims at preventing fire is a component of the AL of maintaining a safe environment. These activities are an essential part of living as fire can cause utter devastation. Health education aims to spread knowledge about fire hazards and to encourage self-discipline in carrying out precautions. Unsafe disposal of lighted cigarette ends has in the past caused many fires in places such as shops, hotels, hospitals and warehouses. The social trend is towards a decreasing number of smokers, but if smoking is permitted in public buildings the provision of adequate means for safe disposal of cigarette ends is a fire-preventing activity.

To some extent fire can be prevented by maintaining equipment in a safe working condition. This includes mending frayed flexes, avoiding trailing flexes, not overloading electrical circuits, guarding fires, and using self-extinguishing devices for movable articles like paraffin lamps and oil-heaters which can be knocked over. Care should be taken also when using gas appliances. The light should be applied to the jets as soon as the supply is turned on to prevent a build up in concentration. Yet another contribution to safety is carefulness when using fat for cooking purposes; should the fat catch fire the most effective way to control it is to cover the pan with the lid or with a metal tray and turn off the supply of heat.

Most countries have a set of fire precautions to which the proprietors of public buildings, including shops and hotels, must adhere. Citizens are encouraged, when their houses are empty even for a few hours, to turn off electric switches, remove plugs from sockets and close the doors and windows of all rooms. Closed doors and windows help to confine fire to one room for about 20 minutes by which time expert help is often available. Most countries have a paid, professional fire brigade who are expert in fire fighting and fire prevention; they play a big part in the education of citizens, helping them to become fire prevention conscious.

Detecting, containing and extinguishing fire are the three main principles when dealing with fire. Detection is often by smell and by seeing smoke and flame. Combustion cannot continue in the absence of oxygen and fire extinguishers work on this principle. If the flame is sufficiently small, merely smothering it with thick material such as a rug will cut off the atmospheric oxygen supply and extinguish the fire. Closed windows and doors help to contain smoke as well as flames and this is an important point to remember because inhaled smoke can immobilise people trying to escape from a building.

In hot dry weather, many countries fear forest fires from carelessly attended picnic fires and inadequate disposal of lighted cigarette ends although ignition can occur outdoors from the heat produced by sun shining through glass carelessly left lying on the ground, especially if it is near shrubland and forest. Spontaneous generation of heat causing fire can occur also when garbage containing organic matter and metal cans is tipped into a land hollow and left to disintegrate and subside. It is evident that knowledge as well as self-discipline is necessary to maintain a safe environment.

Preventing infection

An essential dimension of the AL of maintaining a safe environment is preventing infection. Infection results from the successful invasion of the body by pathogenic microorganisms and, because these are ever-present in the environment, preventing infection is a fundamental issue in disease prevention and health promotion. Much is now known about the biological characteristics of pathogens and the epidemiology of infection, and successful methods have been developed which can inhibit the growth and spread, and harmful effects of these organisms. However, while public health measures at national and international levels can do much to prevent and control infection, the participation of individuals is vital because of the continuing importance of many basic personal and domestic hygiene activities. Therefore, all people require to understand about the sources of infection, the modes of transmission of pathogenic microorganisms, human portals of entry, susceptibility to infection and principles basic to the control of infection. These topics are discussed briefly in the remainder of this section and the main points of the first three subjects are summarised in Figure 7.1.

Sources of infection. The source of infection is the site where the pathogenic organism grows and multiplies. The natural warmth of the human body encourages microorganisms to multiply rapidly. For pathogens to establish themselves in the human body they must be in the right place, in sufficient numbers and be sufficiently virulent. The body's defence mechanisms against infection — immunity (p. 35) — can usually cope with small numbers and the body only succumbs to infection when the invading numbers are large or when, for various reasons, resistance is lowered.

Pathogens are usually species specific and, therefore, the most common sources of infection in man are human beings themselves. A person's skin, mouth and nose have a natural flora of microorganisms, streptococci and staphylococci being the main ones. Esch coli, which is present in the large bowel may pass from the anus to the urethra and invade the urinary tract or may be spread by the hands to other sites. Therefore, a person can infect himself and auto-infection, as it is called, is important to recognise as a source of infection.

Alternatively, a person can be infected by another person and any form of interpersonal contact allows microorganisms to be transmitted from one individual to another. The source of infection may be a person who is incubating an infectious disease, or actually suffering from an infection, or recovering from one, or a carrier who is himself not affected but is harbouring pathogens which can infect others.

Animals provide another source of infection in the environment and, like humans, animals can harbour and spread pathogenic microorganisms. The common house fly can carry many different pathogens; the mosquito carries malaria and yellow fever; brucellosis can be contracted from milk cows; and rabies in man results from a bite by an infected dog. These are just a few examples of animal-borne infection to which humans are susceptible.

A few infections arise from inaminate sources: for example, pathogens that cause tetanus are harboured in the soil.

Modes of transmission. In order to understand how infection is spread, it is necessary to know about the various modes of transmission.

These are noted in Figure 7.1 and are briefly discussed below.

Direct contact is most likely to lead to infection of the skin, conjunctiva or mucous membrane. Skin diseases, such as impetigo or scabies, are transmitted by direct contact. The sexually-transmitted diseases (e.g. syphilis, gonorrhoea and non-specific urethritis) are so-called because they occur as a result of direct sexual contact with an infected partner. Some oral and respiratory in-

SOURCES OF INFECTION: EXAMPLES

• human sources	– auto-infection: a person who contaminates himself at a site other than the original infected source
	– other humans: person who is incubating an infection
	: person who is suffering from an infection
	: person who is recovering from an infection
	: a carrier – person who is not affected but is harbouring pathogens
• animal sources	– e.g. dogs, cows, monkeys
	– e.g. birds, insects
• inanimate sources	– soil

MODES OF TRANSMISSION: EXAMPLES

• by direct contact	– direct transmission from an infected person to another person as in skin disease, sexually-transmitted diseases and some respiratory infections
• by fomites	– indirect transmission from infected person to another via inanimate objects in the environment
• by airborne droplets and dust	– infected person sprays pathogens into the air when breathing/coughing/sneezing/ talking/laughing: pathogens fall to the floor and mix with dust
• by contaminated food and drink	– infection (e.g. from infected food handler) transmitted in food and drink
• by animals/insects	– mechanical transmission (e.g. pathogens carried on the body/legs) or spread of pathogens by blood-sucking insects

HUMAN PORTALS OF ENTRY: EXAMPLES

• by the placenta	– to the fetus from the mother's blood supply, e.g. syphilis, rubella
• by inhalation	– entry of airborne pathogens, e.g. common cold, measles, whooping cough, diphtheria, respiratory tuberculosis
• by ingestion	– pathogens in food and drink are ingested and digested, e.g. dysentery, typhoid, gastroenteritis, brucellosis, and bacterial food poisoning
• by the skin	– infection of skin, and mucous membrane by direct contact, e.g. skin diseases, conjunctivitis, infective foot disorders, sexually-transmitted diseases
• by invasion of tissue	– via a cut in the skin or surgical wound (e.g. staphylococcal infection)
	– via the bite of an animal or insect

Fig. 7.1 Infection: summary of sources of infection, modes of transmission and human portals of entry

fections follow direct contact: for example, infectious mononucleosis (glandular fever) is frequently described as the 'kissing disease'. Direct hand contact can transmit infection from one person to another or, in the same person, from one location to another. For this reason, handwashing is the single most important personal activity in preventing infection, so it is essential that people wash their hands after going to the toilet and before touching food.

Indirect contact involves transmission by fomites. Fomites is the word used to refer to inanimate objects in the environment (such as clothing, bedclothes, crockery and cutlery, instruments and furniture) and these can act as reservoirs for infection. Fomites with smooth hard surfaces (e.g. glass) are easier to clean than those made of fabric. Disinfection by physical and chemical means is important in preventing the spread of infection by fomites.

To prevent the spread of infection by airborne droplets, people should cough and sneeze into a handkerchief, preferably a paper one which can be disposed of by burning or flushing down the toilet. Even during breathing and talking, organisms present in the nasopharynx, throat and mouth are expelled in droplets of secretion. For this reason, masks may be worn by personnel in operating theatres and on other occasions (e.g. wound dressing) when the patient is likely to be at risk of succumbing to infection. Droplets also fall to the floor and contribute to the dust and its microbial flora and this mode of transmission is especially important in streptococcal and staphylococcal infection in hospitals, hence the emphasis on reducing dust by damp dusting and vacuum cleaning in this environment. Adequate spacing of beds also helps to prevent direct droplet spread of infection in hospital, as does good ventilation. A person known to have an infectious disease is usually nursed in an isolation cubicle; barrier nursing is another means of isolation. Many of the common infectious diseases of childhood are transmitted by airborne droplets (e.g. chickenpox) and, therefore, isolation from other children during the period of incubation and infection is a means of preventing spread of these diseases.

Protection of food and drink from contamination, for example by flies, and handwashing before touching food are basic measures to prevent the transmission of infection in food and drink. People who have infected sores, such as boils or styes, should not prepare food, especially when it is to be distributed to large numbers. Contaminated food, water or milk can result in an epidemic outbreak and these infections, such as the salmonelloses and bacillary dysentery, are further spread by hands contaminated with faeces. Milk and food can also be contaminated by infection in the animals which provide them and preventing the transmission of such disease (e.g. brucellosis) involves strict control over the source and supply of animal food products for human consumption. Animals can also transmit infection on their bodies, as can insects (e.g. flies becoming contaminated with faeces) and many widespread epidemic infections are transmitted by blood-sucking insects.

Human portals of entry. The microorganism must invade the body tissues before infection results and, following invasion, infection will develop only if the body defence mechanisms fail to prevent multiplication of the pathogen. As will be apparent already, there are various portals of entry for invasion of the body by infection. Even before birth, infection can gain entry to the fetus from the mother's blood via the placenta. For this reason, pregnant women have their blood tested to detect syphilis so that treatment can be provided to ensure that the baby is not infected. Rubella (German measles) can cause devastating damage to the fetus in early pregnancy and girls who have not had an attack of this disease by the age of puberty are offered immunisation against this virus so that any baby conceived would be protected.

Many microorganims enter the body via the respiratory tract and avoiding inhalation of pathogens would be easy if they could be seen! It may seem trivial to say that people with a cold should isolate themselves but it would help in the maintenance of a safe environment for others. At least sufferers should minimise the spray from their sneezes by using a clean handkerchief and, likewise, when coughing.

Ingestion is another means by which microorganisms gain entry to the body. The pathogens that cause dysentry, typhoid and some forms of gastroenteritis are excreted in the faeces. Hands contaminated with faeces, if inadvertantly put near the mouth, can re-infect the person himself or infect food which may be consumed by others. Strict handwashing routines are imperative to prevent this. Fortunately the technology of the food processing industry is now so sophisticated as to have all but eliminated infection from this source. However, fresh food, and food consumed which has been prepared and cooked by others, must always be regarded as a potential source of infection. Whether in a large institution, a small restaurant, a bakery, a take-away food shop or the kitchen at home, those who handle and cook food must adhere strictly to the rules of food hygiene. Food poisoning is increasing and the main types of bacteria responsible are salmonella (mainly in meat and poultry); staphylococcus aureus (the skin and nose of human carriers is the main source); and clostridium perfringens (which contaminates raw meat, poultry and some dried products). Raw foodstuffs are the most likely source of food poisoning and foods which encourage bacterial growth are meats and poultry (raw and cooked), foods with a meat base (e.g. soups), eggs, milk and milk products (e.g. cream). There are three main principles involved in the prevention of food poisoning. Firstly, the spread of contamination is prevented by separating foodstuffs (to avoid cross-contamination); by cleanliness on the part of the foodhandler; and by cleanliness of cooking equipment. Secondly, pathogens already in food can be prevented from multiplying by cold storage and avoiding delay between preparation and serving of food. Thirdly, thorough cooking and rapid cooking will help to destroy pathogens (Graham & Lee, 1981).

Although the skin provides a barrier against infection, it can be successfully invaded by pathogenic microorganisms, as can the body's mucous membranes (e.g. the conjunctiva). Common examples of infective foot disorders are athlete's foot and verruca, notoriously picked up from public swimming baths and communal bathrooms.

Pathogens can invade the body tissue through a cut in the skin and for this reason even minor cuts and grazes should be attended to properly and observed for signs of infection. Prevention of infection is the objective whenever surgical wounds are cleaned and covered with a sterile dressing. The number of microorganisms on the skin at the time it is cut will depend on how recently the skin was washed or, in the case of surgery, how adequately skin preparation was undertaken.

Invasion of tissue by pathogens may result from the bite of an animal or insect, e.g. rabies is caused by the bite of an infected dog; Marburg disease by the bite of a green monkey; and malaria is caused by the bite of a mosquito.

Susceptibility to infection. People will be less susceptible and more resistant to infection if they have an adequate diet and sufficent exercise, sleep and rest. Tired, malnourished people are prone to infection.

When a person is ill, the body's natural defence mechanisms are already under stress, and therefore, less able than usual to resist the invasion of pathogenic microorganisms. An unfavourable environment may also decrease resistance to infection: for example, prolonged exposure to cold and damp may increase susceptibility to infection. Resistance to specific infectious diseases can be acquired in several ways (p. 35), and, of course, infants during the first few months of life are relatively unsusceptible to many infections because of transplacentally derived immunity.

Prevention of infection. In any scheme aimed at preventing infection, destruction of the pathogenic microorganisms plays a large part. Agents which kill organisms are called disinfectants or antimicrobial agents, and they are physical or chemical in nature. Physical disinfectants include the natural elements like sunlight and freezing as well as generated heat and cold: chemical disinfectants include liquids and gases. A success story of the 20th century is the discovery of antibiotics, substances which can be introduced into the human body to combat pathogenic microorganisms.

Another approach in preventing infection is based on the principle of isolation. Isolating an infected person has long been used as a means of preventing the spread of infection and has been very effective in campaigns against the more serious and highly infectious diseases, such as smallpox and tuberculosis. As well as isolating the person

suffering from the disease it is, of course, important to locate people who have been in contact with the sufferer and, if necessary, they too must be isolated, treated or kept under surveillance. For this reason, 'contact tracing' has become an integral part of the control of infectious disease. Galbraith (1983) outlines the aims and methods of contact tracing which has been used in recent years in the U.K. in relation to sexually transmitted disease and tuberculosis, and during limited outbreaks of typhoid fever, diphtheria and Lassa fever.

Measures to increase people's resistance to infection are also important in prevention, and it is in this context that immunisation has played such a major part (p. 36). In the United Kingdom, parents are advised to have their children immunised against diphtheria, tetanus, poliomyelitis, whooping cough and measles. Immunisation against tuberculosis is given to non-reactors to tuberculin in adolescence (the BCG test). Nurses, particularly health visitors, have an important role to play in encouraging parents to take up immunisation and there is concern about falling rates of acceptance. This may be partly due to the fact that young parents of today are less aware of the seriousness of some of the diseases, as Arnold (1978) points out in her discussion of poliomyelitis. There is no doubt too that parents have become more aware that immunisation carries some risk of adverse reaction and this has been most publicised in relation to the whooping cough vaccine. On the one hand there have been reports suggesting that the vaccine can cause brain damage in some children and, on the other, the whooping cough epidemics in recent years have re-awakened fears of the damage the disease itself can inflict. Miller & Rose (1981) point out that at the turn of the century whooping cough was, after measles, the commonest infectious disease killer of young children in Britain. After introduction of wide-scale immunisation in the late 1950s the incidence reduced, but now the number of babies vaccinated has dropped to 30%, compared with 80% in 1974. Epidemics of whooping cough have occurred in the U.K. in several of the intervening years. Readers who wish to know more about this subject are referred to an article by Pincher (1982) in which she outlines the pros and cons of the vaccine and describes her own investigation into the reasons why some parents omit it from their children's immunisation schedule.

Apart from immunisation of young children, pregnant women are considered to be a priority group because certain infectious diseases can cause serious damage to the developing fetus. Rubella vaccine is offered to all girls in early adolescence and to non-pregnant women of child-bearing age who are found to be serologically negative for this antigen. Cytomegalovirus is a less well-known infection which affects considerably greater numbers of babies than rubella. However, although only a minority affected by it develop microcephaly and other conditions associated with mental handicap, it is common and attempts are underway to develop a vaccine which would prevent potential damage.

Indications for vaccination against other infectious diseases (e.g. enteric fevers, cholera, typhus, yellow fever and rabies) depend on individual risk of exposure and international travel regulations. The nature of immunisation programmes as a means of preventing infection is determined according to the prevailing circumstances of a particular country and readers in countries other than the U.K. should supplement this section with relevant local information.

Nobody now needs to be, nor should be, vaccinated against smallpox. This disease has now been eradicated from the world, an achievement which must rank as one of WHO's greatest successes. Some vaccine is being kept in a limited number of centres in case of resurgence of smallpox.

Control of epidemics. Controlling epidemics is important in preventing infection and, in this age of travel, this is a concern which extends beyond the boundaries of any one nation to international collaboration. Incidence of infection in each country is notified to the World Health Organization so that necessary strategies can be implemented to prevent spread to other countries by travellers, cargoes and animals. An account of the spread of cholera through Asia and Europe in the 1830s is given by Swan (1983) and makes interesting reading even today.

A very real threat of the present time — the problem of rabies — is discussed by Vella (1981). Rabies was indigenous to the U.K. before successful eradication at the turn of the century. However, the threat of importation of the disease has returned, not only on a small scale relating to violation of quarantine regulations by dog owners but because the rabies virus has been spread throughout Europe into France (U.K.'s nearest continental neighbour) by the red fox and concern is rising too about rabies-infected bats in Europe. If the rabies virus were to take roots in the wild life of the U.K., domesticated pets would be at risk and so, in turn, would the population. Concern about rabies seems a somewhat trivial issue in a discussion of the huge topic of preventing infection, but it serves as a reminder that this is a subject which will always be fundamental to maintaining a safe environment, though the precise nature of the concern will vary among countries and over time.

Preventing pollution

One dimension of maintaining a safe environment is preventing pollution. Contamination of water supplies for drinking by untreated human excrement has always been a basic aspect of pollution prevention. In more recent times, urbanisation and industralisation have produced a whole new set of problems and these are man-made. To a great extent air pollution has been brought under control over large populous areas as a result of smoke control measures (p. 145). However, an endless supply of new chemicals is finding uses in industry and agriculture, in and around the home, and in the production of food. Although strict controls are placed on the use of chemicals there is always the possibility that they may prove to be harmful in the long-term. Disposal of industrial waste into rivers and seas is a major source of water pollution.

One pollutant which has attracted considerable concern in recent years is lead. Lead occurs widely in nature, in the soil and in the water. In compound form it has come to be used in paint as a pigment, in plastics as a stabiliser and in petrol as an anti-knock agent. Lead has long been used by man and its toxic properties have long been recognised. Severe lead poisoning is a cause of intellectual impairment. It is widely known that there are harmful effects from inhalation of outfall from a lead works; for children who ingest lead by chewing lead-painted toys; and for families whose drinking water is supplied through lead pipes. Measures have been implemented to control such specific sources of lead poisoning. However, more recently, concern has shifted to the more insidious problem which affects the entire population — pollution of roadside areas by leaded petrol. Fall-out from exhaust emissions is not only directly inhaled but can be ingested because lead settles on the hands and on vegetables, crops and fruit growing near roadsides. In many countries there has been a phased reduction in the lead content of petrol and the U.K. government has announced its intention to move towards lead-free petrol (Healy & Aslam, 1981).

An entirely different kind of problem in modern living is 'noise pollution' and that term is increasingly being used to describe the problem of excessive noise. An environment in which people cannot sleep adequately because of excessive noise cannot be considered a safe environment. People who live near noisy factories, close to flight paths near airports, and in the proximity of busy motorways, all suffer from excessive noise by night and day. During the day, other city dwellers can be disturbed by the noise of traffic, especially heavy lorries going past their homes. People who work in heavy industry are subjected to the noise of machines and measures to minimise the effects include the use of noise-abating apparatus and the wearing of ear muffs. As well as affecting sleep, noise is thought to create tension and fatigue, both of which can contribute to accidents and mental ill-health.

Preventing pollution is one dimension of maintaining a safe environment which is largely a public rather than a personal responsibility. However, there are many ways in which individuals can protect themselves and others from the potentially dangerous effects of pollutants. Washing hands and washing fruit and vegetables before eating are obvious and simple safety measures which all individuals can employ. House owners can ensure that dangerous chemicals are stored away securely and prevented from coming into contact with food and the skin. Lead water tanks and pipes should be replaced with safe alternatives and financial assistance may be available for this. Parents can take care to ensure that children's toys and furniture have not been finished with lead paint which should be avoided for house decorating purposes. Parents can also campaign for children's play areas and school playgrounds to be sited away from busy roads because of the danger of lead poisoning from exhaust fumes. These are just a few examples of ways in which individuals can participate in preventing pollution.

THE PURPOSE OF MAINTAINING A SAFE ENVIRONMENT

The purpose of maintaining a safe environment is virtually inseparable from the nature of this AL and, since that has just been described at length, little more need be added here. Obviously, the first and foremost purpose in all of the activities involved — preventing accidents, fire, infection and pollution — is human survival.

However, in circumstances when life itself is not threatened, the purpose becomes one of preventing, or at least minimising, injury and ill-health. An accident can result in some form of disablement or disfigurement and, even if its effects are only temporary, the human suffering involved can be intense. The effects of fire can be devastating: the pain of burned tissue, the stigma of visible scars and the loss of property and personal possessions. Infection too can involve discomfort and absence from work; and it can mean isolation. Pollution, though often more insidious in its effects, can cause ill-health and even permanent intellectual impairment.

Surely 'prevention is better than cure', but of course prevention demands knowledge and self-discipline and, for these to be applied, requires individuals to develop an understanding of the purpose of maintaining a safe environment.

LIFESPAN: EFFECT ON MAINTAINING A SAFE ENVIRONMENT

The inclusion of the lifespan as one component of the model serves as a reminder that living is a lifelong process, from conception to death. Safety is a basic human requirement for survival, development, health and happiness at every stage of the lifespan.

During prenatal existence, a safe environment is provided by the mother's uterus but, from the moment of birth, a baby becomes instantly exposed to all the hazards in the external environment and is totally dependent on adults for the provision of a safe environment in which to thrive and survive. For young babies, choking and suffocation are major death risks; and protection from accident, infection, and excessive heat or cold is of vital importance. When they become more active and curious, crawling babies and toddlers are increasingly vulnerable to accidents in the home and, as has already been described, falls, burns and accidental poisoning are major causes of injury and death at this stage of the lifespan.

In contrast, school-age children are most at risk to hazards in the outdoors environment, particularly in the roads and in the school playground. Once at school, children cannot be under constant adult surveillance and learning about safety and personal responsibility for maintaining a safe environment is an important dimension of education.

During adolescence bicycle accidents and sporting injuries become more common and, although more aware of danger, rebelliousness or over-confidence may result in lack of consideration for personal safety and the safety of others.

For young adults, hazards in the work environment become an added area of responsibility in the AL of maintaining a safe environment and the degree and type of danger vary according to the nature of the work. Adults, especially when they become parents, develop an increasing sense of responsibility concerning safety and may become involved politically over issues of personal, local or national safety.

The process of ageing, which involves a gradual deterioration of physical and intellectual ability and loss of acuity of the senses, inevitably results in lessened ability to carry out the many activities involved in the AL of maintaining a safe environment. Elderly people become more prone to falls, are vulnerable to pedestrian accidents and at risk to the hazards of infection and fire. Maintaining a safe environment during the final stage of the lifespan may involve dependence on others and on safety aids and require renewed awareness of the hazards which are ever-present in the external environment.

FACTORS INFLUENCING MAINTAINING A SAFE ENVIRONMENT

The AL of maintaining a safe environment is, by nature, multi-dimensional and therefore, not surprisingly, many different factors play a part in influencing the way individuals carry out the activities involved. In keeping with the relevant component of the model, the factors involved are discussed under the following headings — physical, psychological, sociocultural, environmental and politico-economic factors.

Physical factors
If a person is to carry out the AL of maintaining a safe environment, acuity in all of the five senses is vital

because safety hazards are identified through vision, hearing, touch, smell and taste. Obviously any impairment in the nerve pathways associated with the senses will make a person less able to identify hazards in the environment and, therefore, more likely to suffer an accident. For example, impaired vision and impaired hearing are obvious limitations on safety as a pedestrian, making such simple tasks as crossing a road a hazardous undertaking. Impairment can be of the sensory receptor, or of the pathway carrying the impulse to the brain, or of the brain's interpreting ability. Even if there is no impairment in an individual's ability to become aware of a hazard to safety, there may be some reason why he is prevented from taking the necessary avoiding action. A physically disabled person or a frail elderly person are obvious examples of people who may be physically unable to avoid accidental injury in certain circumstances. Also physiological malfunction, like fainting, can cause injury; reduced immunity can render an individual more susceptible to acquiring an infection; and, in general, illness is likely to reduce a person's physical ability to continue to carry out activities aimed at maintaining a safe environment.

Psychological factors

Intellectual processes are involved in learning about maintaining a safe environment and in carrying out the many activities involved. Therefore, people who suffer from intellectual impairment may be unable to acquire adequate knowledge and to respond quickly and appropriately to a threat to safety. For this reason, severely mentally handicapped people depend on others for protection and surveillance and, similarly, parents and teachers accept responsibility for the safety of children in their care.

Attitude to safety and prevention is important and it is desirable that people develop a concept of safety and an awareness of their personal responsibility in maintaining a safe environment, for themselves and for others. Undersirable attitudes include thinking that accidents, fires and infection happen only to others and hoping that someone else will do the campaigning about pollution issues.

Personality and temperament play a part in the attitudes people hold about maintaining a safe environment and affect their efficiency in carrying out the activities involved. Mood is also an important factor. Angry people may become aggressive and violent, possibly causing injury to themselves or to others, and 'non-accidental injury to children' is increasingly recognised as a serious social problem of today. Depressed people may endanger their own safety because tiredness, lethargy and loss of motivation and self-confidence result in a lack of attention to maintaining a safe environment. Worried and preoccupied people are also vulnerable to accidents, perhaps especially on the roads either as drivers or pedestrians.

Stress is known to be an important contributory factor in relation to accidents. For example, research findings suggest that children of families under stress are more vulnerable to accidents, such as ingestion of poisons. Stress factors include circumstances such as serious illness in a family, pregnancy, recent house move, one parent away from home and anxiety or depression in one or both parents (OHE, 1981).

Confidence also plays a part in maintaining safety. The over-confident driver or motorcyclist may overtake without due caution, thus increasing the risk of causing a road traffic accident. Conversely the under-confident person may be hesistant to predict danger or to react to it with sufficient purpose or determination. Therefore, both over-confidence and under-confidence may play a part in creating an environment in which accidents happen more readily.

The complexity of psychological factors involved in the AL of maintaining a safe environment means that publicity campaigns and health education programmes must go beyond simply imparting information about safety, realising that people often know what they should and could do, and yet do not act upon their knowledge. Health education programmes in schools can contribute towards the development of a concept of safety and a responsible attitude towards maintaining a safe environment. In the same way, publicity campaigns and advertising and television documentaries can disseminate knowledge about safety, and attempt to change attitudes and behaviour in a positive way.

Sociocultural factors

Each culture has a unique interpretation of the concept of 'safety' and what is deemed to be responsible, 'safe' behaviour by individuals. This is true largely because the problems associated with maintaining a safe environment are different in different parts of the world. The most obvious of the differences are apparent from a comparison of the problems in so-called developing societies with those which confront the industralised societies.

In many developing societies the lack of basic amenities, such as clean water and proper sanitation, produces an inherently unsafe environment. Infectious diseases, particularly the diarrhoeal diseases, are both difficult to prevent and control in such circumstances and they are largely responsible for the high morbidity and mortality rates in many areas.

In industralised countries, such rudimentary amenities as piped water and sanitation have long been taken for granted and there has been a virtual elimination of major infectious diseases over the past century. However, affluence and technological advances have created new kinds of safety hazards for people who live in Western society. There are all the industrial hazards such as excessive noise, polluted air and contamination of water by industrial waste and, as has already been described in detail, a large-scale problem in the form of accidents.

Within any one society, there are internal differences in relation to the problems of maintaining a safe environment and the particular kinds of hazards to which certain groups of people are exposed. There are social class differences as is apparent, for example, in statistics concerning accidents. Analysis of such statistics pertaining to the U.K. (OHE, 1981), shows that there is a substantial social class difference in childhood mortality from accidents and violence, the overall rate for children of parents in unskilled occupations being nearly five times that for children of parents in the professions. The differential is even greater when pedestrian fatalities are singled out for analysis; and significant class discrepancies have also been observed for specific types of non-fatal accident, such as burns and scalds. Such social class disparities have been linked to a variety of factors, for example, the deficiency of safe play areas for children of the lower social class groups is offered as one explanation for the high rate among them of pedestrian fatalities. Social class inequalities are always difficult to explain precisely but there is no doubt but that they exist in relation to the AL of maintaining a safe environment.

Environmental factors

It is obvious that environmental factors exert a far-reaching influence on this particular AL and, indeed, the concept of 'safety' has no real meaning unless it is considered in relation to 'the environment'. In an earlier section of this chapter, a great range of activities which individuals carry out in maintaining a safe environment were mentioned in relation to preventing accidents in the home, at work, at play and while travelling. Houses, factories and offices, sports grounds and playgrounds, and roads are all 'environments'. In each of these environments there are numerous 'factors', many of which constitute a threat to the safety of individuals and numerous such hazards have been mentioned, as have types of pollution in the environment.

Taking a broader view of the term 'environment', thinking of the 'natural environment', other kinds of factors can be seen to influence this AL: for example, climate and geographical location. It does not take much imagination to appreciate that maintaining a safe environment in high latitudes and high altitudes with the long months of snow, ice and subzero temperatures will differ from maintaining a safe environment in the humid heat of a tropical forest.

The term environment is also often used in a very diffuse way and many people today would describe the environment in which we live as a generally unsafe one. Violence, vandalism, terrorism and hijacking are all too frequently in the news and act as a constant reminder that personal safety is threatened not only by elements, objects and events in the environment, but also by the human beings who live in it.

Politicoeconomic factors

Both political and economic factors influence the AL of maintaining a safe environment to a very great degree. Although many of the activities involved are carried out by individuals, and there is much scope for personal decision-making and responsibility, the business of maintaining a safe environment is very much a political concern and responsibility — at regional, national and international levels. As has been described, many aspects of maintaining a safe environment are controlled by legislation. Laws exist which ensure that as far as possible, accidents, fire, infection and pollution are prevented. Governments also accept a responsibility to increase public awareness of hazards and safety measures and desirable standards of safety through publicity campaigns and education. All such activity is both in the interests of personal and national safety, but also is based on an economic argument.

An unsafe environment will result in accident and ill-health, and both are a burden on a nation's economy. Of course, preventing accidents and promoting safety also costs a great deal of money. Safe houses, roads, vehicles, workplaces and play areas all cost money. So too does the provision of emergency services (such as the fire service) which are sufficiently well-equipped and manned to respond promptly and effectively when required.

The economics of maintaining a safe environment are not just the concern of government for, through taxation, individuals contribute to the national purse. For example, a substantial proportion of the road tax levied on vehicle owners goes towards paying for road maintenance and improvements. For individuals, the costs of maintaining a safe environment are, however, by no means all indirect ones like that. Maintaining safety in the home is an expensive business and, for families with children, the purchase of recommended safety equipment — such as car safety seats, stair gates, a playpen and a cooker guard — adds up to a considerable sum. For families of low income such items are almost certainly prohibitively expensive.

People do not need to be politicians to engage in politics. Individuals and pressure groups can exert a considerable influence on government and have indeed done so very effectively in relation to many aspects of the AL of maintaining a safe environment. For example, the recent introduction of seat belt legislation in the U.K. was at least in part due to persistent lobbying by sections of the community, including the medical profession. Frequently too, people who live in a particular geographic location combine together to form a pressure group if their neighbourhood has been earmarked by government for the siting of, for example, a new motorway or nuclear power station which is considered to constitute a substantial threat to their safety and health. All citizens have a responsibility to be involved in the politicoeconomic decisions which influence the AL of maintaining a safe environment — not necessarily for their own safety, but for that of others and especially that of their children and, indeed, their children's children.

It is perhaps that long-term perspective which is at the root of present-day concern over the increasing international tension and the ever-expanding nuclear arsenal held by the superpowers, making nuclear war seem more and more inevitable. Knowledge of the devastating effect which even a limited nuclear attack would have on the environment and the people in it has motivated increasing numbers to campaign vociferously for nuclear disarmament, either multilateral or unilateral. It is interesting that doctors and nurses, who on the whole prefer to remain apolitical, have become actively engaged in this campaign. Some are members of the CND, others of the Medical Campaign Against Nuclear Weapons. In 1983 the Royal College of Nursing, the professional organisation for British nurses, issued a report on the nursing implications of planning for nuclear war. An examination of the report is presented by Hicks (1983). The report outlines what would happen in the event of nuclear war and maintains that talk of planning for, and training in triage and mass casualty techniques is meaningless, for surviving nurses would be able to do little other than help to provide limited care for casualties and comfort the dying.

Opinion on the nuclear issue is divided and other arguments are involved too, for example economic considerations. Some people think that the vast amounts of money spent by governments on nuclear weapons would be better spent on other needs, such as health care. Protagonists argue that the nation's defence is more important. However, there is no disagreement that preventing nuclear war is vital to maintaining a safe environment for people now, and for future generations.

DEPENDENCE/INDEPENDENCE IN MAINTAINING A SAFE ENVIRONMENT

There are several different aspects of the concept of dependence/independence, which is incorporated in the model, and can be considered in relation to the AL of maintaining a safe environment.

The general principle that dependence/independence status is closely linked with an individual's point on the lifespan was outlined in the discussion of the model of living, and is certainly applicable to this AL. Broadly speaking, there is dependence in the early stages of the lifespan; independence during adulthood; and the likelihood of at least some degree of dependence again in old age.

Without question, babies are totally dependent on others for the maintenance of a safe environment and require to be protected from accidents, fire, infection and pollution. Young children are also to a very great extent dependent upon adults for their safety. They do not have either the mental or physical equipment to be able to carry out the many complex activities involved in the AL of maintaining a safe environment. Neither do they have any real appreciation of the hazards in the environment or a well-developed understanding of the concepts of safety and personal responsibility for maintaining safety.

Throughout adolescence, such attributes develop but, although more independent, people of this age-group are still dependent on adult guidance and surveillance. In contrast, adults are expected to assume independence for maintaining a safe environment and are involved in doing so in the home, at work, at play and while travelling. In old age, there may be the will to retain independence in this AL but circumstances and the effects of the process of ageing may force an elderly person to be dependent on others, at least to some degree. Financial constraints may limit maintenance of safety in the home: for example, an old person may not be able to afford to replace worn carpets or an ageing electricity system and both are potential causes of accident. In addition, loss of acuity of the senses — particularly impaired sight and hearing — will reduce an elderly person's awareness of danger, for example when crossing roads or when cooking in the kitchen. Even if the senses are acute, physical frailty reduces the ability to take the necessary quick action to avoid accidental injuries, such as by falls or burns.

Although independence in the AL of maintaining a safe environment is the norm during adulthood, the fact that by no means all adults have this capacity is important to recognise. People who are mentally handicapped cannot be expected to cope with many aspects of this AL independently. As they may be engaged in a wide range of adult activities, such as cooking and shopping and so on, their dependence upon others for safety is especially important to recognise. Similarly, although many physically handicapped adults are extremely independent in their everyday lives, the AL of maintaining a safe environment is one aspect of living with which they may need considerable help. In addition to dependence on people, a person who is physically handicapped will almost certainly be dependent on aids and equipment; for example, a specially equipped bathroom to minimise the risk of falling while bathing and going to the toilet and special safety gadgets in the kitchen to ensure that cooking can be accomplished without the risk of being cut or burned.

Another group of people who are unlikely to achieve full independence for maintaining a safe environment in adulthood are those who are visually handicapped. To a remarkable extent, blind people do cope with the many hazards to personal safety which exist but they are likely to be more vulnerable in an unfamiliar environment. Therefore, while they may be independent in their own homes, dependence on others may be necessary in other settings, for example when out of doors or when travelling by public transport. It is interesting to reflect on the value of a guide dog to a blind person as an aid to independence in the AL of maintaining a safe environment.

People who are mentally, physically and visually handicapped have been described in terms of their 'dependence' and this has been compared with the 'independence' enjoyed by intelligent, able-bodied adults in relation to the AL of maintaining a safe environment. However, it is worth pausing to question whether 'independence' in this AL is actually attainable by any adult person, irrespective of mental and physical ability. The fact is that no individual has complete independence in this AL. Irrespective of personal efforts to maintain safety, all people are exposed to dangers — natural forces as well as man-made hazards — which are inherent in the environment and which the individual is impotent to control or eliminate. Equally important, the safety of any individual is dependent on the safe behaviour of others. A person can take every precaution to avoid accidents while travelling but cannot guarantee his safety because there are people who drive dangerously, or conditions such as poor visibility, and these factors are outside his control. Similarly, a person can attempt to avoid infection by washing hands before handling and eating food, but nevertheless, is dependent on others as to whether or not the food itself was free of pathogenic microorganisms when it was purchased from the shop. Numerous other examples are easy to think of which support the idea that complete independence in the AL of maintaining a safe environment is just impossible. Every individual is dependent on others — other ordinary individuals as well as people with special responsibilities for maintaining a safe environment who include, for example, politicians, town planners, public transport personnel, employers and manufacturers, firemen and police.

INDIVIDUALITY IN MAINTAINING A SAFE ENVIRONMENT

The purpose of the model is to describe how a particular person develops *individuality* in carrying out the Activities of Living. The following list is a résumé of the topics which have been discussed under the headings of the components of the model in relation to the AL of maintaining a safe environment.

Lifespan: effect on maintaining a safe environment
- Babies — need protection from accident, infection, excessive heat/cold

● Preschool children	— vulnerable to accidents in the home
● Schoolchildren	— vulnerable to accidents on the roads and in the playground
● Adolescents	— vulnerable to road, bicycle and sporting accidents
● Adults	— vulnerable to hazards in the work environment; vulnerable to road traffic accidents; responsibility for safety of children
● Elderly people	— vulnerable to falls in the home, hazards of infection and fire, pedestrian accidents

Factors influencing maintaining a safe environment

● Physical	— acuity of the senses
	— physical ability/disability
	— susceptibility to infection
	— state of physical health/ill-health
● Psychological	— intellectual ability/impairment
	— attitude to safety (home, work, play, travel)
	— personality and temperament
	— mood and motivation
	— level of stress and confidence
	— level of knowledge about safety precautions
	— responsiveness to safety legislation/health education
● Sociocultural	— cultural factors (e.g. concept of safety)
	— social factors (e.g. prevalence of infectious diseases)
	— social class (e.g. risk of accident)
● Environmental	— housing
	— standard of safety in the home
	— exposure to hazards in place of work
	— hazards in play settings
	— risk of accident on the roads
	— exposure to environmental pollution
	— climatic and geographical factors

- Politicoeconomic   — knowledge and attitude to safety legislation
  - — personal spending on safety measures
  - — political awareness/involvement (e.g. pollution, nuclear war)

Dependence/independence in maintaining a safe environment

- Dependence in infancy/childhood/old age
- Constraints on independence in adulthood (e.g. mental/physical/sensory handicap)
- Dependence on others
- Dependence on aids

Maintaining a safe environment: patients' problems and related nursing activities

Each day, throughout the day, although not always aware of it, people are engaged in carrying out numerous activities which have the specific purpose of maintaining a safe environment. As with all of the Activities of Living, there are many similarities in the way different people carry out this AL. However, as the preceding section shows, a variety of circumstances determine an individual's vulnerability to certain hazards in the environment, and result in individuality in the way necessary preventive activities are carried out. The concept of individuality provides the link between the model of living and the model for nursing.

Individualised nursing is based on knowledge of a patient's individuality. Therefore, in relation to the AL of maintaining a safe environment, the nurses need to know about the patient's individual habits and problems. While observing and discussing relevant topics with the patient (along the lines suggested in the résumé above), the nurse might bear in mind the following questions:

- what kind of activities does the individual usually engage in with the purpose of maintaining a safe environment?
- what factors influence the way in which the individual carries out the AL of maintaining a safe environment?

- what is the individual's level of knowledge regarding maintaining a safe environment?
- what is the individual's attitude to maintaining a safe environment?
- has the individual experienced any difficulties in the past with maintaining a safe environment and, if so, how have these been coped with?
- what problems, if any, does the individual have now (or seem likely to develop) with maintaining a safe environment?

The objective in collecting this sort of information is to discover the patient's usual routines; what can and cannot be done independently; what previous coping mechanisms have been employed; and what problems exist or may develop in relation to this AL. By its very nature it is likely that most will be potential problems (though there may be actual problems too), and, therefore, the goals set and nursing intervention decided upon will be mainly preventive in nature. Accordingly, evaluation will be undertaken to ascertain that the preventive measures implemented have been effective. The goal of individualised nursing for this AL will be achieved if assessing, planning, implementing and evaluating all take account of the patient's individuality in maintaining a safe environment.

That, in the most general of terms, describes how the nursing process method is applied. However, in different circumstances, nursing assessment of the AL of maintaining a safe environment would differ in approach, scope and content. For example, assessment by a health visitor of a mother's knowledge about maintaining a safe environment for her young child in the home would obviously be quite different from an occupational health nurse's assessment of an employee's risk of accident at work. Therefore, in different nursing contexts there will be different kinds of problems identified and, accordingly, different types of nursing activities will be implemented. Teaching is one type of nursing activity which is always relevant in relation to the AL of maintaining a safe environment. Exploiting opportunities for education of people of all ages and in various settings (home, school and workplace) is probably the main way in which nurses can contribute to the collective effort to prevent injury and ill-health which is caused by accident, fire, infection and pollution. These subjects were dealt with in detail in the first part of the chapter and, therefore, although they should be recognised as relevant to nursing in relation to the AL of maintaining a safe environment, they are not discussed further.

The remainder of the chapter deals with some circumstances in which nurses are directly involved with assisting patients who have problems in maintaining a safe environment. There are two sections. The first of these is concerned with patients in hospital. Florence Nightingale said 'the hospital shall do the patient no harm'. Yet in most countries there is continual concern about the number of patients who develop a hospital-acquired infection quite unrelated to the reason for their admission; about the accidents which happen to patients while they are in hospital; about the perennial danger of fire in hospitals; and about the dangers associated with the use of drugs in hospital. In a way this is not surprising when one considers the size and function of a hospital, and the fact that hospitals are busy places: 'busyness' increases stress and tension, and errors and accidents are more likely to occur in such an atmosphere. From the patient's point of view, admission to hospital involves a change of environment and routine and that, in itself, creates problems with the AL of maintaining a safe environment.

The second section, with which the chapter ends, may be relevant to the nursing of patients in hospital but is not confined to that context. It considers, in very broad terms, the variety of circumstances which can cause a change of dependence/independence status for the AL of maintaining a safe environment. This section, therefore, provides a direct link between the model of living and the model for nursing.

CHANGE OF ENVIRONMENT AND ROUTINE

Most human beings are conservative and dislike change, particularly enforced change as when a patient is admitted to hospital. Patients can feel insecure and frightened in this new environment and nervousness and anxiety increase the risk of accident. A patient in a nervous state is more likely to bang into, or trip over, objects; shaking or tense hands are more likely to drop things, spill things and so on. Some patients become disorientated, a more likely reaction if the patient is elderly or has already shown signs of mental confusion. Nurses can help all patients by talking with them, keeping in mind the objective of orientating them to the new environment and routine. The sooner this is done the better. Whatever the intended length of the patient's stay, patients report the highest anxiety levels during the first 24 hours (Wilson-Barnett, 1978).

Unfamiliar environment
Familiarity with an environment makes it less hazardous; for example people adjust spatially to avoid objects in their immediate vicinity. Just on admission, a patient has not had time to make any necessary spatial adjustments. This could well relate to the design of the hospital bed which may not be at the same height as the one with which the patient is familiar. For some patients more than others, it is important for the nurses to know that familiar height.

Where mechanically-operated height-adjustment beds are provided and the patient is capable with instruction, of operating the mechanism, he can maintain his independence in this respect. When the patient is not capable, then the nurse is responsible for operating the mechanism to maintain the patient's safety. Several surveys conducted in hospitals have shown that the majority of accidents occur at the bedside. The Scottish Hospital Advisory Service (1978) reported from observation visits to long-stay hospitals throughout Scotland that even when adjustable beds were provided, they were frequently found at a height too high for the patients' safety.

Patients may have to be nursed on a bed with a ripple mattress or an air bed. While providing greater safety from the pressure hazard, they can create spatial problems for the patient. The increased height relative to the bedside locker and bed table may require spatial adjustment. Over-reaching for an article on nearby furniture is a frequent cause of accidents. Patients can be helped by nurses who, before leaving the bedside, test whether or not the patient can comfortably reach articles on the locker.

Disabled and older patients who experience difficulty when rising from a chair will like most people, have their 'special' chair at home, out of which they can rise easily, and on which they may hang a walking stick to help with safe rising. These patients can experience many kinds of problems when in a different environment: such as increased stiffening due to lack of exercise because they find it so difficult to get out of the hospital chair; incontinence for the same reason. Shearing injury to the sacral tissues and the heels can be caused by patients sliding forward on vinyl-covered chairs. Nurses can help, within the constraints of the type of chairs provided, by 'matching' the chair to the patient, not just helping the patient to any chair.

Noisy environment
Unfamiliar noise is more disturbing than familiar noise. One study of noise in hospital (Bentley et al, 1977) used from among the several decibel scales the dB(A) one, because of its close relation to noise that damages human hearing. Measurements were taken in an open Florence Nightingale ward, a cubicle in a cul-de-sac of this ward, and a general intensive therapy unit (ITU). A profile based on pooled data of all observations is shown in Figure 7.2 which has to be studied in conjunction with the following information:

The International Proposal for Noise Abatement with Respect to Community Response suggests the following basic noise limits:

day time	45	dB(A)
evening	40	dB(A)
night	30	dB(A)

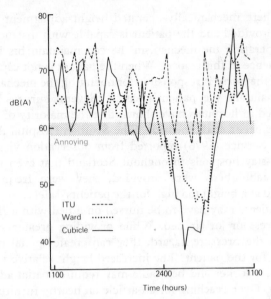

Fig. 7.2 Noise: profile based on pooled data (from Bentley et al 1977 Perceived noise in surgical wards and an intensive care area. British Medical Journal 2: 1503–1506)

Figure 7.3 shows that noise level in the Nightingale ward and in the cubicle during the night was above that in the usual bedroom. During the day the level in the ITU was above the 'annoying' level. There is evidence (Murphy et al, 1977) that nearly all patients who enter hospital for surgery soon accumulate a considerable sleep deficit which must be partly caused by the noisy environment. Equipment and conversations among staff were the main causes of noise and consequently the researchers wrote: 'We recommend that from time to time sound engineers should use the simple methods that we have used ... to show the staff how much they pollute the environment. Furthermore, the staff should be educated against noise pollution as part of good hospital procedure'.

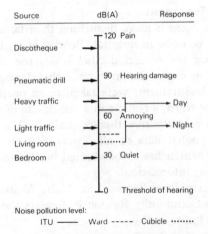

Fig. 7.3 Comparison of noise levels (from Bentley et al 1977 British Medical Journal 2: 1503–1506. Figures 7.2 and 7.3 reproduced by kind permission of the authors and editor of the British Medical Journal)

Nurses can help by modulating their voices when on duty, wearing shoes which do not cause excessive noise when walking; closing doors quietly, preventing them from banging; and handling equipment quietly.

Risk of accident

Some mention of accidents has already been made but further, more specific comment is relevant. If nurses are to attempt to prevent avoidable accidents to patients, then they need to be aware of what and where the hazards are; when accidents are most likely to occur; and which patients are most at risk. For patients who are identified from assessment as being at particular risk, relevant preventive activities should be included in the list of interventions written on the patient's nursing plan. Some of the nursing activities which might be relevant can be deduced from the following discussion, which is based on the reports of two studies of accidents in hospital.

The study reported by Moorat (1983) involved an analysis of accident reports from 1979 to 1981 in an English general hospital. The following information was collected: patient's age and gender; time and place of accident; activity being undertaken at the time; and type of accident and injury sustained. The questions asked and the main results of the study are summarised below:

- How many patients have accidents while in hospital, and is the number increasing?
  Over the 3 years in question, the number of accidents rose from 406 in 1979, representing 3.8% of patients, to 605 in 1981 (5.1%).
- Where in the ward do accidents most frequently occur?
  The findings were in keeping with what is known: that accidents most frequently occur at the bedside. Other main locations were the toilet, dayroom, shower/bathroom and corridor.
- What is the most dangerous time of the in-patient's day?
  Contrary to popular belief that night-time is most dangerous, results dispelled this. Early morning was shown to be the peak period, with most accidents taking place beween 0600 and 1100 hours. Afternoon was a relatively safe time, but a peak occurred in late evening (1900–2100 hours) when patients go to the toilet or commode and get into bed.
- During which activities are accidents most likely to happen?
  The two activities of using the toilet or commode and getting out of bed were responsible for 49% of all accidents. Other main activities related to accidents were getting up from a chair, walking unaided and getting into bed. It is interesting to note that getting out of bed is much more hazardous than getting in;

and that of beds in use in the hospital concerned, 65% were of adjustable height. (This finding appears to corroborate the observations of the SHAS report of 1978, mentioned on p. 99.)

- What kind of patients are particularly at risk?
Of all the accidents reported, 68% involved patients between the ages of 56 and 86 years. Patients over the age of 70 are particularly at risk (44% of accidents involved that age group). Female patients who had accidents were older than the male patients: those at risk being 76 years old or over.

While Moorat's study shows that older patients are especially prone to accidents in a general hospital, Morris et al (1981) concentrated exclusively on a geriatric hospital which is a setting in which falls are common. Adopting the same method, analysis of accident reports (for the year 1979), rather similar findings are reported: for example that the greatest risk of accidents was in the early morning and that, overall, people in the 75–84 years' age group are the most vulnerable. What is particularly interesting about this report is the discussion of findings. The authors stress that, although falls in geriatric hospitals are common, their consequences are seldom serious. They comment that 'a low fall rate in patient areas may merely reflect low patient activity and over protectiveness by the nursing staff.' They consider that routine completion of accident forms in the case of non-injurious accidents may promote anxiety and defensive practices in nurses. Bearing in mind that it is the active and independent patients who appeared to be most at risk to falls, the authors conclude: 'The prevention of all falls is not an appropriate objective of patient management in departments of geriatric medicine. Instead the primary aim should be the promotion of patient activity within acceptable limits of safety.' This does not, of course, imply that nurses should not be concerned with the prevention of unnecessary accidents. However, it is a very relevant consideration and one which ties up with a point made early on in this chapter, concerning the balance between protection and freedom in the context of preventing accidents in childhood.

Risk of fire

Fire is a lethal and perennial menace in hospitals ... It is the nursing staff more than any other category of employee who will bear the burden of the consequences of fire. It is the nurse who will have to decide on whether to evacuate or who to move, how and where. It is a heavy responsibility and the appropriate attitude and degree of awareness should be cultivated.

Dooley, 1981

The following facts presented put the problem in perspective:

- In 1976 in the U.K. there were approximately six hospital fires every day: a fire which involves casualties, rescues, escapes or evacuations occurs on average once every six days.
- The major sources of ignition are smokers' materials, malicious ignition and cooking appliances.
- Most fires occur in the ward area.

Fire precautions are the responsibility of all staff and Dooley advocates that staff training should cover: how to guard against fires; how to react in case of fire; how to raise the alarm; how to help evacuate patients; how to stop fires spreading; and how to help fight the fire. The charge nurse of a ward has a special responsibility to know precisely what action should be taken in the event of a fire; to be aware of any special risks, such as oxygen or cyclopropane cylinders; and to familiarise all new staff to the ward with the routine and the location of fire alarms, exits and fire-fighting equipment. Some patients, perhaps especially those who express anxiety about the risk of fire or who are known to have experienced a fire, may welcome being told about the fire precautions in the ward.

The fact that smoking represents the single greatest cause of fires in hospital is certainly knowledge which nurses should share with patients, as well as act upon themselves. Nurses must constantly be alert to the fire dangers inherent in smoking and should exercise vigilance at all times; enforce rules about where smoking is permitted; and ensure that cigarette ends are not left smouldering, especially at night.

Preventing fire was described in the first part of this chapter as an essential activity of maintaining a safe environment. If this is so in ordinary everyday living, then how much more so it is in the hospital environment. All the money, skill and effort expended on patients in hospital would be in vain if they are not adequately protected from the risk of fire.

Risk of infection

When patients come to hospital they are living in close contact with more people than usual. The human body is a reservoir of microorganisms as illustrated in Figure 7.4 and they are easily transferred to other things and people via the hands. A potential problem for the patient is the risk of infection because he is in contact with greater numbers of pathogenic microorganisms than he was at home. And this at a time when his resistance is likely to be lowered. A large number of organisms and lowered resistance are two of the necessary conditions for infection to become established.

It was to keep down the population of pathogenic microorganisms in hospital that 'damp dusting' of all laying surfaces used to be considered a nursing activity. Nowadays such activities have been designated 'non-nursing' duties, but nurses liaise with domestic management to achieve a safe environment for patients. Dust invariably contains pathogens which have settled out of the atmosphere.

RESERVOIR	MICROORGANISM	TRANSFERENCE TO HANDS
Nose	Staphylococci	Unprotected sneeze→droplets Protected sneeze→handkerchief Blowing nose→handkerchief Touching nose
Skin	Staphylococci Streptococci	Live and multiply in pores and hair follicles Shed with scales into clothing
Bowel	Salmonella — causing typhoid Bacillus — causing dysentery	From faeces
Mouth and throat	Staphylococci Streptococci	Unprotected sneeze, cough→droplets Protected sneeze, cough→handkerchief

Fig. 7.4 The human body as a reservoir of microorganisms

In ordinary breathing droplets are projected 150 to 180 cm; the distance is increased during talking, coughing and sneezing. There is therefore ample opportunity for all surfaces in a ward to be contaminated, particularly bedclothes, bedcurtains, floors and footwear as illustrated in Figure 7.5. It also shows the methods of spread of infection in hospital, an ever present patient's potential problem. Nurses must be constantly vigilant in every activity so that there is no break in infection control. This is especially necessary because the patient can come into contact with pathogens which have become resistant to one or more of the antibiotics.

From studying Figures 7.4 and 7.5 it will be seen that in hospital there are many potential danger points for contamination by direct contact, for example with infected articles or with hands which have been inadequately washed or not washed at all after dealing with contaminated discharges or materials.

Handwashing is undoubtedly the main activity in preventing the spread of infection. All hands are covered with microorganisms particularly between the fingers and under the nails. Even immediately after washing, a few colonies of pathogenic microorganisms can be cultured from them. These are mainly staphylococci, harmless in small numbers because the body's defence mechanisms can deal with them, but disastrous if large numbers are transferred to a patient. The bacteria causing typhoid, dysentery and other forms of gastroenteritis are excreted in faeces and they can only enter the body through the mouth, sometimes referred to as the 'faecal-oral' route of infection. It is therefore imperative that patients and staff practise the habit of adequate handwashing after visiting the toilet and before touching food.

Taylor (1978) provides a useful evaluation of handwashing techniques used by various grades of nurses (Fig. 7.6). She demonstrated that coverage of the skin while handwashing was often inadequate and indications for handwashing were often uncertain. She advocated that nurses should be taught the principles of aseptic and hygienic techniques based on good evidence rather than

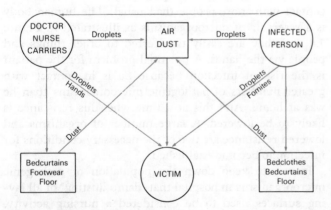

Fig. 7.5 Spread of infection in hospital

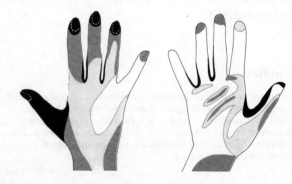

Fig. 7.6 Handwashing Palm (right) Back (left). Key: black = most frequently missed areas; brown and stippled = less missed areas (Taylor, 1978)

ritual procedures. Watson (1978) states that no amount of sterile supplies or antiseptic agents will protect the patient from an attendant with contaminated hands.

Should the patient have a wound, he can breathe staphylococci on to it, or transfer them from his nose to his wound via his hands. This potential problem is called auto-infection; if it is to be avoided, teaching the patient is an inescapable part of nursing.

The patient may have little idea of pathogens and none whatever of asepsis. He may think that the purpose of the dressing and bandage on his wound is 'to keep it clean'. So when the bandage slips and the wound is in contact with the sheet, he might think that it is all right, because the sheet is 'clean'. Purposeful conversation is essential to discover the patient's idea about so many things that nurses take for granted.

The patient may have an infectious condition when admitted and naturally will be anxious about infecting others. Barrier nursing and isolation will help the patient to feel some security that precautions are being taken. However, as Barnett (1983) describes, isolation can have profound emotional effects on the patient: such as disorientation, anxiety, feelings of undesirability and distress due to separation from family. Therefore, it is important for nurses to be aware of the problems of isolation as experienced by the patient, and to attempt to alleviate them. It is essential that the patient is told why he is being isolated and the reason for the various precautions should be explained. Information is needed too about the part the patient is expected to play in preventing the spread of infection. Again, patient teaching is a vital nursing activity.

Just as co-operation between nurse and patient is absolutely essential for infection in hospital to be effectively controlled, so too is co-operation among all members of the multidisciplinary health care team. Henderson (1981) expresses this need in the slogan 'Team up to control infection' and says: 'One profession cannot successfully isolate and combat infection. Only by the co-operation and commitment of all hospital personnel can any infection control programme be really successful; therefore a multidisciplinary approach is logical and must be actively encouraged.' She goes on to discuss the role of the infection control nurse in the multidisciplinary team and concludes: 'Infection control may be only one element in the total care of the patient, but it is a vital one in that it promotes improvement in standards of care and safety.'

There is no disputing how vital this aspect of patient care is when one considers the prevalence of hospital-acquired infection (HAI). In 1980 a large-scale survey, the first for some 120 years, was conducted in England and Wales to ascertain the extent of the problem. An article written by the doctor who masterminded the study (Meers, 1981) provides an account of the method and main findings. A total of 18 163 patients were surveyed in 43 hospitals. From the data obtained, it is now clear that at any one time more than 10 000 patients in the acute hospitals of England and Wales are suffering from hospital-acquired infection (nosocomial). Overall, 19.1% of patients were judged to be infected at the time of the survey. This total was made up of 9.9% community-acquired infections and 9.2% hospital-acquired infections (i.e. previously infection-free patients who contract infection as a direct result of hospitalisation). Respiratory tract infection was the most prevalent type, accounting for 29.3% of the total, but this mainly came into hospital with patients (i.e. community-acquired infection). The most common hospital-acquired infection was that of the urinary tract (which is partly preventable), with respiratory tract second, and surgical wound infection just behind in third place. These results are shown in Figure 7.7.

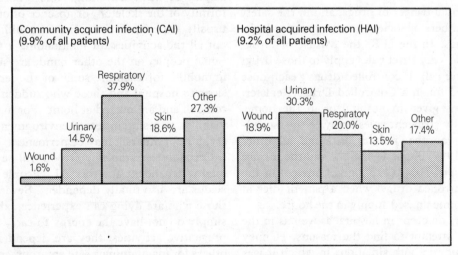

Fig. 7.7 Infection among patients in hospital (Meers, 1981) The prevalence of infection among patients in hospital divided according to the major types of infection concerned, according to a survey of 18 163 patients in 43 hospitals in England and Wales, 1980 (Reproduced from The Times Health Supplement with permission.)

Meers concludes:

A survey is worthless if its results are not put to good use. The information derived in the present one will, it is hoped, justify the allocation of resources to hospital infection control, help locate areas where there is waste, allow rational decisions to be made on priorities, and act as a baseline for further study of the components of and means to be used for preventing HAI. Perhaps its most significant use will be in education. If those who currently suppress the thought of infection in their wards can be made to recognise its presence and realise its importance, a first step will have been taken to control it. There is no hope of progress so long as the existence of infection is denied.

Readers are referred to the text on hospital-acquired infection, which is noted in the additional reading list at the end of the chapter, for further study of this important subject.

Risks associated with medications

At home many patients have a personal medication routine like taking medications orally; inhaling them from a nasal spray; applying them to the skin; putting them in the form of drops or ointment into the eye; injecting them from a syringe; inserting them in the form of a suppository into the rectum or in the form of a pessary into the vagina. Patients are responsible in their own home for maintaining safety in relation to these medications.

It is customary in many hospitals for patients to forfeit this responsibility and to become dependent on medical, nursing and pharmaceutical staff. It is imperative in the interests of patient safety that nurses accept the responsibility of giving to the right patient, the right medication, in the right dose, by the right route, at the right time. Ramsay & Ballinger (1977) report a research study that investigated the problem of identifying psychogeriatric patients; with early ambulation the majority of patients are up in a chair for some part of the day. A suggested safety precaution is to have a photo of the patient on the drug record card.

Due to the potential danger of drugs, and in the safety interests of all members of society, most countries legislate to control drugs. In the U.K. the Misuse of Drugs Act 1971 is in force. Very strict rules apply to those drugs which in the Act are called 'controlled drugs'; each dose has to be accounted for in a Controlled Drugs Register, whether the drug is given in hospital or in the home. Different but equally stringent rules apply to the 'scheduled drugs', those on the 'poisons list' and all other 'drugs'. Hopkins (1977) discusses the law and the misuse of drugs; the *Nursing Times* (1977) gives advice on the destruction of 'controlled drugs' when a patient dies at home and there is some unused supply in the house.

Medication errors do occur in hospital as well as in the community. In an attempt to find the reasons, Henney (1976) reports a study in both situations in which it was found that there are two components of error in the community; non-comprehension and non-compliance. Non-comprehension meant that the patients did not understand the regime and in the case of non-compliance they understood but did not follow the instruction. Nurses can help patients with these problems. Teaching patients in hospital can be accomplished by letting them have, say, their six medicines in a tray at each medicine round. Under supervision they can select the ones that have to be taken at that particular time. In this way patients can gain confidence that they will be able to cope when they go home.

CHANGE OF DEPENDENCE/INDEPENDENCE STATUS

The dependence/independence continuum in the model of living serves as a reminder that all people experience change of dependence/independence status for the Activities of Living in the normal course of the lifespan. In the context of nursing, the concept of dependence/independence is an important one. According to the circumstances, nurses either help patients to cope with enforced dependence (short- or long-term), or help them to regain the level of independence to which they were accustomed prior to the episode of ill-health. There are many different reasons why people can experience difficulty in achieving or maintaining independence for the AL of maintaining a safe environment and, therefore, may require assistance from nurses or others. The main reasons are briefly described under the following headings: physical problems; mental problems; problems due to sensory impairment/loss.

Physical problems

Physical mobility is essential for the many activities aimed at maintaining safety, whether at home, at work, at play or while travelling. Those born with severe deformity of the skeleton, or absence of one or more limbs, usually experience some life-long difficulty in carrying out all the activities for maintaining a safe environment. Some people, on the other hand, are suddenly rendered immobile, for example some of the 'emergency' admissions to hospital and those who suddenly collapse or become ill and are nursed at home. For many of them, their inability to maintain a safe environment is only temporary, but for others it may be permanent.

Certainly, a tetraplegic person will be permanently and totally dependent for this AL. People who are unconscious are also totally dependent. Severely ill people and those who are dying can experience exhaustion and they simply do not have the energy to carry out the necessary preventive activities; they are dependent on nurses and others for maintaining a safe environment.

Even apparently minor problems, such as any enclosure of the hands or restriction of finger mobility, can render a person less independent for this AL. If there is any restriction on movement, however slight, of the spine, hips and lower limbs, the person may be unable to get out of the way of a dangerous moving object with sufficient speed to prevent mishap. Those who are bedfast or chairfast are similarly unable to take avoiding action. Patients with broken bones can be additionally restricted by traction apparatus and they forfeit much of their independence for this AL.

Physical imbalance of any kind can interfere with independence too, for example affecting the patient who has had a limb amputated. Recent anaesthesia and certain medications can cause patients to feel unsteady on their feet. People who take sleeping pills can also be at risk of falling, especially if they rise to void in the night, and the 'hang-over' feeling in the morning can create a safety risk.

Most of the physical problems, therefore, are primarily mobilising problems. These are discussed in detail in Chapter 14 but for each patient, the nurse needs to assess what that particular mobilising problem means in relation to the AL of maintaining a safe environment. She can then identify actual and potential problems and include in the patient's nursing plan whatever precautions are necessary, for example to prevent accidents.

Mental problems

As well as those born mentally handicapped, there are people whose intellect is impaired as a result of infection in, or injury to the brain. They may not recognise when they are in danger, for example when crossing a busy road, or they may not know how to carry out even the most basic safety precautions necessary for the prevention of fire, accidents and infection. In a hospital for the mentally handicapped much of the nurse's time is devoted to maintaining a safe environment for the patients and also to helping them to understand and to put into practice essential safety measures.

Several of the mental illnesses result in a diminished awareness, so that the sufferers are not able to be completely responsible for carrying out the activities to achieve a safe environment. The mental illness of depression can result in suicidal thoughts and there may or may not be expression of intent. Such people need help in maintaining their environment in a condition which is safe for them until their mood improves.

If this cannot be assured, then the person may require admission to a psychiatric hospital. One important role of such hospitals, is that they provide a safe environment for mentally disturbed people, at the same time in severe cases, protecting members of the community from possible harm as a result of violence to persons or property. Nurses are concerned with the AL of maintaining a safe environment in relation to individual patients but, at the same time, must bear in mind the safety of others. The

fact that this AL has a collective dimension in addition to the personal one was mentioned in the early part of this chapter.

Problems due to sensory impairment/loss

All five senses are used in activities carried out with the purpose of maintaining a safe environment and, therefore, impairment or loss of any one can result in problems. Some of the problems can occur so gradually, for example the onset of deafness, that the person adjusts gradually and so is able to maintain his independence for this AL. Sudden impairment or loss, however, is likely to cause dependence, at least temporarily.

Visual impairment/loss
It is unusual for a person to lose the sight in both eyes at the same time, but loss of sight in one can be followed later by loss of sight in the second eye. A student can get some idea about what it means to try to maintain safety using one eye by blindfolding one eye and walking round the classroom noting the several changed perspectives. Similarly she can blindfold both eyes. She will then be more able to establish empathy with patients who have visual problems; she will have some idea about what they might find helpful, and what is required for independence to be maintained or regained.

Aural impairment/loss
Again it is unusual for a person suddenly to become deaf in both ears, but something like a loud nearby explosion can cause sudden deafness in one ear. A student can get some idea of what it means, in terms of maintaining a safe environment, to be deaf in one, then in both ears by

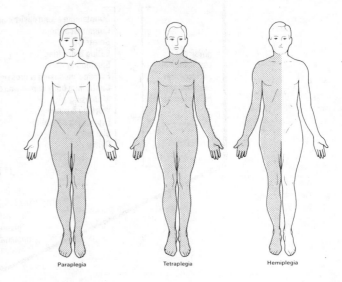

Paraplegia   Tetraplegia   Hemiplegia

Fig. 7.8 Sensory loss in types of paralysis

using earplugs. She can ponder on such questions as: What are the implications for safety if a person does not hear the whistle of the boiling kettle or the sound of a pot of food boiling over or the noise of approaching traffic?

Sensory impairment/loss

The patient with sensory loss has a problem in that he cannot feel heat, cold, pain and pressure. To help anyone who has sensory loss a nurse should try to imagine maintaining a safe environment with no awareness of heat, cold, pain and pressure. Sensory loss sometimes occurs in large areas like the lower limbs and lower trunk; in all four limbs and the whole trunk; in the arm and leg on the same side of the body. Sensory loss frequently occurs with motor loss; the patient is paralysed and it compounds the problem of maintaining a safe environment. The different types of paralysis are illustrated in Figure 7.8.

Smelling and tasting impairment/loss

When cooking, many people check the contents of bottles, packages and the like by smelling or tasting them. When a person is deprived of these sensations he cannot use them as checks when maintaining a safe environment. Nurses can help these patients by first observing tactfully whether or not they can read and write. If so, they can be advised to pay special attention to labelling containers

and paper bags as to their contents. People who cannot read and write could be advised to use a signing system, and could be encouraged to use any available adult literacy programme.

As has been implied from the comments made, the nurse's ability to identify patients' problems with the AL of maintaining a safe environment which result from impairment/loss of the senses, to a great extent depends on her ability to be imaginative and empathetic. Once aware of what the problems are, the nurse can help the patient to develop alternative ways of detecting and responding to hazards in the environment, thereby maintaining maximum independence for this AL.

In the second half of this chapter some of the problems and discomforts which can be experienced by patients in relation to the AL of maintaining a safe environment have been described. This provides the beginning nurse with a generalised idea of these; it will be useful in assessing, planning, implementing and evaluating an individualised programme for each patient's AL of maintaining a safe environment.

This chapter has been concerned with the AL of maintaining a safe environment. However, as stated previously it is only for the purpose of discussion that any AL can

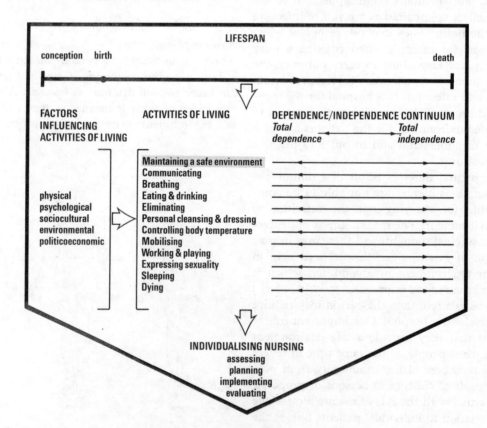

Fig. 7.9 The AL of maintaining a safe environment within the model for nursing

be considered on its own; in reality the various activities are so closely related and do not have distinct boundaries. Figure 7.9 is a reminder that the AL of maintaining a safe environment is related to the other ALs and also to the various components of the model for nursing.

REFERENCES

Arnold A 1978 Poliomyelitis — a present threat. Nursing Mirror 146 (20) May 18: 16–17

Barnett R 1983 Isolated but not alone. In: Infection control in hospital and the community. Supplement to Nursing 20 December: 7

Bentley S, Murphy F, Dudley H 1977 Perceived noise in surgical wards and an intensive care area: an objective analysis. British Medical Journal 2: 1503–1506

Clarke L 1982 Health and safety in NHS premises. Nursing Times 78 (8) February 24: 313–314

Community Outlook 1982 Children and accidents at home. Nursing Times 78 (32) August 11: 212–223

Dooley T P 1981 Fire! The nursing response. Nursing Times 77 (43) October 21: 1845–1848

Finch J 1983a Radiation hazards. Nursing Mirror 156 (23) June 8: 39

Finch J 1983b Employee's obligations (in maintaining a safe and healthy work environment). Nursing Mirror 156 (26) June 29: 21

Galbraith N S 1983 Contact tracing in the control of infectious disease. Nursing Times 79 (23) June 8: 55–56

Graham T, Lee W 1981 The nurse's role in the prevention of food poisoning. 1. Eat, drink and be healthy. Nursing Mirror 152 (13) March 26: 39–40 2. Now wash your hands please. 152 (14) April 2: 31–34

Healy M A, Aslam M 1981 The lead sandwich syndrome. Nursing Times 77 (37) September 9: 1598–1600

Henderson M 1981 Team up to control infection. Nursing Times 77 (12) March 19: 510–512

Henney C 1976 Drug administration. Nursing Mirror 142 (14) April 1: 52–54

Hicks C 1983 Preparing for the unthinkable. (Nursing implications of planning for nuclear war.) Nursing Times 79 (44) November 2: 8–10

Hopkins S J 1977 The law and the misuse of drugs. Nursing Mirror 144 (20) May 19: 25–26

Maddocks G 1981 Accidents in childhood: Growing to independence. Nursing Mirror, Clinical Forum 5, 152 (21) May 20: viii–xiv

Meers P 1981 A dangerous place to be ill. (Risk of infection in hospital.) The Times Health Supplement November 13: 18

Miller D, Rose E 1981 Whooping cough vaccine in perspective. Nursing Times 77 (22) May 28: 937–939

Mitchell R G 1984 Falls in the elderly. Nursing Times 80 (2) January 11: 51–53

Moorat D 1983 Accidents to patients. Nursing Times 79 (20) May 18: 59–61

Morris E V, Isaacs B, Brislen W 1981 Falls in the elderly in hospital. Nursing Times 77 (35) August 26: 1522–1524

Murphy F, Bentley S, Dudley H A 1977 Sleep deprivation in patients undergoing operation; a factor in the stress of surgery. British Medical Journal 2: 1521–1522

Nursing Times 1977 Advice on destruction of controlled drugs. Nursing Times 73 (34) August 25: 1300

Office of Health Economics 1981 Accidents in childhood. Office of Health Economics, Briefing No. 17 (September) London

Pinchen C 1982 Whooping cough. 1. Swings and roundabouts 2. Why not? Nursing Mirror, Clinical Forum 12, 155 (23) December 8: 24–28, 29–31

Ramsay A C, Ballinger B R 1977 Drug distribution and identifying psychogeriatric patients. Nursing Mirror 145 (1) July 7: 21

Sadler C 1983 Healing the hordes. (How occupational health nurses manage accidents in large crowds.) Nursing Mirror 79 (20) May 18: 17–20

Scottish Hospital Advisory Service 1978 New facilities: old practices. Health Bulletin 36 July 4: 152

Smith T 1981 Cause of death: attitude of mind. (Epidemiological perspective on road accidents.) The Times Health Supplement December 11: 12–13

Swan P 1983 Cholera: A visitation on Victorian society. Nursing Mirror 157 (15) October 12: 30–34

Taylor L J 1978 An evaluation of hand washing techniques 1 and 2. Nursing Times 74 (2) January 12: 54–55; 74 (3) January 19: 108–110

Watson K 1978 Medical microbiology. Nursing Mirror 146 (5) January 2: 32–33

Wild D 1983 Old people: Falls in homes. Nursing Times Community Outlook 79 (44) November 9: 320

Wild D, Nayak U S L, Isaacs B 1981 Prognosis of falls in old people at home. Journal of Epidemiology and Community Health 35: 200–204

Wilson-Barnett 1978 Factors influencing patients' emotional reaction to hospitalisation. Journal of Advanced Nursing 3 May: 221–229

Vella E 1981 Rabies: The British point of view. Nursing Times 77 (37) September 9: 1584–1586

ADDITIONAL READING

Ayliffe G A J, Collins B J, Taylor L J 1982 Hospital-acquired infection: principles and prevention. Wright, Bristol

8

Communicating

The activity of communicating

Man is essentially a social being and spends the major part of each day communicating with other people in one way or another. The activity of communicating is therefore an integral part of all human behaviour.

There is now considerable knowledge from research in the behavioural sciences about body or non-verbal language, use of which can enrich the AL of communicating. And even in the more familiar mode of verbal language, research has uncovered some interesting and illuminating aspects.

An understanding of the complexities of both components of communicating is likely to help people to carry out this AL in a manner which is effective and brings satisfaction to themselves and others. But what does 'communicating' mean?

THE NATURE OF COMMUNICATING

Most written languages have an alphabet, and in English everyone is familiar with the 26 letters from which many thousands of words can be constructed, each having a dictionary definition to help the process of communicating. Words however are only symbols and they can have different meanings for different people. Even in the English-speaking countries of the U.K. and North America there are differences as the following pairs of words show: nappies, diapers; lift, elevator; pavement, sidewalk; the bonnet of a car, the hood of a car. So there are occasions when it is important to check the meaning attached to a particular word. Words can also have different meaning according to the context in which they are used. Think of the word 'game' associated with a sports stadium and a butcher's shop; the word 'eye' related to biology and to embroidery.

The arrangement of words can affect meaning. 'Blanket this on child the put' has no meaning. Yet if these six words are rearranged to read 'Put the child on this blanket', the sentence has meaning. However, if they are rearranged to read 'Put the blanket on this child' the sentence has a different meaning. Choice of words and their arrangement in sentences to convey exact meaning are therefore vital in the activity of communicating.

Some words such as 'older' and 'younger', express relativity; to make them meaningful, further information is needed such as 'older than x'. Words can be emotionally neutral and factual like 'black man' and 'illegitimate', whereas others — 'nigger' and 'bastard' — not only indicate a fact but suggest a derisive attitude. Yet other words denote a value judgement assigned by the user — large, medium, small; good and bad being examples. Consequently, especially when recording and reporting information, the need to use neutral, factual words is necessary.

The use of language involves a number of skills, mainly speaking and listening; reading and writing. When *speaking*, it is not only what is said but equally important how it is said. With practice, the clarity, speed, pitch, inflection and tone of voice can all be used to convey exact meaning. In response to a request, the answer 'I don't mind doing it' can be said in a pleasant positive manner, assuring the listener that the task will be done willingly. On the other hand it can be said in a grudging negative manner leaving the listener uncomfortable and possibly guilty at having made the request.

Listening is much more than hearing; it is an active process whereby the listener attends exclusively to the speaker, not only to the words that he is speaking. There are advantages to listening in a face-to-face conversation which communication links such as the telephone and tape recorders do not offer although being in the presence of the speaker is not an absolute prerequisite for 'good listening'. For instance a telephone listening service is offered to people in distress by such associations as the Samaritans and Befrienders. The listeners are trained to hear and interpret silences, sighs, sobs and so on.

Reading is a skill which many people take for granted. Yet even in developed countries there is concern about the extent of illiteracy among adults, and special classes are offered to cope with this problem. Many readers are hindered by inaudibly 'pronouncing' each word rather than scanning a group of words to get the meaning of a sentence. Rapid reading classes are sometimes available and can be helpful in correcting this deficiency.

Again, the skill of *writing* is often taken for granted, yet there are adults who are handicapped because they cannot write their name. Adult literacy campaigns aim to improve writing as well as reading. But even so-called educated people can have difficulty in writing fluently, especially when under stress as for example in an examination setting.

Individuality, and many of the complexities of human beings are reflected in their speaking, listening, reading and writing, so it is useful to consider the total process of communicating.

The process of communicating

The study of cybernetics has contributed considerable information about the process of communicating. Basically communication is said to occur when a person (the sender) has a message which he sends in a particular medium, so that it is received by a recipient in whom it produces a response, followed by feedback to the sender (Fig. 8.1). This seems a simple process.

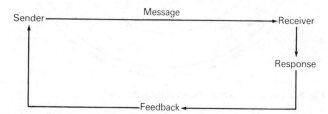

Fig. 8.1 Basic model of communicating

Further thought reveals however that it is not so simple, and that there are several stages, at any one of which error can occur which breaks a link in the chain of communication (Fig. 8.2). At the beginning of a conversation, one person has an idea which he encodes in language

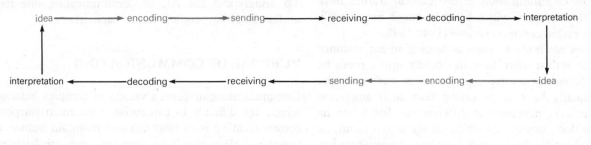

Fig. 8.2 Stages in the two-way process of communicating

symbols and then sends by speaking. The other person (the receiver) hears them, decodes and interprets by attaching meaning to them (interpretation). 'Foreign' words can be heard but meaning cannot be attached to them; they cannot be interpreted. In response to interpretation the sequence is repeated in reverse and so on.

The complexity of the AL of communicating can already be appreciated. Effective communication, of course, is dependent on the communicators' several abilities within the verbal language component, notably those of thinking, speaking, listening, reading and writing (Fig. 8.3). However the necessary skills within the body language component are also of enormous importance.

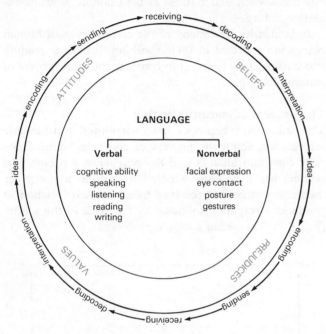

Fig. 8.3 The complexities of communicating

The study of non-verbal communication or body language is now receiving much more attention and the term 'kine' has been adopted for each 'unit' of body movement which transmits a message. The kine is analogous to a letter in the verbal alphabet. Kinetics is still a young science but it would seem that human ability to exert conscious control over body language is less easy than with verbal communication indeed clinical studies have revealed the extent to which body language can actually contradict verbal communications (Fast, 1978).

Man uses his body to express himself in for instance the way he walks; when he walks boldly into a room he may be declaring his feeling that all is well with the world. Equally he may be saying that he is angry, so further cues are necessary to differentiate. But when he opens the door slowly and walks slowly into a room, he may be indicating that he is feeling low or apprehensive. The stance that people take, too, can transmit feelings of boredom, exhaustion, high or low mood and so on.

The effectiveness of facial expression is recognised in such colloquial expressions as 'A look enough to kill' or 'A sour look'. One can transmit feelings such as disapproval, disgust, anger, irritation, pleasure, love and understanding by facial gesture. The eyes reveal mood and they can for instance, by staring, be used to express incredulity. People vary in the amount of eye contact which they make and maintain when communicating. The lecturer who constantly stares out of the window is unlikely to convey to the students much personal interest in them.

While communicating verbally most people move their hands in a manner which they hope will augment what they are saying. But the finger tapper, sitting silently, may be saying 'I am nervous and afraid.' The feet are also used in communication. Some people when sitting with crossed knees have a habit of swinging one leg. At one time it probably was a tension-releaser but may have become habitual. Toe-tapping is more likely to be expressing a current anxious mood.

In the main, the clothes people wear express current mood, state of finance, intent to go to work, preparation to take part in sport and so on. Indeed the term 'language of clothes' is now fairly commonly used and is discussed in more detail in Chapter 12, Personal Cleansing and Dressing.

Most people, at times, are aware of sending contradictory messages. For example, in response to a ring of the door bell the words 'Do come in, I'm pleased to see you' might be spoken while the facial expression might say 'I'm busy, I wish you hadn't called.' People by being frank and honest with themselves can achieve greater congruence of the messages transmitted in these two languages — verbal and non-verbal.

Communicating is a highly individual activity. The communicator brings to the conversation his attitudes, beliefs, values and prejudices, these being fashioned by previous experience which must necessarily be affected by social background. The contribution of each person is affected by their current needs: the need to be dominant or submissive; the need to be talkative or silent and so on. Yet in discussing communicating, it is not the individual that is crucial; it is the interpersonal relationship. To understand the AL of communicating one has to understand how people relate to each other.

PURPOSE OF COMMUNICATING

Communicating involves a variety of complex behaviours which are difficult to categorise. One main purpose of communicating is to establish and maintain human relationships. Most people imagine that they are fairly competent communicators; adults have been doing it all their lives! In fact, it is all too easy to conclude that if one's message is misunderstood, the receiver is at fault; and if the other person's attempt to communicate is not understood, then the other person's mode of expression is deficient in some way. The individual's interpretation of a situation is based on personal beliefs about communication competence — one's own and the other person's — and these beliefs affect how the individual relates to others, and how others relate to the individual. A lot depends on how individuals view themselves. This self-perception is said to start at birth as the infant begins to develop a feeling of trust, and this has already been mentioned in Chapter 4. With a feeling of trust comes, among other things, the ability to recognise personal strengths and weaknesses, the development of self-respect and faith in oneself, the development of respect and concern for others; all of which are essential for the establishment and maintenance of human relationships, and are basic to the AL of communicating.

The simplest form of communication is dyadic, the individual with one other person such as a parent, a marriage partner, a friend, a colleague, but there are extensions of the dyad in the form of small group communication, as indeed happens even with children when they go to school and find opportunities for communicating with different children and adults, beyond the home setting. Eventually adults become members of more and more dyadic, small and large group communication systems. A term often applied to a large group system is an organisation and these are usually created to accomplish a specific purpose, for example a hospital is organised for the treatment of people with disease; and is perhaps within a yet larger organisation, a national health service, which in addition is responsible for maintenance of health, prevention of disease and rehabilitation.

In an organisation such as a hospital, communicating is a means to an end but in some organisations it is an end in itself. For example in schools and colleges and universities, the purpose is communication in a teaching/learning context. The mass media too are concerned essentially with communicating, usually *giving* information although it may also involve *exchange* in the form of readers' letters to a newspaper or phone-in programmes on radio. Of course the mass media are not concerned only with information giving/exchange; they also communicate in order to entertain. And this is true of the theatre, art and music. Music in fact is a universal language of a non-verbal nature which is rich in expression. It can be played, listened to, read and written throughout the world, irrespective of mother tongue and usually brings great satisfaction to sender and receiver.

Whether an end in itself, or a means to an end, communicating in some form or other permeates every aspect of living — maintaining a safe environment, eating and drinking, dressing, working and playing, expressing sexuality and so on. There are a few individuals such as hermits or members of closed religious orders who choose to reduce their opportunities for communication and human interaction to a minimum (and they may find satisfaction in communing with nature, or with a deity) but for most people communicating with fellow humans is essential to living, to survival and to the quality of life.

BODY STRUCTURE AND FUNCTION REQUIRED FOR COMMUNICATING

Already it must be apparent that many physical and physiological activities combine to permit interpersonal communication. The central nervous system is the main co-ordinator of the body functions and will be outlined briefly in this chapter along with the structure and function of the larynx, eye and ear. However we have chosen to include in this section the endocrine system because it also is an integrating system, indeed the production of most hormones is directly or indirectly under the control of the nervous system. Moreover, there is growing evidence that peptides (small molecules made up of just a few of the amino acid sub-units of proteins) now appear to be both neurotransmitters and hormones. Perhaps this is not surprising because morphological studies have shown that most peptide-secreting cells are derived from the neuroectoderm tissue of the embryo (Whitehead 1981). Other sensory organs as well as the musculo-skeletal system, especially the muscles of respiration, are necessary structures for effective communicating but they are described briefly elsewhere in the book.

Probably the most obvious structures associated with communicating are the larynx, the eye and the ear.

The larynx

The larynx contains the vocal cords which are necessary for speaking. The cords are two thickened folds of mucous membrane, and when resting, lie on either side of the tube-like larynx (Fig. 8.4A) which joins the pharynx above to the trachea below. Air on its way to and from the lungs passes through the larynx. For voice production the cords have to be drawn nearer to the centre as illustrated in Figure 8.4B, so that they can be vibrated by the passing air. Taut cords produce a high pitched

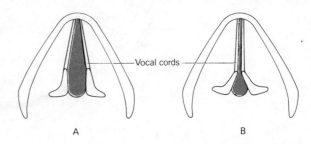

Fig. 8.4 Position of the vocal cords A. when resting B. when speaking

sound and slack ones a sound of low pitch. Length of the cords also affects pitch, longer ones giving a lower pitch and shorter ones a higher pitch. The laryngeal muscles are used in conjunction with the facial and intercostal muscles, together with the diaphragm in the complicated activity of voice production.

The eye

The eye, by receiving visual stimuli, enables observation of body language, and is needed for the reading and writing components of communicating. Furthermore the eyes, eyebrows and eyelids are part of facial expression and are thus transmitters of body language.

Visual stimuli are in the form of reflected light rays travelling from near and distant objects; those from near ones are still divergent as they approach the eyes, whereas those from distant objects are almost parallel. For clear vision all these rays must focus on a particular spot at the back of the eye and this is achieved by the lens. The stimuli are then transmitted by the optic nerve to the occipital lobe of the cerebrum for interpretation.

The shutter mechanism controlling the number of light rays entering the eye is called the iris; it is visible as the coloured part, which is incomplete centrally; the hole so formed is the pupil. When the radial muscle fibres in the iris contract the pupil enlarges to admit more rays (Fig. 8.5A) and when the circular fibres contract, the pupil decreases in size to minimise reception of rays (Fig. 8.5B).

The two spherical eyes are each contained within a bony conical socket called the orbital cavity. To maintain

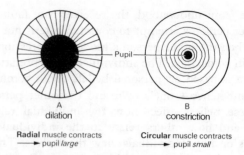

Fig. 8.5 Pupil of the eye. A. dilated B. constricted

their position they rest on a pad of connective tissue which also acts as a store for fat, depletion of which gives a 'sunken' appearance to the eyes. There are two oblique muscles and also four strap-like muscles, each having an anterior attachment to the eyeball, one above, one below and one on either side; and a posterior attachment to the conical socket. They permit the upward, downward and lateral movements of the eye. Any imbalance in these muscles is evident in what is commonly known as a squint or strabismus.

The tear gland. Also called the lacrimal gland it is tucked into the outer upper orbital cavity. The secretion, tears, contains an enzyme, lysozyme, which is bacteriolytic (capable of destroying bacteria); blinking spreads tears over the eyeball thus keeping it moist and protected from infection. Excess tears drain into the nose or spill over on the cheek.

The three coats of the eye. These are illustrated in Figure 8.6. Five-sixths of the outer coat is called the

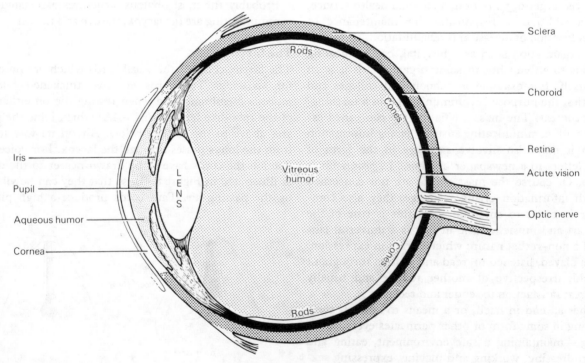

Fig. 8.6 The structures of the eye

sclera, visible as the white of the eye; the anterior one-sixth is named the cornea (window) because it is a transparent structure. It is also highly sensitive and an approaching irritant immediately produces the blinking reflex for automatic protection by the eyelids. The middle coat follows a similar structural pattern. The posterior five-sixths is called the choroid; it is pigmented and absorbs the light rays being likened to the black paint on the inside of a camera; the iris (and the pupil) form the anterior one-sixth. The inside coat, the retina, is only present posteriorly; it is composed of the sensory nerve endings (rods and cones) of the optic nerve. The rods require vitamin A for functioning in dim light, and the cones are active in bright light.

Figure 8.6 not only illustrates the three coats of the eyeball but also shows the other refracting media, that is the aqueous humor and the vitreous humor which as well as the lens play their part in convergence of light rays on the spot of most acute vision on the retina.

The eyebrows are thickened portions of skin and subcutaneous tissue which overlie the orbital ridge of the frontal bone; the hairs are arranged in a characteristic shape for human beings, but also it is individual for each person. Movement of the eyebrows is an important part of facial expression.

The eyelids are two loose folds of skin, which when their free edges are in apposition, cover and protect the anterior eyeball. The conjunctiva, a mucous membrane which covers the cornea and the anterior portion of the sclera is reflected to line the inner surface of both upper and lower eyelids. At the junction of the mucous membrane and the skin are the special hairs, eyelashes. The eyelids, consciously or unconsciously, are transmitters of body language.

Visual perception. Also basic to the activity of communicating is visual perception which involves interpretation of what is seen. It is impossible however, at any one time for a person to perceive all the visual stimuli coming from the environment. The person's attitudes, values, beliefs and prejudices determine what is perceived as 'foreground' and what is relegated to the 'background'. This complicated process of selectivity is highly individual as can be shown by asking people to make a list of the objects observed in a particular room. Similarly if each person were asked to make a list of the things which he observed about other people in the room, the lists would be different and would manifest the selectivity of the observer, fashioned by his previous experience.

The ear

The ear receives aural stimuli and permits the hearing and listening components of communicating. The aural stimuli are in the form of sound waves which pass along the outer canal to vibrate the tympanic membrane (ear drum) which is stretched across the end of the canal (Fig. 8.7). The stimulus is then transmitted via three small bones reaching across an air-containing cavity; the first one is attached to the ear drum and the third one to a membrane covering what is called the oval window. Vibration of this window disturbs the fluid on the other side in the cochlea, and this stimulus is transmitted by the auditory nerve fibres to the temporal lobe of the cerebrum where it is interpreted as sound.

The external ear. The ear lobe and an S-shaped canal form the external ear. Very few human beings can move the ear lobe by voluntary contraction of the muscles, so that it no longer fulfils the function of being a mobile catchment cup for sound waves as it does in animals. The skin of the canal has hairs and contains special glands which secrete wax both of which prevent the entry of dust and foreign bodies such as insects. Wax contains protective substances, various bacteriolytic enzymes, and

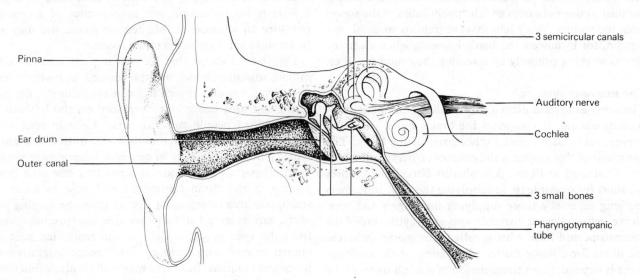

Pinna

Ear drum

Outer canal

3 semicircular canals

Auditory nerve

Cochlea

3 small bones

Pharyngotympanic tube

Fig. 8.7 The structures of the ear

some immunoglobulins which act locally to prevent allergy. The tympanic membrane separates the external ear from the middle ear.

The middle ear is an air-containing cavity bounded on one side by the tympanic membrane and on the other by the oval window with three tiny bones stretching across as mentioned. In order to maintain equal pressure on either side of the tympanic membrane, a pharyngotympanic tube connects the middle ear cavity with that of the pharynx so that any necessary air can pass along during the act of swallowing. Posteriorly the middle ear cavity connects with the mastoid cells and all these structures are lined with mucous membrane continuous with that of the upper respiratory tract, so it is possible for pathogenic microorganisms to pass from the nose and pharynx into the middle ear and mastoid cells and cause infection.

The internal ear is a very complicated series of minute canals hollowed out of the temporal bone. Those dealing with hearing are in the cochlea which is in the shape of a snail's shell. Those accommodating balance are in the shape of three semicircles set in three different planes, separated from the cochlea below by a hollow called the vestibule. All these structures contain fluid as well as nerve endings which transmit the stimulus from movement of the fluid to the brain. The stimuli from the cochlea are interpreted as sound.

Aural perception. Basic to the activity of communicating is aural perception. It is much more than hearing; it involves interpretation of the stimuli by the listener. From previous experience is it possible to make sense of the sound? Is it rain on the window or a dripping tap? The sight of a dripping tap would confirm the latter and would be an example of visual and aural perception complementing each other. Sometimes a person wants to attend exclusively to what he is hearing and closes his eyes to exclude visual stimuli. There is selectivity in aural perception so that at an orchestral concert, a budding violinist in the audience can selectively listen to the sound from the violins. Many jobs involve training in aural perception, for instance a mechanic knowing when a car engine is working properly by assessing the sound it makes.

The nervous system

The nervous system plays a part in all the components of communicating. It comprises the brain, spinal cord, and nerves and connects up all other parts of the body. The basic unit of this system is the neurone, a nerve cell which was illustrated in Figure 3.8, plus its fibres. Some fibres are short for example those supplying the face, and others are long especially those supplying the fingers and toes. Nerve cells collected together appear greyish under the microscope and form what is called grey matter, whereas the fibres form white matter. Awareness of the environment is dependent on transmission of stimuli from all the organs comprising the sensory system via sensory nerves

to the brain for interpretation. Reaction to both internal and external environments is accomplished by transmission of stimuli from the brain via motor nerves which supply not only muscles to produce movement, but also glands to provide body secretions.

To free the brain for concentration on its mental and emotional activities and its voluntary control of body movement, the involuntary muscle in the internal organs and the secretory cells in the glands are supplied with nerves from a special 'automatic' portion of the nervous system. It is therefore customary to describe the nervous system in two parts: the central and the autonomic.

The central nervous system. The word 'central' is descriptive of the placement of the brain and spinal cord. The brain is protected by the bones of the skull, and the spinal cord by the vertebral column. The delicate brain and spinal cord are further protected by being completely covered by three membranes known collectively as the meninges.

The meninges. The first enclosing membrane (pia mater), which dips into all the ridges of the surface of the brain and cord, ensures an excellent blood supply. Between this and a more loosely fitting membrane (arachnoid mater which is said to be like a spider's web in structure, hence its name) is the cerebrospinal fluid to cushion the organs and prevent jarring. More durable protection is provided by a strong outer covering, the dura mater.

The cerebrum. This organ occupies the major part of the cranial cavity. It consists of two hemispheres, each having mainly grey matter on the periphery and white matter centrally. The hemispheres are connected by a bundle of fibres, a sort of bridge under which there are spaces (ventricles) filled with cerebrospinal fluid. It is in the ventricles that the fluid is manufactured from the blood and it flows into the subarachnoid space to surround the brain and spinal cord as illustrated in Figure 8.8. It is for protection and maintenance of a constant pressure on all areas of this delicate tissue and may also be important for nutrition of the tissue.

Figure 8.9A shows that the cells in three cerebral areas initiate impulses which are transmitted in motor nerves to skeletal, eye and speech muscles respectively, the cells in the last area being best developed on the left side in right-handed people and *vice versa*. Cells in four other areas (Fig. 8.9B) interpret stimuli transmitted to them in sensory nerves, the cells in one area interpreting stimuli from all parts of the body as sensation; one area interpreting stimuli from the mouth and nose as taste and smell; one area interpreting stimuli from the hearing part of the ears as sound and another area interpreting stimuli from the eyes as sight. Cells in the remaining area are known to deal with memory, intelligence, cognitive activity and emotions but there may well be other functions.

The cerebellum is a smaller organ lying below the pos-

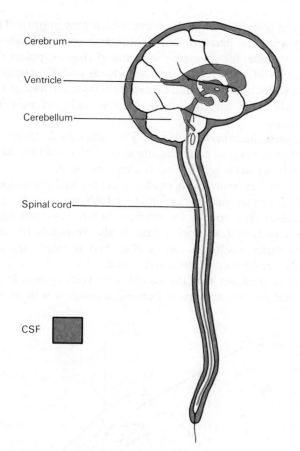

Cerebrum

Ventricle

Cerebellum

Spinal cord

CSF

Fig. 8.8 The distribution of cerebrospinal fluid

terior cerebrum; it also has mainly nerve cells on the outside and fibres on the inside, arranged like the branches of a tree. It too is divided into two cerebellar hemispheres. Its functions are complex and many of them are controlled below the level of consciousness, that is a person is unaware of the functioning of control mechanisms such as those for balance and equilibrium; co-ordination of muscles so that several contract together and in immediate sequence to produce smooth, steady and graceful movement; maintenance of such things as muscle tone; nutrition of all tissues and posture. Many of the complicated muscular movements in everyday living such as walking are at first practised with conscious effort and are eventually taken over at an automatic level by the cerebellum.

The brain stem comprises several structures which lie below the cerebrum and in front of the cerebellum. In the midbrain the fibres from the cerebral hemispheres converge into two bundles to pass under a bridge-like structure the pons varolii which among its functions connects the two cerebellar hemispheres. Below these is the medulla oblongata where most motor fibres from the cerebral hemispheres cross over so that each cerebral hemisphere controls the opposite side of the body; upward travelling sensory fibres also cross over here. A group of nerve cells lie centrally forming the hypothalamus and they control among other functions, the body temperature, the appetite, the sensation of thirst and the cycles of sleeping/wakefulness. There are also reflex centres which initiate sneezing, coughing and vomiting when there is something irritating the respiratory tract or the stomach respectively. The medulla also contains regulation centres for cardiac, respiratory and vasomotor functions. From various parts of the brain, 12

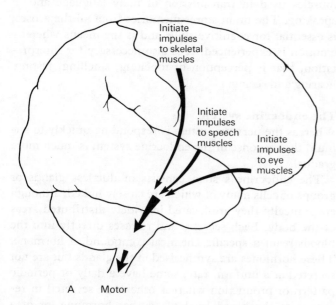

Initiate impulses to skeletal muscles

Initiate impulses to speech muscles

Initiate impulses to eye muscles

A   Motor

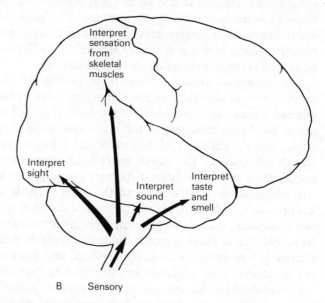

Interpret sensation from skeletal muscles

Interpret sight

Interpret sound

Interpret taste and smell

B   Sensory

Fig. 8.9 A. Motor impulses initiated in the cerebrum B. sensory stimuli received by the cerebrum

pairs of cranial nerves emerge to supply many parts of the face, neck and body.

The spinal cord is a continuation of the brain stem and begins at the level of the foramen magnum in the occipital bone. It is suspended within a protective sac of cerebrospinal fluid inside the vertebral canal and although it ends at the level of the second lumbar vertebra it is safely anchored by a cord-like structure to the base of the canal, further reducing jarring. The 31 pairs of spinal nerves emerging from the spinal cord pass at each side out of the bony canal between the vertebrae to supply tissues throughout the body. The nerve cells are located around the centre of the spinal cord in the form of the letter 'H' and the fibres in four columns are on the outside.

The cord allows transmission of stimuli to and from the brain but it also permits reflex actions which are involuntary responses to sensory stimuli; the example in Figure 8.10 is a motor response, another one is blinking

end in ganglia within the organ which they supply. The responses to parasympathetic innervation are localised and specific, for example the cranial division supplies the muscles of the eye, the salivary glands and the thoracic and abdominal viscera. The sacral division innervates the muscle tissue of the bladder, colon and rectum (Fig. 8.11).

Sympathetic nervous system. The sympathetic thoracolumbar fibres pass from the spinal cord and end in ganglia which are arranged in two chains, one on either side of the vertebral column. It produces generalised physiological responses rather than those which are specific and localised. It responds for example to stress, strong emotions such as fear, anger, pain; it also responds to cold. The varied responses can be described as mobilising the body's resources for defensive action.

It is apparent that the complex nervous system is essential for the activity of communicating as well as the

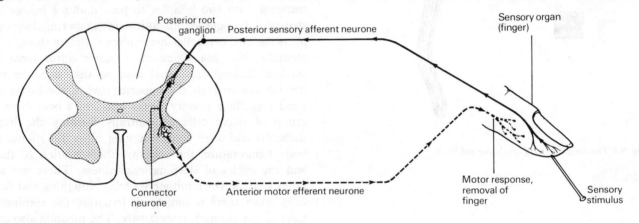

Fig. 8.10 Reflex action

when particles of dust approach the eye. Reflex actions are mainly protective in nature, but it is possible for the brain to override the automatic response. For example, when unprotected fingers grasp an uncomfortably hot plate belonging to the best dinner service they will hold on to it until the nearest laying surface is reached!

The autonomic nervous system. This portion of the nervous system supplies the involuntary muscles in the internal organs and also the secretory cells in glands. The nerve fibres pass from and to the brain and spinal cord often using the pathways of the cranial and spinal nerves already described. To afford control of involuntary muscle there has to be antagonistic nerve supply, that is one which causes contraction and the other relaxation. To provide this dual supply the autonomic nervous system is divided into sympathetic and parasympathetic systems. Neither of these is under voluntary control; their activity is responsive to the body's internal and external environments. They are however influenced by emotion.

Parasympathetic nervous system. The parasympathetic craniosacral fibres pass from the brain and spinal cord to

other ALs to be discussed in this book. It controls all the muscles used in transmission of body language and in speaking. The brain stores memories from all the senses, is essential for cognitive skills and is the means whereby emotion is experienced. It is also necessary for interpretation, that is perception of touching, smelling, tasting, hearing and seeing.

The endocrine system

Whereas the nervous system is responding quickly to stimuli, the response of the endocrine system is much more gradual.

The endocrine system consists of ductless glands or groups of cells many of which are closely linked, although anatomically they are located in widely distributed areas of the body. Each secretes and releases directly into the bloodstream a specific chemical compound, a hormone. These hormones are synthesised in the glands but are not secreted at a uniform rate; some have a daily or periodic pattern of production whereas others are secreted in response to the blood level of another hormone, or of a

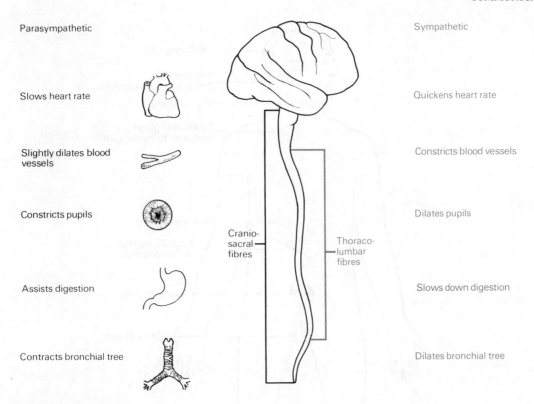

Parasympathetic

Slows heart rate

Slightly dilates blood vessels

Constricts pupils

Cranio-sacral fibres

Assists digestion

Contracts bronchial tree

Sympathetic

Quickens heart rate

Constricts blood vessels

Dilates pupils

Thoraco-lumbar fibres

Slows down digestion

Dilates bronchial tree

Fig. 8.11 Autonomic nervous system

specific substance such as sodium, sugar or water. Hormones are lost from the body by excretion or by metabolic inactivation.

Current knowledge of hormonal mechanisms is still incomplete and this chapter contains only a brief outline of what is known about the main endocrine glands and their actions:

pituitary gland
thyroid gland
parathyroid glands
adrenal or suprarenal glands
islets of Langerhans (in the pancreas)
pineal gland
testes in the male
ovaries in the female.

The testes and ovaries secrete hormones related to the reproductive system and are described in Chapter 16 which is concerned with the AL of expressing sexuality. The positions of the main endocrine glands are shown in diagrammatic form in Figure 8.12.

The pituitary gland or hypophysis. The oval-shaped pituitary gland is situated in the hypophyseal fossa (sella turcica) of the sphenoid bone at the base of the brain. It has important connections by nerve fibres and blood vessels to the hypothalamus which lies above it. Sometimes it is referred to as the master gland in the endocrine system because it influences secretion from most of the other endocrine glands. The pituitary gland consists of

three lobes — the anterior, middle and posterior lobes — each having different functions (Fig. 8.13).

The anterior lobe of the pituitary gland secretes:

somatotrophic or growth hormone
thyrotrophic or thyroid stimulating hormone (TSH)
adrenocorticotrophic hormone (ACTH)
lactogenic hormone (prolactin)
gonadotrophic hormones
● follicle stimulating hormone (FSH) in the male and female
● interstitial cell stimulating hormone in the male only
● luteinising hormone (LH) in the female only

The *growth hormone* has its highest concentration during childhood although it is still necessary after reaching adulthood in order to stimulate the constant repair and replacement of body tissue. Growth hormone promotes mainly protein anabolism, the conversion of glycogen to glucose, and the absorption of calcium from the intestine.

The *thyrotrophic hormone* (TSH) controls the growth and activity of the thyroid gland, its target organ, which produces thyroxine. The secretion of TSH is influenced by the concentration of thyroxine in the blood as it flows through the hypothalamus.

The *adrenocorticotrophic hormone* (ACTH) stimulates the cortex of the adrenal glands, its target organs, and similarly is influenced by the concentration in the blood flowing through the hypothalamus of the adrenal cortex hormone.

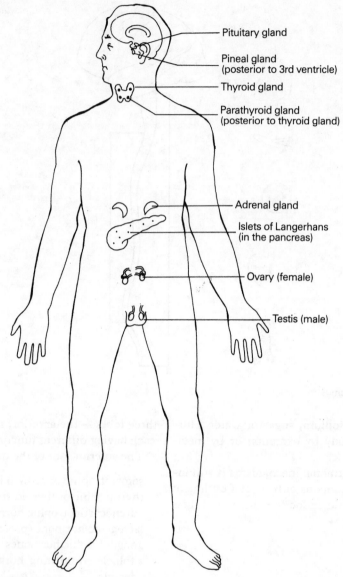

Pituitary gland

Pineal gland
(posterior to 3rd ventricle)

Thyroid gland

Parathyroid gland
(posterior to thyroid gland)

Adrenal gland

Islets of Langerhans
(in the pancreas)

Ovary (female)

Testis (male)

Fig. 8.12 The sites of the main endocrine glands

The *lactogenic hormone* acts directly on the mammary glands or breasts following delivery of the baby and the placenta (see p. 298 in Chapter 16 on Expressing Sexuality). Along with other hormones, it stimulates the breasts to produce milk (the actual development of the breasts during pregnancy is influenced by the ovarian hormones).

The *male gonadotrophins* are the follicle-stimulating hormone which influences its target organs, the testes, to produce spermatazoa; and the interstitial cell stimulating hormone which acts on the interstitial cells of the testes to stimulate the production of testosterone.

The *female gonadotrophins* are the follicle stimulating hormone which influences the development and ripening of the ovarian follicle which in turn produces oestrogen; and the luteinising hormone which influences the maturation of the ovarian follicle, ovulation, and the formation

of the corpus luteum which in turn produces progesterone.

The middle lobe of the pituitary gland does not appear to have many functions; it is thought to affect the development of melanocytes which give the skin its colour.

The posterior lobe secretes pituitrin, containing two hormones:

pitocin or oxytocin
vasopressin or antidiuretic hormone (ADH)

Pitocin affects the cells of the lactating breasts pushing milk down into the ducts behind the nipple. Although acting on the uterus in late pregnancy, the secretion of pitocin is increased just before and during labour and is further stimulated by the baby sucking at the breast.

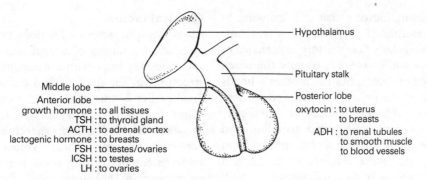

Fig. 8.13 The pituitary gland, its main hormones and their main target organs

Vasopressin or antidiuretic hormone (ADH). Its secretion is influenced by the osmotic pressure of blood circulating through the hypothalamus. A rise in osmotic pressure increases the secretion of ADH and more water is absorbed from the kidney tubule, whereas a fall in pressure reduces ADH so more urine is produced. Vasopressin also affects involuntary muscle in the blood vessel walls causing contraction and thus raising the blood pressure.

The thyroid gland. This two-lobed gland is situated in the neck and produces three hormones. *Thyroxine* and *triiodothyroxine*, which to function adequately require iodine ingested in food, are regulated by TH from the pituitary gland. Their influence is wide-ranging — they are essential for physical and mental development; for utilisation of oxygen (they affect the basal metabolic rate, BMR); for carbohydrate absorption, energy and heat production; for nerve stability; and for the maintenance of healthy skin and hair. The third hormone, *calcitonin*, inhibits the reabsorption of calcium from bones so reduces the blood level of calcium.

The parathyroid glands. These four glands on the posterior aspect of the thyroid gland secrete the hormone called *parathormone* which can mobilise calcium from the bones. Along with calcitonin, which has an opposing effect, it maintains the blood concentration of calcium within normal limits.

The adrenal glands. The two adrenal glands are situated on the upper pole of each kidney and each has two distinct parts, a cortex and a medulla.

The outer cortex produces three types of hormones. The *glucocorticoids*, influenced by ACTH from the pituitary regulate carbohydrate metabolism; and the *mineralocorticoids* help to maintain the electrolyte balance of the body. The *sex hormones* — testosterone, oestrogen and progesterone — are controlled by ACTH and are produced in both males and females; they influence the development of the secondary sex characteristics.

The inner medulla of the adrenal glands is made up of tissue similar to the sympathetic nervous system and some of its functions are similar. The medulla produces the hormones *adrenalin* and *noradrenalin*. These, as does

the sympathetic nervous system, prepare the individual to react quickly to fear and danger, popularly described as preparation for fight or flight. Their secretion dilates the coronary arteries to improve the flow of blood to the heart, dilates the bronchi, and dilates the blood vessels of muscles; constricts the peripheral arteries to the skin so the person is pale; converts glycogen to glucose; reduces the secretion of saliva; dilates the pupils of the eye; increases the action of the sweat glands; and inhibits micturition and defaecation.

The islets of Langerhans. These ductless glands are dispersed throughout the pancreas and secrete their hormone directly into the bloodstream, the α cells producing *glucagon* and the β cells producing *insulin*. They have opposing actions with glucagon raising the blood glucose level and insulin lowering it; the former converting glycogen to glucose and the latter converting glucose to glycogen.

The pineal gland. The exact functions of this small gland situated near the 3rd ventricle of the brain are still a matter for conjecture but it is thought that they are associated with the release of gonadotrophic hormones from the anterior pituitary gland.

Any dysfunction of the endocrine glands causes a decrease or an increase in the secretion of its hormones. Because of the diverse physiological functions under hormonal control, the signs and symptoms of endocrine disorders may be reflected in many parts of the body. They control some of the body's vital functions, and deviations in their concentration outside the range of normal can be serious.

It is fascinating how these endocrine glands, widely separated from each other and with no anatomical connection, can have such a widespread effect on other tissues in the body, and sometimes opposing actions in the process of maintaining homeostatic balance.

LIFESPAN: EFFECT ON COMMUNICATING

The lifespan component of the model is particularly relevant to the AL of communicating. Even in the prenatal period the fetus is communicating that it is growing in size; and in the later months of pregnancy that it is capable of movement. The baby's first worldly experience of non-verbal communication, however is usually the touch of the midwife's hands or sometimes the mother's hands and everyone present at the delivery is relieved to hear the initial cry, the first verbal communication. Thereafter the infant experiments with cooing and babbling and soon can sense the 'meaning' of words and phrases from how they are spoken, and by the volume, intonation and so on. The baby is then ready to associate words with objects or people, and later begins to utter the correct word in response. By a long process the child gradually learns and uses an increasing vocabulary. A vital aspect of this learning is the stimulation from other people in the environment especially the mother or mother substitute who by speaking and singing to the child, and touching and cuddling, provides the basic experiences for interpersonal communication. Indeed, children deprived of such stimulation may grow up to have difficulty with human relationships.

During adolescence, the teenager may develop special meanings for certain words known only to the peer group and not understood by adults. However as well as this private communication channel, most adolescents extend their vocabulary and modes of expression, verbally and non-verbally, as they move away from the constraints of home and school contacts, and explore new environments with different types of relationships.

It is estimated that the majority of adults have a speaking vocabulary of 3000 to 5000 words although their reading vocabulary may well be more. On the other hand there are those whose speaking vocabulary contains only a few hundred words of not more than three syllables and their reading vocabulary not many more. Often current slang and colloquialisms make up the bulk of such people's language. These factors will naturally have their effect on acquisition of writing skills.

In old age, deterioration of vision and hearing can lessen the ability to communicate effectively by causing distortion of sensory input. Also there is a gradual loss of function of some brain cells which can result in forgetfulness and sometimes confusion. Swollen finger joints can make writing difficult. Frailty can interfere with body posture and gesture. All these factors may contribute to problems in the older person's AL of communicating.

FACTORS INFLUENCING COMMUNICATING

Like all other ALs, communicating is influenced by a variety of factors. In keeping with the relevant component of the model, these are described under the following headings — physical, psychological, sociocultural, environmental and politicoeconomic factors.

Physical factors

Many physical factors influence a person's ability to communicate by means of verbal and non-verbal language, and especially important are adequately functioning body structures in the nervous and endocrine systems as outlined earlier in this chapter. For example, for the acquisition of speech there has to be at least adequate hearing, an adequately functioning speech apparatus and the opportunity to hear others' voices for imitation. The achievement of reading skills requires at least minimal vision, and the accomplishment of writing skills is further dependent on an adequately functioning preferred hand. Communicating by body language is dependent on adequately functioning nervous and musculoskeletal systems.

Hormone production is also related, although less obviously, to communicating. The sex hormones are responsible for the distinguishable difference between the male and female voice. Structurally the male larynx is on average longer anteriorly/posteriorly so that the male voice after puberty is lower in pitch than that of the female. However both males and females differ in the control which they have over the many muscles, including the diaphragm, used in voice production. Thus some people have low, monotonous voices and others can modulate the voice for effective and varied expression. There are also differences related to patterns of physical contact as a means of communicating between males, between females, and between males/females; and these are mentioned in Chapter 16 when expressing sexuality is discussed.

Psychological factors

Level of intelligence affects communicating in that it influences learning ability. It therefore plays an important part in the extent of the vocabulary acquired for use in everyday living. A person with a limited vocabulary can usually manage well in familiar surroundings but may experience difficulty, for instance when filling in many of the forms which have become a feature of our modern society such as an insurance form. Problems can arise even for intelligent people with an extensive vocabulary, for example when they are communicating with someone on a subject other than their own speciality.

Nervousness affects communicating as people going for an interview know only too well. Anxiety may make it difficult to respond fluently and interviewees may come away feeling annoyed that they have not done themselves justice. For others, in spite of adequate content in their conversation, the non-verbal behaviour of tremulous hands, dilated pupils, perspiration on brow and upper lip, can inform the interviewer of the state of nervousness.

Current mood also has its effect on communicating. Excitement usually increases the rate of speech, raises the voice pitch and there may be more than usual gesticulation. Anger is usually expressed in a loud voice. Depression flattens the voice almost to monotony; movement is slowed, and a dejected facial expression is characteristic of many people when they are in a low mood. In comparison, cheerfulness lightens the voice, and is likely to produce a smiling expression. Of course communication is two-way, and the mood of the recipients is also important for effective communication. It is not uncommon to refer to a 'hostile audience' or a 'receptive audience'.

Loss of self-respect and faith in self may make communicating a problematic activity. In such circumstances, an event which normally would be considered insignificant might produce a reaction of worthlessness, guilt or shame. A person might be overly critical of others, probably a subconscious effort to raise self-esteem. Those who have not experienced some type of long-term, warm, trusting relationship in their early years may find it difficult to communicate effectively and confidently with other people.

Psychological factors certainly affect both verbal and non-verbal communicating.

Sociocultural factors

Now more than ever, an increasingly mobile and multiracial society demands that consideration be given to sociocultural factors in communicating (Henley & Clayton, 1982). As far as verbal language is concerned, even within one language there can be several local vocabularies which strangers cannot understand. Accent or dialect can communicate place of residence during acquisition of language; and it may take time for the listener to become accustomed to a different dialect. Social status can also be conveyed by language. For example in the U.K., the range of vocabulary can be indicative of level of education attained; this can influence the type of job procured which determines economic bracket of income and in turn determines the person's social class according to the Registrar-General's classification (p. 278).

Apart from dialect or accent or social class indicators, the specialist vocabulary in certain occupations and professions is almost a 'language culture'. Technical expressions which are in everyday usage within an occupational group, can be totally alien to outsiders. For example, despite the computer revolution, the language of computer users still has to be interpreted to the uninitiated; and for clients in the health care system, the vocabulary of staff is often unintelligible or, when only snatches are overheard and understood, is open to misinterpretation and can cause the client and family great distress.

Other sociocultural differences affect body language. Mode of dress can communicate such diverse information as a person's ethnic origin, religious affiliation, or occupation. Although communicating by touch is the most primitive mode, there are culturally determined touching patterns for adults. Some cultures permit a reciprocal hug to signal welcome on arrival, and again on departure to signal appreciation of the visit. The accepted practice in other cultures on these occasions is a kiss on each cheek; yet in others a kiss on the lips: in some it is nose-rubbing; and in others only reciprocal hand-shaking is acceptable. There are also differences regarding the amount of gesticulation and mobility of the lips when communicating which are culturally determined. There are culturally determined practices related to eye contact, for example certain aborigines, to be polite, do not look into each other's eyes as they talk, whereas in the Western world, it is polite to maintain eye contact during conversation.

Environmental factors

The appropriateness of the physical environment can certainly contribute to the effectiveness of the AL of communicating. Poor ventilation in a room and extremes of temperature can be conducive to discomfort and interfere with concentration when communicating. Lighting, too, is important. Excessive light and glare can make a person feel too uncomfortable to converse, and poor lighting can mean that important non-verbal cues are missed. Soft lighting is deliberately used for example by restaurateurs to induce a feeling of relaxation, enhance the enjoyment of the meal, and promote pleasurable conversation. Environmental noise can have an effect on communicating. Some people find it easier to speak about personal matters if there is background noise, be it music or the hum of conversation, while others find even the slightest noise distracting. Rooms which afford aural privacy usually help when personal matters need to be discussed, for example, an interview or consultation with a member of health care staff. In such a setting too, conversation is more likely to be encouraged if the furniture is so arranged that the interviewee and the interviewer are not physically separated by a desk; that the chairs are reasonably comfortable and in a position to allow eye contact; and that there are no unplanned interruptions.

Apart from personal interviews, the physical layout of a room is important for any group work; chairs with desks in serried rows for example are not so conducive to discussion as chairs arranged in a circle or round a central table. This type of arrangement allows all members of the group to see who is speaking, to have eye contact, to observe body language and to maximise the impact of non-verbal cues which are so important to the AL or communicating.

Politicoeconomic factors

The economic status of an individual will almost certainly be communicated to others in a variety of ways, for example by the choice of neighbourhood for purchase of a house, the choice of social circle and the type of occupation — at least in Western cultures.

Communicating can also be influenced by the economic status of the Local Government group which serves a neighbourhood. For example it may influence the availability of such services as play-groups and nursery schools when young children have wider opportunities to practise communicating; new types of activities and different relationships can be explored in these settings which add to the child's capacity to communicate and are critical at this stage of development.

Of course, technological advances have greatly enhanced the individual's capacity to communicate. In industrialised societies, even in lower economic echelons, most people have access to and are influenced by mass media communications in the form of newspapers, radio and television. Then at national and international levels there is an elaborate network of telecommunication, sometimes incorporating the use of satellites, which permits rapid transworld communication.

The availability of telephone, radio and television is often dependent however on services provided by government, so politicoeconomic decisions are involved and some would even maintain that the mass media provide opportunities for political pressure, and for communicating in the form of propaganda.

Nowadays all large organisations — including hospitals or indeed a whole health service — are aware of the need for effective communication within and between different levels and grades of staff in order to achieve efficient management. There is widespread use of informal meetings, circulation of reports, notice board announcements, newsletters, in addition to the communication associated with committee structures and official correspondence. Many organisations in fact are overwhelmed by a superabundance of communications and some are looking to computerisation to solve some of the problems created by information bombardment.

The rapidly growing use of computers in many areas of everyday living is often referred to as the computer revolution, similar in scale to the 19th century industrial revolution. In the Western world, the use of computers is no longer novel in, for example, industry, commerce and banking, and the need for computer literacy is recognised to the extent that education for the computer age now begins at primary school level.

Of course, new technologies bring new problems and one cause for anxiety is the ease of retrieval of data. This is especially true of personal data but also of enormous importance when research data or top secret intelligence are stored in computers. Usually one is advocating ease of communication and almost paradoxically it is the ease with which large amounts of data can be communicated by computers which is at issue. In the U.K., in 1984 a bill was introduced in parliament seeking legal safeguards which will ensure that computerised personal health data about patients will be available only to health professionals and not to groups such as the police, tax authorities, industry, and social services personnel.

Politicoeconomic and legal factors have enormous potential to influence the AL of communicating.

DEPENDENCE/INDEPENDENCE IN COMMUNICATING

Communicating is an AL where movement along the dependence/independence continuum has a direct relationship with the lifespan component of the model. Even when a baby is born with the intact body structures required for communicating, it is necessary to learn to use those structures, to perceive, and to attach meaning to discrete sounds. Stimulation from parents enhances the speed of learning, and great patience is required to perceive and decode the communicating done by babies and children, both verbally and non-verbally. On the other hand, adults can be curiously lacking in perception. An extreme example would be an instance when there are signs of child abuse and the cues are not picked up by people outside the home setting. The young are certainly dependent on others for the AL of communicating and likewise, sometimes, the elderly.

Physical body structure of course, influences the degree of dependence in communicating. Intact physical structures which enable one to see, hear, taste, smell and touch, and those which permit speech and body language are basic to independence, although some degree of impairment can often be compensated for or coped with. However, mechanical aids can do much to lessen the disability of impaired body structure. The problem of diminished sight can be reduced or corrected by using spectacles or an illuminated magnifying glass: and for those who are severely handicapped the use of specially prepared large-print books or of braille or of tape-recordings can help considerably in retaining a measure of independence. For those who have impaired auditory structure and function, it is possible now to have quite sophisticated, unobtrusive hearing aids which dramatically improve their quality of living and there are also amplifiers available for telephone conversations and public meetings. For those who are dumb, a sign language is useful and especially for mentally handicapped people who have speech difficulties, there are symbolic languages such as the Bliss Symbolic Communication System and the Makaton Vocabulary Language Programme which have greatly improved their capacity for communicating (Kiernan, Reid & Jones, 1983).

A few years ago, it was quite revolutionary to provide an aid, called Possum, for those who were quadriplegic;

it enabled the paralysed person, by blowing on a type of keyboard, to manipulate light switches, radio and television sets, telephone and so on. However, recent technological advances have made possible a robot which can be programmed to carry out a range of services on command. These developments hold great promise for severely disabled people who although dependent on a machine, would have a feeling of relative independence; their range of control in communicating and getting an appropriate response would be increased and they would be less dependent on people to carry out a number of everyday living activities.

INDIVIDUALITY IN COMMUNICATING

One of the fascinating things about individuality in communicating is that each person develops a distinctive voice, instantly recognisable, for instance, on a telephone. Given the individuality of voice, it is little wonder that people also vary enormously in their communicating habits. Any description of individual habits in this AL is influenced by the interplay of the four components of the model already discussed and how these focus on the fifth component, individuality in communicating. The following is a résumé.

Lifespan: effect on communicating
- Fetal growth and movement/birth cry
- Infancy and childhood — increasing skills/forming relationships
- Adolescence — extension of skills/relationships
- Adulthood — variety in performance
- Old age — gradual loss of activity/reduction in skills and relationships

Factors influencing communicating
- Physical
  - intact body structure and function
  - speaking/voice pitch
  - hearing
  - seeing
  - reading
  - writing
  - gesticulating
- Psychological
  - intelligence/range of vocabulary
  - self-confidence
  - self-respect
  - prevailing mood
- Sociocultural
  - mother tongue
  - dialect/accent
  - vocabulary
  - personal appearance/dress
  - patterns of touching/eyecontact/gesticulation
- Environmental
  - temperature/ventilation
  - light
  - noise
  - type/size of room
  - arrangement of furniture
- Politicoeconomic
  - income
  - occupation
  - communication channels/mass media
  - computers
  - legislation to protect data/individual

Dependence/independence in communicating
- Unimpaired body structure and function
- Seeing aids
- Hearing aids
- Speech aids
- Possum/robots

Communicating: patients' problems and related nursing activities

Unless they are detrimental to health, it is important that, during an episode of illness, the patient's individual habits of living are changed as little as possible. It is therefore important that the nurse should know about these habits and use the knowledge to devise an individualised plan of nursing. In order to discover what the patient can and cannot do, the nurse will be seeking answers to the following questions:

- how does the individual usually communicate?
- what factors influence the way the individual carries out the AL of communicating?
- what does the individual understand about communicating?
- what are the individual's attitudes to communicating?
- has the individual any long-standing difficulties with communicating and how have these been coped with?
- what problems, if any, does the person have at present with communicating, or seem likely to develop?

The nurse will find answers to these types of questions in the course of conversing with the patient and his family and observing their behaviour; and there may also be relevant information in other records such as medical records to which the nurse has access. The collected information can then be examined, in collaboration with the patient when relevant, to identify any problems being experienced with the AL. The nurse may recognise potential problems and it may be appropriate to discuss them with the patient. Mutual, realistic goals can then be set to prevent potential problems from becoming actual ones; to alleviate or solve the actual problems; or to help the patient cope with those which cannot be alleviated or solved. Bearing in mind what the patient can do for himself, the nursing interventions to achieve the set goals can then be selected according to local circumstances and available resources. These interventions should be written on the nursing plan along with the date on which evaluation will be carried out in order to decide whether or not the stated goals have been, or are being, achieved. All these activities are necessary in order to provide individualised nursing.

Communicating is the only means a patient has of getting information about his illness, telling staff of his problems, keeping in contact with relatives and relating with fellow patients. However effective his communicating skills, it is highly probable that he will experience some problems in the course of adjusting to a new environment for instance when admitted to hospital.

Most hospitals send to those who are to be admitted from the waiting list some type of preparatory material ranging from a leaflet to an illustrated brochure, the latter in particular for children. But this type of communication presupposes that the receivers have the necessary vision and can read. When this is not so, they are deprived of this initial preparation, as are all those who are admitted under the label 'emergencies'.

Nurses are becoming more aware of the need for effective communication and many articles have been written in recent years about its importance. There is also a considerable amount of evidence to indicate that patients themselves see communication as a crucial part of their care. Cartwright (1964) and Raphael (1969) did some early work on this issue yet a later report (Reynolds, 1978) does not give reassuring results; in a surgical ward more than 50% of the patients were dissatisfied with the amount of information they received. When such a high percentage consider information to be inadequate, it is apparent that the pattern of nurse/patient communication needs to be reviewed. Relatives, too, seem concerned about lack of communication and the 'unavailability of the nurses'. Information collected about the relatives of cancer patients showed that only a minority have anything more than superficial contact with the staff caring for the patient, and a number of these relatives would have welcomed an opportunity to share their anxiety, not only about the patient but about their own feelings (Bond, 1982).

Many patients have the highest praise for the effectiveness of communication with hospital staff but there is also a lot of criticism, and it is useful to outline some of the problems which can arise when a patient is admitted to hospital. The remainder of this section is a general discussion of the types of patients' problems related to communicating and the relevant nursing activities. They are grouped under headings which indicate how the problem can arise:

Change of environment and routine
Change of dependence/independence status
Discomforts associated with communicating.

CHANGE OF ENVIRONMENT AND ROUTINE

Once the patient is inside the ward several dimensions of his communicating have changed, for example the social dimensions. Members of the group with whom he lives, usually the family, are no longer present; the people with whom he communicates at work are absent; and likewise the people with whom he chooses to spend the leisure part of each day.

Unfamiliar people
The patient's problem is that he has joined a group of unfamiliar people, some of whom, the patients, are present all the time; others, the nurses, are in his vicinity for some of the time; and a whole variety of others appear 'to come and go'. It is little wonder that even the most confident individuals experience some difficulty in trying to make sense of such an environment, one which is alien to most people.

Admission. In some instances the patient is very ill on admission and in these circumstances explanations and introductions have a lower priority than life-sustaining treatment and nursing. So what can the nurse do to help the patient with the AL of communicating? Initially only essential information need be communicated — that he is in hospital, that relatives have been informed, how to summon the nurse and so on. As the condition improves there can be gradual and fuller exchange of information between nurse and patient.

For a patient admitted from the waiting list, the nurse who 'admits' him (that is the initial showing of the patient to the bed and the space which he will occupy) should help with the inevitable quandary of meeting new people in somewhat unusual circumstances. It should be remembered that an anxious person, even an intelligent one, does not retain as much new information as normally. The nurse should therefore attempt to communicate only the information necessary for the patient to manage say, the next 24 hours. In one study, patient anxiety was measured and found to be highest in the first 24 hours of a hospital stay (Wilson-Barnett, 1978).

Introduction of nurse and patient. The first nursing activity is introduction of the nurse, by name, to the patient. If name badges are worn, it should be indicated to a sighted person that it would not be considered rude for him to read name badges. However nurses need to remember that people who wear bifocal spectacles have difficulty in reading at that level, and any cues regarding inadequate vision should be noted. The patient should be told of the mode of address used in that particular hospital for professional staff. It is important to remember that the patient needs some information about the different members of the health care team so that he can relate satisfactorily to them. If uniforms distinguish the different grades of nursing and domestic staff, then this is useful information for the nurse to communicate to the patient.

Introduction to other patients. For all but the very ill or those admitted as an emergency the nurse can help the patient with his problem of being among unfamiliar people by introducing him to the other patients in his immediate vicinity. These are the people who will be present throughout each day and they help to give the new patient a feeling of 'belonging'. Several studies report that other patients are a great support and source of information to new patients (Franklin, 1974). Only factual information like how long each patient has been in the ward should be given. It is important for the nurse to remember the professional responsibility of maintaining confidentiality so the medical diagnosis and any personal details about the other patients must not be divulged.

Communicating staffing patterns. The nurse who admits the patient needs to explain whether or not he has been allocated to her in a patient allocation scheme; if so, for how long she will be on duty; and the staffing arrangements that will be made for the other two shifts. If team nursing is the pattern, then this has to be explained and the other members of the team for that shift can introduce themselves as and when necessary. If the work pattern is neither of these, again the patient needs to know this. He should be encouraged to express any particular anxieties and queries until the nurse assesses from verbal and non-verbal interaction that he has a reasonable grasp of the staffing pattern as it applies to him, and knows from whom he can seek any further help. He cannot be expected to feel safe and secure without this information.

Empathy. All the foregoing, and all activities carried out in the vicinity of the patient, offer the nurse an opportunity to establish empathy with him. Empathy is described in various ways. Irving (1978) maintains it is ... that degree of understanding which 'allows one person to experience how another feels in a particular situation ...

Empathy implies knowledge and understanding of the other person's feelings, the situation he is in, and a positive feeling toward him.' In practising empathy a nurse shows that she 'cares' about what is happening to a patient. She conveys this by what she says and how she says it, by what she does and how she does it. She shows respect for him as a unique human being by taking every opportunity to reinforce his individuality. This can be accomplished by addressing the patient at each encounter using the name he prefers; remembering for example at meal times that he prefers coffee to tea; that he prefers to bath in the morning and so on. She shows empathy by acquiring knowledge of the patient and his needs, and having a sense of responsibility in helping the patient to fulfil his needs.

In a small study in the U.S.A. empathy scores were recorded for male and female students in nursing, and male and female students in other disciplines. Macdonald (1977) found that the male nursing students scored highest; male non-nursing students lowest; and falling in a band between these, the female non-nursing students scored higher than the female nursing students. As it seems that some nursing students have less empathy than some members of the public, there is obviously need for improvement in nurse education to ensure the acquisition of empathy. Ability to establish empathy can be improved with persistent sensitive practice as outlined above and as described by Marson (1979).

Nurse/patient relationship. The relationship between nurse and patient is essentially a human one (p. 110). However each patient is in the health care system for a purpose, getting help with health problems, actual or potential. The nurse is there to make the nursing contribution to the solution, amelioration or prevention of the patients' actual or potential problems. She therefore is not in the individual patient/nurse relationship from choice, but in the capacity of making a professional contribution. A consideration of what she brings to the relationship is therefore necessary.

The nurse brings to the relationship herself as a unique human being, the culmination of her particular life experiences. She also brings compassion for people and a commitment to nursing, together with nursing knowledge and skills. Her emotional maturity should be such that she does not have to gratify personal needs at the patient's expense. For example a need to be dominant and make decisions may deprive patients of practice which they require in order to deal with, for example, their problem of indecision, common in some mental illnesses. A strong mothering need may motivate a nurse to dress patients when it would be in their best interest to re-learn dressing skills.

The nurse brings to the relationship a maturity which permits toleration of frustration: a patient is not at home when she makes a house call; a patient does not take his medication; another removes his dressing or falls out of bed. The trigger points are innumerable but a nurse should have the maturity to deal with the resultant feelings in a constructive way that avoids reflecting any annoyance on to the patient. Nobody expects the nurse to be a paragon of virtue but the nurse is meant to be realistic, is meant to have self-knowledge because she has to use herself in the relationship. Her personal needs have to be met by other supporting staff, by counsellors or by the significant others in her life.

The patient is also a unique human being who has been fashioned by life experiences. Something is wrong, so already his image of himself has changed. Change is uncomfortable at the best of times and he is discomforted. If the diagnosis is uncertain and an array of diagnostic tests is required, then the patient is bound to be anxious both about the tests and the potential results, and inevitably, he is worried if surgery is prescribed. Worried people do not concentrate, hear or understand so well as usual. However, if the nurse takes the time to give information to the patient, it has been shown in various studies to be beneficial (Hayward, 1975; Wilson-Barnett, 1978; Boore, 1980; Bond, 1982). By becoming a patient, not only treatment is sought; comfort is also sought from nursing staff, and information-giving seems to be an important component of comfort.

Psychological comfort is inextricably related to physical comfort although some interactions are deliberately planned to contribute to psychological comfort. It may be as fleeting as a look of acknowledgement when passing the patient's bed; or it may be less transient for example helping the patient through the stages of accepting and coping with chronic illness; or when a patient has a mental illness, it may be the major emphasis for most interactions.

Every nurse needs to develop psychological and social skills as well as manual skills in order to maintain an effective nurse/patient relationship while the patient requires it; and these skills are also required to relinquish the relationship when appropriate.

Discharge. Providing patients with information on admission to hospital and throughout their stay may be acknowledged as an important part of nursing but frequently, discharge is a very rushed affair. All too often patients and their families are not given enough information about planning the convalescent period, about continued medications and treatments, expected rate of progress, and return to employment. Several studies have shown that this type of information does not seem to be communicated and, for example, Mayou et al (1976) discuss the great need for it following myocardial infarction. In *Using a Model for Nursing* (Roper, Logan & Tierney, 1983), the third year student nurse contributing to the study in a surgical ward, commented that the model approach helped her to appreciate the need for planned discharge goals; even when admitting the patient, she was alerted to consider what the patient required to know on discharge in order to resume her usual Activities of Living.

Staff-to-staff communicating between hospital and community services is another important aspect when considering a patient's discharge and Parnell (1982) highlighted some of the problems in her study. For example available information was not being sent; there was reluctance to put certain items in writing; telephone messages left with a third party could be distorted; there was incomplete information; there was a lack of feedback. She concluded that although her findings showed considerable improvement since previous studies, there were still problems and she makes proposals to rectify at least some of them.

Unfamiliar place

A patient newly admitted to the hospital environment will naturally be anxious about keeping in touch with family, friends and work associates. Anxiety may be lessened by information about such things as a mobile shop where stationery and newspapers can be bought; ward arrangements for collection and delivery of mail; for making and receiving telephone calls, and for visiting. Gradually the patient's new environment seems less strange and threatening as he becomes aware of the possibilities for communication between hospital and his familiar environment. But he also needs information to permit the continuance of his other everyday activities. It can be communicated to him by adequate labelling of, for example, toilets and bathrooms. The letters should be sufficiently large and should be placed so as to cater for patients with poor vision. This is especially helpful to the older patients who may have difficulty in learning and remembering, and who may require to visit the toilet during the night. Labels are less anxiety-provoking and easier to see from the corridor if they project at right angles to the door than if they are on the doors.

As the days pass in this unfamiliar environment, some patients (particularly those with deficient vision and hearing, and those who for one reason or another do not read a daily newspaper) can lose track of the time of day, the day of the week and the day of the month. Patients can become distressed as they ask visitors what day it is. The provision of a large calendar and clock in each ward can be useful in preventing this apparent disorientation and nurses can mention these factors each day to patients who are experiencing difficulty of this kind.

Unfamiliar language

The new patient who probably has the biggest problem with communication is the one who does not speak the national language. With increasing multiracial societies in most countries and the speed of modern-day travel such patients are found in hospitals throughout the world. This is recognised as an international problem and voluntary organisations such as the League of Red Cross Societies have produced helpful translations in many languages. At a local level, voluntary help is usually available; there is often a list of people speaking other languages who are willing to act as interpreters. Failing this, nurses can help by using empathy, ingenuity and miming.

Even when the same national language is spoken by patient and nurse, both can experience problems in aural perception when their attention has to be directed to listening because of accent or dialect. The nurse can help to avoid this problem by speaking clearly and slowly, stopping for clarification when this seems necessary.

A problem can also be experienced when there is a difference in the vocabulary used by patient and nurse. This can operate in both ways — the patient might use words which the nurse does not readily understand and vice versa. Take the words used for the place for eliminating: bathroom, convenience, lavatory, loo, toilet, water closet (W.C.) and where there is no sewage system, simply 'the closet'. But in North America the word closet is the term used for a wardrobe. There are countless other examples but the above should serve to alert nurses so that they can prevent patients' problems in this area. This is accomplished by becoming expert at observing and interpreting non-verbal cues indicating incomprehension, and by exploring with the patient the cause of the break in the chain of communication and correcting it.

Further differences in vocabulary can produce problems for patients when words with a medical definition are used in the process of communicating: insomnia, migraine, diarrhoea. Nurses should therefore discover from patients what meaning these words have for them, so that they can be sure that they and the patients are talking about the same conditions. This naturally applies also to specific medical words, and when it is necessary to use them the nurse may find it necessary to correct inaccuracies and add explanations.

Some patients experience difficulty when talking with nurses about activities such as eliminating and expressing sexuality. They may fear that they are not using the 'right' words. It is therefore helpful if nurses start by saying that people use different words, and asking the patient to give the information in his own words. Yet another type of vocabulary can have difference in meaning for patient and nurse and thereby give rise to difficulties — words describing parts of the body, though having a particular anatomical reference, do not necessarily have that reference for lay people, even intelligent lay people. Where appropriate, pointing to the area on one's own body is helpful or using visual aids, which can be as simple as drawing a diagram while explaining the location of the part.

Even the use of ordinary vocabulary can result in problems for patients. An example is given by Lelean (1973). The surgeon instructed a patient not to bend her back after an operation. When she was allowed out of bed the nurses (who presumably had not received the instruction) no longer assisted in washing her and the patient said that she would be glad to get home so that her legs and feet could be washed.

Unfamiliar activities

Nursing, medical and other activities, taken so much for granted by the staff, are strange to the patients. Franklin (1974), in her study of patient anxiety on admission to hospital, found that most patients disagreed with the statement 'The nurses tell me what will happen to me'. The value of giving information to the patient about nursing procedures was already mentioned on page 125 to illustrate that information giving was an important component of comfort to a newly-admitted patient. However explanations about nursing activities also seem to be able to reduce pain and decrease the incidence of infection. Hayward (1975) investigated the results of giving adequate preoperative information to patients and in his monograph *Information — A Prescription against Pain* he concluded that 'informed' talking is more effective in this context than 'just talking'. Boore (1979) also investigated the effect of preoperative preparation of surgical patients on postoperative stress, and called her monograph *Prescription for Recovery*. She demonstrated that giving information about prospective treatment and care, and teaching exercises to be performed postoperatively, reduced stress in surgical patients after operation. Moreover, the incidence of infection was decreased in these patients.

Change of role

In the adult patient's familiar world many parts are played and there is communication with many people: spouse, offspring, other family, friend, acquaintance, coworker, employer and club-member. He had control over when, how and where he communicated with them. Now he finds himself in hospital, and he has to continue this AL of communicating while assuming the sick role or patient role discussed on page 56.

Family relationships. In hospital, the spouse's communication with the patient, and the reciprocal communication of the patient with spouse, in a setting that includes nightclothes, bed, single or multiple room/ward, is essentially different. Should the visiting spouse be accompanied by offspring or other family members, further modification of the partners' behaviour may be perceived to be necessary. At this sensitive period in these people's lives, such modification can be misinterpreted by any one or more members of this group and may have repercussions in family relationships. Nursing includes 'caring' about the family and what they mean to the patient. Indeed family disruption may have contributed to the illness. After visitors have departed, nurses should pay attention to a patient's non-verbal behaviour as well as to what is said. Nurses should not pry for prying's sake but they need to be sensitive to any cues that all is not well and sensitive to the patient's desire to discuss anxieties.

Reversal of roles. The reversal of roles can cause the patient anxiety. Should the patient be the breadwinner and the person who had attended to the business and financial side of family life, then there will have to be a reversal of roles; these items will have to be attended to by a responsible other person, usually the spouse. And the previous level of frankness and freeness in communication between the spouses about these matters can narrow or widen the possibility of stress between them during these communications in a hospital ward. Money in present-day society is equated with power, consequently few people can bring themslves to communicate their financial hardship because of one family member being in hospital. The added anxiety of unpaid bills can be a result of hospitalisation and can have long-term effects.

Visitors. The reaction of friends to the change of role can be a sensitive matter. A patient may find it difficult to come to terms with which of his friends, co-workers and employers did, or did not, communicate with him during his indisposition. Some of these people may not have found it convenient to visit but may have phoned; some may have 'visited' but not gained access to the ward. It is therefore important that the patient's lines of communication are kept open by relaying these enquiries to him — they are easily jotted on a memo pad to be given to him at a convenient moment.

Information-giver. Another potential problem for the patient is that he finds himself in the role of information-giver, and it is often information of a very personal nature. It is therefore important to understand at the outset that anything communicated to members of the professional staff will be treated as confidential. Members of the public in general are concerned about personal information held by computers. Where health information is stored in computers, it is important that the patient understands the safeguards against unauthorised people gaining access.

Patients may not see the relevance of giving information about their social history when their problem is a physical one. When it is relevant, great sensitivity is required in eliciting such information and telling patients how it helps in planning their nursing. For example, if the person is severely incapacitated and has difficulty in mobilising, it can be important to know whether, when at home, it is necessary to go upstairs to the toilet, or even to an outdoor toilet.

Information-receiver. As already mentioned, an increasing number of research reports shows that a frequent complaint made by patients is lack of information. Some-times the required information is about what tests are going to be performed and why; the results of tests; the medical diagnosis, particularly if for example heart disease or cancer are suspected; how long to expect to be away from work and so on. Whatever the nurse staffing arrangements, several nurses will help the patient during every 24 hours. Each one needs to know what the pateint has been told and what he currently appears to understand. This is an essential part of nursing, not only to reduce patients' complaints but to permit nurses to be accountable to the patients whom they serve.

CHANGE OF DEPENDENCE/INDEPENDENCE STATUS

It is understandable that with an Activity of Living which has so many dimensions, a number of variables can affect the individual's capacity to be independent. Any change in status can be influenced by the age of onset, perhaps congenital; the type of onset, sudden or gradual; and degree of difficulty, ranging from partial to complete; and whether or not the problem is reversible. Some of the main problems which patients can encounter in relation to the AL of communicating are outlined below.

Cognitive problems. Children who are born mentally handicapped frequently do not possess the necessary intellectual ability to communicate verbally. However with patient teaching, many can learn to respond to verbal messages such as greetings and simple instructions, and some are able to learn to speak. For children who are mentally handicapped, non-verbal communication assumes greater importance than usual. Through play, physical contact, hand language and body language, mentally handicapped people can be encouraged to achieve their optimal level for communicating.

Sometimes there is impaired cognition following an illness or an accident. Prior to the event, communication had not been a problem, and this loss of mental acuity may involve drastic changes in lifestyle related to employment and loss of earning capacity, as well as loss of self-respect and hardship to the family. The nurse needs to know how aware such patients are of the impairment, how they experience the impairment, what they feel about it, and so on. They need to talk about what the change means in their lives; whether or not they will be able to communicate sufficiently to continue at work and carry out their leisure time activities. If the patients do not recognise their assets, it is important that they are helped to do so, and positive comment on whatever they accomplish will help them to regain self-respect.

In declining years some people show signs of diminishing skills in thinking and remembering, for instance by giving inappropriate replies while talking with another person. Nurses should continue to talk to these patients as if there were no deterioration, because they do have unpredictable rational periods and at those times they can be mortified at being spoken to as if they were children. Should these patients be at home there must be surveillance to be sure that they can manage the AL of communicating at a safe level.

Speaking problems. Physical dysfunctions can lead to distortion of the voice and cause communication problems. Enlarged tonsils and swollen glands for example may make speaking mechanically difficult. These conditions are usually temporary in nature and reversible. A distortion of longer duration occurs when a child is born with congenital hare lip or cleft palate. These can be corrected by surgery but a considerable amount of speech therapy is required in the post-surgery period to ensure that such children can communicate in a way which is understandable to others.

There are occasions when one is at a loss for words but most people find it difficult to imagine what it would be like to be unable to speak. Certainly one could still see, listen, read, write and communicate non-verbally. So these are the modes which have to be exploited when a patient suddenly loses his ability to speak, whether it be temporary or permanent in nature.

Temporary loss can be produced by for instance a surgical incision of the trachea and insertion of a metal tracheostomy tube to maintain patency. Where possible it is important that the patient understands the nature of the operation, but sometimes it has to be performed in an emergency. The patient will almost certainly be conscious and needs considerable support which the nurse can supply by the manner in which activities are carried out, continuing to talk even although there is no verbal response. A pad and pencil is an alternative means of communicating, and it is important that some means, such as a bell, is within the patient's reach in order to attract the nurse's attention when help is required.

Permanent loss can be induced by surgical removal of the larynx, a laryngectomy. Again the patient needs to understand the permanency of the loss of natural voice production. Usually every encouragement is given to develop oesophageal speech. Air is purposely swallowed into the upper gullet, from whence its gradual release, while using all the other speaking muscles, produces intelligible speech. The nursing contribution involves encouraging the patient to carry out the speech therapist's instructions; not showing impatience as he practises; and not showing embarrassment at the changed voice. The patient can be advised to join one of the self-help groups — Laryngectomee Clubs — which exist to give support and encouragement to people with similar problems.

Aphasia is loss of ability to speak; it is experienced by some though not all people who have a stroke. Depending on the exact location in the brain of the cerebrovascular accident (CVA), so the patient's problems are different. (Miller & Dobson, 1984).

Expressive aphasia is the term used when people know what they want to say, and even though able to move the mouth, simply cannot say it. It is the right-handed person's problem when there is a CVA in the left motor speech area, because the speech area is best developed in the left cerebral hemisphere. It is frustrating because intelligence is unimpaired. Also hearing has not changed, although strokes tend to occur in the older age group who may already have some impairment, so it is important to collect information about hearing ability.

It is also important for the nurse to note whether the patient does manage to speak any word or words. With the objective of the patient speaking an increasing number of words, the nurse puts into practice advice given by the speech therapist. This usually consists of encouraging the patient to say particular words, separately at first to ensure success, then short sentences and so on. Nursing time is much better spent on these exercises than on long one-sided conversations, which may only produce frustration when the patient cannot talk. Indeed great distress can be caused when nurses and relatives do not appear to understand the disability and talk as if to a child. It is more emotionally satisfying if the nurse just stays with the patient from time to time during each day, providing company, a way of showing that he is still valued as a person.

Receptive aphasia is the term used when there is impaired comprehension of spoken and written words, although the patient can still say the words aloud. According to the patient's previous reading ability and hearing acuity, (and this information must be collected) the words can still be seen and heard but there is difficulty understanding and remembering. Receptive aphasia is difficult to recognise as the patient's correct responses may result from practice rather than comprehension. Fox (1976) gives an account of this complicated disability and a useful comparison of expressive and receptive aphasia. The right-handed person can have receptive aphasia when there is a CVA in the left sensory speech area, again because it is best developed on the left side and the fibres cross over. The ability to think and vocalise words is retained, but the words spoken may be out of context. One can imagine being in a foreign country where not a single person speaks your language. That is how life seems to the patient with receptive aphasia and sometimes the resulting distress is expressed as outbursts of anger and tears. The nurse really does need to demonstrate comfort and concern in ways other than vocally.

The patient requires to re-learn association of words with things — the things he needs in everyday living — toothbrush, toothpaste and so on. It is useful to keep these articles on a tray near the patient so that the nurse can encourage extra repetition whenever opportunities are available to spend time with the patient.

Hearing problems. The congenitally deaf or hard of hearing baby has difficulty in acquiring vocal communication skills because of the inability to hear. One of the early assessments of all babies is a simple hearing test so that, should any impairment be identified, specialist advice can be sought early.

Recurrent middle ear infections can produce a problem for young children who are still acquiring basic communication skills; the resulting reduction in hearing capacity can retard the learning process. Of course at any stage on the lifespan an ear infection or even the presence of excessive wax may interfere with hearing. However these are usually transient impediments. It is a different matter when there is a sudden loss of hearing; the person is now in a silent world, and even in the midst of people, there is intense loneliness. Nevertheless visual cues are still received as others glance in the deaf person's direction while talking and, bereft of hearing, the reaction varies. There may be signs of paranoid behaviour; there may be loss of self-respect; the person may become more easily cross and irritable. On the other hand, deaf people may feel so uncomfortable in the company of others that there is physical withdrawal which may well increase the feeling of loneliness.

Everything possible must be done by the nurse to convey to the patient that although deaf, he is still valued as a person and it is worth noting that in Stockwell's study (1972) deafness was one reason for patients being 'unpopular' with nurses. The nurse must use non-verbal language as much as possible paying attention for example to the manner in which she sets down a meal tray. The patient has no loss in cognitive ability or speech and can still pass an opinion about the meal, indeed should be asked to do so. If nurses persevere, patients who are deaf will begin to lip-read and can be encouraged to join a class for development of this skill. To help lip readers, the nurse's face should be at the same level as the patient's, at a comfortable distance to accommodate the patient's vision, and in a good light.

The patient and members of his family may decide that use of a hand language would solve their communicating problem. With practice it can be quicker for the other members than writing the input part of conversation with the deaf person — but of course he can still speak in reply! With tolerance and good humour the problem of communicating can at least be reduced, if not overcome.

If there is even minimal hearing, to help the patient use it when communicating, it may be possible to augment it with a hearing aid. However the aid magnifies every sound and at first some sounds can be startling until the patient learns to filter them out. It needs a lot of encouragement and support during the learning period to use the aid to best advantage. If it is the 'body-worn' type, most people find it works best if worn near the midline on the chest with the microphone facing outwards. It is clipped on to an article of clothing. Nurses should speak slowly and clearly 'to' the exposed microphone and encourage lip reading. With technological developments it is now possible to have small unobtrusive aids which are effective as well as being aesthetically acceptable. In the U.K. the Department of Health and Social Security has produced an excellent booklet, *General Guidance for Hearing Aid Users.*

Seeing problems. A baby may be congenitally blind and from the outset, the parents require careful specialist advice so that other communication channels are exploited to the optimum. When a patient becomes suddenly blind, the problem is different.

People who lose the sense of sight change from a world of light and colour to a world of perpetual darkness. They cannot see their environment or the person to whom they are speaking, so miss all the visual communication cues. They cannot write letters although may still be able to write a signature if the hand is placed exactly where it is required. They cannot read letters and the friendships maintained in this way are no longer 'private' because a nurse or volunteer has to read them to the patient. Of course there are tape recordings, but again they are less 'private'. A phone at home can be modified, but it may be less easy to use the hospital telephone.

When there is a sudden loss of sight the nurse can give more effective help if she understands that people suffering any form of loss go through similar psychological stages to those of grieving (p. 335). The nurse therefore needs to help such patients to deal with, and not deny, the feelings of anger and frustration, and must convey the intended message by voice alone since it is not complemented by visual cues. However the patients still have visual memory of colour, shape, size and so on and can be helped to develop mental images if the nurse describes the environment and what is going on, and encourages others to do likewise. This is particularly important if any treatment is going to be carried out so that the patient knows what to expect but it is also helpful for the patient to have ordinary activities such as a food tray described while the nurse is helping the newly blind patient with a meal. For anyone whose sight has been suddenly impaired, it is important that nurses indicate their approach before touching the patient and that they speak in a normal voice; sudden loud speech will startle the patient.

Some patients may have sudden loss of sight in only one eye and although the human body is amazingly adaptable, it takes some time to adjust to visual communication when half of the usual visual field has been lost. For those who have undergone certain types of ophthalmic surgery the covering of both eyes in the immediate postoperative period, although transient, can be alarming. If such patients are in the older age group, they are usually less adaptable and inability to see can add to the confusion at being in the strange environment of a hospital; in fact, some can become disoriented.

Problems related to impaired sensation. When a person loses the sensation received via the skin the AL of communicating is robbed of the touching component for that area of the body. Touching is an activity which people do not readily talk about. Only when deprived of sensation does a person realise what an important and indeed pleasurable part of communicating it can be.

If the hand is affected such things as handshaking, of course, become merely perfunctory. Loss of sensation also affects the person's ability to receive cues which prevent injury and contribute to maintaining a safe environment. Without the sensation of touch, it is not possible to detect excessive heat, and the skin area may be burned; or the person may bump into sharp objects without realising the damage. It is important that the nurse allows such patients to talk about these problems and help them to work through the stages of 'loss' until they learn to cope with a dysfunction of this type, especially if it is irreversible.

Problems related to impaired movement. When a patient loses the ability to move, the affected area of the body can no longer be used to convey non-verbal messages. According to the extent of the paralysis (Fig. 7.8), so the change in mode of communicating is different as are the compensatory needs to maximise the remaining components of verbal language.

A hemiplegic patient can be deprived of up to 50% of his ability to communicate non-verbally. Hemiplegia is most commonly associated with stroke, a condition caused by a cerebrovascular accident (CVA). When it occurs in the right cerebral hemisphere there is a left hemiplegia because the nerve fibres cross at the base of the brain. A left CVA results in a right hemiplegia, and since the majority of the population is right handed, many people with a left CVA are also deprived of the writing component of communicating.

Furthermore hemiplegia can be accompanied by facial paralysis. The lip lies limp and down-drawn on one side but it may not be conveying the sadness and depression which body language experts associate with down-drawn lips. Facial paralysis may include a drooping eyelid which minimises the eye contact component of body language and the visual input component of verbal language. A left hemiplegia can also interfere with speaking.

Again it is a case of the nurse helping the patient to work through the various emotional stages of coming to terms with lost abilities in the several components of communicating. The patient can be encouraged to write with the other hand. Nurses need to become skilled at recognising cues (other than down-drawn lips) of sadness and depression and dealing with these as seems appropriate. The nurse when communicating with the patient

should be on the same side as the unaffected eye both for the pateint's comfort and to maximise visual input.

Whatever the extent of the hemiplegia, nursing activities include provision of emotional support, and encouragement to re-learn control of the paralysed muscles — as advised by the physiotherapist — so that there will be improvement in the patient's AL of communicating non-verbally and by writing.

The *paraplegic patient* is also deprived of up to 50% of the ability to communicate non-verbally, but it is a different distribution from the 50% of the hemiplegic patient, so the problems are different. The most common cause of the condition is accident and a preponderance of the victims are young males. They cannot move from the waist downwards so they are deprived of their characteristic walk and the other information conveyed by this portion of the body, one of the greatest anxieties usually being related to the communicating elements of expressing sexuality.

Helping the patient with the AL of communicating includes several of the nursing activities given for the hemiplegic patient. However as soon as possible the paraplegic patient is rehabilitated to a wheelchair life, which in itself can present communicating problems. Just as a small child's eye level when standing is at the adult's leg level, so the wheelchair patient's eye level is at most people's waist level. Nurses can help by offering same level eye contact to prevent a feeling of being talked down to — physically, of course!

The *tetraplegic patient* is deprived of most of the ability to communicate non-verbally; retaining only the function for facial expression and eye contact. It is not possible to use a hand to write; otherwise the function for communicating by verbal language is intact. Some of these patients can be encouraged to write holding a pen in the mouth and sometimes they can be encouraged to use a special typewriter by tapping keys with a rod held in the mouth. They too can be rehabilitated in a wheelchair, and same level eye contact helps.

Body langauge problems. Much of present-day knowledge about body language is the result of research on 'normal' subjects. However, there are people who do not have a 'normal' body either in structure or function, with which to transmit such a language. Not only is there a problem in transmission of body language but there is a problem in interpreting the body language transmitted by these people. For example, a congenital curvature of the spine can result in several types of 'hunch back', sometimes accompanied by a drooped shoulder or shoulders. One of the patients' problems is an inability to assume the 'upright' posture with braced shoulders which is characteristic of a confident, cheerful and optimistic mood. They have therefore to express these needs in other ways. Nurses should learn to recognise that the body language of mood and attitude cannot be expressed in the usual way by people who have structural or functional defects which affect posture and gait.

Generalised overactivity is often an expression of anger and frustration. However there are patients who, while not being angry or frustrated, simply cannot relax and sit still; it is characteristic of hyperactive children and some mental illnesses, and can be a problem to the individual and to others in the family. It is usually inadvisable to restrain forcibly such patients as this can make them angry or even violent. Special attention therefore needs to be paid to the environment so that they do not harm themselves or others, as they pace restlessly back and forth or indulge in meaningless movement.

Some patients have a problem with localised overactivity seen as an inability to control one or more muscle groups. For example the arms might swing in purposeless movement, so the patient is unable to communicate by pointing to something that is wanted. Because frequently there is an associated low level of intelligence which precludes acquisition of verbal skills, nurses need to observe these patients' body movements closely, to discover whether or not any message is being transmitted.

Though there may not be structural abnormality, enforced posture such as lying in bed, sitting in a wheelchair or chair can produce body language problems. This is particularly so for eye contact, which is more likely to occur when eyes are at the same level. Nurses can help by being seated when talking to these patients.

Changes in various modes of communicating have been discussed separately in order to give each its importance but in reality, the patient may be adapting to change in several modes simultaneously. For example a patient with a left hemiplegia may have both a sensory and a motor loss; and may have either a receptive or expressive aphasia, or a mixture of both. Because such a patient is likely to be in an older age group, there may also be lessened visual and auditory input, so helping with the AL of communicating is an enormous challenge to the nurse.

Patients in intensive care units also have problems with communicating. Some distressing event has led to their admission; they are surrounded by strange equipment and unusual sights and sounds, including other critically ill patients; and staff carry out frequent investigations and treatments. They may feel too ill or too drained of energy to ask appropriate questions or may get the impression that the staff are much too busy to listen, or may have an injury which impedes conversation or makes it difficult to receive a communication. When patients have difficulty in responding, research has shown that they often receive limited deliberate communication (Ashworth, 1980).

For a patient in coma (p. 326) there is no communication by any mode. However any gradual return to consciousness is often observed as a response to touch. The manner in which a nurse communicates her concern

while for instance bathing an unconscious patient, is obviously important. The stimulus of a constant familiar voice or repetition of a familiar tune — and nowadays these may be utilised in the form of tape-recordings — may eventually produce a response and help to re-establish the patient's AL of communicating.

Of course, a number of patients who are admitted to hospital may have been blind or deaf or dumb or partially paralysed for a period of time. It is particularly important that the nurse discovers what the individual's usual coping mechanisms have been so that as far as possible, the patient can continue these practices and use his limited capacities for communicating to the optimum level.

Obviously communicating is not easy. Patients need and enjoy the human interest of social conversation and this is usually an effective way of establishing the basis of a relationship. But planned purposeful communication is also required. Observing and listening, as well as asking appropriate questions, can help the nurse to assess the timing of planned communication and the level at which the information is given. The nurse's control of non-verbal cues will determine the type of approach and Bridge (1981) in *Speaking without Words* discusses the importance of positioning, posturing and gesturing.

Although effective communicating is not easy, it is possible for the student nurse to learn the skills. A research project carried out by Clark (1981) involves audio tapes and video tapes of actual nurse-patient conversations and underlined the importance of teaching nurses the basic interpersonal skills. It would seem that U.K. students are inadequately prepared for this role (Briggs & Wright, 1982).

DISCOMFORTS ASSOCIATED WITH COMMUNICATING

When there is dysfunction of any of the body structures required for communicating, the patient may experience discomfort. No attempt will be made to give an exhaustive list of discomforts; the following are merely examples. A number of discomforts can arise because of minor injury or infection in the area of the nose/throat, ears or eyes and interfere, in varying degree, with the three more obvious aspects of communicating — speaking, hearing and seeing.

Speaking, for example, can be affected when there is inflammation of the larynx causing laryngitis. Apart from the throat being painful, there may be discomfort on swallowing, and there probably will be accompanying hoarseness or even loss of voice until the infection is brought under control by the body's natural defence mechanisms or use of drugs. Likewise, external pressure over the area of the larynx, caused by parotitis, may affect the voice. In such circumstances communication by means of speech may therefore be affected. Dryness of the mouth also interferes with speech. It may be due to a variety of causes such as reduced fluid intake; or associated with excitement or anxiety; or infection; or it may be caused by the use of certain drugs for example certain anti-emetics and anti-depressant drugs. Dryness of the mouth, of course, is deliberately caused pre-operatively when a drug such as atropine is given to dry up secretions prior to general anaesthesia. Mouth dryness is frequently a feature, too, when parenteral feeding has been prescribed (p.175) and among other things, can inhibit verbal communication at a time when the patient particularly requires interpersonal contact. Unless contraindicated, a drink will relieve dryness of the mouth, a mouthwash may prove helpful, and something as simple as sucking a sweet or medicated lozenge may stimulate salivation sufficiently to relieve discomfort.

Hearing may be affected because of inflammation which is present when there is a boil in the external meatus or when there is a middle ear infection. The associated pain may be relieved by analgesic drugs, and sometimes the application of a suitably protected hot water bottle or electrical heating pad over the area of the ear. The reduced hearing capacity may also be a major problem for the patient.

A discomfort which sometimes accompanies hearing impairment is tinnitus. The intra- and extra-cranial blood vessels in the head and neck, the molecular motion of air within the middle ear, as well as circulating blood in or near the organ of Corti, are all possible explanations of tinnitus (Lindsay, 1983). Almost everyone can hear noises in the ear if in quiet enough surroundings but environmental noise usually masks it. However the tinnitus which accompanies impairment of hearing is said by sufferers to be worse than hearing loss, and the monotonous buzzing or ringing sounds can cause insomnia and depression and total distortion of their living pattern. Drugs do not seem to bring relief; surgery can correct some problems; electrical stimulation of the cochlea may give substantial improvement; but so far, portable masking devices such as an ear-level hearing aid which delivers a continuous masking sound, often closely imitating the distressing tinnitus sound, has proved most successful. Biofeedback techniques have also shown improvements in this distressing condition for some sufferers.

The capacity for *seeing* can be affected by, for example, inflammation of the conjunctiva, or by infection of the eyelash follicle causing what is commonly termed a stye. Bathing the eye, and the topical application of eye drops or antiseptic/antibiotic eye ointments may help to relieve the discomfort but the patient will also be concerned about the accompanying reduced vision. Non-verbal cues may be missed while communicating and the person's usual facility for reading and writing may be impaired.

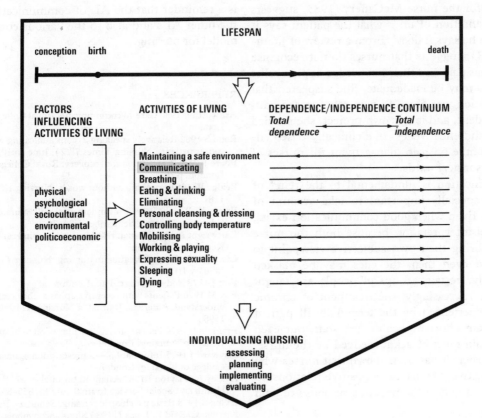

Fig. 8.14 The AL of communicating within the model for nursing

The discomforts mentioned above are only examples but serve to illustrate the general point. Although mostly transient, they do interfere with communicating. A number of these discomforts involves some degree of pain which is specific to the area affected indeed, it may be possible to see the cause of the pain. However patients may complain of pain in any part of the body and in many instances, it is not possible for the nurse to see the cause. In some instances the pain may be associated with a specific AL, for example a respiratory infection causing a pain in the chest. However the pain may be non-specific, for example a patient complaining of headache a few days after abdominal surgery. In such circumstances the patient's communication about pain is apparently unrelated to the current reason for hospitalisation and is entirely subjective regarding site and degree of severity.

Pain is a complex phenomenon experienced by many people but difficult to define. It has already been discussed in Chapter 3 and is also mentioned in relation to each AL. In the proforma for documentation suggested by Roper/Logan/Tierney (p. 349) the nurse would normally chart the incidence of pain in relation to the AL if it is AL-specific, but non-specific pain would appropriately go under the AL of communicating.

Pain has been the centre of a considerable amount of research in a number of disciplines and is acknowledged to have physiological, psychological and sociological aspects. However for the nurse McCaffery (1983) suggests an operational definition. 'Pain is what the patient says it is, existing when he says it does'. From a review of literature, Sofaer (1983) suggests that nurses do not recognise when a patient has pain and their knowledge of pain relief and of analgesics may be inadequate. She suspected that insufficient attention was given to pain relief in the education of the student, and in her own project, she studied the practicality and effectiveness of a clinically-based educational programme on pain management for nurses of all levels in four surgical wards.

Good communication is fundamental to the relief of pain and it is especially important to take account of non-verbal cues. Even when good communication exists, there may be misinterpretation because both the nurse and the patient bring their own subjective viewpoint to the situation and even then, the cues may be masked because culturally, certain groups of people are taught not to complain. Increasingly, the treatment of chronic pain and pain experienced by the terminally ill patient has become a team effort by health care staff, but even more transient pain must be acknowledged by the nurse. As mentioned earlier, it has been shown that nurses who communicate effectively by having a positive relationship with the patient, can affect the patient's response to pain relief.

Not only in pain relief but in all forms of therapy, the communication between nurses and patients plays a vital role. George Eliot, the 19th century novelist, once wrote 'We are all islands, shouting lies to one another across seas of misunderstanding!' Perhaps this is a somewhat jaundiced view but nurses should bear it in mind when considering their approach to patients. In the therapeutic situation, it is the patient who is disadvantaged and nurses must make more positive efforts to improve their communication skills. Effective communicating is a crucial element in assisting patients to cope while regaining or retaining their optimal level of functioning in everyday activities of living.

In the second half of this chapter some of the problems and discomforts which can be experienced by patients in relation to the AL of communicating have been described. This provides the beginning nurse with a generalised idea of these; it will be useful in assessing, planning, implementing and evaluating an individualised programme for each patient's AL of communicating.

This chapter has been concerned with the AL of communicating. However, as stated previously it is only for the purpose of discussion that any AL can be considered on its own; in reality the various activities are so closely related and do not have distinct boundaries. Figure 8.14 is a reminder that the AL of communicating is related to the other ALs and also to the various components of the model for nursing.

REFERENCES

Ashworth P 1980 Care to communicate. Royal College of Nursing, London

Bond S 1982 Relatively speaking 2: communicating with families of cancer patients. Nursing Times 78(24) June 16:1027–1029

Boore J 1979 Prescription for recovery. Royal College of Nursing, London, p 76

Bridge W 1981 Speaking without words. Nursing 1(27) July:1178–1181

Briggs K, Wright B 1982 A fundamental skill. Nursing Mirror 155(9) Education Forum 1 September 1:34–36

Cartwright A 1964 Human relations and hospital care. Routledge and Kegan Paul, London

Clark J 1981 Communication in nursing. Nursing Times 77(1) January 1:12–18

Fast J 1978 Body language. Pan, London

Fox M 1976 Patients with receptive aphasia: they really don't understand. American Journal of Nursing 76(10) October:1596–1598

Franklin B 1974 Patient anxiety on admission to hospital. Royal College of Nursing, London

Hayward J 1975 Information — a prescription against pain. Royal College of Nursing, London

Henley A, Clayton J 1982 Asians in hospital — what's in a name? Health and Social Service Journal July 15: 855–857

Irving S 1978 Basic psychiatric nursing. Saunders, Eastbourne, p 32

Kiernan C, Reid B, Jones L 1983 Signs and symbols. Heinemann Educational, London

Lelean S 1973 Ready for report, nurse? Royal College of Nursing, London, p 14

Lindsay M 1983 The roaring deafness. Nursing Times 79(5) February 2:61–63

Macdonald M 1977 How do men and women students rate in empathy? American Journal of Nursing 77(6) March:998

Marson S 1979 Nursing — a helping relationship. Nursing Times 75(13) March 29:541–544

Mayou R, Williamson B, Foster A 1976 Attitudes and advice after myocardial infarction. British Medical Journal 1:1577–1579

McCaffery M 1983 Nursing the patient in pain. Harper & Row, London

Miller M, Dobson M 1984 Stop, look and listen. Nursing Mirror 158(3) January 18:40–41

Parnell J 1982 Continuity and communication. Nursing Times Occasional Paper 78(9) March 31: 33–40

Raphael W 1969 Patients and their hospitals. King Edward's Hospital Fund, London

Reynolds M 1978 No news is bad news. British Medical Journal 1:1673–1676

Roper N, Logan W, Tierney A 1983 Using a model for nursing. Churchill Livingstone, Edinburgh

Sofaer B 1983 Pain relief — the core of nursing practice. Nursing Times 79(47) November 23:38–41

Stockwell F 1972 The unpopular patient. Royal College of Nursing, London

Whitehead S 1981 The puzzle of peptides — neurotransmitters or gut hormones? Nursing Times 77(3) January 15: 122–123

Wilson-Barnett J 1978 Factors influencing patients' emotional reaction to hospitalisation. Journal of Advanced Nursing 3 May:221–229

ADDITIONAL READING

Bridge W, Clark J 1981 Communication in nursing care. Macmillan, London

Calnan J 1983 Talking with patients. Heinemann, London

Scottish Health Education Group 1981 Health teaching: a nursing activity. SHEG, Edinburgh

Smith V, Bass T 1982 Communication for the health care team. Adapted for U.K. by Faulkner A. Harper & Row, London.

9

Breathing

The activity of breathing

'Taking the first breath' is of crucial importance at the birth of every baby and determines whether or not the infant will have a viable existence as a human being. From then on breathing seems effortless and people are not usually consciously aware of the act of breathing until some abnormal circumstance forces it to their attention.

THE NATURE OF BREATHING

Physiologically speaking, breathing in is called inspiration, breathing out is expiration and the whole process is referred to as respiration. Inspiration is concerned mainly with the intake of oxygen from the atmosphere, and expiration with the expulsion of carbon dioxide.

In a simple, one-celled organism such as an amoeba, the oxygen passes from the air through the cell membrane to permit metabolism within the cell. Complex animals like man, however, with millions of cells, require more oxygen than can readily be taken in by diffusion through an unmodified body surface, hence the need for the respiratory system and its close link with the cardiovascular system.

THE PURPOSE OF BREATHING

The whole point of breathing is to convey oxygen (O_2) from the atmosphere to each cell in the body so that it can create the energy to engage in its various activities. The cell is the basic unit of all life and respiration is the most fundamental of its processes; respiration is needed for all cell activities.

Man, however, is a multicellular organism so the human body must have suitable structures to convey oxygen from the atmosphere to every single cell. This is achieved by the respiratory and cardiovascular systems. Oxygen is breathed into the lungs and there is a transfer point between the thin-walled air sacs (alveoli) in the lungs and the thin-walled blood vessels (capillaries) in the cardiovascular system. Once into the cardiovascular system, O_2 combines with the haemoglobin in the red blood corpuscles and is transported around the body in the bloodstream. In the vicinity of every cell the haemoglobin releases the oxygen and it is transferred from the blood capillary to the cell.

The cell uses oxygen to provide energy for its activities, and in the process carbon dioxide (CO_2) is formed, a waste product of combustion. The CO_2 is conveyed by similar means back through the cardiovascular and respiratory systems to be breathed out as expired air. This whole process of ventilation therefore has several requirements:

- adequate oxygen in the atmosphere
- a functioning respiratory system
- a large moist surface in the lungs where the oxygen and blood are in close proximity to allow exchange of O_2 and CO_2
- a physical 'bellows' arrangement (the thoracic cage) with muscles to operate it and nerves to control the muscles
- a 'transport' system, the blood
- a 'carrier' in the transport system, the haemoglobin
- thin-walled capillaries in close proximity to the cells where O_2 and CO_2 can be exchanged
- healthy cells which are capable of using the O_2 and releasing CO_2

This complex integrated activity is in constant use to collect O_2 from the atmosphere; transport it in the blood to the cells; collect the cells' CO_2; and transport it to the lungs where it is released to the atmosphere. It is evident that the action of the heart and blood vessels are complementary to breathing. It is therefore logical to expect that impairment at any point in this complex sequence of the cardiopulmonary system is going to affect the exchange of gases and the individual's ability to 'breathe'.

BODY STRUCTURE AND FUNCTION REQUIRED FOR BREATHING

As has already been described, the activity of breathing involves two separate body systems — the respiratory system and the circulatory system. To emphasise that the two systems are so inextricably linked, the respiratory system will be discussed as the 'pulmonary aspects of the cardiopulmonary system', and the circulatory system as the 'cardiovascular aspects of the cardiopulmonary system'.

Readers are reminded that the presentation of body structure and function here, as throughout the book, is no more than an outline.

Pulmonary aspects of the cardiopulmonary system: the respiratory system

This system is made up of the following organs (Fig. 9.1):

- the nose
- the pharynx   } upper respiratory tract
- the larynx

- the trachea
- the two bronchi   } lower respiratory tract
- the two lungs and their covering, the pleura

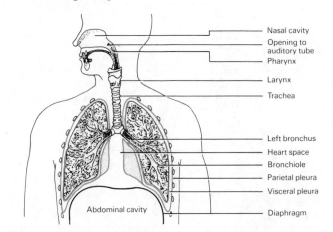

Fig. 9.1 The respiratory organs

Nasal cavity
Opening to auditory tube
Pharynx
Larynx
Trachea
Left bronchus
Heart space
Bronchiole
Parietal pleura
Visceral pleura
Abdominal cavity
Diaphragm

In health the upper respiratory tract is concerned with what might be termed 'air-conditioning'; it is designed to ensure that air which enters the lower respiratory tract is warmed, moistened and filtered.

The nose is the sensory organ for smell and is a funnel-shaped cavity divided by a septum into two nostrils. The openings into the nose are called the anterior nares and when a patient has respiratory distress, it can be observed that the small muscles in the area are dilated in an attempt to get more air into the respiratory system. The rich blood supply in the nose ensures that inspired air is warmed and saturated with the water vapour while the cilia, aided by a layer of sticky mucus help to trap foreign matter.

The pharynx is a muscular, funnel-shaped cavity lying behind the nose and mouth and is a common pathway for both air and food. Posterior to the nose are two openings, the auditory tubes, through which air is conveyed to the middle ear and pathogens may spread from the mouth along this route causing middle ear infection.

Situated in the pharnyx are areas of lymphoid tissue called the tonsils and adenoids which trap pathogenic microorganisms thus helping to prevent infection, but in the presence of severe infection they may become inflamed and cause tonsilitis. Spaces within the bones of the face called sinuses communicate with the nasal cavities by means of narrow openings, and when the above protective mechanisms are ineffective, the sinuses may become infected causing the condition known as sinusitis.

The larynx is made up of several pieces of cartilage, the most prominent of which is the thyroid cartilage (Adam's apple). It is large and more prominent in men than in women and can be easily seen and felt under the skin (Fig. 9.2). Another leaf-shaped cartilage, the epiglottis, is

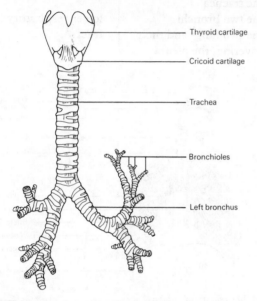

Fig. 9.2 The trachea, bronchi and bronchioles

situated behind the tongue and when saliva, mucus and food are swallowed, the epiglottis closes the larynx so that these substances are directed into the oesophagus (Fig. 9.3). This reflex action prevents particularly food from entering the air passages and when, on rare occasions,

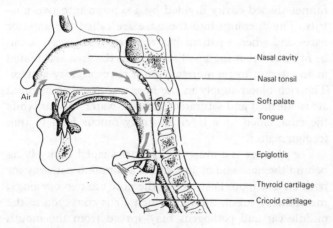

Fig. 9.3 The airflow from the nose to the larynx

something does 'go down the wrong way', a coughing reflex is activated in an attempt to eject this food which is foreign to the air passages.

Stretching across the larynx are the vocal cords and as air is forced through them, sounds are produced so the larynx is sometimes called the 'voice-box', and the tongue is used to convert these sounds into words. In the condition called laryngitis, where the cords are inflamed, the air flow is impeded and the voice may be reduced to a whisper.

The trachea begins at the cricoid cartilage then branches into two main bronchi, one bronchus to each lung. Each bronchus then divides and subdivides and ends in terminal bronchi which communicate with a cluster of alveoli (Fig. 9.4). These alveoli are small air vesicles

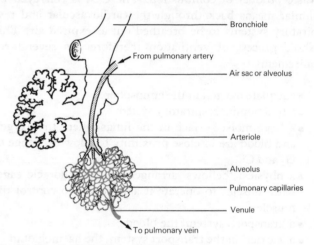

Fig. 9.4 Alveoli with arterioles and venules

bounded by a single layer of epithelium which are in direct contact with the pulmonary capillaries. It is here that the exchange of oxygen (O_2) and carbon dioxide (CO_2) takes place between air in the alveoli and blood in the pulmonary capillaries.

Each lung is enveloped in serous membrane called *the pleura*. Visceral pleura encapsulates the lung substance and it is reflected as the parietal pleura which lines the thoracic wall. In health, the two layers glide on each other but if, for some reason, the pleural space contains air (pneumothorax) or fluid (pleural effusion or hydrothorax), the lung may partially 'collapse' and cause difficulty in breathing.

Pulmonary or external respiration

These terms are used to describe the interchange of oxygen and carbon dioxide within the lungs and there are three aspects to this complex process.

Respiration: muscle control. The lungs themselves have no muscles. They are forced to expand and permitted to contract by the movement of the ribs (achieved by the intercostal muscles) and the diaphragm, a muscular partition between the thoracic and abdominal cavities (Figs. 9.5 and 9.6). Since breathing continues rhythmically even during sleep, these muscles might seem to have an inherent rhythm but this is not so; the intercostal and diaphragmatic muscles are controlled by nerves.

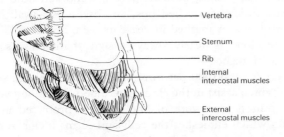

Fig. 9.5 Section of the internal and external intercostal muscles: ribs, sternum and vertebrae

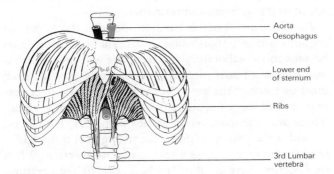

Fig. 9.6 The diaphragm

Respiration:nerve control. The rhythm of breathing is maintained not in the lungs themselves nor in the related muscles but in a nerve centre which is situated at the lower part of the brain, in the medula oblongata (Fig. 9.7). This is the respiratory centre (really an inspiratory centre and an expiratory centre) and from this site rhythmic impulses go to the intercostal and diaphrag-

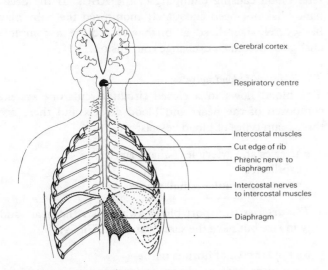

Fig. 9.7 The nerve control of respiration

matic muscles controlling alternately contraction and expansion. The respiratory centre is connected to other parts of the central nervous system (brain and spinal cord) and to the other parts of the body so impulses to the centre can modify the rate of breathing in response to body activities. Breathing stops, for example, when swallowing and when speaking because of impulses from the throat which are conveyed to the respiratory centre.

Table 9.1 The mechanism of external respiration: inspiration and expiration

Inspiration	Expiration
1. The diaphragm contracts on impulse from the phrenic nerve; the intercostal muscles contract on impulse from intercostal nerves.	1. The diaphragm relaxes on cessation of the impulse; the intercostal muscles relax on cessation of the impulses.
2. As the diaphragm contracts it moves down enlarging the size of thoracic cavity from top to bottom; as the intercostal muscles contract they raise the ribs and push the sternum forward, so enlarging the size of the thoracic cavity from side to side and front to back.	2. As they relax, the thoracic cavity is reduced in its three dimensions.
3. The thoracic cavity is enlarged in three dimensions, so there is lower pressure in the lower respiratory tract.	3. As the thoracic cavity decreases in size, the pressure in the lungs is above atmospheric pressure.
4. The lungs are connected to the outside air so it enters the lungs until the pressure equals atmospheric pressure.	4. The lungs are connected to the outside air so air is forced out.

Respiration:chemical control. The rate of breathing, however, is controlled not by lungs, nor by the muscles, nor by the nerves; it is controlled by the amount of CO_2 in the blood. CO_2 acts on the respiratory centre and causes it to send out impulses to the muscles of respiration. The more CO_2, the faster the rate of breathing. If the breath is held, CO_2 builds up in the blood stream and its effect is so powerful that, in spite of himself, the person recommences breathing. It is an inevitable cycle. Utilization of O_2 in the cells leads to the production of CO_2 which circulates in the blood which leads to an increase in the depth and rate of breathing, which leads to an increase of O_2 in the blood for use by the cells, and so on. The mechanism of external respiration is presented briefly in Table 9.1, indicating the sequence in inspiration and expiration.

As already mentioned, the respiratory tract deals only with the mechanism of external respiration; the interchange of oxygen and carbon dioxide at cellular level (internal respiration) is dependent on the existence of the cardiovascular system.

Cardiovascular aspects of the cardiopulmonary system: the circulatory system

The circulatory system has two main parts which communicate with each other and are intimately associated. The blood circulatory system consists of:

- the blood
- the heart and blood vessels

The lymphatic system consists of:

- the lymph
- the lymphatic vessels

The lymphatic system is not involved in the activity of respiration (although all of its cells, like any others, require oxygen) and the circulatory system has many other functions besides the transport of oxygen and carbon dioxide. Nevertheless, these systems will be described briefly at this point.

The blood

Blood is a warm, red, sticky fluid, salty to the taste and one can learn these facts from one's own observations. Examined under the microscope, however, the blood is seen to consist of cell-like objects floating in a clear, slightly yellow liquid called plasma. There are about 6 litres (10 pints) of blood in the adult body.

Plasma is a clear straw-coloured fluid. About 90% is made up of water and in it are dissolved all the food substances; waste products of metabolism; hormones from the endocrine system; antibodies for protection against materials foreign to the body; and anti-coagulant substances which prevent the blood from clotting while in circulation.

Blood corpuscles are the cell-like objects floating in the plasma and there are three types:

- red blood corpuscles
- white blood corpuscles
- platelets

Red blood corpuscles (RBC: 5 000 000 per c mm of blood). These are formed mostly in the red bone marrow and contain an important substance called haemoglobin which combines loosely and reversibly with O_2 so when there is an oxygen-rich environment as in the capillaries in the lungs, haemoglobin combines with O_2. Blood is brighter in colour when the haemoglobin is combined with O_2 so blood in arteries on the way to the tissue cells is bright red while blood in veins returning from tissue cells with the CO_2 is a darker red.

Iron and vitamin B_{12} are needed to form haemoglobin. Iron deficiency anaemia occurs if the individual does not have enough iron in the diet and he complains among other things of tiredness because the RBCs are less able to carry O_2 to the muscles. Lack of B_{12} in the diet causes a condition called pernicious anaemia.

White blood corpuscles (WBC: 8000 per c mm of blood). Some of these corpuscles can squeeze through the walls of the capillaries into the tissues to combat invading microorganisms. They surround and digest materials foreign to the body and in the process, living and dead organisms, WBCs, dead tissue cells, and cell fluid form a semi-fluid mass called pus; an abscess is a walled-off mass of pus. A marked increase in the number of WBCs in the blood is nearly always a sign of infection somewhere in the body.

Platelets (300 000 per c mm of blood). These are small cells which assist in the clotting of blood. If a blood vessel is ruptured a network of fine fibres is produced in the blood which enmeshes the cells and forms a clot to plug the vessel and prevent haemorrhage.

Blood withdrawn for transfusion and for certain tests must be kept fluid and has a chemical, sodium citrate, added to it to prevent clot formation.

Blood groups. When it has been decided that a patient requires a blood transfusion, a specimen of blood must be sent to the laboratory for grouping and cross-matching. Before a transfusion is commenced, a careful check must be made of the group of the donor's blood to ensure that it will be compatible with the recipient's blood. There are four main blood groups named A, B, AB and O, and if the patient is given the wrong group the RBCs tend to clump and cause a severe adverse reaction. When this occurs there is likely to be a rise in temperature, there might be a rigor, the person probably becomes jaundiced and the clumped cells may occlude the kidney tubules and lead to renal failure or even death.

The Rhesus factor is another important constituent of blood. When present, the individual is described as having blood which is Rhesus positive (Rh + ve), and when absent, Rhesus negative (Rh − ve). The Rhesus factor is important in pregnancy. When the mother is Rh − ve and the fetus is Rh + ve there can be an adverse reaction in fetal blood causing clumping of the RBCs. If the pregnancy has not been adequately monitored the baby may be severely jaundiced at birth and require a complete change of blood: an exchange transfusion.

The heart and blood vessels

The blood flows in a closed-circuit circulatory system composed of the heart and blood vessels and there are three main types of blood vessels:

- arteries and arterioles (small arteries)
- capillaries
- veins and venules (small veins)

The arteries transport blood away from the heart and vary in size but have the same structure (Fig. 9.8):

- an outer coat of fibrous tissue
- a middle coat of elastic and muscular tissue which

varies according to the size of the artery; in arterioles there is more muscle and elastic tissue and this is important for the maintenance of blood pressure

- an inner lining of epithelial cells, a 'surface' tissue

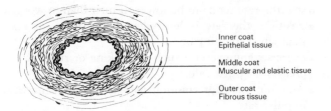

Fig. 9.8 The structure of an artery

The capillaries have walls which are one cell thick and permit the passage of fluid with substances in solution but not the outflow of RBCs or plasma proteins.

The veins transport deoxygenated blood from the tissues to the heart and although like arteries they have three coats, there is less muscular and elastic tissue. Most veins possess valves which prevent a backward flow of blood (Fig. 9.9).

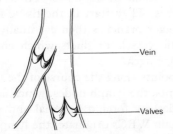

Fig. 9.9 Section through a vein showing valves

The heart. Maintenance of a constant flow of blood through the body requires the application of pressure at some point in such a closed-circuit circulatory system. This is provided by a very efficient pump, *the heart* (Fig. 9.10). In the human, the heart has two distinct parts: the right side of the heart pumps blood to the lungs to collect

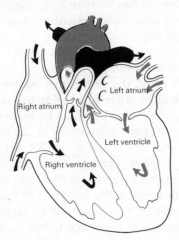

Fig. 9.10 The heart

oxygen and discard carbon dioxide (the pulmonary circulation, concerned with external respiration), and the left side of the heart pumps blood to all tissue cells including its own and those in the lungs (the cellular or systemic circulation, concerned with internal respiration).

The blood coming into both sides of the heart first enters smaller, weaker, upper chambers: the R. atrium and L. atrium. When the heart relaxes, blood surges from the R. and L. atria into the larger, stronger chambers below: the ventricles. The muscles of the filled ventricles then contract, pumping blood out of the heart from the L. ventricle into the aorta and from the R. ventricle into the pulmonary artery. Flaplike valves between the atria and ventricles close automatically and prevent blood moving back into the atria. Similarly, crescent-shaped valves in the aorta and pulmonary artery close and prevent the flow of expelled blood back into the ventricles.

From the very large artery, the aorta, repeated branching distributes blood through the arteries and arterioles to the capillaries, the walls of which allow the passage of O_2, CO_2 and nutrients between the blood and cells: cellular or internal respiration (Fig. 9.11).

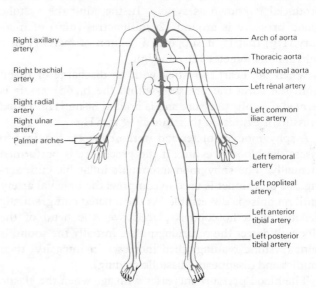

Fig. 9.11 The aorta and the main arteries of the limbs

From the capillary network, the blood moves into venules, the small veins, and progressively larger ones and finally to the two large venae cavae which deliver it into the R. atrium (Fig. 9.12). Once in the R. atrium it goes to the R. ventricle then to the lungs via the pulmonary artery and its branches to discard carbon dioxide and pick up oxygen. From each lung the blood returns via two pulmonary veins to the L. atrium then to the L. ventricle, and so the circuit continues.

Blood pressure
The blood exerts pressure on the walls of the vessels in which it flows. In the living body, arteries are full of

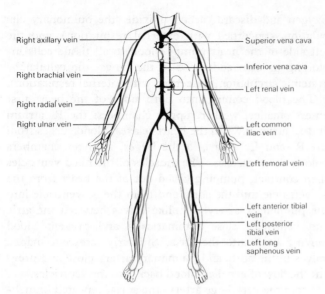

Right axillary vein

Right brachial vein

Right radial vein

Right ulnar vein

Superior vena cava

Inferior vena cava

Left renal vein

Left common iliac vein

Left femoral vein

Left anterior tibial vein

Left posterior tibial vein

Left long saphenous vein

Fig. 9.12 The venae cavae and the main veins of the limbs

blood which causes a continuous stretch in their elastic walls. When the L. ventricle contracts and discharges blood into an already full aorta, the increased pressure produced is known as systole. In the adult the systolic blood pressure is around 120 millimetres (mm) of mercury (Hg) that is, it supports a column of mercury in a sphygmomanometer 120 mm high.

When the heart is resting with no discharge of blood from the aorta the pressure within the blood vessels is termed diastolic pressure and is around 80 mm Hg. Blood pressure is expressed therefore as $\frac{120}{80}$ mm Hg.

A sphygmomanometer and stethoscope are required to assess the blood pressure, if the procedure is performed manually. The sphygmomanometer's inflatable cuff, acting as a tourniquet is used to compress the brachial artery until no pulse is discernible. As the inflated cuff gradually deflates, a stethoscope is placed over the bend of the elbow to detect the returning pulse. Initially the sound is faint (systolic reading) then increases in intensity, then muffles and disappears (diastolic reading).

The blood pressure increases with age when the elastic tissue in the blood vessel walls is less resilient. It also rises during strenuous exercise or when there is an increase in the anxiety level. The reading should normally be recorded, therefore, when the person is at rest and relaxed.

Pulse
Every time the left ventricle contracts, it sends a surge of blood through the arteries under great pressure and a wave passes along the walls of the arteries which can be felt at any point where an artery can be pressed against a bone. The wave travels more rapidly than the blood and in the healthy adult occurs about 70 times per minute. It is most easily felt at the wrist, the site most frequently used for recording the pulse rate.

In health many factors affect heart beat and hence the pulse rate:

- age: the pulse rate in the small baby may be around 140 beats per minute
- sex: the rate tends to be lower in men than in women
- position: the rate is less when lying down, at rest, than when standing up
- exercise: any exercise such as walking or running increases the pulse rate
- emotion: stress or emotion usually cause an increase in pulse rate

As with the blood pressure recording, the pulse rate usually is counted when the person is at rest and relaxed.

Lymph and lymphatic vessels
Fluid and its dissolved substances pass from the blood capillaries into the tissue spaces and hence into the cells and vice versa. However, not all the fluid finds its way back into the blood capillaries directly. In most of the body there is another set of capillaries quite separate from those through which blood flows. These are the lymphatic capillaries. They start in the tissue fluid and join up to form bigger branches then eventually become two large lymphatic vessels or ducts which empty into the large veins of the neck.

At various points along the course of the lymph vessels are enlargements, the lymph nodes, which act as filters to remove and destroy foreign material and it is in these areas that certain WBCs originate: the lymphocytes. The lymphatic system therefore has several functions:

- to return fluid from the tissue spaces to the blood circulation (to the veins in the neck)
- to filter out material which is foreign to the body
- to manufacture lymphocytes which help to combat infection

There are other masses of lymphatic tissue in the body with a similar protective function: the tonsils, the adenoids and the spleen.

Cellular or internal respiration
The main parts of the circulatory system have been briefly described in order to provide the framework for understanding the means by which O_2 is transferred from the pulmonary system, transported in the blood then released to the cells in exchange for CO_2 — the process of cellular or internal respiration. The pulmonary and circulatory systems are inextricably linked as the cardiopulmonary system to allow the full cycle of pulmonary respiration and cellular respiration, and a knowledge of the normal mechanism is necessary before it is possible to understand deviations from normal.

LIFESPAN: EFFECT ON BREATHING

Unlike most of the other Activities of Living, growth and development throughout the lifespan have little effect on breathing. However, the fact that there is a direct relationship between age and the rate of breathing (and also pulse rate and blood pressure) is relevant knowledge in the present context.

Rate of breathing is measured by counting the number of times the chest wall rises and falls over a given period. An infant's rate of breathing may be up to 44 per minute but in children it is about 20 per minute and the range of normal for adults is 12 to 18 breaths per minute. In the older person, however, the breathing rate increases and respirations are shallower. These changes are due to the decreasing elasticity of the lungs and less efficient gaseous exchange between the alveoli and the pulmonary capillaries.

The pulse rate, as has been mentioned (p. 142), also varies in relation to age, the average of 140 beats per minute in the small baby decreasing gradually to around 70 beats per minute in adulthood. Males tend to have a slightly lower rate than females. The pulse rate tends to remain stable at the adult level for the rest of a person's life, unless altered by disease processes.

Blood pressure increases with age. In infancy the blood pressure is around 90/60 whereas in adulthood the average is 120/80, with little change in the later years unless due to the effects of disease. Adults with pressures above 140 mmHg systolic and/or 100 mmHg diastolic are referred to as hypertensive; adults with pressures below 100 systolic are considered to be hypotensive.

FACTORS INFLUENCING BREATHING

Commonly occurring activities such as speaking, laughing and eating cause minor alterations in the breathing pattern, though rarely is the individual really aware of these adjustments. Even in the healthy person, however, a number of factors can in a more obvious way influence the rate, depth and regularity of breathing — such as a degree of physical activity (physical factors); changes in mood and emotion (psychological factors); and, of course, the composition of inhaled air and the presence of abnormal constituents in the atmosphere (environmental factors). The fourth group of factors included in this component of the model — sociocultural factors — is not relevant to this AL and, is therefore, omitted. Under the fifth heading, politicoeconomic factors, control of pollution is mentioned and the problem of smoking is discussed.

Physical factors

During vigorous exercise in the healthy adult an increase in rate is quite normal, because the muscles are requiring more oxygen. To transport the oxygen more quickly, the heart beats faster so the pulse rate is simultaneously increased; in fact, respiration and pulse rates are related in a ratio of 1:4, and an alteration in one is usually accompanied by an alteration in the other. Conversely when the body is resting, particularly when sleeping, the respiratory rate is usually decreased.

Not only rate but the rhythm of breathing can be affected during such physical activities as talking, laughing, eating, singing, yet seldom are these variations given conscious thought. Even sneezing and coughing, if transient, are rarely pondered over as a deviation in the normal pattern of breathing.

In contrast, however, breathing is noticeably affected by smoking. Shortness of breath, persistent cough (sometimes productive) and chest pains are common everyday complaints in people who smoke. Most people are now aware that cigarette smoking is dangerous, causing physical damage to the body systems required for breathing — the respiratory system and the circulatory system. Long-term effects on the respiratory system include narrowing of the bronchioles, ciliostasis, increase in the production of mucus, epithelial changes and decreased gaseous exchange. Short-term effects on the circulatory system include rise in blood pressure; increase in pulse rate; increase in carboxyhaemoglobin causing lowered blood oxygen levels; and disturbed electrical activity of the heart. In the long-term there is increase in free fatty acids causing increased blood viscosity and tendency to platelet clumping, and increase in atheroma formation. The variety of effects occurs because tobacco smoke is made up of many different compounds (Table 9.2).

The three main physical diseases related to smoking are:

- coronary heart disease
- cancer of the lungs or bronchus
- chronic bronchitis and emphysema

Table 9.2 Composition of tobacco smoke and effects of the compounds (Based on HEC 1983)

- Nicotine
A powerful alkaloid which arouses or stimulates in small doses and depresses in large doses. Acts on the central and autonomic nervous system. Effects vary according to the individual and the amount inhaled.

- Carbon monoxide (*CO*)
A gas with a high affinity for haemoglobin. Up to 15% of haemoglobin can be converted to carboxyhaemoglobin, thus preventing it from carrying oxygen. Related to atherosclerosis because CO increases permeability of arterial walls to cholestrol.

- Carcinogens
Mainly found in the 'tar' (condensate from smoke) which is deposited in the smoker's lungs. The tar has been shown to cause cancer in animals (believed it can have same effect on humans).

- Irritants
In the 'tar'. Cause lung damage (e.g. narrowing of bronchioles, ciliostasis).

The risk of heart disease is evident in the fact that the average smoker is about twice as likely to die of a heart attack than a non-smoker. Smoking can also increase the severity of asthma (the effect of carbon monoxide) and hypertension. Many other disease processes are also related to smoking: these include congestive cardiac failure, respiratory infection, angina, atherosclerosis, cancers (mouth, pharynx, larynx, pancreas and bladder) and peptic ulceration. Smoking in pregnancy has harmful physical effects on the fetus, mainly due to a diminished oxygen supply because of the effects of the carbon monoxide.

It is important to recognise that there are two routes for smoke produced by burning cigarettes — 'mainstream smoke' which is inhaled by the smoker and 'sidestream smoke' which goes directly into the air that others breathe. The latter is not filtered and is potentially dangerous to non-smokers, hence increasing concern about what has come to be called 'passive smoking'. People who are chronically exposed to sidestream smoke may have a decreased lung function and may have an increased risk of lung cancer. There may be added danger for people who suffer from lung or heart disease. Children are also affected by sidestream smoke and in smoking households are more prone to chest problems and upper respiratory tract infections.

There is no doubt about the fact that cigarette smoke causes widespread damage to the physical well-being of people, not only to those who smoke but also to those who do not.

Psychological factors

There is a psychological aspect to smoking. One of the problems about smoking is that it produces a state of dependence.

Dependence on tobacco is a form of addiction. In an attempt to help people to recognise the complex set of circumstances which precede the state of absolute dependence on any chemical substance be it tobacco, alcohol or drugs, the World Health Organization has defined three types of dependence:

- *social dependence:* the person depends on a chemical in order to conform to the behaviour patterns of his particular community
- *psychological dependence:* the person depends on a chemical to provide enjoyment and/or suppress or come to terms with mental or emotional conflicts
- *physical dependence:* the person becomes dependent on a chemical for normal functioning

It seems that dependence on tobacco grows insidiously over the years. In many instances it starts as social dependence perhaps even at an early age while at school. It may be that there is oral gratification in having a cigarette between the lips; or the act of inhaling gives a special pleasure; or the feeling of relaxation may be associated with exhaling; or perhaps the greatest attraction lies in having something to do with the hands which would otherwise fidget. Sooner or later there is physical dependence, and many people in spite of determined effort to give up smoking find that they have lost their independence in this action.

Those who do manage to give up smoking may suffer from unpleasant psychological symptoms for several weeks: for example, depression, irritability, anxiety, restlessness and lack of concentration. These are symptoms which result from the withdrawal of nicotine.

Leaving aside the specific subject of smoking, in very general terms the AL of breathing can be seen to be influenced by a variety of psychological factors. Certain emotional events in life can affect the individual's breathing habit. Sadness and grieving, for example, may affect the rate and depth of respirations resulting in audible and visible activities such as sighing and sobbing.

And at some time or another, everyone has had the experience of being suddenly startled; fright is often accompanied by an indrawn, gasping respiration followed by an increase in breathing and pulse rates. The two quite different emotions of anxiety and pleasurable excitement may also cause an increase in breathing and pulse rates and even minor, fairly transient pain can have a similar effect. Emotions, such as anxiety and fear, and circumstances which produce stress, can also increase the blood pressure. High blood pressure (hypertension) is sometimes thought to be caused by stress and anxiety; but the part played by temperament and emotional factors is difficult to assess. However there is no doubt that worry about high blood pressure is only likely to exacerbate the problem.

Environmental factors

The aspect of the environment which is obviously most relevant to consider in relation to the AL of breathing is the atmosphere. It is logical to expect that the composition of inspired air will affect the rate, depth and rhythm of breathing. Atmospheric air is a mixture of gases, it has a variable humidity, it contains microorganisms and it has a temperature characteristic of an area's geographical location and altitude (Table 9.3). But how do these factors affect breathing?

Oxygen. Every cell in the human body requires oxygen and each time a person breathes, 4% of the oxygen content of inspired air is retained for cell metabolism.

At high altitudes, the air has a lower oxygen content than at sea level and even at moderate heights, the human respiration rate will increase in an attempt to compensate. On the other hand, too high a concentration of oxygen would support combustion too readily and be incompatible with life.

Table 9.3 Composition of atmospheric air

Constituent	Inspired air	Expired air
nitrogen	78%	78%
oxygen (O_2)	20%	16%
carbon dioxide (CO_2)	0.04%	4.04%
rare gases	1%	1%
water vapour	variable	saturated
microorganisms	variable	variable
temperature	variable	body temperature 37°C (98.4°F)

Nitrogen. Although present in atmospheric air, it cannot be used by the human body; it is in the form of an inert gas and acts as a diluent to the oxygen.

Carbon dioxide. Exhaled air contains 4% more carbon dioxide than inhaled air. In the process of preserving the ecological balance, plants and other vegetation, during photosynthesis, utilise carbon dioxide by retaining the carbon as a form of food and releasing the oxygen into the atmosphere and so the cycle of gas exchange between humans/animals and the plant world goes on.

Water vapour. The air breathed by humans is moistened by the water vapour in the atmosphere, thus preventing irritation of the respiratory mucous membrane. On the other hand, expired air has picked up some of the body's water so has a higher water content than inspired air, and saturation is reached when the water vapour begins to condense, visible on the breath when atmospheric temperature is low.

If the atmospheric humidity is very high, perspiration lies on the skin and the body cannot cool itself by the process of evaporation. For this reason, living in a very hot climate where there is high humidity can cause discomfort and in extreme cases heat exhaustion, one of the features being respiratory distress.

Environmental temperature. In a temperate climate, at sea level, the environmental temperature is usually lower than body temperature and consequently, some heat is lost from the body with each breath. Most people find this a reasonably comfortable environment for living, working and playing. When the environmental temperature is considerably higher, it is more difficult to maintain a comfortable balance between the human body and the atmosphere and, in extreme cases, heat exhaustion will result. Conversely, when the environmental temperature is low, the loss of body heat may cause chilling of the whole body and hypothermia (see Ch. 13) will result.

Microorganism content. Dispersed throughout the atmosphere are many millions of microorganisms; most are non-pathogenic but some, when inhaled, can cause infection in the respiratory tract, for example the common cold. Microorganisms fall to the floor or settle on objects in a room by force of gravity, and convection currents can recirculate them in the atmosphere and perpetuate the possibility of inhalation by man.

Pollutants. While out-of-doors in and around an *urban area*, man is frequently exposed to possible abrasion of the tissue in the respiratory tract by inhalation of smoke containing minute particles which are the products of combustion in domestic heating systems, industrial furnaces and transport vehicles. Condensation around the solid particles produces fog, often referred to as smog, a reminder that the smoke is the real hazard.

In many large cities, attempts have been made to reduce this health hazard by encouraging the use of smokeless fuels for household purposes. Some governments have passed legislation making it obligatory that grit is extracted before furnace smoke is released into the atmosphere; that street-cleaning machines spray water on the dust before sweeping; that garbage collection vehicles have mechanisms to prevent dust from dispersing into the atmosphere. At an international level, the World Health Organization is studying and monitoring the problem of atmospheric pollution and assisting with the exchange of information about prevention on a worldwide scale so that the air, so necessary to human life, will be less of a health hazard.

In the *work situation*, there may be exposure to respiratory abrasion from industrial waste particles, organic and inorganic, for example from linen, hemp, wool, metal, stone and coal. The coal-mining industry has a long history of protective practices to prevent the onset of the dreaded disease, pneumoconiosis, which develops when coal-dust particles become imbedded in the lung tissue and eventually cause gross impairment in the capacity to breathe. More recently it has been confirmed that inhalation of minute particles of asbestos can cause cancer of the lung and a detailed Code of Practice has been designed in the U.K. to help workers protect themselves from the hazard. In this instance, even more widespread education is necessary because articles such as ironing boards and cooking pot stands have asbestos insets, and householders sometimes use asbestos for lagging pipes and insulating roofs.

Workers who are at risk in these types of industries are encouraged to use the appropriate preventive measures provided and to have regular chest X-rays so that any adverse effects will be promptly detected and treated. At international level, the International Labour Organization (ILO) has taken measures to encourage governments to provide employees with protection from several types of respiratory health hazards.

At *home*, householders can pollute the air by failing to provide good ventilation, thus increasing the concentration of products from expired air. The oxygen and carbon dioxide content does not reach dangerous levels but the increased temperature and humidity is conducive to rapid multiplication of microorganisms. If poorly ventilated, the household atmosphere may also be permeated with unpleasant odours from the kitchen or toilet accommodation. Inhalation of leaking gases from appliances and from paraffin stoves can cause headaches, drowsiness or indeed, in large quantity, may render the occupants unconscious.

One of the most recent and interesting areas of research into ways of combating the ill effects of pollution concerns the use of ionisers (Lim, 1982). In the atmosphere there are positive ions (molecules which contain an electrical charge and which adversely affect human beings, for example causing headaches) and negative ions (which have a stabilising effect on both body and mind). It has been shown that negatively ionised air, for example in the office or classroom, results in improved performance and a feeling of well-being. Lim cites examples, and goes on to discuss some of the various medical settings in which ionisers have been tried out: for example, in burns units; in efforts to combat infection in hospital; and for patients suffering from anxiety and associated stress symptoms. Work on the effects of ionised air is in its very early stages but there appears to be possible application in combating pollution in urban areas, in the work situation, at home — and in health care settings too.

Politicoeconomic factors

Many of the topics discussed in the preceding section have an obvious politicoeconomic dimension: for example, the problem of atmospheric pollution. That problem is primarily a responsibility of government and in many industrialised countries legislation exists to control and reduce the hazards associated with atmospheric pollution for city dwellers and workers at risk. However, individuals have responsibilities too; for example, to comply with the requirement to burn smokeless fuel or to wear a protective breathing mask at work. In such ways individuals minimise risks to others and avoid hazards which might affect their own breathing.

The remainder of this section will focus on the problem of smoking. Mention has been made already of this problem, in terms of its physical effects on the body (see physical factors) and in relation to the development of dependence (see psychological factors). Consideration of smoking as a politicoeconomic issue is yet another perspective on the problem. Most governments are concerned that smoking is a recognised and serious threat to health and are only too aware of the fact that treatment of smoking-related disease is a drain on the finances available for health care. However, at the same time, the government obtains revenue from the tax on cigarettes and so there are two sides to the economics of the problem. From an individual's viewpoint too, smoking has an economic dimension because it is an expensive habit in which to indulge.

The costs can be calculated in human terms too. Over the past two decades there has been an accumulation of evidence which demonstrates that smoking is a prime cause of premature death, disease and disablement in Western society. In the United Kingdon it is estimated that every year 50 000 people die before their time because of smoking, and these deaths account for 1 in 6 of all premature deaths. Cigarette smoking greatly increases the risk of lung cancer which kills over 38 000 people in the U.K. every year. The association of smoking with heart disease, chronic bronchitis and emphysema has previously been mentioned.

The effect of smoking on women's health has become an issue of particular concern. Over the past 20 years it has become more socially acceptable for women to smoke and this trend is reflected in the statistics. Between 1969 and 1978 lung cancer rates in women in the U.K. rose by more than 50% (compared with only 8% in men), and the risk of circulatory and heart disease is especially high for women over 35 and on the contraceptive pill. The effects on the fetus of smoking during pregnancy have already been described (see 'physical factors'). Almost twice as many mothers who smoke have low birth-weight babies (less than 2.3 kg/5 lb at birth) than non-smokers and there is a higher perinatal mortality rate in the first month among babies born to smokers. The harmful effects of smoking during pregnancy must be a cause of concern to any government which, through its health care system, seeks to provide effective prenatal care.

Smoking among children is an equally worrying problem. A number of studies have shown that experimentation with cigarettes may begin as early as 5 years of age (North, 1983). Mention was previously made of the harmful effects of sidestream smoke on children (see 'physical factors'). Children whose parents smoke are more likely to smoke themselves in the future. Any country which invests effort and money in child health services and in education must consider seriously the problem of smoking as it affects children.

Many of the facts about smoking which have been presented in this chapter are derived from information made available by the Health Education Council (HEC, 1983). The fact that the HEC (and its Scottish counterpart, the Scottish Health Education Group) is a government-funded body provides evidence that the U.K. government is concerned to publicise the dangers of smoking and to promote health education activities aimed at encouraging people to stop smoking. Many other groups with health education interests engage in education and mount vigorous campaigns against smoking: for example, ASH (Action on Smoking and Health) which was set up by the Royal College of Physicians, and the National Society of Non-smokers which was founded in 1926 and may be best known for its instigation of an annual National 'No Smoking' Day.

However, the money spent on prevention by the government and all the various organisations is infinitesimal compared to the millions of pounds spent on sales promotion by the cigarette companies. Anti-smoking advertising campaigns play a part in bringing about changes in smoking behaviour but a variety of approaches is needed, aimed at both the individual and at society as a whole. Programmes in schools have a crucial role in attempting to stop people ever starting to smoke; advice and information by doctors and other health professionals remain important, both for healthy people as well as those suffering from smoking-related disease; improved methods to help people to give up smoking are being developed, for example the use of nicotine gum and behavioural techniques; and, for the protection of non-smokers from sidestream smoke, there has been a gradual increase in restriction on smoking, for example in public buildings (e.g. cinemas), places of work and on public transport.

There has, in fact, been an overall decline in the prevalence of smoking in Western countries since the 1950s. In Britain, the prevalence of smoking among men fell from 61% to 46.5% between 1960 and 1975 (although there was a slight increase among women). Smoking has declined most rapidly among the higher social classes of the population and, most notably, among members of the medical profession.

According to Daube (1977) a survey carried out in 1974-75 on the smoking habits of health professionals and school teachers showed that large numbers of doctors have given up smoking. At some time 66% of general medical practitioners had smoked but, at the time of the survey, only 21% continued to do so; 33% of midwives and health visitors were smokers and 48% of hospital nurses. The high prevalence of smoking among this section of the nursing profession has become a matter of considerable concern.

However, to put it into perspective, it is only fair to point out that the rate is much the same as that in the general population. It is disturbing, however, that it appears that many nurses take up smoking during their training (Small & Tucker, 1978). The reason why many nurses smoke, in spite of their direct contact with victims of smoking-related disease, and their knowledge of the harmful effects of smoking, is unclear.

A survey of hospital nurses was conducted by Murray et al (1983) to determine whether certain aspects of nurses' working and living conditions could explain their smoking practices. The proportion of nurses in that sample who smoked regularly was much smaller than that found in other British surveys (e.g. Small & Tucker, 1978), possibly resulting from the higher social background and low rate of parental smoking; and the majority of smokers had started smoking before commencing training. However, the prevalence of smoking and heavy smoking was substantially higher in the final year of training than in the first 2 years. Stress at work was most frequently reported by third year students and was the most important work characteristic related to the nurses' smoking practices.

Hawkins et al (1982) discuss the assumption that the reason for the prevalence of smoking among nurses is the high level of stress exerted on them by their job. They point out that there is no conclusive evidence that nursing is more stressful than other jobs, and that it is extremely difficult to investigate this suggested relationship because of the difficulty of identifying and quantifying occupational stress. Hawkins et al report the preliminary results of a large-scale nationwide survey into smoking and stress among nurses. The smoking incidence among all nurses was found to be 33.6%, ranging from 42.2% among psychiatric nurses down to 14.5% among health visitors. Respondents in the questionnaire survey suggested a variety of sources of stress in their work and relief of stress did emerge as a main reason for smoking. Further research is being undertaken to try to identify those aspects of nursing which are most stressful and, by understanding more about stress in nursing, it may become possible to reduce pressure on nurses and lower the smoking rate within the profession.

In nursing, and in all walks of life, the problem of smoking remains an important health issue of the time. Those who work in the health care services must recognise that they have a responsibility to contribute to the efforts underway to discourage and reduce smoking. Increasingly, governments are recognising that smoking is not just a health problem but one which must be considered an important politicoeconomic issue. How best to combat the habit of smoking and prevent its deleterious effects remains unanswered however and, according to one survey (De Moerloose, 1977), legislative action does not seem to be particularly effective.

DEPENDENCE/INDEPENDENCE IN BREATHING

The dependence/independence continuum in the model of living, which is closely related to the lifespan, serves as a reminder that for all people there are times when a state of dependence is the norm. Breathing is perhaps the only AL which individuals perform independently right from birth throughout the entire lifespan, until the moment of death. In health, changes in dependence/independence status for breathing do not occur and therefore further discussion of this component in the context of the model of living is not required. However, certain illnesses do cause loss of independence for breathing and some of the reasons for dependence (on nursing care, oxygen and mechanical aids) are outlined in the second part of this chapter (p. 151) in the context of the model for nursing.

INDIVIDUALITY IN BREATHING

The purpose of the model of living is to describe how a particular person develops individuality in the Activities of Living. The following is a résumé of topics which have been discussed in the opening sections of the chapter and in the sections concerned with the components of the model of living. These topics are relevant when considering a person's individuality in relation to the AL of breathing.

Lifespan: effect on breathing
- Age vis à vis rate of breathing
  pulse rate
  blood pressure

Factors influencing breathing
- Physical
  - characteristics of breathing (rate, depth, rhythm, sound)
  - level of activity
  - cough (if any)
  - smoking (habits if smoker; exposure to sidestream smoke if non-smoker)
- Psychological
  - dependence on tobacco
  - motivation to stop smoking } smokers
  - knowledge of and attitudes to smoking
  - effects of emotional status on breathing
- Environmental
  - exposure to air pollution
    at home
    at work
  - knowledge of and attitudes to air pollution
- Politicoeconomic
  - knowledge of and attitudes to air pollution
    prevention of smoking-related disease

Dependence/independence in breathing
- Independence normal in health
- Dependence associated with ill-health

Breathing: patients' problems and related nursing activities

Knowledge of the patient's individual habits in the Activities of Living is the basis on which individualised nursing can be developed. Whereas some of the ALs are characterised by tremendous variation in individual habit, this is not so with breathing because it is primarily a physiological function which requires minimal activity on the part of the person. However, as has been described, many different kinds of factors — psychological and environmental, as well as physical — can influence breathing. Ashworth (1979), using three case histories, illustrates the importance and relevance in nursing of this broader perspective on breathing and concludes by saying: 'Good care requires a proper assessment of all the factors relevant to an individual patient.' Therefore, the initial nursing assessment of a patient should elicit relevant information about a person's individuality in breathing, and the various topics noted in the preceding section can be borne in mind by the nurse. Certainly in all cases the patient's age has an important bearing on the characteristics of breathing. If the patient is a smoker, then detailed information about smoking habits should be collected. This may be relevant in the context of understanding the patient's disease; and would be utilised in the context of health education concerning smoking (see suggested reading list, Nursing Times 1983). The kinds of questions which the nurse can bear in mind when assessing the AL of breathing are:

- does the individual breathe normally?
- what factors influence the individual's breathing?
- what knowledge does the individual have about breathing?
- has the individual experienced any difficulties with breathing in the past (or a longstanding breathing problem) and, if so, how have these been coped with?
- does the individual appear to have any problems (actual and/or potential) with breathing at present and are any likely to develop?

The objective in collecting this information is to discover the patient's usual habits in relation to the AL of breathing; whether there is any impediment to independence in breathing; previous coping mechanisms in relation to breathing difficulties; and any current or incipient problems with breathing.

Of course, for patients admitted specifically for investigation or treatment (medical or surgical) of an actual breathing problem, in other words, when there is dysfunction of either of the body systems required for breathing (respiratory system and circulatory system), nursing assessment would require to be much more detailed. In making observations and asking questions, the nurse would bear in mind the patient's medical diagnosis and any information already obtained from the medical records or medical staff. However, it is not within the scope of this text to deal with specific disease processes or their medical treatment. That is not to imply, however, that such knowledge is not necessary — for it is, and many nursing interventions for patients with breathing problems are medically prescribed. Rather, here, the intention is to provide only a general introduction to patient's problems with breathing and related nursing activities, mainly for the benefit of the beginning student.

The healthy individual gives very little conscious thought to the vital, life-long activity of breathing. But when for whatever reason there is some interference with respiratory function, there is need for competent treatment of the cause. The cause may lie in the respiratory system itself, or in the heart; or it could be excessive loss of blood (haemorrhage), resulting in 'air hunger'. Whatever it is, the interference may be sudden and dramatic calling for rapid emergency action and if the difficulty is more than transient, there is a need to provide support for a very anxious, distressed person. The feeling of suffocation and the inability to control such a vital function as breathing can be terrifying. The person with less sensational respiratory difficulty must have equally competent, supportive care because a reduced capacity to breathe can disrupt the function of many other activities of everyday living; and if the incapacity is prolonged, may necessitate a considerable change in lifestyle.

A good nurse can help someone to 'breathe freely' or 'get his breath' in more senses than one, not least by caring for him in such a way that it restores or reinforces the way he sees himself as a worthwhile individual who is respected and valued by others.

Ashworth, 1979.

CHANGE OF ENVIRONMENT AND ROUTINE

Irrespective of the individual's diagnosis, merely coming into hospital can alter the patient's normal breathing activity. The ward temperature may be so warm that the patient feels he is 'suffocating'; or the central heating may reduce the atmospheric water content causing irritation to the nose and mouth; or the odours peculiar to hospital may be unpleasant to him; or the strangeness of the surroundings may be so overwhelming as to produce the rapid, shallow breathing which often accompanies anxiety.

Unless occupying a single room, the patient may also have problems about smoking. If a heavy smoker, he may feel restricted and irritated by rules about limitations on indulging in this activity. If a non-smoker, he may abhor the enforced stay in an atmosphere of stale smoke or may be apprehensive about the fire hazards when fellow patients seem careless about extinguishing cigarettes.

The nurse must be alert to these circumstances and within the constraints of communal living attempt to accommodate the requirements of both non-smokers and smokers, as far as is possible. The risk of fire in hospitals on account of smoking has previously been mentioned (p. 88) and nurses should be vigilant on this account.

CHANGE IN BREATHING HABIT

Many people erroneously believe that problems associated with breathing indicate only disorders of the lungs or upper airways. As mentioned earlier in the chapter, it can be deduced that any alteration to the cardiopulmonary sequence of events associated with respiration will have an effect on the individual's capacity to breathe and the patient may experience problems related to change in rate, rhythm and character of breathing.

Rate
Apart from atmospheric changes, the *rate* of respiration may be increased if there is:

- obstruction in any part of the respiratory tract such as a fragment or a swelling which narrows the lumen of respiratory passages
- loss of functioning tissue in the respiratory tract because of injury or disease
- defect in the intercostal muscles or diaphragm perhaps because of injury, or of the nerves serving those muscles as in poliomyelitis
- defect in the circulatory system such as impaired cardiac action which impedes circulation, or reduction in the size of the blood vessel lumen because of the deposit of fatty plaques as in atherosclerosis
- decrease in the number of red blood corpuscles as in haemorrhage, or reduced haemoglobin in the red blood corpuscles which occurs in iron deficiency anaemia

Usually these defects cause an increase in respiration rate as the body tries to make up for the O_2 deficit by breathing faster but in some instances such as head injury, brain tumours, or meningitis when the respiratory centre is depressed because of oedema, the respiration rate is slower. A decrease is also associated with toxic conditions or with the intake of certain drugs (such as morphine) which depress the respiratory centre; indeed overdosage will cause respiratory arrest.

Rhythm

The *rhythm* involves the time interval between each respiration (which should be equal) and the depth of respiration. Usually deep slow breathing occurs when a patient is in coma, and shallow restrained breathing occurs in for example pleurisy when the patient is attempting to diminish the sharp stabbing pain caused by inflammation of the pleura. In a type of breathing known as Cheyne-Stokes breathing there is a marked and somewhat eerie change of rhythm found in a variety of conditions where the patient is critically ill. It begins slow, shallow and quiet, becomes deeper and noisier then dies away; and may be followed by a short period of apnoea (cessation of breathing), then the cycle recommences.

Character

The *character* of the patient's breathing may also be altered. Loud snoring or stertorous breathing is associated with brain injuries and alcoholism; a harsh grating sound called stridor occurs when there is obstruction of the larynx; a grunting note on expiration may occur in pneumonia; and wheezing is associated with asthma.

These are all subjective assessments and can be detected by the ear unaided, but by using a stethoscope various sounds can be identified which are indicative of the state of the lung tissue: constrictions, consolidation and the presence of excess mucus and fluid.

Moderate change in habit

There are various self-care remedies for mild forms of respiratory distress. Even a common cold causes discomfort when breathing because of congestion in the upper respiratory tract. Distress may be more marked in those who have asthma but bronchodilator drugs prescribed in spray form and self-regulated can bring rapid and dramatic relief during an acute spasm.

Another remedy which can be used at home is the steam inhalation to which menthol crystals may be added; it helps to loosen abnormal secretions in the respiratory tract and thereby eases breathing. A Nelson's inhaler may be used but an ordinary spouted domestic jug and towel serves the same purpose (Fig. 9.13). Whether in home or hospital, care must be taken to ensure that steam inhalation equipment is handled carefully to prevent spillage and scalding, and to prevent irritation to the eyes. When use of steam is dangerous, specially designed apparatus such as a croupette (with canopy) or a croupaire (without canopy) may be used to humidify the atmosphere; they can be used continuously without the exertion of holding equipment and without the anxiety of scalding so are particularly useful for children who have respiratory problems, or for confused patients.

Marked change in habit

For the patient, severe difficulty with breathing (dyspnoea) is a distressing symptom which requires imme-

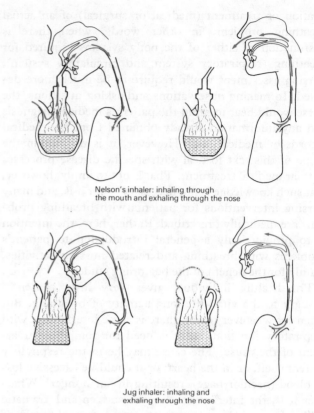

Nelson's inhaler: inhaling through the mouth and exhaling through the nose

Jug inhaler: inhaling and exhaling through the nose

Fig. 9.13 A steam inhalation

diate attention. Though distressing it does in fact indicate that a compensatory body mechanism is attempting to convey more O_2 to the cells. Every movement of the body uses up O_2 and produces CO_2 so it is obvious that everything should be done to spare the patient unnecessary activity. Lying flat, normally the most restful position, is however contraindicated as it further embarrasses breathing; when flat the abdominal organs slide against the inferior aspect of the diaphragm and inhibit its movement and the rib cage also has limited expansion.

The patient must therefore sit up in a well-ventilated room and indeed often requests to be near an open window. In hospital, special beds may be available which help to maintain the sitting position and are often more comfortable for the patient and easier for the staff, but if these are not available, the nurse should be skilful in helping the patient to find a comfortable sitting position well supported by pillows. A bedtable with a pillow on which the patient may lean forward supported on his arms sometimes gives considerable relief and is restful. Many patients find it more comfortable however to sit well supported in an armchair and, at home, a person with chronic breathlessness usually prefers to do so. The inability to breathe except when in the sitting position is called orthopnoea.

Breathing is such a vital activity of daily living and marked difficulty causes the patient great anxiety and distress so the nurse must adopt a quiet, calm manner when carrying out procedures and should anticipate his needs as much as possible.

There are occasions when the breathless patient cannot be lifted out of bed for bed-making, and changing a bottom sheet with the patient in the sitting position is more difficult than when lying flat so every move in the procedure should be planned beforehand so that he is spared unnecessary, oxygen-consuming exertion.

Because he is gasping for air, the patient is breathing through his mouth as well as his nose, and the mouth can become very dry so a drink in a covered container should be at hand, and should a reduced fluid intake be prescribed, a pleasantly flavoured mouthwash can be comforting. Milky drinks may have to be followed by oral hygiene if the mouth is to be kept clean and comfortable and cracked lips require an application of cream or glycerine.

Apart from the change in rate, rhythm and character of breathing associated with respiratory distress, other effects on total body functioning may cause the patient distress. Nervous tissue is particularly sensitive to oxygen deficit and the patient with respiratory problems may show signs of impaired brain function: headache, dizziness, drowsiness, restlessness, faulty judgment, disorientation. The nurse must therefore be on the alert for indications of abnormal behaviour and remember that such symptoms are often reversible if the O_2 supply is improved.

The patient's colour may also be altered. Cyanosis, a bluish tinge in the skin, the lips, the nail beds and in mucous membrane is indicative of respiratory distress. The muscular system too reacts to oxygen deficit and the person tires easily and feels exhausted on very slight exertion. A person who is breathless requires skilful nursing. Activities and relatively minor anxieties with which he would normally cope unaided assume abnormal importance when he is fighting for breath and the nurse must not be irritated by his frequent attempts to seek attention, and to seek reassurance of her presence.

In an attempt to hasten the transport of available O_2 to O_2-deprived cells the heart beats faster to keep up with demand, so the pulse rate as well as the respiratory rate may be greatly increased during respiratory distress. If distress proceeds to imminent respiratory failure, it is a medical emergency and after ensuring that the airway is

clear, mechanical ventilation must be instituted as described in the next section.

CHANGE OF DEPENDENCE/INDEPENDENCE STATUS FOR BREATHING

Obstructed air passages

To maintain independence in the crucial activity of breathing, the most obvious need is the maintenance of a *clear airway* in the upper respiratory tract. A conscious patient will cough to remove obstructions but the semiconscious and unconscious patient must be carefully observed as the cough reflex is depressed and it may be necessary to clear the patient's air passages mechanically. In emergency situations the nurse may have to do this with her finger, suitably protected in case the patient clenches his teeth, but in a hospital setting, clearance may be achieved using a catheter and suction to the mouth or nose, or by inserting an *artificial airway* into the throat in order to keep the tongue forward and the airway patent (Fig. 9.14). The semiconscious and unconscious patient

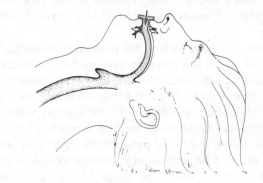

Fig. 9.14 An airway in position

should remain in the semiprone position to facilitate drainage from the mouth and prevent accumulation in the pharynx (Fig. 9.15).

Obstruction due to excessive secretion may however be beyond the reach of an artificial airway or a catheter inserted via the mouth/nose and a *tracheostomy* may be required. An incision is made into the trachea, and a tube inserted and secured in position by tapes tied at the back of the neck (Fig. 9.16). The air entering a tracheostomy is not warmed, moistened and filtered as normally occurs

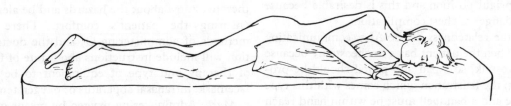

Fig. 9.15 Positioning of an unconscious patient

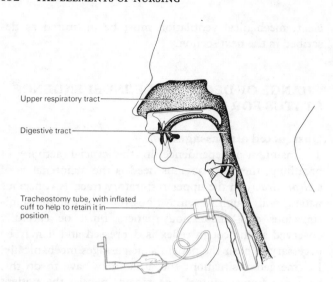

Upper respiratory tract

Digestive tract

Tracheostomy tube, with inflated cuff to help to retain it in position

Fig. 9.16 A tracheostomy tube in position

in the nose and upper respiratory tract so the patient is more liable to infection. The removal of secretions by suction is therefore performed using a sterile catheter and gloved hands and the inner cannula of the tube can be removed for cleansing and replaced by a sterile substitute cannula.

To the conscious patient, tracheostomy suctioning can be a most alarming procedure and must be carefully explained, although when the use of a tracheostomy is a long-term measure, the patient may eventually be taught to suction himself. If this is done, he is often relieved to be in control of the situation and less dependent.

In the initial stages the patient may develop an irritation of the skin around the tracheostomy but a soothing keyhole dressing under the flange of the tube usually brings relief. The tapes holding the tube in position may cause distress and should be checked to ensure that they are sufficiently tightly tied to hold the tube securely without causing skin irritation. When soiled, the tapes should be changed not only for comfort but for prevention of infection, and the patient may be concerned about the appearance. It is not common but there are occasions when air gets into the tissues around the tube and it causes a rapidly spreading puffiness in the surrounding tissue which crackles when touched. The surgeon must be informed so that he can relieve the obstruction and ease the patient's discomfort and distress.

Usually the patient who has a tracheostomy will want to sit in an upright position and this is desirable because it lessens the danger of chest complications.

Reflecting the relatedness of the ALs, communicating is a problem when the patient has a tracheostomy because he is unable to talk, so a pad and pencil should be provided to lessen the frustration which comes with this type of dependence and a handbell must be within hand reach so that he can summon help (see also Ch. 8). Sometimes

a light gauze dressing is placed over the opening of the tube and when the patient is shown how to place his finger over the dressing, it is possible though difficult to speak.

Initially there may be difficulty with feeding and sometimes thickened fluids are easier to manage than thin liquids. Mouthwashes and mouth care are comforting and also help to prevent infection.

With the aid of a tracheostomy, excessive secretions which are reachable by insertion of a catheter can be removed but there may be secretions at a lower level in the respiratory tract, impeding the passage of O_2 from the alveoli to the capillaries. *Postural drainage* may be needed for this problem.

It is important in the first instance to teach deep breathing exercises. The patient is then helped into a position, depending on the site from which secretions must be drained, which will encourage the excess mucus and pus to move by gravity into contact with healthy tissue and initiate coughing. Postural drainage usually involves leaning over the side of the bed then coughing and spitting into a large receptacle placed on the floor which is suitably protected by a disposable paper sheet so the nurse must ensure privacy as this is a somewhat undignified position to adopt, and most people dislike coughing and spitting in public. The physiotherapist in these circumstances can be an important member of the health team and may assist with vibration and percussion movements over the affected lung area, but the nurse usually has to assist the patient. The appearance and odour from the sputum may cause the patient distress and the receptacle should be removed as soon as possible.

The exertion involved in this technique of postural drainage usually leaves the patient exhausted and the nurse must help him into a comfortable position in bed to recover then provide facilities for sponging his face and hands and for rinsing his mouth. Despite the unpleasantness to the patient, postural drainage can bring quite dramatic relief especially in the morning after wakening: secretions gather during sleeping hours when there is relatively little change in body position.

Oxygen insufficiency

When there is prolonged reduction in the O_2 content of the patient's blood, the lack must be corrected by the addition of O_2 to the inhaled air and if the nurse is to give intelligent sensitive care she must understand the therapy, know about the hazards and be alert to means of ensuring the patient's comfort. There are various methods of administering O_2 and the doctor's prescription will include instructions about rate of flow, duration of therapy and type of equipment to be used usually facemask, intranasal apparatus or oxygen tent.

Mask. Administering oxygen by means of a face mask allows a high concentration to be reached rapidly and maintained, so it is often used in emergency situations. A Polymask is reputed to give a 60% concentration when flowing at 6 litres per minute and is useful for most acute episodes of respiratory distress (Fig. 9.17). For chronic conditions, a much lower concentration of O_2 is desirable and the Venturi mask gives about 25% concentration when oxygen is supplied at 4 litres per minute; the mask is designed so that the patient breathes in atmospheric air mixed with the pure oxygen.

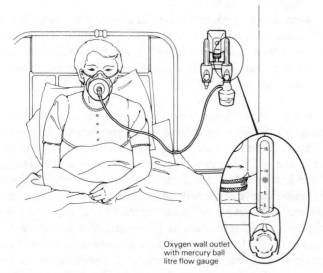

Oxygen wall outlet with mercury ball litre flow gauge

Fig. 9.17 Administering oxygen from a piped supply using a flowmeter, humidifier and mask

If it is a patient's first experience, the placing of a mask on the face of a person who is already breathless can be frightening and the nurse must remain with him until his anxiety is at least diminished if not completely allayed, and encourage him to control the rate and depth of inspiration. The mask is positioned over the bridge of the nose and mouth and secured lightly by means of retaining straps over the back of the head. It must be checked frequently to ensure that it is as comfortable as possible and not chafing the skin.

While the mask is in position, it is not possible for the patient to talk and this barrier to communication increases his anxiety so a call bell must be within reach to summon assistance. Understandably, the mask must be removed for eating and drinking, so during meals, it should be dried and the patient should be given facilities to sponge his face before the mask is replaced. Attention should be given to mouth care and cracked lips.

Intranasal apparatus may be used for O_2 administration by means of a catheter, or oxygen spectacles with nasal attachments, or a nasal mask which leaves the mouth uncovered. This type of equipment is less restricting and permits speech, eating and drinking without removal but it can be irritating to the nasal cavities which should be cleansed and lubricated at frequent intervals.

Intranasal apparatus can be just as frightening to the patient as an oxygen face mask, and even more so, an oxygen tent can create tension and anxiety.

Tent. When a patient requiring oxygen is restless or confused, it may be necessary to use an oxygen tent which is placed over the top of the bed allowing the patient to sit in an O_2 enriched atmosphere. All practical nursing procedures are performed through zipped slits in the tent.

Not surprisingly the patient feels very dependent, isolated and apprehensive because although the tent is made of transparent material, he feels cut off from people and from ward activities. The nurse must therefore use every possible opportunity to communicate with the patient.

Except when the Venturi-type mask is used for chronic respiratory conditions, the oxygen must be moistened before it reaches the patient and this is achieved by passing it through a humidifier. The oxygen supply may be piped to the ward or it may be stored in cylinders which stand at the bedside and cylinder changes should be effected outside the ward as the noise involved in changing a cylinder head can be acutely distressing to an already anxious patient.

Emergency O_2 equipment in the ward should be checked daily to be ready for use, and empty cylinders must be clearly marked and removed from the ward precinct as quickly as possible.

Any supply of oxygen presents a fire hazard. It is the nurse's responsibility to ensure that when oxygen is in use, a warning notice is placed on the cylinder and the dangers explained to the patient, his visitors and to fellow patients. Smoking is forbidden; mechanical toys, electric bells and heating pads are removed; bedmaking and hair combing should be done with care to avoid creating static electricity; and every member of staff should know how to use the nearest fire extinguisher and raise the fire alarm.

A more detailed account of the various methods of delivering oxygen to the spontaneously breathing patient is provided in an article by Levi (1979). Some of the equipment in common use is illustrated, and there is an outline of the advantages and disadvantages of each piece of equipment. Methods of humidification in common use are also described.

Many nurses express anxieties about the prospect of having to use equipment for administering oxygen, humidification or for assisted ventilation (which is the topic of the next section). Most of the equipment is in fact relatively straightforward to use if manufacturer's instructions are followed carefully, and opportunity for supervised practice following demonstration is provided. It is essential for nurses to know how to check that the equipment is functioning properly, how to clean it after use and, most importantly, how to minimise the patient's discomfort while it is in use. After all, the nurse's primary responsibility and concern is for the patient and not the machine, but that priority is only possible if the nurse feels familiar and confident with the equipment concerned.

Mechanical defects

Anything which interferes with the mechanics of breathing is going to cause problems for the patient. A defect in the respiratory muscles or the nerves supplying them means that the patient cannot breathe without mechanical assistance. Artificial ventilation can be divided into two groups; those operating on the principle of negative pressure on the outside of the chest (the traditional 'iron lung', though now modified) and those operating on the principle of positive pressure which forces air into the lungs by means of a power driven source causing the lungs and chest to expand. Levi (1979) describes these two types of ventilators (referring to them as 'external body ventilators' and 'lung ventilators') and their uses. Some of the machines in common use are illustrated in photographs, providing a useful source of material for nurses who are not familiar with ventilators.

Patients who require artificial ventilation are highly dependent for the AL of breathing and they and their families require considerable emotional support.

Ashworth (1979) considers that of all types of respiratory problems, the greatest difficulties are experienced by the patient whose breathing is being maintained artificially via a tracheal tube and who is also paralysed by drugs or the pathological condition which caused the respiratory failure. She says:

Speech and other forms of communication may be impossible except perhaps blinking of the eyelids and other small movements. It can be very frightening to be unable to indicate needs or feelings, and also very frustrating. To add to the problem, even experienced nurses may find it very difficult to go on talking to someone who appears unresponsive, who cannot talk, move, smile or perhaps even open their eyes.

In a small study in five intensive care units it was found that there was a correlation between the amount of communication by the patient and by the nurse: the less the patient communicated, the less intentional communication there was by the nurse. An awareness of this should encourage nurses to seek to maintain communication (and to encourage relatives to do so too) even with apparently unresponsive patients, for the reason Ashworth gives:

To someone who is aware yet totally helpless and unable to control even his own breathing, it is essential to have people to talk to him by name about things which interest and concern him, if he is not to lose his sense of identity and to feel like 'just another body in a bed'.

Respiratory failure

Acute respiratory distress, whatever the cause, may progress to respiratory failure which can result in cardiac arrest because of the functional interdependence of the two systems. Cardiac arrest is characterised by absence of pulse, blood pressure and heart beat, and by dilatation of the pupils. Irreversible damage to the brain and cardiac tissue may take place in 4 to 6 minutes so assistance must be summoned immediately and cardiac arrest emergency procedures commenced without delay. Every hospital has its own policy but the principles are identical:

- ensure an adequate airway; remove obstructions manually or by suction
- extend the neck and insert an airway if available, then commence artificial ventilation; mouth-to-mouth or mouth-to-nose ventilation or use a resuscitation bag
- commence artificial circulation by external cardiac massage (Skeet, 1978)

Episodes of respiratory/cardiac failure and its treatment inevitably raise ethical issues associated with resuscitation. When, for example, the person is terminally ill, or in the older age group, or for some reason is suffering from irreversible brain damage, the case for resuscitation is sometimes questioned; also, if it is unlikely that the person will survive without the aid of sophisticated life-support techniques such as prolonged mechanical ventilation. These instances can only be judged on individual criteria. The decision to commence resuscitation techniques and to discontinue them is usually made by a team of health professional staff, and often close relatives of the patient are involved in the decision.

DISCOMFORTS ASSOCIATED WITH BREATHING

Cough

Coughing can cause considerable distress to the patient, may interfere with many daily activities and may even prevent him from sleeping. If sputum is produced the patient should be helped to cough in order to remove the excess secretions and reduce the possibility of superimposed infection. Postoperatively, especially after thoracic and abdominal surgery, the patient is encouraged to do deep breathing exercises and to cough for this very reason. It is reassuring for him if the nurse 'splints' the surgical incision with her hands as the patient has a great fear that the sutures will give way because of the muscular effort involved.

Coughing is a frequently encountered respiratory discomfort and is really a reflex protective mechanism used by the body to expel foreign material from the respiratory tract. There are various observations which the nurse should make:

Character. A 'dry' cough has little expectoration; a 'loose' cough is associated with the production of sputum; a short restrained, suppressed cough accompanies pleurisy and pneumonia; there is a short, frequent, dry cough in early tuberculosis; a breathless, distressing cough is associated with cardiac conditions.

Duration and frequency. A cough is described as continuous in untreated pneumonia for example, and as spasmodic in asthma.

Time. With many disease conditions coughing is worse in the morning when the patient awakens and changes body position.

Effect on the patient. A cough can be irritating but shallow, or it may involve strenuous effort and leave the patient exhausted.

Expectorant drugs may be prescribed when a cough is productive of sputum, but when it is unproductive, irritating and preventing sleep, soothing cough syrup can be given to reduce discomfort and permit longer periods of rest.

Sputum

Sputum is usually the outcome of coughing. It is a secretion poured out from the irritated lining of the respiratory tract and consists mainly of mucus but if associated with an infection, pathogens will also be present.

The patient can be very distressed by the appearance of sputum and by having to spit in front of other people. If the amount is small, he may prefer to spit into a tissue which is folded and placed immediately into a disposal bag at the bedside. Otherwise he may use a disposable sputum mug which has the lid replaced when not in use.

There are several observations of the sputum which the nurse should make:

Quantity. The daily amount may have to be measured.

Consistency. In acute conditions sputum is sticky and tenacious; in long-term conditions it is often more fluid; if associated with infection it is purulent.

Colour. Sputum is usually greenish-yellow in the presence of pus; blood stained in mild tuberculosis and pneumonia.

Odour. Malodorous sputum is usually associated with infectious conditions such as abscess of the lung, bronchiectasis or pulmonary gangrene and large quantities of foul-smelling sputum are expectorated (it is this type of condition which often requires postural drainage).

Haemoptysis

Coughing up blood is called haemoptysis and may vary in severity from mere streaking of the sputum, a common symptom in bronchitis, to a massive haemorrhage. Coughing up frank blood is alarming to the patient and to those in the vicinity, so the bed should be screened. The nurse should remain with the patient and he should be helped into a comfortable position, which usually by choice will be sitting up supported by pillows. Unless massive and resulting in sudden death, the bleeding will stop provided the patient can rest quietly. Usually a se-

dative is ordered immediately and the calming effect of the drug enables the patient to control the cough and to use it effectively instead of dissipating energies in useless coughing bouts which merely aggravate the bleeding. Soiled linen should be changed and removed as quickly as possible, the face and hands should be sponged and a mouthwash offered. Careful observation is subsequently required and restlessness may be an indication that a further episode will occur.

However small in amount, haemoptysis should be considered as potentially serious and should be reported. Carcinoma of the lung and pulmonary tuberculosis are common causes of haemorrhage.

Allergy

Allergy can cause discomfort in breathing. Substances in the atmosphere which have no obvious adverse effect on most people can cause acute discomfort to those who are allergic. Attacks of sneezing with profuse watery nasal discharge, nasal obstruction and watering of the eyes are associated for example with the condition known as hayfever, which is probably an antigen-antibody reaction. The usual antigen is pollen from grasses, flowers, weeds and trees and as grass pollen is the most common cause in the U.K., the disorder is at its peak during May to July. Allergies may however also be due to odours or fumes or sudden changes in temperature. The episode usually lasts for a few hours and can be controlled by drugs such as decongestants and antihistamines although often a complete cure cannot be found. Allergies are an inconvenience rather than a disease but can be disrupting to social life and to domestic/work activities.

Pain

Chest pain may be caused by injury to the thoracic cage and muscles or associated with cardiac conditions, and pain in any part of the body may cause alterations in the normal breathing pattern. But pain in relation to the respiratory tract itself is of two main types:

a. pain made worse by coughing and experienced behind the sternum — the type of pain associated with inflammation of the trachea
b. sharp, stabbing pain made worse by deep breathing and coughing and caused by inflammation of the pleura

Note should be made of the site, onset, duration, and intensity and any precipitating factors. As with pain of any kind every attempt should be made to remove the cause or minimise the effect and if these measures are unsuccessful, to help the patient to handle pain. In many instances, assisting the person into a comfortable position will help and someone with pleuritic pain will usually lie on the affected side. If an unproductive cough is the cause, soothing cough syrup may alleviate the discomfort and if antibiotics are prescribed for an inflammatory condition they will counteract the infection and therefore relieve the pain-producing inflammation.

Pain is common to most chest injuries particularly when ribs are fractured. It is usually experienced in the back and is aggravated by movement especially deep breathing and coughing. Often the patient feels less distressed if supported in a sitting position. In most instances where the pain is a result of fracture it decreases within about 5 days of the injury but during these painful days it is important for the patient to know that he will be handled gently and that he will be offered analgesics when necessary. It may be adequate to give them by the oral route but if the pain is severe, analgesics by injection are indicated and in some instances the intercostal nerves are infiltrated with local anaesthetic to control the pain level.

There are instances when chest pain which affects the activity of breathing is really cardiac pain sometimes referred to as angina; the site is characteristically behind the sternum or across the chest. It is usually described as being crushing in character and there may be radiation down one or both arms or even into the neck and shoulders or through to the back. The patient is profoundly shocked and cardiac arrest may occur. This pain which is a feature of myocardial infarction must be relieved so that the shocked state may be reversed. A number of patients with this condition are admitted to intensive coronary care units which have highly specialised health teams skilled in emergency treatment.

Anxiety about investigations

Sometimes investigations which are carried out to assess dysfunction in the respiratory system cause discomfort or pain. Probably the most commonly used investigative technique is X-ray which is not in itself painful, although it may cause discomfort if performed in conjunction with the introduction of an opaque dye to outline the bronchi and bronchioles, a bronchogram. Respiratory function tests are sometimes prescribed and they may cause discomfort. A bronchoscopy on the other hand, may be painful and can be alarming; a tube is passed into the upper respiratory tract and the tissue lining can be viewed by means of a lens in the eyepiece. In all these procedures, the patient will have some anxiety about what he will be expected to do, how he will react and what the result will be.

The nurse must therefore take time to explain any preparation involved prior to the procedure, and what to expect during and after. Any relevant instructions about the patient's expected behaviour should be stated clearly and simply. Factual information about the preparation and technique will be found in the ward procedure book

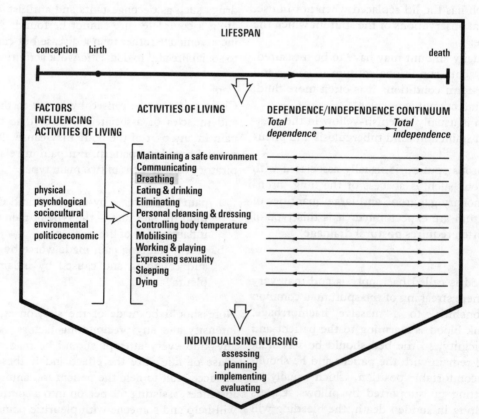

Fig. 9.18 The AL of breathing within the model for nursing

but the nurse must interpret it to the patient according to her perception of his preparedness to receive the information; and on the basis of assessed level of comprehension, perhaps most important of all, in response to the patient's own expressed fears and anxieties.

In the second half of this chapter some of the problems and discomforts which can be experienced by patients in relation to the AL of breathing have been described. This provides the beginning nurse with a generalised idea of these; it will be useful in assessing, planning, implementing and evaluating an individualised programme for each patient's AL of breathing.

This chapter has been concerned with the AL of breathing. However, as stated previously it is only for the purpose of discussion that any AL can be considered on its own; in reality the various activities are so closely related and do not have distinct boundaries. Figure 9.18 is a reminder that the AL of breathing is related to the other ALs and also to the various components of the model for nursing.

REFERENCES

Ashworth P 1979 Psychological and social aspects of respiratory care. Nursing 1st Series (November) 7: 295–299
Daube M 1977 No smoke without fire. Nursing Times 73(10) March 10: 330–331
De Moerloose J 1977 Legislative action to combat smoking around the world. WHO Chronicle 31: 362–372
Hawkins L, White M, Morris L 1982 Smoking, stress and nurses. Nursing Mirror 155 (15) October 13:18–22
Health Education Council 1983 The facts about smoking: what every nurse should know. HEC, 78 New Oxford Street, London WC1A 1AH
Levi T 1979 Breathing equipment Part 1 (Oxygen therapy and humidification) Part 2 (Ventilators and humidifiers) Nursing 1st Series (September) 6:260–263 and (November) 7:336–339
Lim D (1982) Clearing the air. Nursing Times 78 (6) February 10:256–257
Murray M, Swan A V, Mattar N 1983 The task of nursing and risk of smoking. Journal of Advanced Nursing (March) 8:131–138
North N 1983 Smoking: stopping them starting. Nursing Times Community Outlook 79 (44) November 9:343–347
Skeet M 1978 Principles and practice of first aid. (Cardiac arrest.) Nursing Mirror Supplement February 23 146:8
Small WP, Tucker L 1978 The smoking habits of hospital nurses. Nursing Times 74(49) November 16 :1878–1879

ADDITIONAL READING

Allan D 1984 Patients with an endotracheal tube or tracheostomy. Nursing Times 80(13) March 28:36–38
Bailey R 1979 Drugs and the respiratory system. Nursing 1st Series (November) 7:315–318
Brown SE 1979 Respiratory physiotherapy and the nurse. Nursing 1st Series (September) 6:257–259
Faulkner A 1983 Nurses as health educators in relation to smoking. Nursing Times Occasional Paper 79(8) April 13:47–48
Howe P 1979 The respiratory effects of surgery. Nursing 1st Series (November) 7:324–327
Jackson H 1979 Nursing care of patients with chest injuries. Nursing 1st Series (November) 7:303–309
Knepil J 1983 The control of breathing. Nursing Mirror 156(19) May 11:44–45
Maxwell M 1983 Everything you need to know about shock. Nursing Mirror 156(12) March 23:17–19
Nursing Mirror 1982 Respiratory emergencies. Clinical Forum 3 154(11) March 17:i–xvi (A pull-out supplement containing 6 articles to present an overall picture of medical and nursing care required by patients admitted to hospital with acute respiratory illness.)
Nursing Times 1983 Helping people to stop smoking. Nursing Times 79(23) June 8: 63–65 A description of, and extracts from, the teaching packs produced for nurses (one for hospital nurses, one for nurses working in the community) by the Health Education Council, PO Box 415, London SE 99 6YE (or in Scotland, from SHEG Network, PO Box 4000, Glasgow G12 9JQ.)

10

Eating and drinking

The activities of eating and drinking

Human life cannot exist without eating and drinking, such is the essential nature of this activity. It takes up a considerable part of each day since apart from the time involved in eating a meal, food has to be procured and prepared; indeed in some instances it has to be grown by the individual family. In most cultures it is the women who select, buy and cook the family's food. However in many industrialised societies, with the movement towards a greater sharing of parental and domestic activities, this is beginning to change and men are playing a much more active part in matters related to food and feeding.

THE NATURE OF EATING AND DRINKING

The human body is a highly complex collection of millions of cells. The cycle of each cell's growth and development as well as the constant cell activity requires an energy source, and the source of all energy used by the body is obtained from eating and drinking. At subsistence level, human beings will eat almost any available food, often in its raw state, in order to meet the basic need for sustenance. In more affluent societies however, it is possible to make a choice about what will be eaten; there probably will be a mix of cooked dishes and food in its natural state; and quite elaborate rituals may be associated with the setting, the utensils used, the presentation of the meal, and the choice of accompanying drinks.

Nearly all solid food has a high water content but as most of the body consists of water, an additional intake of fluid is essential to continued human existence. Actually the newborn baby's diet is entirely fluid in the form of milk or water but as children get older, they quickly learn that fluid intake can consist of a wide variety of beverages.

Human milk of course is the natural food for infants, and the sucking reflex is present at birth. As the baby grows, milk on its own does not supply enough nutrients to satisfy appetite so semi-solid and solid foods are introduced to the diet; and the child becomes proficient in chewing as the teeth appear. The sense of taste is developed too. Milk is somewhat bland in flavour and as solids are added, the child learns to experiment with a variety of tastes. Nevertheless even in the same family, there are individual differences related to food and drink; there may be marked likes and dislikes, some of the family may have large appetites and some small, some may be quick eaters, some may be slow. Even at a young age, each individual is consciously aware of this essential AL of eating and drinking; indeed throughout life, the waking day is punctuated by meals — breakfast, lunch, supper or some variation on these words — and many other Activities of Living are arranged around them.

THE PURPOSE OF EATING AND DRINKING

The basic purpose of eating and drinking is to provide the fluids and the nutrients necessary to permit growth of body cells until adult stature is reached. Thereafter, throughout life, the water intake and nutrients replenish the substances needed in all the cells to maintain an adequately functioning body. An original view that the number of cells capable of storing lipid as white fat can be increased by overfeeding during infancy but remains constant thereafter, has been modified (Ellenborgen, 1981). Recent studies indicate that the estimated 30 billion cells capable of storing fat can increase at any age. It has been found that, in animals, what has been termed 'brown' fat — it contains cytochrome oxidase — makes up about 1% of the total fat and until recently, the maintenance of body temperature during hibernation and in the newborn was believed to be the chief function of brown fat. Some studies by Rothwell and Stock raise the possibility that it may play a critical role in the prevention of obesity during increases in calorie intake, but for humans, according to Ellenborgen, this has not yet been proven. The study of food and the associated biological processes of growth, maintenance and repair is known as the science of nutrition and an outline of this subject is given.

Providing nutrients is the biological reason but eating and drinking also serve several other purposes in everyday living. During family mealtimes, for example, eating plays an important part in learning about the culture. The meal provides an opportunity for the young child to learn about the rituals of serving food, about the vessels from which different foods are eaten, and about the utensils used for certain items in the diet.

As the child explores relationships with people both within and outside his family circle, he begins to appreciate that food can have considerable social significance concerned with interpersonal relationships. In almost all cultures, eating and drinking are considered social occasions and offering a meal to visitors is one overt way of expressing friendship and hospitality. Eating and drinking in most societies are also an integral part of such diverse family ceremonies as birth, marriage and death; and of some national holiday festivities and religious festivals.

It is not surprising therefore that deep-rooted beliefs and attitudes are associated with the AL of eating and drinking.

BODY STRUCTURE AND FUNCTION REQUIRED FOR EATING AND DRINKING

As a member of the health team, the nurse is in a strategic position to educate the public in the community and in the hospital about the principles of healthy eating and drinking habits. But to utilise available opportunities, it is necessary to have a background knowledge and in this section there is a brief outline of the basic constituents of food followed by an outline of the digestive system.

Nutrition
From every country in the world comes an enormous variety of foodstuffs but when analysed, they can be classified into a few essential constituents:

- carbohydrates
- proteins
- fats
- vitamins
- mineral salts
- dietary fibre
- water

To function effectively each cell in the body requires these substances, and to maintain health and efficiency the individual must have a balanced intake daily of all these constituents. Carbohydrates, proteins and fats are oxidised in the body to provide it with energy and the amount of energy produced by these different nutrients can be measured. In many countries, it is assessed in heat units called Calories — the weight-watcher frequently maintains that he is 'watching his Calories'. Since 1975 however, the United Kingdom has adopted the kilojoule (kj), the SI (Système International) unit for dietetic calculations (see Appendix 4). The kilojoule requirement for an individual varies with height, weight, age, sex, climate and occupation but roughly speaking, the daily intake for an adult female with a sedentary job might be around

8000 kJ (2000 C), for a pregnant woman around 12 000 kJ and for a man doing heavy physical work 16 000 kJ. To provide a balanced diet, a person on a diet of 8000 kJ (2000 C) might have:

about 4400 kJ (1100 C)
    carbohydrates   = 55% of the total
about 1200 kJ (300 C)
    proteins   = 15% of the total
about 2400 kJ (600 C)
    fats   = 30% of the total

Vitamins, mineral salts, dietary fibre and water are essential to health but do not provide kilojoules of energy.

Carbohydrates. The starches and sugars are composed of carbon, hydrogen and oxygen and are found in foods such as sugar, potatoes, cereals, fruit and vegetables. Before they can be used by the body they must be reduced to glucose.

1 gram of carbohydrate yields 16 kJ (roughly 4 C)

Carbohydrates provide heat and energy and can be stored in the liver as glycogen but when eaten in excess are deposited in the fat depots of the body as adipose tissue.

Proteins. The body relies on proteins for its supply of nitrogen, but they also contain carbon, hydrogen, oxygen, sulphur and phosphorus; they are broken down to amino-acids prior to absorption. Protein foods are, for example, meat, fish, eggs, milk products, soya beans, peas, beans and lentils.

1 gram of protein yields 17 kJ (roughly 4 C)

These foods supply the essential amino-acids for building and repair of body tissue. For this reason, children require a higher proportion of protein foods than adults, and people who have been ill may be prescribed a high-protein diet to replace damaged tissue and to replace weight loss.

Fats. Carbon, hydrogen and oxygen are present in fats but in different proportions to carbohydrates and before they can be absorbed they must be broken down to fatty acids and glycerol. There are two main groups: animal fats and vegetable fats. Animal fats are present in dairy products and in bacon, oily fish, meat; vegetable fats are found in, for example, margarine and nuts. The fatty acids present in most 'hard' fats like butter and lard are called saturated fats and it is thought that if there is a high content in the diet, they are a factor in causing high blood pressure, arteriosclerosis and other circulatory disorders.

1 gram of fat yields 37 kJ (roughly 9 C)

In the body, fatty deposits are found around delicate organs like the eye or kidney to protect and maintain their position, and fats also have an important function in transporting fat-soluble vitamins but the general function of fatty foods, as with carbohydrates, is to provide heat and energy.

Vitamins. Good health is dependent on vitamins and most cannot be manufactured in the body so they must be obtained from food. Vitamins are chemical compounds which are classified into two main groups:

fat-soluble vitamins: A   D   E   K
water-soluble vitamins: B   C   P

Vitamins are required in only small amounts. In many instances this function is catalytic, as components of enzyme systems involved in essential metabolic reactions. Although not supplying energy to the body, some are needed for the regulation of energy; and some are needed for the regulation of tissue synthesis. They are required therefore for the general health of tissues and gross deficiency can lead to specific disease conditions for example rickets (lack of vitamin D); scurvy (lack of vitamin C); beri-beri and pellagra (lack of vitamin B). Vitamins are found in many foods; the fat-soluble are mostly in dairy products, fat meat and fish oils; and the water-soluble in fresh fruit and vegetables, nuts and the germ of cereals.

Mineral salts. Although required only in small quantities, these inorganic elements have many essential roles. They are components of body tissues and fluids, and of many specialised substances such as hormones, transport molecules and enzymes. For example, calcium and phosphorus are required for teeth and bone production; iron is required for red blood corpuscles; iodine is needed for the hormone secreted by the thyroid gland, an endocrine gland; sodium is important in the maintenance of the fluid volume in the body.

Sodium is an example of an electrolyte and the balance of the various electrolytes in the body is of critical importance. An electrolyte is formed when an inorganic compound such as salt (sodium chloride) is dissolved in water and dissociates into two or more electrically charged particles. For example, in the body, sodium chloride (Na Cl is the chemical symbol) is present in solution as sodium (Na^+) and chlorine (Cl^-). The desired range of the different electrolytes in the cell fluid and in the extracellular fluid is known. When, because of disease or loss of fluid from the body this electrolyte balance is upset, the function of body cells may be grossly impaired. Mineral salts are widely dispersed in foods — meat, fish, dairy products, vegetables — and are needed in very small quantities.

Dietary fibre. The cellulose part of food which passes through the digestive tract and is excreted as part of the faeces is called dietary fibre. It does not at any time become part of the body structure but its bulk helps to stimulate muscular movement in the large intestine and promotes defaecation thus preventing constipation. There is also evidence that the breaking down of fibre by colonic bacteria makes the stool more acid and this is one of the reasons why fibre is believed to reduce the amount of possible carcinogens (Burkitt, 1983).

Water. The chemical symbol H_2O represents water and signifies that each molecule is composed of two parts hydrogen to one part oxygen. Water is essential to life and makes up about two-thirds of the body weight. Death will follow if there is water deprivation for more than a few days as many body processes are dependent on its presence: water is the main constituent of all body fluids; many physiochemical changes take place in the environment of the body fluids; most nutrients and cellular waste products are soluble in water.

In a 24-hour period the adult human requires about 2500 ml of water and if the intake is inadequate or if the loss of water is excessive (urinary output does not usually exceed 1500 ml per day) the person will experience the sensation of thirst.

In most instances, food and fluid intake is controlled by appetite and thirst. There are centres in the brain which are sensitive to changes in the levels of blood glucose and other nutrients and to the body fluid content.

But to understand how the foods we eat and drink are transformed into substances which can be absorbed into the body and used by the cells, it is necessary to know about the basic structure of the digestive system.

Digestive system

Many complex activities take place within the digestive tract which is virtually a tube, about 10 metres in length, stretching from the mouth to the anus. As food passes through this tube it is broken down by physical and chemical agents until it is reduced to a form suitable for absorption: glucose, amino-acids, fatty acids and glycerol.

The activities of the system can be classified as:

- *ingestion:* taking food into the system
- *digestion:* breaking down the food physically into small particles so that it can be acted on effectively by chemical substances called enzymes, which are produced by various glands in or close to the tract
- *absorption:* absorbing the end products of digestion into the bloodstream mainly in the area called the small intestine for transportation to all the body cells
- *elimination:* excreting non-absorbable substances and the waste products of the breakdown processes

Elimination will be discussed in Chapter 11 and here the digestive system will be described only as it relates to the first three functions: ingestion, digestion and absorption. The structures involved in these activities are:

- the mouth
- the pharynx
- the oesophagus
- the stomach
- the small intestine

and to assist with these activities, various secretions are released into the system from:

- the salivary glands
- the gastric glands
- the pancreas
- the liver
- the intestinal glands

The mouth. This cavity is involved in the reception, mastication and swallowing of food (Fig. 10.1). Various structures in the mouth are sensitive to stimuli which are interpreted as texture and temperature of food, but the main organ of taste is the tongue. Its taste buds pick up stimuli from dissolved foods which are interpreted by the brain as flavour and help to make eating and drinking a pleasurable activity.

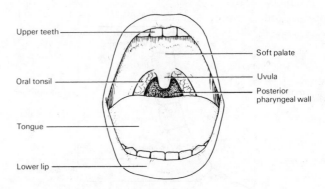

Upper teeth

Oral tonsil

Tongue

Lower lip

Soft palate

Uvula

Posterior pharyngeal wall

Fig. 10.1 Structures seen in the open mouth

The mechanical breakdown of food is commenced by the teeth (Figs 10.2, 10.3 and 10.4); because of their shape and arrangement they can bite, chew, tear and grind food. Then the muscles of mastication in the mouth and tongue contract and relax alternately to break down large particles of food into small particles thus providing a large surface area for the action of saliva.

Normally, three pairs of salivary glands (Fig. 10.5) constantly produce the watery fluid called saliva and it keeps the mouth healthy and sufficiently moist to facilitate speech. In response to the sight, smell and thought of food however, the glands produce more saliva in order to lubricate, moisten and soften the food and to release an enzyme. This enzyme begins the chemical digestion of

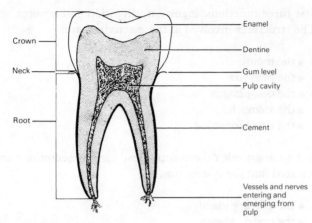

Fig. 10.2 Structure of a tooth

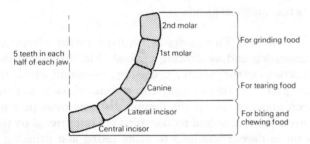

Fig. 10.3 The milk teeth

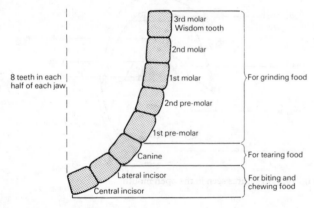

Fig. 10.4 The permanent teeth

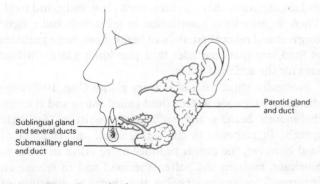

Fig. 10.5 The salivary glands

food by acting on complex carbohydrate molecules so that they are reduced to a less complex form.

The pharynx. This is a tube-like structure which receives the food when it has been sufficiently moistened by saliva and formed into a soft mass or bolus; it is then ready for swallowing. By an upward movement of the tongue, the bolus is pushed backwards into the pharynx, a muscular funnel-shaped cavity behind the nose and mouth. The bolus is gripped by the muscles of the pharynx and propelled into the oesophagus but on its way it passes over the top of the larynx. The mechanism whereby food in the pharynx is simultaneously prevented from regurgitating through the nose and from being inhaled into the larynx is illustrated in Figures 10.6 and 10.7.

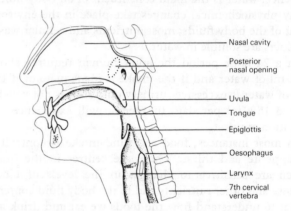

Fig. 10.6 The pharynx

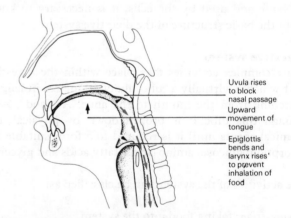

Fig. 10.7 The pharynx during the act of swallowing

The oesophagus. This is the muscular tube which passes from the pharynx down through the diaphragm into the stomach. The mucous membrane which lines the oesophagus produces mucus to lubricate the food as it goes down into the stomach by peristalsis, a movement produced by contraction and relaxation of the muscular wall. At the lower end of the oesophagus the muscle fibres form a sphincter, at the cardiac orifice. The presence of food in the upper oesophagus stimulates the peristaltic action which eventually propels the bolus through the cardiac orifice into the stomach (Fig. 10.8).

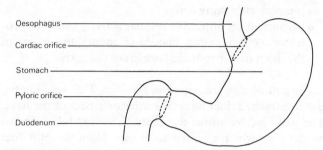

Fig. 10.8 The stomach

The stomach. Lying below the diaphragm, the stomach is a muscular sac where food is mechanically broken down by the peristaltic action of the muscle wall and mixed with the gastric juice produced by the glands in the stomach lining. Gastric juice consists of water, mucin, hydrochloric acid, mineral salts, enzymes, and the intrinsic factor. The water and mucin lubricate and liquefy the food; the acid has a disinfectant effect; the enzymes assist the chemical breakdown especially of protein foods; the intrinsic factor is needed for the formation of red blood corpuscles and lack of intrinsic factor causes the condition called pernicious anaemia. The stomach acts as a temporary food reservoir allowing the gastric juice time to act on the foodstuffs; then eventually food passes through the sphincter called the pylorus and enters the small intestine (Fig. 10.9).

The small intestine. About 7 metres in length, the small intestine lies in the abdominal cavity rather like a coiled tube and is surrounded by the large intestine. The first part is called the duodenum. It is C-shaped with the curve enclosing the head of the pancreas and into it flows

pancreatic juice from the pancreas and bile from the liver. Bile is important in that it emulsifies fats, but apart from this participation in the digestive process, bile is needed for the absorption of vitamin K; it also colours the faeces and has an aperient action.

Like the rest of the digestive tract, the small intestine has muscular walls and is lined with mucous membrane. But in this region, the mucous membrane is thrown into folds which increases the surface area, and projecting from the surface are myriads of small finger-like processes called villi, each containing blood capillaries and lymph capillaries (lacteals) into which food is absorbed. Between the villi are the glands which produce the intestinal juice (Fig. 10.10).

The alkaline pancreatic and intestinal juices (a contrast

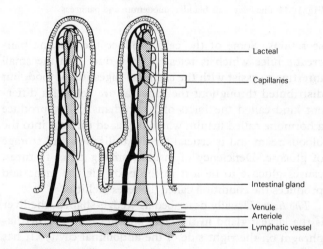

Fig. 10.10 Two villi

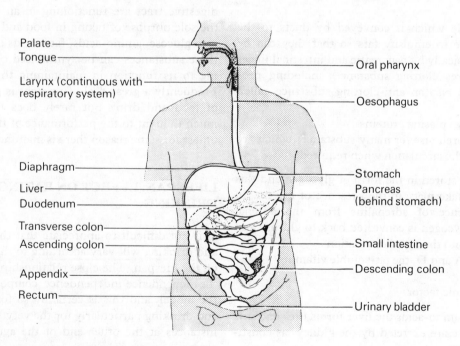

Fig. 10.9 Anterior aspect of the organs in the digestive system

to the acidity of the gastric juice) complete the chemical breakdown of foodstuffs into glucose, amino-acids, fatty acids and glycerol ready for absorption into the villi.

The pancreas is an organ which lies in the abdominal cavity behind the stomach with the head lying in the curve of the duodenum (Fig. 10.11). It produces two

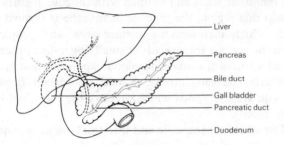

Fig. 10.11 The liver, gall-bladder, duodenum and pancreas

secretions. Some of the cells produce the alkaline pancreatic juice which is released via a duct into the small intestine to assist with the chemical digestion of food, but distributed throughout the pancreas are cells of a different kind called the Islets of Langerhans. They produce a hormone called insulin which is passed directly into the bloodstream and is crucial for the utilisation and storage of glucose. Deficiency of insulin, among other features, causes glucose to be lost to the body via the urine and produces the condition called diabetes mellitus.

The liver. Usually described as wedge-shaped, the liver is the largest gland in the body and lies beneath the diaphragm on the right side of the abdominal cavity. It has many important functions which necessitate intensive cellular activity:

- it secretes bile which is conveyed by ducts to the small intestine to emulsify fats so that they can be acted on chemically by pancreatic and intestinal juices
- it manufactures clotting substances including pro-thrombin and also an anti-clotting substance called heparin
- it manufactures plasma proteins
- it acts as a storehouse for many substances which are released into the circulation when required:
  a. glucose is stored in the form of glycogen and this can only take place in the presence of insulin. In the presence of adrenaline from the adrenal glands, glycogen is converted back to glucose and released into the blood circulation
  b. vitamins A and D, the fat-soluble vitamins
  c. iron
  d. anti-anaemic factor
- from excess amino-acids the liver forms urea and uric acid and these are excreted by the kidneys as constituents of urine

- it inactivates many drugs
- because of the intensive cellular activity the liver produces a considerable amount of energy and is one of the main heat-producing organs of the body

The gall-bladder and common bile duct. This small organ and its attached duct lie on the inferior aspect of the liver. The gall-bladder stores the greenish yellow bile secreted by the liver which at intervals passes down the bile duct to the duodenum to emulsify fats, then passes on in the small and large intestines to colour and deodorise the faeces. When for some reason the duct becomes blocked (by a gall-stone within the duct or an external neoplasm compressing the walls of the duct) and bile is unable to enter the duodenum, it passes into the blood circulation and colours the skin; the patient looks yellow and is said to be 'jaundiced'. If this occurs, the faeces are pale, fatty and foul-smelling and as the bile is then excreted by means of the kidneys, the urine has a dark orange appearance.

The peritoneum. A serous membrane lines the abdominal cavity; it is called the peritoneum and it is reflected over the organs within the cavity. It secretes serous fluid to prevent friction, yet at the same time it gives support to abdominal organs and also provides support for blood vessels and nerves. A long loose fold of peritoneum, rather like an apron, dips down from the stomach and lies in front of the abdominal organs. This omentum, as it is called, contains lymph nodes and fatty deposits so helps to protect abdominal organs against infection, and is also a physical protection and a fat depot.

These complex structures in the upper part of the digestive tract are functioning in an integrated way for the sole purpose of taking in food and fluid and reducing it to glucose, amino-acids, fatty acids and glycerol so that these substances can be synthesised by each cell according to its function in maintaining the body's activities. Frequently a great deal of thought is given to the choice of food and drink but rarely does the individual give much thought to the performance of the digestive system unless for some reason there is malfunction.

LIFESPAN: EFFECT ON EATING AND DRINKING

It is not difficult to appreciate that the activity of eating and drinking will vary according to the individual's stage on the lifespan. The close relationship of the lifespan and the dependence/independence component is integral to the model, and this is certainly so for the AL of eating and drinking particularly for the very young, and in some instances at the other end of the age spectrum for the elderly.

The AL commences *in utero*. The physical growth and development of the fetus is dependent on nutrition received from the mother via the umbilical cord, so the quality and quantity of the maternal diet is important throughout pregnancy and features highly in health education during the prenatal period. Nevertheless it is incredible how a woman with a very low nutritional intake can still provide nourishment to a growing fetus — admittedly at the expense of her own strength and health.

Currently, if the mother has decided to breast-feed, it is customary to put the newborn infant to the breast almost immediately after delivery. It is said that attitudes to food are influenced by the baby's early experiences with feeding and if these were associated with warmth, pleasure and satisfaction, then attitudes will probably remain positive throughout life. In the infant stage of the lifespan, breast milk provides nutrition for the baby in the form which is most suited to human infants. Provided the mother is taking a reasonable diet, the constituents of breast milk are present in the correct ratio for the infant's digestive system; and the milk is sterile, at the correct temperature, and available without elaborate preparation. Breast feeding is also considered desirable for the baby's emotional growth as the close proximity to the mother promotes a feeling of security.

For a variety of reasons however, artificial feeding may be the method of choice. In these instances, dried milk preparations are frequently used. It is most important that the amount is carefully calculated using the measuring spoon provided in the packet, and the prescribed measure of liquid. Otherwise the baby may develop an electrolyte imbalance which can lead to a dramatic disruption of his physiological processes. Provided the feed is accurately prepared and the bottle and teat are scrupulously cleaned and then sterilised, the mother can provide a feeling of security for her child by, among other things, cradling the baby in her arms during the feed.

As the infant grows, milk is no longer adequate for nutritional requirements and the process of weaning from breast or bottle-feeding begins. Semisolid foodstuffs, usually cereals, possibly fortified with minerals and vitamins, are offered on a spoon. The baby therefore has to develop a different eating skill; instead of sucking he has to cope with food on a spoon and manipulate the semisolid in his mouth before swallowing. Not surprisingly there is initial awkwardness and time must be given to experiment.

Eventually he begins to handle the spoon himself and lift the food to his mouth. He experiments with gripping and controlling the spoon and tracing the spatial pathway from plate to mouth. The resultant 'messiness' is inevitable but patience and the presence of a warm supporting mother or mother substitute permit him to acquire the necessary dexterity. Gradually, solid foods such as egg, fish, meat and cheese are introduced into the diet and eventually the child becomes independent in the necessary skills for eating and drinking.

During adolescence, abnormalities of appetite are believed to be more common and in extreme cases may lead to anorexia nervosa with a severe slimming regime, weight loss and vomiting after eating. Conversely, there may be excessive appetite (bulimia) leading to obesity. Usually, however, adolescents expend a great deal of energy and have large appetites which, in the Western world, increasingly seem to be satiated by high energy snacks rather than traditional meals.

The variation in food and drink preferred by adults is legion and the variety becomes more obvious when there is a multiracial society. Health education related to food and drink is currently popular in most Western cultures and has prompted numerous commissions to investigate what should be recommended as a 'balanced' diet or 'prudent' diet or 'healthful' diet — the latest term favoured by the U.S.A. Food and Nutrition Board of the National Academy of Sciences. There is considerable concern about the 'balance' of the various constituents because, apart from the extremes of undernutrition and excess, certain diseases are reputed to be directly related to dietary intake. For example in affluent countries, coronary heart disease, sometimes even in young adulthood, is a major problem and various investigations have pointed to dietary causative factors especially high cholesterolaemia and the excessive intake of foods rich in saturated fatty acids. Controversy still exists however and in a report published in 1983 'Proposals for nutritional guidelines for health education in Britain' (Health Education Council) a government paper is cited which makes no recommendations about cholesterol reduction in the diet, or about the substitution of polyunsaturated by saturated fatty acids.

Going to the end of the lifespan the elderly person often has less appetite for food; there is usually less physical activity so there is not the same requirement for the energy-giving foodstuffs. There may also be less interest in cooking and preparing a meal for one, if the person is living alone, and hastily prepared snacks often do not provide the necessary vitamins, minerals and dietary fibre. It is a sad reflection on the welfare state that many elderly people admitted to hospital are suffering from malnutrition either as a primary or secondary reason for admission. The most frequently occurring manifestations of malnutrition are severe weight loss and cachexia, iron deficiency anaemia, folate deficiency, scurvy and osteomalacia. Being housebound may be due to apathy or dementia but a physical disability also may make it difficult or impossible to go out for shopping. There is usually an increasing dependence on others as the old person moves to the end of the lifespan and this will probably influence the choice of food and drink, and perhaps reduce the pleasure usually associated with this Activity of Living.

FACTORS INFLUENCING EATING AND DRINKING

Eating and drinking play a significant part in the everyday living pattern of all age groups and for most people they are pleasurable activities. However, there are many factors which can influence this AL and affect the individual's reaction to food and drink. The various factors are described, using the categories which appear in the model under the headings of physical, psychological, sociocultural, environmental and politicoeconomic factors.

Physical factors

To benefit from the nutrients in food and drink, a functioning digestive system is needed but most of its functioning is not seen and is rarely given much thought by the healthy person. Most obviously, a normally formed mouth is required for eating and drinking. There are problems for babies who for example are born with what is called a hare-lip and/or cleft palate which diminishes the sucking action; usually a flap is fitted to the teat or the baby is spoonfed until surgical repair is undertaken. Adequate natural teeth or dentures are also required if solid foods are to be properly chewed although edentulous people can remain well-nourished by taking nutrients in semisolid and fluid form.

Apart from the digestive tract itself, if independence in feeding is to be achieved and maintained, at least one functioning upper limb is needed. Even a transient loss of function in one hand emphasises the dependence most people have on two normally-functioning upper limbs to shop for, prepare, cook and eat a meal. Having sight usually adds considerably to the ease and enjoyment of eating and drinking although it is not imperative for physical independence in this AL; blind people usually master the spatial problem of lifting food from the plate to the mouth, often with astonishing dexterity.

The physiological aspects of appetite are important when considering the AL of eating and drinking such as the amount of food in the stomach, and the concentration of nutrients in the plasma as it flows through the hypothalamus, the appetite regulating centre in the brain. Irrespective of cause, anorexia or a prolonged lack of appetite will cause loss of weight, and conversely, excessive appetite will usually lead to obesity. So weight is a visible physical aspect of eating. There are also sex differences. By and large, women of the same height and age are less heavy and eat less than their male counterparts although of course there are enormous individual differences.

In the industrialised world, very few people know what hunger means but most people have experienced thirst. Water represents about two-thirds of the body weight, and after oxygen, is the most important constituent for the maintenance of life. People can live for several days without food but only for a few days without water. It is available to the body from many sources and although drinking water and beverages are the most obvious form of intake, the water content of food also makes a significant contribution.

Water balance is directly related to the homeostatic function in the body's internal environment — electrolyte concentration, osmotic pressure, acid-base balance and body temperature. And as with appetite, the sensation of thirst is associated with the plasma concentration as it flows through the hypothalamus; osmoreceptor cells are sensitive to the osmotic pressure. When the body tissues, for whatever reason, are deprived of water, the person will experience thirst; if unrelieved, the individual will develop a dry furred tongue, will complain of fatigue and in later stages, the tissues will appear loose and flabby, the eyes sunken, and there will be obvious weight loss. If this condition of dehydration is not reversed, the pulse and blood pressure fall, the temperature is raised, the person goes into shock, then coma and death will ensue. Such is the essential nature of eating and drinking for the intake of water.

Psychological factors

A minimal level of intelligence is necessary to master the skills used in the process of eating and drinking. This is apparent when observing a young child as he experiments intellectually as well as physically with the development of mealtime skills, and likewise it is apparent when observing mentally handicapped children whose intellectual development is retarded; they often have great difficulty in acquiring eating and drinking skills (Caunter & Penrose, 1983).

A certain intellectual level is also required for the acquisition and application of the knowledge needed to select and prepare a diet which will maintain health, and a great deal of time and effort are expended by the government, the health professions and the media in health education to interest the general public in desirable eating practices. The acquisition of knowledge is required also to apply appropriate food hygiene practices when handling food; and to dispose of food waste in such a manner that it will not attract vermin and flies which have the potential to harbour and spread pathogenic microorganisms to humans.

The individual's emotional state may sometimes affect food intake. The child's excitement prior to a holiday, the anxiety associated with examinations, the stress of a change of job may well reduce the accustomed intake for that individual. These however are usually transient. Loss of appetite or lack of desire for food over a prolonged period can be indicative of a more serious disturbance in emotional states and is referred to as anorexia nervosa. It has a peak incidence in adolescence especially among girls. Despite evidence to the contrary, the individual views herself as fat and will refuse to eat or will deliberately vomit following food intake. Anorexia nervosa is usually considered to be a disturbance in personality development, often in the relationship with one parent, and becoming aware of personal feelings and impulses then learning how to cope with them is part of the slow process back to a normal pattern of eating and drinking.

In contradistinction, some people use food as a source of comfort and security and may eat compulsively to compensate for lack of fulfilment in the basic needs of love and belonging. Some writers have certainly attempted to explain obesity in terms of personality factors related to anxiety, apprehension and tension but Kaplan (1979) maintains that obesity may stem from lack of hunger awareness. This may result from, for example, an overprotective mother who may impose what she considers the child needs, disregarding the child's own sensation of hunger and fullness.

Compulsive overeating is seen as a form of dependence on food and a parallel in drinking would be excessive intake of alcohol resulting in dependence on alcohol. Currently, alcoholism is a major problem in many countries of the world. Usually the onset of dependence on alcohol is insidious, starting with social drinking but when out of control, the habit can lead to irresponsible behaviour, petty crime or even assault, and bring distress not only to the individual but to family and friends.

Sociocultural factors

Food and water are essential to man's survival but it is fascinating to consider the sociocultural and religious practices associated with this AL.

In certain cultures it is customary to take meals in the home in a special room set aside for the purpose but there are many variations, and it may be accepted practice to eat under a tree, round a camp fire or in a tent. Not only the setting but the style of eating may vary considerably. Some societies make use of fingers, others use chopsticks, or knives, forks and spoons; some eat food from a communal bowl, others from individual plates; some sit cross-legged on the floor, others customarily use a chair. In a few cultures there may even be segregation of the sexes at mealtimes with adult males eating together but separately from adult females eating together. More commonly, however, the meal is an occasion when all members of the family are sharing news about the day's activities although in some industrialised countries, the increasing use of 'fast' foods and the consuming dominance of TV-viewing are altering the pattern of mealtime socialising.

Certain religious groups have definite rules about the choice and preparation of specific items on the menu. For example the orthodox Jew must prepare and serve dairy products and meat dishes separately, while the Koran forbids Muslims to touch pork and alcohol, and the devout Hindu will not eat animal products. There are however other groups who, not for religious reasons, are vegetarians and will not eat animal products.

Apart from these constraints, each culture has its own traditional dishes and a look at the restaurants in most large cities is a measure of the fascinating variety.

Environmental factors

Physical environmental factors can affect the choice of food. Obviously geographical position, soil fertility, climate and rainfall will determine the type of food which can be grown locally, and will also influence the meat, fish and poultry content of the diet. Nowadays, for industrial nations with their extensive import/export networks, reliance on local food is not such a dominant feature of everyday living but it is crucial for about two-thirds of the world who are dependent on local produce.

Availability of fuel is also a consideration. Although certain groups such as Eskimos eat raw fish and seal, it is customary in most countries to improve the palatability of food by cooking many of the vegetables and fruit fibres, and the flesh of fish, fowl and animals. Also some form of fuel is needed for preservation of food for example in bottling, canning or deep freezing, and making storage possible.

Food is imperative for human existence but an adequate supply of water is even more important. Three-quarters of the world's surface is water but getting an adequate supply of fresh, clean water which is safe to use for drinking and cooking is one of the world's pressing problems. Most of the world's water is salt and in the oceans; only 3% is fresh and only a small amount of that is accessible as a public water supply. Many of the world's women and children have to walk miles to draw water from a stream or well which may be inadequate for all the Activities of Living; when a safe supply is available on tap, water is so much taken for granted. Accessibility and distribution of food and water in the local environment certainly contribute to the ease of eating and drinking.

In a slightly different sense, the environment is obviously taken into account by restaurateurs who consider that the ambience of the environment can contribute to food and drink enjoyment. Noise, hustle and bustle are not thought to be good for digestion and many hoteliers give considerable thought to the provision of carpeting, lowered lights and soft background music as an environmental aid to both the physiological and psychological enjoyment of eating and drinking.

Politicoeconomic factors

Any consideration of eating and drinking presupposes that food and drink are available. This is not always the case, indeed, about half of the world's population is hungry. In certain areas even now, hundreds of people die every day due to starvation, and many thousands of others are undernourished because they have insufficient food to eat. There are many complex reasons for this maldistribution of food throughout the world, such as infertile soil, inferior seed, inadequate crop rotation, overgrazing, soil erosion, lack of irrigation, lack of knowledge and lack of finance, all of which contribute to a poor yield. Some parts of the world, too, are more liable to suffer from natural disasters such as drought, floods or pestilence which result in crop failure or even large-scale famine. When this occurs, scarcity creates an increase in the price of food which often takes it beyond the financial reach of lower income groups so the people are undernourished or may in fact 'starve to death'. Considerable attempts have been made at national and international levels to redress these gross inequalities but still the problem remains, much of it due to economic and political constraints (Brandt Report, 1980).

Sometimes however the problem is not undernutrition but malnutrition; a problem of quality not quantity. There is enough food but the diet is not balanced in terms of the essential food nutrients. Malnutrition is one of the major causes of ill-health in the world and contributes to premature death or reduced economic productivity because of physical debility. Not only does it lead to specific vitamin deficiency diseases (p. 160) such as scurvy, rickets, beri-beri and pellagra but it reduces resistance to communicable diseases which in turn further deplete the body's resources. To give some idea of the enormity of the problem Habicht (1983) reckons that 1000 million human beings show evidence of malnutrition due to inadequate intake of protein, iron, vitamin A and iodine and at least 12 million are permanently disabled from the consequences. Eleven million die of malnutrition each year.

Protein is the most expensive food nutrient to process and protein-calorie malnutrition is a widespread and serious problem especially in the first years of life. Very young children are highly susceptible to lack of adequate nutrients, and in developing countries babies who have initially been breast-fed may suffer severe nutritional deficiencies, especially of protein, when they are weaned. One of the gross manifestations of protein deficiency in young children is kwashiorkor.

The WHO (World Health Organization) collaborates with the FAO (Food and Agricultural Organization) and UNICEF (United Nations Children's Fund) in the Protein-Calorie Advisory Group set up by the UN and it is paying particular attention to the development of low-cost, protein-rich weaning foods suitable for local production in developing countries. Enhancing self-help is a much more enduring policy than encouraging import of foreign-produced foodstuffs to an undernourished or malnourished nation.

It is not only in the developing countries that malnutrition is found. Vagrants, young people living away from home for the first time, and people living alone — often in the older age group — are at risk of becoming malnourished because of the quality of their diet. A diet of bread, pastry and cups of tea is grossly lacking in, among other things, the much needed minerals and vitamins which are so necessary to health and vitality. To help to prevent malnutrition in the older person, some countries have instituted a 'meals-on-wheels' service. At a small cost or free of charge in cases of financial hardship, a cooked meal is delivered in the middle of the day to the home of those who, because of physical disability or frailty, are unable to go shopping for food or are disinclined to cook for themselves.

Of course malnutrition can exist in the midst of plenty, and indeed is associated with obesity. Insurance companies are becoming hesitant about issuing policies to grossly overweight people because statistics show that compared with their slim contemporaries they are more susceptible to, for example, coronary disease, bronchitis and diabetes mellitus.

Because of the link with disease and dysfunction, a number of industrialised countries are greatly exercised about the need to change their national dietary habits and are attempting to adopt a standard approach to recommendations for the whole population. By and large they include proposals to reduce fat intake to around 30% of total energy intake (of which 10% should be saturated fatty acids); to reduce average sucrose and salt intakes; and to increase dietary fibre. A recent report of this type produced in the UK for the Health Education Council (1983) concludes with a comment on the timescale needed for such changes. It acknowledges that changes of the type proposed cannot be achieved rapidly and suggests a 15 year timespan not only for public attitudes to alter but for agricultural practices, food manufacturing techniques and Government and ECC regulations to change. These adjustments have economic and legal implications, and require not only political decisions but also political will to encourage their implementation.

DEPENDENCE/INDEPENDENCE IN EATING AND DRINKING

Independence in eating and drinking obviously is associated with the individual's stage on the lifespan. Apart from age with the obvious dependence of the young and the potential dependence of the elderly, there are some people who may have a hand or arm defect or who have diminished sight and can still be independent for eating and drinking, provided they have the use of mechanical aids. These aids may be in the kitchen for preparing food, or used when cooking and eating food and allow the individual to retain the maximum self-esteem and dignity despite a physical handicap. For a quite different reason mentally handicapped people too will often have eating and drinking problems and the importance of good positioning with a suitable size of chair and table, in a relaxed atmosphere, are basic to progressive independence.

There is now a range of feeding aids, not necessarily expensive, and a considerable literature (Caunter & Penrose, 1983) with collective ideas which have proved useful to physiotherapists, occupational therapists and speech therapists who have studied the problems of handicapped people so that they can achieve optimal independence in eating and drinking.

INDIVIDUALITY IN EATING AND DRINKING

Individuality is the final component of the model to be introduced. From the preceding discussion it is evident that there are many dimensions of the other components of the model which contribute to the development of individuality in the AL of eating and drinking. Below is a résumé of the main points in the discussion.

Lifespan: effect on eating and drinking
- Nutrition *in utero*
- Breast/bottle-feeding and weaning in infancy
- Increasing skills in eating and drinking during childhood
- Prudent diet during adolescence and adulthood
- Reduced appetite/potential nutritional deficiency in old age

Factors influencing eating and drinking
- Physical
  - state of mouth and teeth
  - intact digestive system
  - physical proficiency in shopping for/preparing food
  - physical proficiency in taking food and drink
  - appetite/thirst regulation

- Psychological
  - intellectual capacity to procure and prepare food and drink
  - knowledge about diet and health
  - weight control
  - alcoholism
  - food hygiene
  - disposal of food waste
  - attitude to eating and drinking
  - emotional status
  - likes and dislikes

- Sociocultural
  - family traditions
  - cultural idiosyncrasies
  - religious commendations/restrictions

- Environmental
  - climate and geographical position
  - facilities for procuring/growing food
  - distance from home to shopping area
  - availability of transport
  - means of cooking
  - means of storage

- Politicoeconomic
  - finance available
  - choice of food and drink
  - quantity and quality of food and drink

Dependence/independence in eating and drinking
- Special utensils
- Mechanical aids
- Kitchen gadgets
- Special transport for shopping

Eating and drinking: patients' problems and related nursing activities

Unless they are detrimental to health, it is desirable that during an episode of illness, the patient's individual habits of living are changed as little as possible. It is therefore important that the nurse should know about these habits and use the knowledge to devise an individualised plan of nursing.

In order to individualise nursing for this AL, it is necessary to assess the activities of eating and drinking insofar as they are relevant to the particular person. Assessing involves observing the patient; acquiring information about eating and drinking habits by asking appropriate questions, and by listening to the comments and questions raised by the patient and family; and using relevant material from available records such as medical records. The nurse would be seeking answers to the following questions:

- how often does the individual usually eat and drink?
- what does the individual usually eat and drink?

- when does the individual eat and drink?
- where does the individual eat and drink?
- what factors influence the way the individual carries out the AL of eating and drinking?
- has the individual any long-standing difficulties with eating and drinking and how have these been coped with?
- what problems, if any, does the individual have at present with eating and drinking and are any likely to develop?

Of course the nurse does not necessarily ask these actual questions because much of the information can be acquired in the course of conversation with the patient.

The information can then be examined to identify, in collaboration with the patient when possible, any problems being experienced with the AL and these can be arranged if necessary in priority. The nurse may recognise potential problems and these can be discussed with the patient. Mutual realistic goals can then be set to prevent potential problems from becoming actual ones; to alleviate or solve the actual problems; or to help the patient cope with those which cannot be alleviated or solved. Keeping in mind what the patient can and cannot do, the nursing interventions (and any action the patient has agreed to undertake) to achieve the set goals can then be selected according to local circumstances and available resources. These interventions should be written on the nursing plan along with the date on which evaluation will be carried out, in order to discern whether or not they are achieving the stated goals.

Other members of the multidisciplinary health team are usually involved in the care programme such as doctors and dietitians and perhaps occupational therapists; and it is important that the individualised nursing plan is congruent with the team's mutually agreed objectives for the patient. On the Nursing Plan proforma suggested by Roper/Logan/Tierney (p. 351) there is a section for appropriate entries of this type in order to indicate the relationship between nursing interventions derived from medical/other prescription and nurse-initiated interventions.

However before nurses can begin to think in terms of individualised nursing, they require a general idea of the conditions which can be responsible for, or can change, the dependence/independence status for the AL of eating and drinking and which can be experienced by the person as a problem in carrying out the AL. The remainder of this section is a general discussion of the types of patients' problems related to eating and drinking and the relevant nursing activities.

They are grouped under headings which indicate how the problems can arise:

- Change of environment and routine
- Change in eating and drinking habit
- Change in mode of eating and drinking
- Change of dependence/independence status
- Discomforts associated with eating and drinking.

Many factors can influence the highly individualised activity of eating and drinking. Disease or injury to the digestive system itself may interfere with the activity, or with the individual's capacity to benefit nutritionally from the activity. In addition, disease and pain affecting other body systems can cause disturbance of the appetite and may well alter the individual's intake of food and drink. Admission to hospital however, irrespective of cause, almost always produces some degree of stress and anxiety and can create poblems related to this important activity of eating and drinking.

CHANGE OF ENVIRONMENT AND ROUTINE

Most people are well accustomed to changes of diet while on holiday or during business trips but in these instances, they are usually in control of their decisions about eating and drinking. In hospital however this is not usually so, and mealtimes and their associated activities often come to have increased significance. The individual may be hypersensitive to alterations in the timing of meals and the methods of serving them; he may be apprehensive about the availability of facilities related to hygiene activities; he may be easily irritated by distracting influences; he may be much more apprehensive about fluctuations in appetite. For the young child, in particular, the change in environment and routine in hospital will be bewildering and his developing mealtime habits therefore may be considerably disrupted.

Timing of meals

The patient newly admitted to hospital often has no idea of the mealtime programme: whether to expect a cooked or a continental breakfast; whether the main meal is served in the middle of the day or in the evening; whether he will be allowed to have snacks between meals. Some patients may have heard of the need to fast prior to surgery and certain tests, and be concerned about the discomfort of feeling hungry or thirsty.

The nurse can allay some of the anxiety by offering information and also by providing opportunities for the patient to ask questions so that he can feel reassured about what he is expected to do in continuing this important AL. Most patients understand that in an establishment as complex as a hospital, it is usually necessary to have set mealtimes; indeed, some find that meals give a certain degree of order to the day, providing stable time-points in an otherwise bewildering situation. There are some patients however who consider that the evening meal is served much earlier than in their normal routine, and they choose to keep in the bedside locker some food for a snack. In any case, visitors frequently take food to patients sometimes to tempt a poor appetite but often also as a gesture to indicate concern for their welfare.

Serving of meals

In hospital, patients may find that the way of serving meals is a problem because it is so different from their usual routine. Even though most people are accustomed to 'tray' meals in self-service restaurants, few are used to having all meals served in this manner.

People do not usually choose to be in bed while taking a meal, so for patients who are bedfast, eating and drinking may become a formidable task especially if they must remain in a recumbent position, or attached to various pieces of equipment associated with their treatment.

If bedfast patients can sit up at mealtimes, the nurse should help them into a comfortable position and ensure that adequately supported with pillows before placing the bedtable in an appropriate position ready for the meal-tray. Many people like to drink with a meal and, unless it is contraindicated, most patients have a water-jug and glass on the bedside locker so the nurse should check that it is within easy reach.

Nowadays, many patients in hospital are not bedfast and most will enjoy meals more if sitting at a table; in fact, in new and upgraded wards, a dining area is frequently included in the design of the ward unit.

Meals should be served in a calm, unhurried manner if patients are to enjoy what is really a social event in their day. The nurse should appreciate the symbolism attached to food, indicative of hospitality and caring. Associated with this symbolism, the very acts of serving and accepting food provide an opportunity for establishing and maintaining the important relationship between nurse and patient. A great deal has been written about the patient's loss of identity while in hospital, and when he is addressed by name as food is served it helps to reinforce his individuality and personal importance. Particularly in a psychiatric hospital, group dining may be a deliberate therapeutic measure to give the patient an opportunity to solve some of his problems by practising the social behaviour associated with mealtimes.

Alteration in appetite

Most people have personal idiosyncrasies about food choice and even when an appropriate, attractive meal is served, the patient may not feel inclined to eat. If he is feeling unwell, or homesick, or unused to the type of food served, he may not eat adequately and the nurse must be interested in the 'used' tray. Over a century ago (1859) Florence Nightingale observed:

A nurse will often have patients loathing all food and incapable of any will to get well who just tumble over the contents of the plate or dip the spoon into the cup to deceive the nurse and she will take it away without ever seeing that there is just the same quantity of food as when she brought it, and she will tell the doctor too that the patient has eaten all his diets as usual when all she ought to have meant is that she has taken away his diets as usual.

When a patient consistently fails to eat, the nurse must discuss with him the possible reasons for lack of appetite (anorexia) and also ask herself some critical questions. Perhaps a bedpan is required before meals; perhaps the helpings are too large or the serving is unattractively arranged on the plate; perhaps patients in the immediate vicinity are causing distress and distraction; perhaps the patient craves some particular food item. Nowadays in hospital, there is usually a choice of menu, and dietetic staff may be called in to advise on individual problems, but the nurse should use her initiative in helping the patient to solve the problem of lack of appetite.

As nutrients are essential for the repair of body tissue, it is imperative that nurses know about the therapeutic value of food and observe and report accurately what the patient has eaten.

'Inadequate' hospital meals

One of the problems about observing dietary intake is that in many hospitals, the responsibility for serving food has been transferred from nursing staff to a waitress service.

Following research done in the 1950s, it was concluded that nurses spent considerable time preparing for meals, serving them and collecting trays, and it was suggested that these were non-nursing duties. As a consequence, over the last 20 years, many hospitals have developed 'hotel services' using non-nursing staff, so many different patterns have evolved for the service of meals. Somehow, the responsibility for observing what was eaten by each patient was dissipated and among others, Tweedle (1978) voiced his concern about what he termed 'malnutrition in surgical patients' because it was 'increasingly difficult to ascertain what patients had eaten'. Coates (1984) was also concerned about inadequate nutritional intake in hospital and reviewed some studies done on surgical patients, on long-stay and elderly patients, and on medical patients, commenting on the effects of malnutrition — increased susceptibility to infection, the incidence of more complications, delayed wound healing, the formation of pressure sores. She quotes her own study investigating the total nutrient intake of a random sample of patients taking an ordinary hospital diet in four medical words, and compares it with the recommended DHSS (1975) daily amounts for the healthy individual of related age and sex. The nutrient intake of the hospital diet was significantly lower.

However apart from the concern of individual members of staff, some authorities are becoming exercised about the meal service in hospitals particularly about the nutrient content and particularly about the bad example set by current hospital menus. Brent Health Authority in the London area (1980) has instituted a Food and Health Policy. As well as providing for health education about nutrition to patients and staff, the hospital menus now include for example a higher percentage of wholemeal bread; a proportion of fibre-rich breakfast cereals; a reduction in the amount of fat especially saturated fat; a reduction in the amount of sugar used in cooking, and the addition of fresh fruit. The nutritional value of the menus is being closely monitored by a team of experts.

Even when food is adequate however, some patients will complain about hospital meals. There may be cause for dissatisfaction but grumbling about food may be a manifestation of some more covert need, for example lack of information about the treatment programme, upset of usual routine, lack of attention; the discerning nurse will investigate the significance of dietary complaints.

Pre- and post-meal activities

The majority of patients who are not bedfast will be able to continue their habitual pre- and post-meal routines such as handwashing, visiting the toilet and cleaning the teeth. The bedfast patient may experience considerable concern because he is no longer independent for these activities but the nurse can reduce anxiety by ensuring that these facilities are made available.

Patients will be reassured if they actually see members of the nursing staff wash their hands in preparation for serving meals and/or helping with feeding activities. This is important for general hygiene reasons but it is also important in order that food will be free from contamination by pathogenic microorganisms. Prior to meal-serving, the nurse may have been dressing wounds, or helping a patient who is vomiting or she may have been handling a bedpan. In an establishment such as a hospital, it is crucial that all food-handlers should be scrupulously careful about hand cleanliness because potentially they can infect the food of many people, and people who are more susceptible to infection because they are already suffering from some disorder which has precipitated entry to hospital.

As a pre-meal activity, it is important for nurses to plan their work so that unpleasant sights, sounds and smells will not ruin the patient's appetite for food and drink. As far as possible, treatment appointments in other departments of the hospital should be scheduled for other times of the day, and doctors' rounds should avoid meal-times.

The child in hospital

Admission to hospital can adversely affect the eating and drinking pattern of people in any age group but for the young child, the trauma of separation from mother is compounded by the bewilderment engendered by a change of environment. He is unhappy and confused. In addition, the food will probably be different and will almost certainly be differently served, so recently cultivated home routines for eating and drinking will be broken and his social learning in this AL may be interrupted. It is not surprising if his eating and drinking habits are affected and this may manifest itself as loss of appetite, or refusal to eat, or regressive behaviour with loss of independence in feeding himself. The nurse can often help to prevent this by asking the parents about the child's likes and dislikes, and his previous eating and drinking routines. It is often helpful to the child if a parent remains with him during mealtimes.

CHANGE IN EATING AND DRINKING HABIT

Dietary habits often change during illness. Usually the change is transient but sometimes a patient may have to be helped to re-educate himself about eating and drinking habits on a life-long basis.

Modification of habitual food intake

During illness appetite may range from extreme hunger as is found in uncontrolled diabetes mellitus to utter lack of interest in food when for example a patient has a high fever. When in hospital, the range of need is catered for by providing menus which vary in texture and quantity. The variations can be described broadly as normal diet; light diet which contains no fatty, highly-seasoned foods; soft and fluid diets which are 'light' but are in semi-solid or liquid form and used for ill patients or those who have ingestion, digestion and absorption problems.

Some patients however, whether at home or in hospital, are advised to accept modifications in diet as part of the treatment for a specific disease condition and some may rebel against this suggested restriction of food choice. When patients are grossly overweight for example, they must be willing to accept a diet which is reduced in its daily kilojoule value, perhaps as low as 4000 kJ, and although this entails an overall reduction in dietary intake it usually involves a gross reduction in foodstuffs which have a high carbohydrate content. Patients often find great difficulty in altering life-long eating habits which involve shunning foods they enjoy, and also they feel hungry. They need much encouragement to resist unsuitable food and drink, and need help to learn about a balanced food intake even after a successful loss of weight. The amount of self-discipline required by patients to maintain a *low carbohydrate/low kilojoule* diet should not be underestimated and their efforts require frequent reinforcement. The weight chart is a visible reminder of progress.

Young patients who are diagnosed as having diabetes mellitus, however, will usually require a *high kilojoule* diet which is *low in carbohydrate* because the pancreas is not producing enough insulin to deal with carbohydrate metabolism. Initially these patients may be brought into hospital for tests but once diagnosed and on a regime where they understand the need to balance diet/insulin/exercise, the injections of insulin will deal with the defective carbohydrate metabolism provided the carbohydrate intake is kept low. These people can lead a normal life once they are educated to cope with the diabetic state — and it is a lifelong state. Those who develop diabetes when in the older age bracket are usually obese and the diabetic state can often be contained with a *low carbohydrate/low kilojoule* diet.

Obesity and diabetes mellitus are examples of conditions which necessitate modification in carbohydrate/kilojoule intake but sometimes the fat intake presents a problem. Patients who have infective hepatitis (a form of jaundice) have this type of problem so a *low fat* diet is indicated until the liver recovers from the infection. The problem may be with a specific aspect of fat metabolism, however. People with coronary artery disease may be advised to omit a particular form of fat from the diet, namely saturated fat which is found in lard, butter and other animal fats. It has been found that when dietary intake of saturated fats is greatly reduced the level of blood cholesterol is reduced. High blood cholesterol seems to be associated with the deposition of fatty plaques in the arterial wall and this is conducive to coronary artery disease and myocardial infarction. Those who have had 'heart attacks' are therefore advised to take unsaturated rather than saturated fats in the diet and as with diabetics, this diet is usually advocated for the remainder of the patient's life.

There are occasions when *food and fluid intake is prohibited*; before an anaesthetic and before certain investigations, the patient may be asked to fast for 6–8 hours. An explanation with clear instructions about timing is usually all that is required for most adult patients though in *Nil by Mouth?* Hamilton-Smith (1972) deplores the great variations in practice many of which have no scientific basis. In a paediatric ward as well as explaining the reason, any food or drinks on the bedside locker should be temporarily removed. It is important to check whether or not a patient may have a snack on return from an investigation: it may be some time before the next meal is scheduled. If the nurse does not make and serve the snack herself she should make sure that the dietary staff have been requested to do so and that the patient receives it.

Prior to surgery, a patient is often given by injection a drug called atropine which reduces secretion in the mouth and respiratory tract and therefore reduces the danger of inhalation of fluid during anaesthesia. Patients should be told to expect that they will feel thirsty and experience a feeling of dryness in the mouth.

Modification of habitual fluid intake

Problems with fluid intake are often more urgent than those associated with food intake. Fluid deprivation can only be tolerated for a few days and in a 24-hour period the adult human requires about 2500 ml of water.

There are obvious reductions in fluid intake when it is impossible to procure drinking water — in dramatic shipwreck and desert rescues for example — but excessive fluid output from the body is the usual cause of *dehydration*. It may be found in any condition featuring high fever, vomiting or diarrhoea and also occurs when there is severe haemorrhage, severe burns, untreated diabetes mellitus and untreated diabetes insipidus. It may occur in milder form. Some elderly people with weak bladder control may deliberately reduce their intake in the hope that it will reduce the need to ask for a bedpan; or the patient who is mentally handicapped may be unable to make decisions about the adequacy of intake; or intake may be depleted during prolonged unconsciousness.

In the early stages of dehydration fluid is withdrawn from the skin and tissues in order to maintain the blood volume while simultaneously the kidneys excrete less urine in order to conserve body fluid. If the cause of dehydration is not treated effectively however, more serious effects ensue. The patient will complain of a dry tongue and it will look leathery in appearance; he will be dull and lethargic; the skin will lose its natural elasticity and have a wrinkled appearance; and the urinary output will be grossly reduced and highly concentrated. In extreme cases, blood volume is reduced causing deficient circulation, and in turn the kidneys fail to excrete waste products. Renal failure and death may ensue.

Where there is mild dehydration, the nurse should encourage the patient to drink and ensure that freshly procured drinks of a desired flavour, perhaps with ice, are available. When there is gross dehydration, intravenous fluids will be required usually in the form of a saline infusion as salt will have been lost along with body fluid.

Any gross loss of fluid is accompanied by a dramatic loss in body weight and records must be maintained of weight, fluid intake, all forms of output — urine, faeces, vomitus — and note made of excessive perspiration.

In contradistinction to dehydration the patient's body may retain an excess amount of fluid and the condition is called *oedema*. Oedema is most commonly seen when the heart, as a pump, is not functioning normally. The resulting swelling — it is recognisable by the way the skin in affected areas 'pits' on pressure — is most obvious in the dependent parts of the body such as the feet, ankles, legs and if the patient is sitting in bed, in the sacral area. The patient may be distressed by the ugly appearance of swollen ankles, the discomfort, the reduced mobility. If pressure sores are to be prevented, the stretched 'devitalised' skin in affected areas requires special care. When there is gross imbalance fluid will also collect in the pleural and peritoneal cavities causing respiratory difficulty and the patient will then be breathless and uncomfortable, so a procedure to aspirate the fluid may be needed to alleviate the distress.

It is logical to expect that a patient who has oedema should take a *low fluid/low salt* diet. Again, individual likes and dislikes regarding time and content of fluid intake should be discussed with the patient and a suitable regime adopted. These patients often appreciate a pleasant tasting mouthwash at hand even during the night. Regarding salt intake, condiments are removed from the food tray but salt substitutes may be used for flavouring.

Only a few examples have been cited which involve changes in eating and drinking habits, but in all instances it must be remembered that merely imparting information to the patient does not guarantee advice will be followed. Explaining the reason for a special diet is essential and should take into account the patient's socioeconomic, cultural, religious and moral values. Wherever possible advice should be related to the usual dietary habits of the individual and modifications rather than drastic change should be attempted.

If the patient must continue a special diet for some time, advice may be required in relation to purchase of certain foods, perhaps unaccustomed foods, and home budgeting may need to be adjusted. When a dietitian is not available to provide such a service, the nurse must inform and assist the patient and is thereby provided with an excellent opportunity to offer health education related to nutrition and food handling. It is important to remember too that a long-term dietary alteration may affect not only the individual but the family, and the nurse should be able to make helpful suggestions about food preparation so that the patient does not feel he is ostracised at meal times or creating extra work because of changes in his daily activity of eating and drinking.

CHANGE IN MODE OF EATING AND DRINKING

Nasogastric feeding

When considering the body's nutritional needs it is usual to think of the ingestion of food and fluid by the oral route. There are circumstances, usually transient, when it is not possible for the patient to take nourishment by mouth and parenteral fluids may be prescribed. When a patient suffers from persistent vomiting, for example, it may be necessary to pass a nasogastric tube via the nose/mouth into the stomach (Fig. 10.12) so that he can be fed artificially (Royal Marsden Hospital 1984). The method may also be used when there is physical difficulty with ingestion and swallowing, for example when a patient has a fractured jaw. Quite frequently this method is used also for a patient who is unconscious.

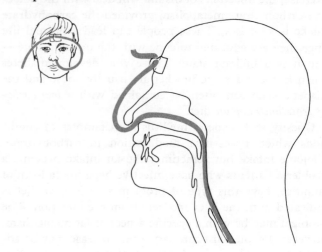

Fig. 10.12 Nasogastric tube *in situ* for feeding

When the patient is conscious, the procedure should be explained and it may help him to feel in control of the situation if he assists with the manipulation of the equipment. Premature babies are sometimes fed in this manner using a very finely calibrated catheter and it is important to explain to the parents why this feeding technique is used.

Until recently, nasogastric feeding was thought to be without risk of infection unless the mixture given became contaminated during or after preparation by enteric pathogens or toxin-producing bacteria; and bacteriological monitoring was rarely carried out. However a study was prompted in one hospital when a patient having nasogastic feeding suffered from profuse diarrhoea and vomiting. Subsequently, pathogens were isolated from the feed, and after meticulous 'sampling and monitoring of a number of feeds, the catering, dietetic and infection control staff recommended that a commercially manufactured product should be used in future to give a better guarantee of microbiological safety than those mixed in the hospital diet bay' (Gibbs, 1983). Where commercial packs are not used, the nurse must ensure that nasogastic feeds are given with scrupulous care in order to avoid adding to the problems of an already disadvantaged patient.

As a route for providing nutrition, a gastrostomy is not so common as nasogastic feeding but the same meticulous handling of feeds is required.

Gastrostomy feeding

When there is an obstruction in the upper part of the

digestive system, it may be necessary to use another technique. The surgeon passes a gastrostomy tube (Fig. 10.13) through the abdominal wall into the stomach so that fluid feeds can be introduced to maintain adequate body nutrition. Again, the patient may wish to help with the procedure once the technique is established.

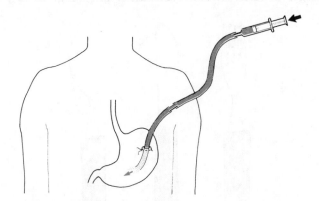

Fig. 10.13 Gastrostomy feeding

Intravenous (parenteral) feeding

These above methods, although not using the usual oral route for the ingestion of food and fluid, do involve direct entry of nourishment to some part of the digestive tract. In some instances when it is not possible to provide nutrition via the tract itself, food nutrients dissolved in fluid may have to be administered straight into the blood stream by means of an intravenous infusion (Fig. 10.14) in order to prevent dehydration and malnutrition. Owing to the cost and potential danger of intravenous feeding, it should not be undertaken lightly and Flannigan (1982) emphasises the importance of ascertaining the need and indications for it, and the investigations which should be

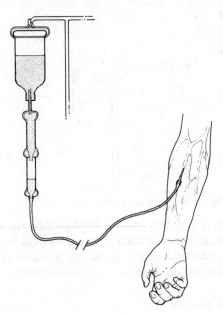

Fig. 10.14 Intravenous feeding

undertaken before proceeding with this mode of providing nutrition. It certainly causes the patient some discomfort and makes mobility more difficult.

Using this method, the potential for infection is even greater than for nasogastric and gastrostomy feeding. As well as contamination of the fluid, there is concern about the possibility of pathogens gaining entry directly into the bloodstream via the cannula site. Smith (1981) discusses these problems and also the anxiety about the patients being inadequately fed, both in quantity and quality, by present-day standards. She describes the use of a nutritional team including biochemist, dietitian, bacteriologist, doctor, pharmacist and nurse who now monitor enteral and parenteral feeding as a group rather than contributing in isolation to patient nutrition. The nurse has a central role in the team and must have knowledge about potential complications in the patient's metabolic status in order to reduce the risk of fluid overload, hyperosmolar states, electrolyte imbalance and hyperglycaemia.

When intravenous infusion is selected as the appropriate method of feeding, the patient, as well as having the discomfort of an intravenous infusion, is often anxious about the need for it, the content, the frequent monitoring, the replenishment at the correct time; and looks to the nurse for suitable explanations and support.

Usually intravenous feeding is used as a short-term measure to assist a patient over a crisis. Sometimes however, failure of absorption due to disease or extensive bowel resection requires longer term therapy. Nowadays if there are problems with peripheral venous feeding or if the nutrient solution used is irritant to peripheral veins, it is possible to provide parenteral nutrition through a catheter, the top of which lies in the superior vena cava or even the right atrium. Wood (1982) describes how cardiac catheterisation is performed under strict aseptic conditions using a local anaesthetic. Apparently most patients experience only a feeling of pressure although the head-down position which is necessary to increase venous filling and avoid air embolism is uncomfortable. Careful explanation of the procedure usually helps to alleviate the patient's anxiety but sometimes sedation is given prior to commencement. The patient and the infusion must be carefully monitored as there may be quite major complications including pneumothorax, damage to the brachial plexus and injury to the subclavian artery.

With any type of artificial feeding, as well as a degree of physical discomfort, there may be emotional problems about the inability to eat normally. Wood (1982), a Clinical Nutrition Sister, maintains that removing the oral stimulation of food may lead to craving for certain foods and also to strange dreams and hallucinations of a most alarming nature. Hunger may or may not be present, and mealtimes in the ward can cause such patients considerable distress. The presence of the tube, too, causes anxiety especially for those with a central venous feeding catheter and participation by the patients (and family), perhaps merely charting the intake, has been found to assist by reducing the distress of dependence. The removal of the oral stimulation of food and fluid, of course, makes it necessary to be vigilant about mouth care (p. 206). Mouthwashes can help to keep the tissue moist, and prevent the accumulation of pathogenic microorganisms. A mouth infection and an unpleasant odour from the breath only add to the patient's problems and increase distress.

CHANGE OF DEPENDENCE/INDEPENDENCE STATUS

For a variety of reasons a patient may require assistance with the actual activity of eating and drinking, and this should be given graciously and with dexterity so that he will be protected from needless embarrassment resulting from his lack of independence in this AL. The ability to help oneself to food and drink is usually taken so much for granted until circumstances occur which interfere with this activity of everyday life and result in problems of dependence.

Problems associated with physical dependence

Posture
Even something apparently simple such as a change of physical posture may create ingestion and swallowing problems, for example when the patient is forced to lie flat when eating. The distress, difficulty and even indignity suffered by the patient in such circumstances should be appreciated by the nurse and dealt with sensitively.

The patient may have to be fed by the nurse, and it is almost impossible for him to feel relaxed if the nurse is standing over him. She should be seated and facing the patient and he must be given time to enjoy what he eats. Sometimes it is more pleasant for the patient if small helpings of solid food are given on a spoon rather than a fork, although he should be consulted about his preference; and liquids may be interspersed throughout the meal or offered at the end according to his wish. Liquids can be given from a spouted feeding cup but a drinking straw usually allows him to control the flow more easily, and nowadays, angled straws made from materials which can withstand warm fluids make mealtimes less difficult for people who require help with feeding.

Oral hygiene is often required before and after the meal and it is a cardinal rule that, unless contraindicated (for example when a patient is unconscious, or has a nasogastric or gastrostomy tube *in situ*, or is on restricted fluids) anyone who needs special oral hygiene, needs also to be helped to take oral fluids in order to keep the mouth tissues in a healthy, comfortable state.

Physical handicap
There are occasions when a patient requires assistance because he is physically disabled or because the preferred hand is out of action due to injury or surgery. Many aids are available to deal with such circumstances, for example larger handles on cutlery to assist grip (Fig. 10.15); a

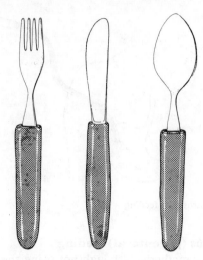

Fig. 10.15 Cutlery with foam-covered handles allowing easier grip for people with upper limb handicap

'tip-up' stand for a teapot (Fig. 10.16); non-spill cups; plate guards; unbreakable crockery; and often the occupational therapist can make useful suggestions which will help the patient to retain independence and dignity at mealtimes. Spilling of food and soiling of clothes are distasteful to most people, especially when eating in the company of others who are not at a physical disadvantage.

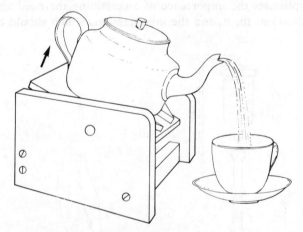

Fig. 10.16 Tip-up teapot stand for 'one-handed' users

For people who are grossly handicapped such as those with spasticity or dysarthria, helping them to be independent in eating and drinking can be a major exercise in skill and adaptation (Caunter & Penrose, 1983).

Respiratory distress
Understandably, breathless patients will appreciate soft

foods which do not require unnecessary effort in chewing. Foods such as steaks and vegetables are obviously contra-indicated and dry foods such as biscuits can be dangerous if inhaled during a breathless episode so should either be avoided or accompanied with fluid to moisten them. Breathless patients need extra time to eat and should be spared the effort of speaking during a meal though not ignored; any verbal communication can be done mainly by the nurse. It may be necessary to give smaller amounts of food more frequently and every attempt should be made to provide interesting meals which are easy to digest but nutritious.

Impaired vision
Occasionally blind patients are admitted to hospital, or as a result of an accident or operation (for example, for removal of a cataract) a patient may temporarily have the eyes bandaged. In these circumstances the food should be cut into mouth-size pieces and the type of food described when served. In most instances, the patient should be helped to retain independence in eating but where necessary the nurse should give assistance.

Problems associated with emotional/psychological dependence

Stress
At some time or other in their lives, most people have experienced emotional stress and one of the manifestations of anxiety can be loss of appetite. The stress and the accompanying upset of the AL of eating and drinking are usually transient. When a person persistently refuses food and fluid however, skill, tact and perseverence are required by the nurse to discover the motive. Disruption of eating and drinking activities may be due to neurotic or psychotic disorders.

Neuroses and psychoses
Many depressed patients are too apathetic and listless to eat. The patient is not hungry, he has no desire for food, he does not want to be bothered with eating and drinking activities. In some instances, he may be merely passive and uninterested and may respond to spoon-feeding, when it is relatively easy to ensure an adequate food and fluid intake.

Some disturbed patients, however, refuse to eat. The patient suffers from delusions and although they seem bizarre the delusions are very real to him: he has no money to pay for food; he is unworthy; his 'bowels are blocked'; his food has been poisoned; a voice is telling him not to eat. At every mealtime, therefore, the patient requires persuasion to eat and having done so, may vomit in order to avert the awful consequences he thinks will ensue if he retains the food in his body.

Apart from bizarre delusions, there are other disorders where the patient refuses to eat and drink and actively resists all persuasion to take nourishment. Anorexia nervosa (aversion to food) is a disorder which occurs mostly in adolescents and more commonly in females than males. In extreme forms it can lead to gross loss of weight, emaciation and even death. The cause is not clearly understood so opinions vary about methods of treatment but some opinions attach a great deal of importance to the relationship between the patient and the nurse who offers the nourishment.

Far from being apathetic, the manic patient is much too active to eat. Frequently, attempts to persuade him to remain seated at a set table for a meal are only marginally successful and a sandwich in his hand may be a more effective way of introducing nourishment.

Alcoholism
It is not possible to talk about eating and drinking without mentioning alcoholism. Currently it is a major problem in many countries of the world, so much so that in 1982 the World Health Organization held a Technical Discussion on Alcohol Consumption and Alcohol-Related Problems which was attended by 100 countries (WHO, 1982). In preparation for the meeting, member states of WHO were asked to provide information on alcohol problems and existing national policies and programmes. The resulting background document revealed that between 1960 and 1980, the increase in global production for beer was 124% and for wine 40%; and between 1960 and 1972, the production of spirits had increased by 61%. Trends in alcohol consumption were also upward. Per capita consumption levels in a number of countries doubled for spirits, wine and beer between 1950 and 1972, and statistics available to 1980 for several countries, show that levels had continued to rise.

The background document highlighted some of the alcohol related problems which affect the community. For example, in several countries, alcoholism or alcoholic psychosis accounts for 20–30% of all first admissions to psychiatric hospitals, as well as accounting for a considerable proportion of admissions to general hospitals. Prolonged drinking can cause cirrhosis of the liver, indeed the incidence of cirrhosis is sometimes used as an index of the magnitude of alcohol problems; in a number of countries, cirrhosis ranked as among the five leading causes of death among males aged 25–64 years. Consumption of alcohol also increases the risk of developing cancer in the larynx, pharynx, mouth and oesophagus. Figures from a Report by the Organisation for Economic Co-operation and Development (OECD) were quoted in the WHO document and indicated that in industrialised countries 30–50% of fatal traffic accidents involve drivers with a high level of alcohol or other drug in the blood. These are some of the effects on the community which, if there is a national health service, has to pay for the health services which are sought as a result of these outcomes, but of course, the individual and family also suffer when there is alcohol abuse.

The development of alcoholism is usually insidious. In some countries, wine drinking may be a normal part of mealtimes and in many societies, people can enjoy a drink socially without experiencing any compulsion to take liquor. Some people, however, come to be dependent on alcohol and this may manifest itself in behaviour which is atypical for that person such as disregard for personal appearance, unpunctuality, irritability or absence from work. Excessive drinking may also lead to irresponsible behaviour, petty crime, casual sexual activity and even disorderly behaviour amounting to assault, perhaps involving police custody. All these deviations bring attendant distress to family and friends.

Sometimes the problem is less easy to detect because the person appears to function adequately in everyday activities yet needs to imbibe at increasingly frequent intervals during the day in order to cope with his commitments. As might be expected, the affected individual begins to suffer from malnutrition because the appetite for food decreases; he then loses weight and his health deteriorates. Eventually there are economic overtones as more and more money is spent on procuring alcohol to the detriment of the family budget, and work capacity may become impaired, often to the point of loss of employment.

In the U.K., various voluntary associations work in conjunction with the National Council for Alcoholism. One is for ex-alcoholics and is called Alcoholics Anonymous (AA), a world-wide association. Members of local branches meet frequently to give each other moral support in the long and continuous process of refraining from drinking alcohol. Another is called the A1–Anon Family Group which is for the spouse, friends and relatives of the alcoholic, and they help one another to cope with the many problems of alcoholism which impinge on family life and cause untold upset.

Despite efforts to provide treatment for alcoholism, the problem seems to be growing. There is evidence to suggest that alcohol intake is increasing among all groups in our society but particularly among women and particularly among women in the 18–25 age group (DHSS, 1980). These findings have considerable significance not only because drinking is starting in a younger age group but because excessive drinking during pregnancy can have adverse effects on fetal development resulting in a range of abnormalities termed Fetal Alcohol Syndrome (Dowdell, 1981). Although most studies about FAS come from U.S.A., it occurs in many parts of the world and in many races. Even in the postnatal period, the effects of alcohol abuse during pregnancy can be exhibited in the newborn. Symptoms of alcohol withdrawal have been observed within 6–12 hours of birth.

Symptoms of 'withdrawal' are perhaps more easily identified when an alcoholic is suddenly deprived of alcohol as may occur after an accident requiring immediate surgery and a stay in hospital. Withdrawal symptoms featuring restlessness, agitation, hallucinations, delirium and disorientation may occur, together with tremor and shaking; the term used for the condition is delirium tremens. The patient may decide to use the incident to seek treatment and if so requires sensitive handling and a great deal of encouragement to proceed. Help may be obtained in one of the special centres which have been created for those who are highly motivated to overcome the uncontrollable craving for liquor. However there is a movement away from intensive therapeutic intervention and prolonged inpatient stay. It is often considered preferable to help the alcoholic and the family within their own environment, mobilising community resources. In this context, inpatient care is seen as a phase within an overall treatment plan, and not sufficient in itself (Brown, 1984).

Currently in the U.K. there are vigorous campaigns to educate the public about the dangers of alcoholism in an attempt to prevent the distress associated with dependence on alcohol and all its sequelae.

DISCOMFORTS ASSOCIATED WITH EATING AND DRINKING

Usually mealtimes are pleasurable occasions but some people may suffer from various kinds of discomfort related to eating and drinking.

Stomatitis
Inflammation of the mouth (stomatitis) can be a severe impediment to appetite and to the physical activity of eating and drinking. The gums and mouth are painful and except in the teething infant, usually dry. The mucous membrane is reddened, the tongue swollen and covered with a dry fur, and in severe cases, the breath is foetid. Stomatitis can be prevented but when it does occur, it requires careful oral hygiene.

There are several causes of stomatitis. It occurs in poorly nourished children, in adults who over-indulge in smoking and alcoholic drinking, during the course of febrile diseases and in ill people whose mouths are not regularly given care. Dehydration and the lack of salivary flow from mastication of food are contributory factors.

Stomatitis also occurs when there is a deficiency in nutrients such as vitamin B, and in iron-deficiency anaemias. It may occur in specific infections such as scarlet fever, diphtheria, syphilis, measles and smallpox, and in a condition called thrush which is caused by a fungus, candida albicans.

Often the tongue is inflamed as well as the mouth because of trauma from the sharp edge of damaged teeth or badly fitting dentures. Quite frequently elderly people have such problems as the gums shrink; relatively simple dental care can add considerably to their enjoyment of eating and drinking.

Nausea

This condition is easily recognised by the person experiencing it but difficult to describe. It occurs in waves, may be accompanied by excess salivation, pallor and sweating, and is often a precursor of vomiting. Almost always there is loss of appetite. Nausea may merely be a manifestation of over-indulgence in food and drink but can also occur associated with anxiety states, post-anaesthesia, jaundice, dysfunction in the digestive tract, or the ingestion of drugs which irritate the lining of the digestive tract, or pain anywhere in the body. It may also be a symptom in the early months of pregnancy probably due to hormonal changes in the mother's body. It may also occur as an undesirable side-effect after administration of, for example, morphine or digoxin, in which case the drug may be stopped, or given in a reduced dose.

Nausea is distressing to the sufferer and the nurse should be comforting and supportive. Some people find it helpful to suck ice when feeling nauseated, others prefer a peppermint flavour, still others find it helpful to lie down in a quiet, well ventilated room. For some a modification of diet, avoiding the nausea-producing food or drink is all that is required. For others an anti-emetic drug may be prescribed to relieve the discomfort until the cause is isolated and treated.

Vomiting

Nausea may be followed by expulsion of the stomach contents. In instances where vomiting is persistent it can lead to dehydration because of the excessive loss of body fluids. It is important for the nurse to observe:

a. time of occurrence
   — early morning: related to pregnancy, renal disease
   — soon after a meal and giving relief from pain: related to gastric ulceration
b. character and appearance
   — containing undigested food: related to indiscretion of food and drink
   — containing red blood: related to rupture of a blood vessel in the upper digestive tract
   — containing dark red digested blood ('coffee grounds'): related to gastric ulceration
   — containing brown foul-smelling material ('faecal vomit'): related to intestinal obstruction
c. manner of ejection
   — effortless and in small quantities: related to intestinal obstruction
   — with much pain and retching: related to gastric ulceration

   — projectile and without warning: related to head injuries, pyloric stenosis (obstruction due to narrowing of the pyloric orifice)

Whatever the form, the nurse should procure, and help the patient to hold the vomit bowl, and assist by wiping his mouth with a tissue. The bed should be screened. Usually the patient will find it comforting if the nurse places her hand on his forehead and assures him by her behaviour that she is sympathetic and not disgusted by such episodes which are undoubtedly unpleasant for both patient and nurse. Most people find it easier if in a sitting position with the head over the basin but if it is necessary to lie flat, the head should be turned to one side and supported, and the patient should be helped into a side-lying position.

It is important to remove vomitus and any soiled linen from the vicinity of the patient as quickly as possible and to provide facilities for the patient to sponge his face and hands and have a refreshing mouthwash. A specimen of vomitus should be retained for inspection however, as it may be helpful in diagnosis of the cause.

Observation of a patient who is semi-comatose or recovering from an anaesthetic is of critical importance. Death can readily result because of respiratory obstruction caused by vomit being sucked into the airway during semi-consciousness. The semi-conscious patient should be turned on to one side in the semi-prone position with all pillows removed until consciousness is regained and with it, the cough reflex.

Heartburn

A burning sensation behind the sternum, often accompanied by regurgitation of an acid-like fluid into the mouth is called heartburn. Usually it occurs following meals and is frequently associated with a gastric ulcer or a hiatus hernia (herniation of abdominal contents into the thorax) but clears up when the ulcer heals or the hernia is repaired. It may be alleviated however by maintaining a sitting position following meals and sometimes, taking an oral alkaline mixture effectively prevents its occurrence. If these measures are unsuccessful a mouthwash helps to counteract the discomfort.

Flatulence

Some patients complain of 'wind' or flatulence. Inevitably some air is swallowed when eating and sometimes when the stomach contracts, the air can be expelled up the oesophagus and produces what is termed belching. In some cultures it is a mark of appreciation following an enjoyable meal; in Western culture belching is usually considered to be an embarrassment. As a single feature, flatulence is not generally considered to be pathological but can cause a great deal of discomfort or even pain and may be relieved by taking a peppermint sweet, or a drink of peppermint water which is usually more effective when given in hot water.

Halitosis

A disagreeable odour from the mouth may cause considerable distress to the patient and to those in his vicinity. Halitosis may be caused by infected gums or decayed teeth and dental attention may be indicated. It also occurs in very ill patients or those who are not taking sufficient fluid and food to keep the mouth clean and healthy. In such instances, the mouth and tongue become coated with a film consisting of bacteria, dead cells and decaying food and it is a nursing responsibility to provide frequent mouth care which will prevent or reduce halitosis and help the patient to feel more comfortable. Unless contraindicated, the patient should be helped to drink as much fluid as possible.

Food allergy

Many authors of scientific papers prefer to retain the term 'allergy' for reference to immunological mechanisms only, and suggest the use of 'idiosyncrasy' or 'food intolerance' to describe an adverse reaction to food (Lindsay, 1984). For the people who suffer, the terms will seem irrelevant. They may experience swelling in different parts of the body; heavy perspiration unrelated to exercise: fatigue not helped by rest; bouts of tachycardia; fluc-

tuations in weight; and the symptoms come and go. Although some patients will have strong suspicions as to which foods provoke the symptoms, says Lindsay, history alone should not be relied on and is no substitute for controlled clinical observation, 'elimination dieting' and challenge with suspected food allergens.

The problems of food allergy can be more dramatic in a baby and may involve for example vomiting, diarrhoea, abdominal colic, rash, respiratory distress, irritability and general failure to thrive (Community Outlook, 1981). Diagnosis is difficult but identification of the cause and treatment may be life-saving.

Pain

Pain in the digestive tract may occur because of an inflammatory condition, an obstruction, a hiatus hernia, an unusual growth, and may be accompanied by vomiting.

Varying degrees of pain occur in most diseases of the upper gastrointestinal tract, often related to the intake of food and often at a specific time interval after meals. Foods which are difficult to digest — fried foods, rich carbohydrates and highly spiced foods — are particularly liable to cause pain and most frequently it is experienced in the epigastric region. The degree or duration of pain from gastric ulceration can often be reduced by taking an oral dose of an alkaline mixture, but in principle, pain should be dealt with by treating the cause.

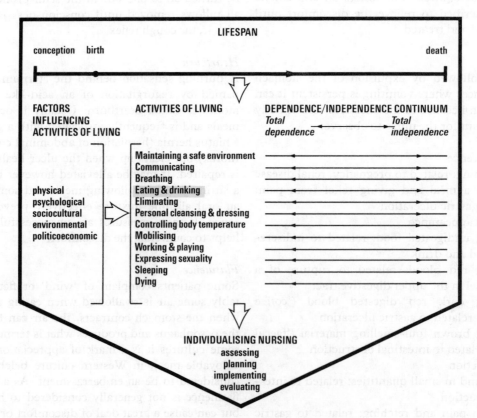

Fig. 10.17 The AL of eating and drinking within the model for nursing

Pain in a hollow muscular tube like the digestive tract can be experienced as *colic*, a severe sharp shooting pain. Colic is a discomfort not uncommonly experienced by babies and it may accompany many types of disorder affecting the digestive tract.

Referred pain (p. 40) can be a feature of gall-bladder disease, and the patient feels the pain in the region of his scapula (shoulder blade).

Anxiety about investigations

To assess deviations in the capacity to eat and drink, and any pain/discomfort in the digestive tract, various investigations are carried out, some of them very elaborate and requiring sophisticated equipment. The most commonly used in relation to this AL of eating and drinking are probably X-ray, which may or may not be combined with a barium swallow or barium meal; gastric secretion tests, and gastroscopy, with or without a biopsy. The actual technique of X-ray is not painful; the barium swallow and barium meal are distasteful; the gastric secretion test causes discomfort but the gastroscopy can be alarming and may even be painful. Nevertheless in all circumstances, the patient will have some anxiety about what he will be expected to do, how he will react and what the result will be.

The nurse must therefore take time to explain any preparation involved prior to the procedure and what to expect during and after. Any relevant instructions about the patient's expected behaviour should be stated clearly and simply. Factual information about the preparation and technique will be found in the ward's procedure book but the nurse must interpret it to the patient according to her perception of his preparedness to receive the information.

Feedback about the results of tests are usually of crucial importance to the patient and are given by the doctor or the nurse in charge of the ward/clinic/health centre.

Whatever the nature of the illness, all patients require a healthful diet delivered in the manner most suitable to the circumstances. The nutrition of patients must be seen as part of the total care and may well determine the success or failure of other treatments. Maintaining or regaining appropriate nutritional status is a crucial aim of treatment, and although it is the responsibility of a health care team, nurses are important members. Nurses are with the patient when meals are served and have the opportunity to note if they take the food and fluid, enjoy eating and drinking or if, as quoted earlier, the patients 'just tumble over the contents of the plate or dip the spoon into the cup to deceive the nurse'.

In the second half of this chapter some of the problems and discomforts which can be experienced by patients in relation to the AL of eating and drinking have been described. This provides the beginning nurse with a generalised idea of these; it will be useful in assessing, planning, implementing and evaluating an individualised programme for each patient's AL of eating and drinking.

This chapter has been concerned with the AL of eating and drinking. However, as stated previously it is only for the purpose of discussion that any AL can be considered on its own; in reality the various activities are so closely related and do not have distinct boundaries. Figure 10.17 is a reminder that the AL of eating and drinking is related to the other ALs and also to the various components of the model for nursing.

REFERENCES

Brandt W 1980 North-South: a programme for survival. Pan Books, London

Brent Health Authority 1980 Food and Health Policy for Brent. Central Middlesex Hospital, London

Brown C 1984 Inpatient treatment. Nursing Times 80(12) March 21:59–60

Burkitt D 1983 Don't forget fibre in your diet. Dunitz, London, p66–68

Caunter M, Penrose J 1983 Solving feeding problems. Nursing Times 79(51) December 21:24–26

Coates V 1984 Inadequate intake in hospital. Nursing Mirror 158(5) February 1:21–22

Community Outlook 1981 Special foods for special babies. Nursing Times 77(11) March 12:85–86

DHSS 1975 Recommended daily amounts of food energy and nutrients for groups of people in the U.K. HMSO, London

DHSS 1980 Drinking in England and Wales. Press Release, London

Dowdell P 1981 Alcohol and pregnancy: a review of literature 1968–1980. Nursing Times 77(43) October 21:1825–1831.

Ellenborgen L 1981 Controversies in clinical nutrition. Churchill Livingstone, New York

Flannigan M 1982 Food for thought. Nursing Mirror 154(16) April 21:44–46

Gibbs J 1983 Bacterial contamination of nasogastric feeds. Nursing Times 79(7) February 16:41–47

Habicht J 1983 Nutrition: a health sector responsibility. World Health Forum 4:5–9

Hamilton-Smith S 1972 Nil by mouth? Royal College of Nursing, London

Health Education Council 1983 Proposals for nutritional guidelines for health education in Britain. HEC, London

Kaplan S 1979 Some psychological and social factors present in the condition of obesity. Journal of Rehabilitation 45:52

Lindsay M 1984 Food allergy or food allergic disease. Nursing Times 78(20) May 19:830–832

Nightingale F 1974 Notes on nursing. Blackie, London (original 1859)

Royal Marsden Hospital 1984 Procedures for nasogastric feeding. Nursing Mirror Clinical Forum 158(20) May 16:i–viii

Smith E 1981 Total parenteral nutrition — a team concept. Nursing Times 77(34) August 19:1464–1465

Tweedle D 1978 How the metabolism reacts to injury: tissue repair. Nursing Mirror 147(21) November 23:34–38

Wood S 1982 Parenteral nutrition. Nursing 2(4) August:105–107

WHO Technical Discussion 1982 Alcohol problems: a growing threat to health. WHO Chronicle 36(6):222–225

ADDITIONAL READING

Anis Kowicz S 1984 Anorexia nervosa. Nursing Mirror 158(15) April 11:42–43

Community Outlook 1983 Diabetes update. Nursing Times 79(19) May 11:115–130

Division of Family Health 1983 The dynamics of breast-feeding. WHO Chronicle 37(1):6–10

Holmes S 1983 You are what you eat. (James Report). Nursing Times 79(48) November 30:8–10

Holmes S 1984 Chemotherapy and the gastrointestinal tract. Nursing Times 80(8) February 22:29–31

Houston M, Howie P, McNeilly A 1983 Infant feeding. Nursing Mirror 156(17) April 27:i–ii

Howard J, Patten S 1981 Nutritional assessment and metabolic profile. In: Wesdorp R, Soeters P (ed) Clinical nutrition '81. Churchill Livingstone, Edinburgh

Khatib H 1984 Allergy in childhood. Nursing Times 80(12) March 21:28–31

McKenna G, Wright M 1983 The hazards of affluence. Nursing Mirror 157(23) December 7:22–24

Mental Health Nursing 1984 Focus on alcoholism: caring for the problem drinker. Nursing Times Supplement 80(12) March 21:55–60

Oliver M 1984 Coronary risk factors: should we not forget about mass control? World Health Forum 5(1):5–18

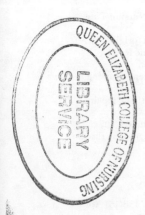

11

Eliminating

The activity of eliminating

Eliminating is an activity of living which all individuals perform with unfailing regularity throughout life. Whatever a person is doing, wherever he is, and regardless of the time of day, he responds to the need to eliminate and this response is an integral activity of everyday life. One of the most interesting characteristics of this AL is that, by custom, it is performed in private. In public buildings, and even in the family home, the provision of a place affording privacy to the individual for eliminating is considered to be essential. Even in societies which emphasise the communal nature of activities of living, eliminating is normally a private activity and the products of elimination are concealed from the public eye.

For the excretion of these waste products quite separate systems of the body are involved. However, they are being discussed together as one activity of living because, as far as the individual is concerned, they are virtually inseparable. The AL of eliminating comprises *urinary elimination* and *faecal elimination*.

THE NATURE OF ELIMINATING

So essential is the nature of eliminating that even a unicellular organism must eliminate the waste products of the metabolic processes which are constantly going on within it. In many multicellular organisms however, separate systems deal with the elimination of urine and faeces. In human beings the urinary system produces and excretes urine; whereas the large bowel or colon produces and excretes faeces — the colon has customarily been described as part of the 'digestive system' but in this text is called the defaecatory system. Eliminating is so necessary that the newborn baby excretes waste matter (meconium) from the bowel, and urine from the urinary bladder shortly after birth by reflex (involuntary) response to a stretch stimulus from fullness in the bowel and bladder. Eventually voluntary control over reflex evacuation of the bladder and bowel is achieved. When necessary though, the desire to eliminate can be suppressed for a considerable time until there is a suitable time and place.

THE PURPOSE OF ELIMINATING

Whereas the AL of eating and drinking is for the sole biological purpose of providing the essential nutrients for living, the AL of eliminating is for dealing with the waste products from utilisation of food and drink. The main purpose of eliminating urine is to dispose of unrequired fluid intake; dissolved chemicals which the body cells are not immediately requiring (and which cannot be stored) so that the body is correctly hydrated, in electrolyte balance and thereby in overall acid/base balance. The main purpose of excreting faeces is to rid the body of indigestible cellulose and unabsorbed food but faeces also contains shed endothelial cells, intestinal secretions, water and bacteria.

BODY STRUCTURE AND FUNCTION REQUIRED FOR ELIMINATING

Early on while learning about the AL of eliminating it is necessary for nursing students to have an overview of the body structure and function required for eliminating. Later on in the programme, students will need to learn more detail about this subject so that they can understand the pathological conditions which can occur in these systems and the effect which they can have on the AL of eliminating: what follows is an introduction to the subject.

The urinary system
This system comprises two kidneys, two ureters, the bladder and the urethra (Fig. 11.1).

The kidneys. It is in the million cellular units called nephrons of which the kidney is formed that the processes of filtration and selective reabsorption takes place, resulting in the formation of urine. *Filtration* is the process whereby fluid is filtered from the body's blood as it circulates, and about 170 litres each day undergo the process. But because of the process of *reabsorption*, only 1 to $1\frac{1}{2}$ litres are eventually excreted as urine. Reabsorption occurs in the long tubules of the nephron (Fig. 11.2); it is selective and as a result, important nutrients (such as glucose and amino-acids) are retained, salts are taken up

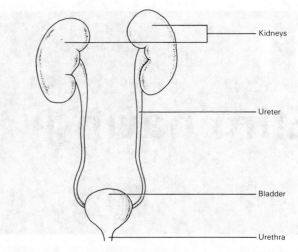

Fig. 11.1 The urinary system

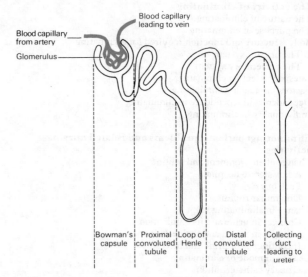

Fig. 11.2 A nephron

according to the body's requirements and waste products (particularly urea, uric acid, creatinine and drug toxins) are excreted. To accomplish this the nephrons are highly specialised structures.

Each nephron begins as a small tuft of tiny blood capillaries encapsulated in the structure known as Bowman's capsule. This glomerulus leads into the end of a tubule which has three sections; the proximal convoluted tubule, the loop of Henle and the distal convoluted tubule. Several tubules lead into collecting ducts which in turn lead to the ureter which leaves the kidney.

The kidneys are situated at the back of the abdominal cavity, one on either side of the spine (Fig. 11.3). They are covered by peritoneum and are embedded in fat. The kidney tissue is arranged as in Figure 11.4 and the blood is supplied from the renal artery.

The ureters. The urine is conveyed from the kidneys to the urinary bladder by the ureters. These are two long muscular tubes which enter the bladder obliquely at its

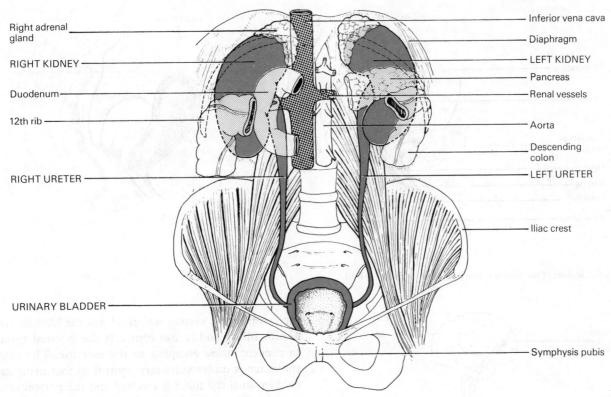

Right adrenal gland

RIGHT KIDNEY

Duodenum

12th rib

RIGHT URETER

URINARY BLADDER

Inferior vena cava

Diaphragm

LEFT KIDNEY

Pancreas

Renal vessels

Aorta

Descending colon

LEFT URETER

Iliac crest

Symphysis pubis

Fig. 11.3 Position of the kidneys, ureters and bladder

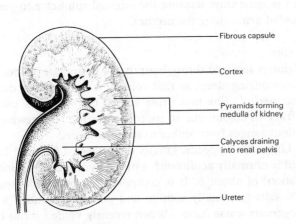

Fibrous capsule

Cortex

Pyramids forming medulla of kidney

Calyces draining into renal pelvis

Ureter

Fig. 11.4 Structure of a kidney

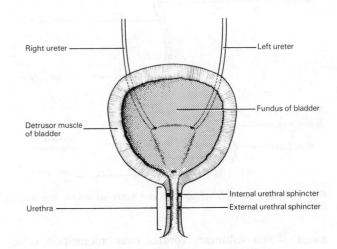

Right ureter

Detrusor muscle of bladder

Urethra

Left ureter

Fundus of bladder

Internal urethral sphincter

External urethral sphincter

Fig. 11.5 The urinary bladder, showing entry of the ureters

posterior base so that reflux of urine is prevented (Fig. 11.5).

The bladder. This is a distensible organ within the pelvic cavity. When full, it protrudes into the abdominal cavity and lies against the anterior abdominal wall (Fig. 11.6, p. 186). In the male the bladder lies in front of the rectum and in the female it is separated from the rectum by the uterus.

The urethra. This conveys the urine from the bladder to the exterior. It is a tube in which the circular fibres of the muscle layer are gathered into two sphincters. The internal sphincter of plain muscle fibres is at the exit from

the bladder and the external sphincter of skeletal/voluntary fibres lies just below. In the female the urethra is very short and opens just in front of the vagina. In the male the urethra is longer, running the length of the penis to open at its tip.

Micturition
Micturition is a complicated process by which, at intervals, the stored urine in the bladder is eliminated. In infancy the process occurs as a reflex act; fullness of the bladder triggers off the specialised voiding centre in the spinal cord (Fig. 11.7) and urine is automatically elimi-

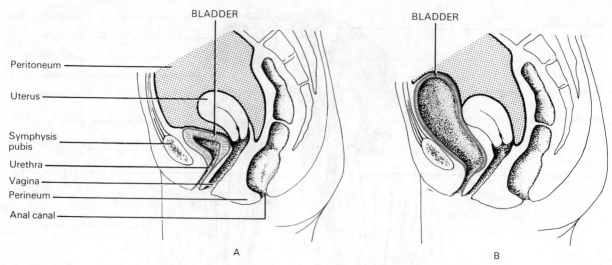

Fig. 11.6 Positions of the female urinary bladder: A Empty B Full

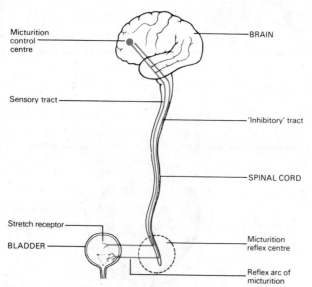

Fig. 11.7 The bladder, spinal cord and brain structures involved in micturition

nated. When voluntary control over micturition is acquired, the brain also becomes involved in the process.

When roughly 100 to 150 ml of urine has collected in the bladder, stretch receptors in its muscle wall are stimulated and impulses are transmitted via the voiding reflex centre along the sensory tract to the micturition control centre in the brain's cortex. The individual becomes aware that his bladder is becoming full. Able to exercise control over the process, the person can choose either to empty his bladder or to inhibit micturition. However, when more than 500 ml or so of urine has collected in the bladder, it becomes difficult to prevent automatic expulsion of urine.

The smooth muscle wall of the bladder has a double nerve supply, one nerve derived from the sympathetic nervous system and one from the parasympathetic. It is the sympathetic system which relaxes the bladder wall to permit filling and it also contracts the internal sphincter to prevent urine escaping to the exterior. The external sphincter is under voluntary control so that urine can be held in until the toilet is reached and the person is ready to void. The parasympathetic nervous system stimulates contraction of the bladder muscle to squeeze urine out, at the same time relaxing the internal sphincter to permit flow of urine along the urethra.

Urine
Urine is secreted throughout the 24 hours but production slows during sleep, so that voiding is unnecessary during that period. The first urine voided on waking is usually darker in colour due to its concentration. Otherwise the colour ranges from amber to straw-coloured.

Urine has a specific gravity of between 1.015 and 1.025 and is normally acidic with a pH (a hydrogen ion concentration) of about 6. It is composed of about 96% water, 2% salts (especially sodium and potassium) and 2% nitrogenous waste (urea). When recently voided it has only a slight smell but after exposure to air, it decomposes and begins to smell of ammonia.

A high fluid intake results in a high urine output and vice versa. However, the normal urine output is around 1 to 1½ litres in 24 hours; the usual frequency of micturition is from 5 to 10 times in that period.

The defaecatory system
As already mentioned the organs involved in the production and elimination of faeces (Fig. 11.8) are usually described as part of the digestive system. However, because of their specific purpose they are being grouped together here and called the defaecatory system.

The food residue, a volume of 500 ml or so per day, passes from the small intestine through the ileocaecal

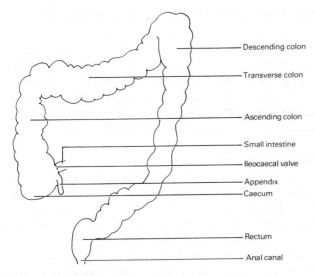

Descending colon

Transverse colon

Ascending colon

Small intestine

Ileocaecal valve

Appendix

Caecum

Rectum

Anal canal

Fig. 11.8 The large intestine

valve to the *large intestine*. After absorption of water, the volume is reduced to about 150 ml of faeces. The large intestine acts as a storage organ for the accumulation of faeces before defaecation. In addition, the bacteria which live there act to synthesise several vitamins, notably those of the B group and vitamin K.

The muscle layer of the large bowel has its longitudinal fibres collected into bands which gather the bowel into puckers in the abdominal cavity. In the mucous membrane, goblet cells are numerous to produce the mucus required to lubricate the passage of the drying faecal matter. The faeces pass through the large intestine (comprising the ascending, transverse and descending colon) to *the rectum* and are eliminated from the body via *the anal canal*. In the anal canal, the circular muscle fibres are collected into the internal and external sphincters. As in the urinary system, the internal sphincter is not under voluntary control whereas the external is. Again, the nerve supply is both sympathetic and parasympathetic.

Defaecation

This is the activity by which faeces are expelled from the bowel to the exterior. The desire to defaecate is initiated by the gastrocolic reflex (the contraction of the colon as food enters the stomach) and by the distension of the colon and rectum due to the presence of faecal matter. Defaecation is brought about by the action of the para-sympathetic nervous system which contracts the bowel and relaxes the internal anal sphincter. This allows the faeces to be expelled if the external sphincter is also re-laxed under *voluntary control*. Expulsion of faeces is as-sisted by the individual contracting the abdominal and chest muscles as this 'sets' the diaphragm and increases intra-abdominal pressure. Squatting is the position which most easily allows the faeces to be discharged but leaning forward while sitting on the toilet best approximates this natural position.

Faeces

The first stool of the infant is a sticky, greenish-black substance called meconium which has accumulated in the bowel from about the fifth month of prenatal develop-ment. This consists of mucus, endothelial cells, amniotic fluid, bile pigments and fats. Meconium is passed several times in the first days of life. Then a brownish-green stool is passed and, a few days later, the baby's excreta become yellow in colour. A breast-fed baby has softer, brighter yellow stools than a bottle-fed baby whose stools are paler, more formed and with a slightly offensive smell. Once the infant is weaned and beginning to have a balanced diet of normal foodstuffs, the faeces begin to take on their familiar composition.

Faecal matter in the adult is normally brown in colour, soft in consistency and cylindrical in form. There is an odour from faeces due to the action of bacterial flora in the intestine and the smell varies according to the bacteria present and the type of food ingested. Faeces are nor-mally composed of water (75%) and solid matter (25%) made up of quantities of dead bacteria, some fatty acids, inorganic matter, proteins and undigested dietary fibre. With regard to number and size of stools, the collection of epidemiological information shows that people in rural third world countries excrete two stools a day with a total weight of between 300 and 500 g, whereas the average for people in Western society is one stool daily weighing between 80 and 120 g (Burkitt, 1983). However on page 190 a study carried out in the U.K. is discussed: it re-vealed that the frequency of defaecation ranged from three times per day to three times per week.

In Burkitt's reference it is also stated that the time taken from ingestion of food to its output as faeces is termed 'intestinal transit time'. Again there is difference in this time between people in rural third world countries and Western societies — approximately 1–1½ days in the former; and about 3 days in young healthy adults in the latter, the time increasing in the elderly to 2 weeks. If car-cinogens are formed in the bowel, their contact with the lining membrane will be minimised by rapid transit time.

An acid stool is produced by bacteria breaking down the unabsorbed dietary fibre, and faecal acidity is thought to be one of the factors which reduce the amount of potential carcinogens in the bowel.

It is likely that in the next few years more information will be available about the function of faeces in prevent-ing not only bowel disease but also disease in other parts of the body. This shows very clearly the importance of constant updating of knowledge.

LIFESPAN: EFFECT ON ELIMINATING

The lifespan clearly has relevance to eliminating and as a component of the model of living will now be focused to this AL. The lifespan starts with conception: in the prenatal stage the placenta does the work of fetal organs such as the bowel and kidneys which do not function fully during this period. Fetal waste products diffuse across the placenta to the maternal blood and are then excreted by the mother in addition to her own waste products.

It has already been pointed out that even the newborn infant voids both bladder and bowel involuntarily. An important milestone in childhood is the acquisition of voluntary control over elimination. Although toilet training helps the child to learn to recognise the signals of the need to eliminate, it cannot really hasten the development of voluntary control because this is dependent on maturation of the required components of the nervous and musculoskeletal systems.

The time to start toilet training a child depends partly on age, and partly on each individual child's 'readiness' to begin. One of the first indicators of 'readiness' for toilet training is the child's awareness of having a full bladder. Soon he begins to warn his mother when he needs to use the potty and at this stage can begin to do without nappies during the day. Control over defaecation is gained before control over urinary elimination.

By 3 years of age many children can go to the toilet on their own and are beginning to be able to do without toileting during the night. Children of 4 are usually competent in the social skills associated with elimination and, by school age, have developed independence and also a feeling of desire for privacy while eliminating.

Gradually when the child has gained control of both activities he can make decisions for himself about where and when he will eliminate. Sometimes the child may misuse these newly acquired skills to manipulate the parents, for example by 'wetting' to attract attention, or by referring to eliminating activities in company to cause embarrassment. Attitudes develop not only to the activities, but also to the products of the activities. Whereas society's attitude to ingestion of food is that it is pleasant, desirable and in the main carried out in the company of others; its attitude to elimination of the waste from food, faeces, is that it is unpleasant, sometimes offensive, intensely personal and carried out in privacy.

At the other end of the lifespan, eliminating habits established in childhood may undergo change. Often in the process of ageing the bladder loses its tone, and the kidneys become less efficient, so that older people sometimes need to eliminate smaller amounts of urine at a more frequent time interval than when younger. The process of ageing can also manifest in the bowel as sluggishness of muscular action and there can be decrease in the volume of faeces as many older people eat less; these conditions can predispose to chronic constipation.

FACTORS INFLUENCING ELIMINATING

Various concepts can help us to describe individuality in eliminating. They incorporate the physical, psychological, sociocultural, environmental and politicoeconomic factors which all contribute to the development of such individuality and in keeping with the model of living will be used as headings in the following discussion.

Physical factors

To be able to eliminate in the normal way a person has to have fully functioning urinary and defaecatory systems. This not only means intactness of the organs comprising these systems but also of the sensory and motor nerves supplying them. Sex influences this AL since usually men stand while passing urine and women sit; this is taken into consideration when providing facilities, particularly in public buildings.

Currently everyone is being exhorted to eat more dietary fibre. It increases the bulk of faeces which in turn increases the motility of the bowel resulting in a soft stool that is easy to excrete regularly. By definition a low-residue diet is non-bulk forming and has the opposite effect. Changes in diet can therefore alter an individual's established defaecation pattern (p. 190).

However, the AL of eliminating involves much more than simply the physical acts of micturition and defaecation. The person must be able to reach the toilet (which often is situated upstairs in homes and public buildings), to undress and dress, to sit on a toilet and rise from it. Post-elimination hygiene too, including the use of toilet paper and handwashing, has to be carried out. It is apparent that eliminating is closely related to the equally complex AL of mobilising.

Psychological factors

A minimum level of intellectual ability is required to learn the many skills involved in eliminating. If the learning is started too early or is very strict some people think that it can contribute to a rigid personality. The development of concepts of modesty and privacy are also important to enable a person to appreciate and conform to the prevailing social customs.

If people are to achieve and maintain a healthy state of eliminating they require knowledge about the relationship of this AL to the amount of fluid taken into and lost from the body; the amount of fibre in the diet, and the type of exercise to keep the abdominal and pelvic floor muscles effective in the act of eliminating.

A person's attitudes and beliefs about this AL may well influence the way it is carried out. For example in a public toilet some people never sit on the 'communal' seat, as they believe that it can carry infection; others flush the cistern to drown the noise of their own eliminating.

Certain emotions may affect the AL of eliminating. Most people have experienced the urgent need to empty the bladder when facing a stressful situation such as an examination. Depression often causes apathy and sluggishness and this can influence eliminating, usually resulting in constipation.

Sociocultural factors

The fact that different words are used in different cultures for things to do with eliminating is interesting. Alternatives such as nappy or diaper tend to be perpetuated from one generation to the next. Likewise the names used for the products of elimination are important, and those used by one cultural group might be considered vulgar by another. Indeed even within a culture, different words may be used by those in different social classes; and in many instances it is family convention which influences the words used. When children first start school they may well be exposed to those from a mix of social classes and as they discover some of these differences they may need help in continuing to use the words selected as family convention.

The child is eventually able to go to the particular place provided for eliminating and gradually there is socialisation according to the concept of privacy and modesty for this AL. There can be difference in the name given to this place, and while the word 'toilet' has a wide acceptance, others such as lavatory and bathroom are used. In most cultures there are 'public toilets' or 'conveniences' for use by people who are away from home and they are usually labelled separately for males and females.

Some strict post-elimination activities are specified by several religions and are transmitted to each succeeding generation. Of course it is desirable that everyone is socialised into acquiring adequate and safe hygiene activities related to eliminating in the interest of preventing infection, particularly the diarrhoeal diseases.

Environmental factors

It is all too easy for those who are used to flush toilets which are attached to a water carriage system of sewage disposal to think that these are the norm. But in some parts of the world people are fortunate if they have chemical toilets, or indeed latrines (earth toilets) which will be discussed in the politicoeconomic section. All three types are designed so that the person can sit on them, but in some countries it is customary to provide a toilet which is a hole in the ground filled with water, on either side of which are foot plates, and elimination is achieved in the squatting position which is functionally an efficient position.

Whether or not an inside toilet is available in a home will obviously influence several aspects of this AL. Most homes have only one toilet and it may be within the bathroom or separate from it. If separate, unless the room has handwashing facilities within it, it may be less easy to uphold standards of hygiene. This applies equally if members of several households have to share a toilet which is not within the home. If to reach the toilet one has to go right outside, then in bad weather the feeling of the need to defaecate may go unheeded which could predispose to constipation.

Politicoeconomic factors

It is difficult for us to realise that only a little more than 100 years ago cholera was rife in the U.K. and still is in some parts of the world. Mortality and morbidity from the diarrhoeal diseases of typhoid, paratyphoid, the dysenteries and enteritis was, and in some countries still is, high. The realisation in the first half of the century that there is a faecal-oral route for spread of such infection led to the increasing introduction of water carriage systems of sewage disposal resulting in a gradual reduction in the incidence of diseases spread by this route. Of course such schemes cost money, and they are dependent on decisions made by a country's government.

In developing countries where the financial budget is not considered sufficient to warrant the implementation of an extensive water carriage system of sewage disposal (the water may not be available), local people in the villages are being encouraged to construct earth toilets. Some countries are using their economic aid from other countries to accelerate this programme in an attempt to achieve the World Health Organization's goal 'Health for all by the year 2000'.

In many countries there is legislation about for example the sanitary requirements for campsites, public toilets, and toilets in public buildings. Minimally, cold water has to be provided for post-elimination handwashing in an attempt to prevent outbreaks of the diarrhoeal diseases.

DEPENDENCE/INDEPENDENCE IN ELIMINATING

The lifespan component of the model of living which was discussed previously is clearly relevant to the concept of dependence/independence for eliminating. For everyone there is a *natural dependence* in the early years and for some there is a return to a varying level of dependence in the later years. There are others who are not capable of achieving independence as they progress through the stages of the lifespan because of congenital conditions as diverse as abnormality of the bowel or bladder, of the nerves supplying them, or physical abnormality of the limbs, or mental handicap. Anywhere along the lifespan people's dependence/independence status can change because of trauma to, or disease of, the bowel or urinary system, or indeed the cause may be in the nervous system. Because the AL of mobilising is a necessary part of eliminating, trauma or disease affecting the musculoskeletal system can also change a person's status on the dependence/independence continuum for the AL of eliminating.

The concept of 'aided independence' is applicable to eliminating. People who for example experience physical decline in advancing years can be helped to retain their 'independence' by provision of a grab rail near the toilet to help them regain the standing position. Should there be stiffness of the hips which makes sitting difficult, a removable raised toilet seat can be used.

INDIVIDUALITY IN ELIMINATING

There are many different factors responsible for shaping each individual's personal eliminating habits. Childhood training and the customs of the person's family and society are important among these.

The actual times of voiding urine vary according to the individual's personal daily routine. Most people void on waking, before going to sleep, and before or after meals. Children and elderly people often make sure they go to the toilet regularly at 2 or 3 hourly intervals in view of their lesser bladder capacity and control.

For most people, defaecation is performed at a set time of the day when time and privacy are available. To find out what actually constitutes 'normal bowel habit' a study was carried out in the 1960s and it was reported by Wright (1974). Two samples of people were taken: patients of family doctors and factory employees. Bowel habits were found to be very similar within the two groups; 99% of them had a frequency of defaecation within as wide a range as three bowel actions per day and three per week! The study concluded that only habits outside this range would be regarded as unusual.

The many people who firmly believed that daily evacuation of the bowel was essential for health, were reassured that this was not so, and there was a general lessening of tension. However, epidemiological information was being collected from underdeveloped third world countries and those in which economic development had led to adoption of a Western way of life, particularly related to diet (Burkitt, 1983). Based on this epidemiological evidence there is a return to the belief that daily evacuation of at least 150 g, and preferably 250 g of faeces is desirable. It can only be achieved by increasing the dietary intake of fibre, but it will take time to convince members of the public that a somewhat drastic change in eating habits is necessary in the interest of health.

The purpose of the model of living is to highlight a person's individuality in living. It can be seen from the discussion so far that there are several dimensions to each of the components of the model of living which can influence the acquisition of individuality in eliminating: and a résumé of the variables described at each component of the model follows:

Lifespan: effect on eliminating
- Involuntary voiding in infancy
- Childhood training for continence
- Loss of muscle tone in old age

Factors influencing eliminating
- Physical
  — fully functioning urinary and defaecatory systems
  — ability to reach the toilet, manipulate clothing, carry out post-elimination toilet, wash hands
- Psychological
  — intellectual ability
  — concept of modesty, privacy
  — response to toilet training
  — attitude to eliminating emotions
- Sociocultural
  — knowledge about diet/eliminating
  — word for products of elimination
  — cultural group/social class/family convention
  — word for place of eliminating
  — post-elimination hygiene/religion
- Environmental
  — type of toilet
  — handwashing facilities
- Politicoeconomic
  — money available for prevention of diarrhoeal diseases

Dependence/independence in eliminating
- Relevant to lifespan
- Congenital conditions
- Disease/trauma
- Dependence on aids/on people
- Total dependence

Eliminating: patients' problems and related nursing activities

It is important that during an episode of illness the patient's individual habits of eliminating are changed as little as possible, unless they are detrimental to health. It is therefore imperative that nurses know about these individual habits and use this knowledge to carry out an individualised nursing plan. The information can be gleaned by nurses bearing in mind the topics noted in the preceding résumé while discussing the AL of eliminating with the patient. It is useful, particularly during the initial assessment phase of the process of nursing if the nurse has in mind the following questions:

- how often does the individual eliminate urine/faeces?
- when does the individual eliminate urine/faeces?
- what factors influence the way the individual carries out the AL of eliminating?
- what does the individual know about eliminating urine/faeces?
- what is the individual's attitude to eliminating?
- has the individual any longstanding problems with eliminating urine and faeces, and if so, how have these been coped with?
- what problems if any does the individual have at present with eliminating urine/faeces and are any likely to develop?

The emphasis during assessment is on the discovery of the patient's usual routines, what can and cannot be done independently, and any coping mechanisms that have been used previously for problems or discomforts which might well be of a chronic or recurring nature. Relevant information from medical records will be noted. In collaboration with the patient whenever possible, any actual problems with the AL of eliminating will be identified. The nurse may well recognise potential problems which may or may not be recognised by the patient and these will of course be discussed with the patient. Mutual realistic goals will be set, to prevent potential problems from becoming actual ones; to alleviate or solve the actual problems; or help the patient cope with those which cannot be alleviated or solved. The nursing interventions and when relevant any activities which the patient agrees to do to achieve the set goals will be selected according to local circumstances and available resources. These will be written on the nursing plan together with the date on which evaluation will be carried out to discern whether or not they are achieving or have achieved the stated goals. All these activities are necessary in order to carry out individualised nursing related to the AL of eliminating.

However, before nurses can begin to think in terms of individualised nursing they need to have a generalised idea of the kind of problems which patients can experience related to the AL of eliminating. These will be discussed together with relevant nursing activities which are encountered early in a nursing career. They are grouped together under five headings:

- change of environment and routine
- change in eliminating habit
- change in mode of eliminating
- change of dependence/independence status for eliminating
- discomforts associated with eliminating.

CHANGE OF ENVIRONMENT AND ROUTINE

From time to time most people experience some disruption to their individualised eliminating habits as a result of a change in environment and routine. Going on holiday inevitably means adapting to a different timetable, doing different things, and making do with whatever toilet facilities are available, even if sometimes these are unfamiliar and unsavoury! If the holiday is a lazy one, it is possible that the less active routine will cause constipation; on the other hand, diarrhoea may be the result of sampling unfamiliar foods. The same sort of problems can be experienced by people who are admitted to hospital.

Admission to hospital

Disruption to established eliminating habits seems to be a common consequence of admission to hospital.

When patients are admitted because of problems associated with urinary elimination or faecal elimination, doctors and nurses ask all sorts of questions about these activities; specimens of urine or faeces are collected and tested and sometimes special procedures such as catheterisation are a necessary part of treatment. Certain communications between patients and staff centre round eliminating. These body functions are no longer private and personal; they seem to the patient to have become everybody's business and not unnaturally he may feel anxious and embarrassed.

Even those patients whose reason for admission is not specifically related to eliminating problems may at assessment be found to be experiencing a problem with this AL. Other patients may encounter difficulties with this AL because of the hospital environment. In particular many patients become bothered by the lack of privacy.

Lack of privacy

Previously in the patient's adult life no-one has asked daily whether or not he has had a bowel movement. This is a routine in many hospitals and some patients who have not been admitted because of a bowel complaint may well consider this an invasion of their privacy.

Curtains round beds may provide visual privacy but they do not provide aural privacy for those patients experiencing urinary or defaecatory problems when giving related information to doctors and nurses. Nurses can help by modulating their voices; choosing to talk with the patient when the beds on either side are empty; or inviting the patient into a room in which nurse and patient can talk without interruption.

For ambulant patients, in many hospital wards which were built in the days when the majority of patients were nursed in bed, toilet facilities are inadequate for the needs of today. Often there are too few toilets or those available are too far away to be readily reached; many are too small for wheelchairs or walking aids; and some are too cold for comfort, or so public they deny any real privacy.

Nurses may not be able to do much about the inadequacy of facilities in the ward, but they can make the most of what exists. For example, toilets should be kept clean and free from the clutter of sluice equipment, and aerosols can be used to keep the air fresh. Patients using the toilet should be allowed as much privacy as possible. How often do nurses thoughtlessly 'pop in' to ask the patient if he is ready to be helped back to bed when a call system could be provided which would avoid this situation?

Unfamiliar routine

If the imposed ward routine for the patients' AL of eliminating is not the same as their individual habit then they are more than likely to have a problem. For example, an individual who usually has a bowel movement immediately after breakfast may find this is not possible because he is expected to stay in bed awaiting the doctor's round. Some people, accustomed to getting up during the night to pass urine, may feel apprehensive about continuing this routine for fear of disturbing other patients.

When showing the newly admitted patient where the toilet facilities are, and discussing things such as when it may be necessary to use a bedpan or provide a specimen of urine, the nurse can take the opportunity to find out as much as possible about the patient's eliminating habits and later to record any relevant information. It is only when an assessment has been carried out that potential problems can be identified and the necessary nursing planned.

As far as possible, patients should be enabled to maintain any deeply ingrained individual habits of eliminating. Bedpan or urinal 'rounds' impose a routine on all patients and it is much better to accommodate each individual's accustomed routine whenever possible.

CHANGE IN ELIMINATING HABIT

Even if conscious, deliberate attention were not paid, for example to how frequently the bladder was emptied, a person probably would notice a marked increase or decrease in the frequency of passing urine and faeces. Should there be a marked change in the colour, odour or consistency of either urine or faeces a person would be likely to notice it too.

As changes in eliminating habit are often indicators of some dysfunction of the urinary or defaecatory systems (or even other body systems) nurses have a responsibility to be able to recognise any change in a patient's urine or its elimination, and faeces and their elimination. Recognition of changes is only possible if the nurse understands what constitutes 'normal' and has data from assessment on the individual patient's norm.

Changes in urine and its elimination

Change in colour. Several factors can cause a change in colour, sometimes transient and not necessarily pathological.

Pale urine may be due to temporary diuresis as a result of excessive fluid intake, or it can result from taking a diuretic drug, or it may be of a continuous nature as in the condition of diabetes mellitus.

Dark urine may mean that it is concentrated as a result of dehydration (p. 173) when less urine is excreted; the colour will lighten as the patient increases his fluid intake. Or it may be caused by the presence of bile pigments (urobilin or bilirubin) due to disease of the liver or gallbladder. The urine will become pigment-free as the disease responds to treatment.

Coloured urine can result from the intake of some foods. Carotene contained in carrots as well as other vegetables and fruits can make urine a bright yellow; beetroot and blackberries can make the urine red.

Medications can also change the colour of urine; an antibiotic called rifamycin makes it an orange-red colour. Naturally, patients should be warned about this.

A smoky colour is indicative of 'occult' (hidden) blood from high in the urinary tract; it is so mixed with the urine that it has lost its identity as blood. On the other hand, urine which is red from frank blood usually means that the bleeding is lower in the urinary tract.

Change in odour. The characteristic odour of urine may change to sweet-smelling, a manifestation of diabetes mellitus. Part of the treatment of diabetic patients is teaching them to test their urine to make sure that it does not contain excess glucose. Decomposing urine smells like ammonia. An infected urine has an offensive fishy smell, and there may be frank pus (pyuria) in the case of severe urinary infection. The patient may need to increase perineal hygiene and be meticulous about changing underwear to prevent odour. In the case of dependent patients this of course would be a nursing activity.

Change in frequency. A change in the number of times a patient passes urine may or may not be accompanied by an alteration in the total amount of urine voided in 24 hours and accurate data are required to establish this.

Increased frequency can vary from that due to the anxiety associated with admission to hospital, and special procedures, tests and so on, to a totally demanding 'urgency' that dominates the patient's life, even disturbing sleep. This type is a very disabling condition. It is often a manifestation of urinary infection (cystitis), a common problem of women and older people.

The frequent voiding of small amounts of urine, although an inconvenience to the person, is actually helpful in combating the infection. The pathogenic micro-organisms are not allowed to remain for long in the urinary tract and so excessive multiplication is prevented. When increased frequency of micturition in an older person is not due to urinary infection, usually it is attributed to deterioration in cerebral function (Lowthian, 1977).

Decreased frequency is closely associated with decreased output and it can result from obstruction, water retention (oedema), kidney disease and dehydration. It is particularly important for nurses to recognise decreased frequency in older patients, since impairment of their thirst mechanism can put them at risk of dehydration. If suspected, the nurse can examine the lips and mouth for dryness, another clue to dehydration.

Change in quantity. Marked deviation from the patient's norm is dangerous because it can result in fluid imbalance. As soon as the change is recognised the patient's fluid intake and output will probably need to be measured and this is a nursing responsibility but depending on the patient's competence, he may be able to help with the measuring and recording on a fluid balance chart.

A decreased output (oliguria) or total absence of urine (anuria) indicates that either urine is not being produced normally by the kidneys as in renal failure, or that its excretion from the bladder is being blocked. In the case of blockage which can be caused by prostatic enlargement, there is retention of urine in the bladder causing a midline abdominal swelling over which there is a dull sound on percussion. It is potentially dangerous and most uncomfortable; indeed, it can be very painful. Sometimes the pressure in the overfull bladder forces urine through the urethral sphincters when the condition is referred to as 'retention with overflow'. Because of the mechanical nature of the blockage, the bladder has to be drained by a catheter (p. 198). The condition can arise postoperatively when some patients experience difficulty in re-establishing micturition and the nurse should report whether or not the patient has passed urine early in the postoperative period.

An increased output can be expected when patients are taking diuretic drugs, their purpose being to increase urinary output in people with oedema. Several of the hypotensive drugs are combined with a diuretic, and nurses need to be aware of this when nursing patients with high blood pressure. Over 2 litres in 24 hours constitutes a pathologically increased output of urine (polyuria). This condition is often associated with excessive thirst (polydipsia) and increased fluid intake, characteristic of the diabetic condition.

Collecting urine specimens. Some changes such as the presence of glucose in the urine in diabetes mellitus are only recognisable from certain urine tests. If urine is to be tested, specimens of urine are collected by the nurse. A 'mainstream' urine specimen is collected into a clean glass measuring jar from urine voided into a clean bedpan or urinal. Such a specimen may be used for biochemical testing for protein, bile, ketones, glucose or blood and is usually done with special dipsticks, the active end of which contains a chemical which changes colour when the urine has in it the substances being tested for. If bacteriological examination is to be performed in the laboratory, a specimen not contaminated with micro-organisms from the lower end of the urethra is necessary — a 'midstream' specimen. It allows the early part of the stream to wash away contamination before collecting the specimen to be tested. In females a proper stream must be established to avoid collecting urine which has flowed over the heavily contaminated areas of the labia and perineal skin. It is not necessary to wash the perineum, and a disinfectant must not be used as some might get into the sample and kill any bacteria present (Meers & Strong, 1980). Of course sterile containers must be used throughout the procedure. King (1980) illustrates and discusses an automatic midstream urine collector which resulted in more reliable specimens. Collecting urine specimens is a common nursing activity but the nurse should remember that it is probably a new experience for the patient. Careful instruction is therefore necessary and ascertainment of whether or not it has been understood. Explanation of the reason for the procedure will help the patient to accept it, and of course privacy and dignity should be maintained throughout.

Changes in faeces and their elimination

Changes in appearance. A disorder of the digestive system may be indicated by a change in the appearance of faeces. Absence of bile, as in biliary obstruction, produces putty-coloured stools. Some obstructive, infective, inflammatory or malignant diseases can cause the faeces to contain blood, which if not visible to the naked eye but detectable by chemical testing is called 'occult blood'. If blood is mixed with the faeces, causing it to look black and shiny, it is known as melaena and comes from a distal site such as the stomach or small intestine. Or it may be evident as frank red blood which, if on the surface of the stools, comes from a local site, and most commonly from bleeding haemorrhoids. Steatorrhoeaic stools, those mixed with mucus and fats, occur in some metabolic disorders. Bulky stools containing undigested food material indicate faulty absorption. Drugs may affect the colour of faecal matter; iron products stain the stool black. Malformed stools, often pencil-like, are indicative of obstruction in the bowel.

Changes in frequency. A healthy person normally has a fairly regular pattern of defaecation. A deviation from this to a decreased frequency is called constipation; change to an increased frequency is diarrhoea.

Constipation. Lack of unabsorbable fibre in the large bowel results in constipation. Dietary fibre is important because it adds bulk to the faeces, making defaecation easy and more frequent. It appears that the diet of Western societies contains much less fibre than is common in societies in rural Africa; consequently the faeces of Western adults have much less bulk and constipation occurs frequently as a result (Burkitt, 1983).

This observation of distinct cultural differences leads to the conclusion that increasing the amount of dietary fibre is likely to prevent constipation. Cereal fibre is more effective than fruit or green vegetable fibre and the easiest way to improve the diet is to take a bran cereal or add small amounts of millers' bran to fruit or cereal.

In a published interview (Swaffield, 1979), Denis Burkitt a well known gastroenterologist was asked 'How does the average person tell if he's constipated?' and the reply was 'Simply by weighing the stools. All you have to do is have some letter scales in the bathroom, and some bits of newspaper or old margarine tubs or whatever and weigh the stools for about four days. ... We should excrete *at least 150 grams daily*, preferably 250 grams.' In the article it states that the average daily stool in Western society is about 120 grams, and as low as 50 grams in some old people.

Whether constipation is an actual or a potential problem, the goal on the nursing plan will be to re-establish the patient's usual frequency of defaecation (unless it was unsatisfactory), and promote ease of defaecation. The nursing intervention would be to ensure that the patient understands the following preventive activities:

- eat a balanced diet which includes fibre-containing foodstuffs (e.g. wholemeal bread, bran cereals, green vegetables, salad and fruits)
- maintain an adequate fluid intake
- take as much exercise as possible
- maintain usual habits of defaecation or establish satisfactory habits
- respond to the sensation of a full bowel
- avoid undue worry about bowel habit
- promote ease of defaecation by using abdominal and pelvic floor muscles

Nurses can do a great deal to prevent constipation by educating all patients to follow this routine. They also need to update their knowledge according to current research findings.

For the treatment of constipation it may be necessary to use laxatives as a short-term measure to re-establish bowel regularity but they should be used as a last resort, and never when a person has abdominal pain, nausea or vomiting. They are prescribed by the doctor but their administration and the subsequent observation and reporting about the patient is a nursing activity. Prolonged use is dangerous because normal bowel function becomes permanently impaired. Unfortunately taking laxatives is a widespread practice in Western countries. A pharmacist (de Mont, 1984) classified laxatives as bulking agents and chemical agents — stimulants, lubricants and saline compounds.

If laxatives fail to remedy severe constipation, suppositories and enemas are treatments which are medically prescribed and thereafter they are a nursing function. Ractoo & Baumber (1983) carried out a randomised trial to compare the effectiveness of two Dulcolax suppositories with one Micralax Micro-Enema on a busy male surgical ward. Out of a total of 176 patients, 82 received the suppository and 94 had the enema. They found that there was no significant difference in effectiveness: it was marginally quicker and simpler to give the enema but the enema was 'very expensive' compared to Dulcolax suppositories.

Duffin et al (1981) ask 'Are enemas necessary?' In a district general hospital 1120 patients were admitted to the geriatric medical wards in a 6 month period, during which 3428 enemas were given. Most of these were the small ready-packaged enemas and it seemed that several were necessary to relieve faecal impaction. The study concluded that the drawbacks were sufficient to warrant a study of other methods of treating constipation and faecal impaction. A suggested 'other' method was whole bowel irrigation which is also termed 'total colonic lavage' (p. 203).

Constipation postoperatively is common, particularly after surgery affecting the gastrointestinal tract. This occurs because there is temporary loss of peristalsis. If this loss persists longer than the initial postoperative period, it develops into a serious condition called paralytic ileus.

However, a much more common complication of constipation is faecal impaction.

Faecal impaction. This is the condition in which faeces harden and accumulate in the colon and rectum, making defaecation difficult or impossible. It is a distressing condition for the patient because, although he may feel the need to defaecate, he is unable to, and abdominal distension and rectal pain cause severe discomfort. Sometimes small amounts of liquid faecal matter bypass the hardened faeces and leak from the anus and this may be wrongly diagnosed as faecal incontinence. Treatment of faecal impaction aims at removal of the impacted faecal matter. This can be accomplished by laxative therapy, a rectal wash-out procedure, manual evacuation or colonic lavage (p. 203).

Diarrhoea. This is yet another change in eliminating habit; it is the condition in which faeces contain excess water and the frequency of defaecation is markedly increased. Gibson & Wilson (1976) comment that 'diarrhoea is a common symptom and may be the result of something as benign and self-limiting as pre-examination nerves or something as serious as carcinoma of the colon'.

Acute diarrhoea has a sudden onset and usually ends rapidly. It is often the result of an infection such as food poisoning, or it may occur from an infectious disease such as typhoid which affects the digestive tract. Chronic diarrhoea exists when the symptoms persist. Ulcerative colitis is an inflammatory condition of the bowel which causes chronic diarrhoea. People who suffer from this often become very debilitated and their lifestyle may be completely dominated and disrupted by this unpleasant disease.

Over time, diarrhoea poses a danger to health because of the excessive loss of fluids and salts, incomplete absorption of nutrients from food, and incomplete synthesis of vitamins. If untreated, the patient will suffer from a multitude of problems. He will become dehydrated and suffer from fluid and electrolyte imbalance, and will lose weight and strength. Medical management may include intravenous administration of fluids and dietary supplements.

Nursing activities, based on assessment of the individual, vary according to the severity and duration of the diarrhoea. Feeling the need to defaecate urgently can be distressing for the patient and, to alleviate fear of soiling, availability of a toilet or commode is essential. The patient should be encouraged to drink more than usual in order to replace fluid lost and to take a nourishing diet which is reduced in fibre-containing foods. Washing of the perianal area and the application of cream can help to alleviate skin soreness around the anus which is caused by the liquid faeces.

Because diarrhoea is often caused by infection, great care must be taken in the disposal of the patient's faeces. Regular handwashing (p. 102) is necessary by both patient and nurse to prevent spreading the infection. Of course, handwashing is necessary whenever faeces are dealt with, such as when collecting a specimen of this excrement.

Collecting a specimen of faeces. A specimen for bacteriological laboratory examination is obtained by asking the patient to defaecate (without also passing urine) into a clean bedpan and, using a spatula or disposable spoon, a small portion of faeces is put into a special sterile container. Stool collections for several days may sometimes be required, for example in cases of steatorrhoea when estimations of amounts of fat in the faeces are made while fat intake in food is controlled. Whenever the nurse is involved in the collection of specimens of faeces she must take care to avoid contamination of herself and her clothes, and adopt a meticulous handwashing technique.

Incontinence of urine and faeces

Incontinence means inability to control the excretion of urine and or faeces. Used without qualification it customarily means urinary incontinence (enuresis) probably because it is a more frequent condition than faecal incontinence (encopresis). When there is both urinary and faecal incontinence, the term 'double incontinence' is used.

When considering the subject of incontinence, few people give any thought to the very complicated phenomenon whereby throughout the day and night most children achieve continence by the age of 3. Norton (1983) gives an account of the complexities which all continent adults have mastered, yet about which the majority of both lay and professional people know very little. However there are some children who do not achieve continence and 1–2% of adults continue to be bed wetters.

If a healthy child continues to wet himself after the age of 5, or regresses to this behaviour after a period of dryness, he can be described as incontinent of urine. Professor Meadow (1981) says that 15% of 5-year-olds and 1% of 15-year-olds wet the bed (nocturnal enuresis). Disease of the central nervous or genitourinary systems is responsible in only a minority of cases. The vast majority of cases of childhood incontinence are viewed either as a deficiency of learning due to absence or ineffectiveness of toilet training, or as a manifestation of anxiety or emotional upset. Whatever the cause, incontinence in childhood is usually a transient condition which disappears without special medical treatment. However, enuresis is disturbing for the child and taxing on his parents, and community nurses can do much to help to treat this problem in the home. Norton (1983) describes two simple but effective treatment approaches. Firstly, the adoption of a very systematic schedule of toileting, with the child being encouraged and praised and perhaps keeping his own progress chart which can build confidence and result in rapid improvement. Secondly, the problem of nocturnal enuresis can be treated using the 'buzzer alarm' apparatus (which was designed on the basis of operant conditioning principles) and this has been found to be a very reliable form of management. The parents may buy the equipment or the nurse may be able to borrow one from the family doctor or health centre for the duration of treatment.

Over the last decade the plight of many incontinent adults has received some publicity but incontinence is still a taboo subject even in many professional circles. Moors (1984) entitled an article 'Confusion, ignorance and inconsistency' and in it she reviewed two reports — *The problem of promoting continence* published by the Royal College of Nursing and *Action on incontinence* a report of a working group (King's Fund project paper, no. 43). These two reports contain up-to-date information and they make it clear that incontinence is a condition which all nurses will have to deal with at some time in their career, since such patients are to be found in geriatric, gynaecology, medical, mental handicap, paediatric, psychogeriatric, surgical and urology wards as well as in their own homes and wherever disabled and handicapped people might be.

The idea of using the term 'promoting continence' is not only an attempt to counteract the stereotype of geriatric wards, and that being old is synonymous with being wet and soiled, but also to incorporate the fact that not all incontinent people are old. There is now evidence that there is considerable incontinence (defined as an episode occurring twice or more per month) in people who are not old: the figures in Table 11.1 are the result of a 5 year study in London, Bristol and South Wales (Thomas et al, 1980). Faecal incontinence in adults aged 15 and over was shown to be 0.5%. Egan (1984) in a short question and answer article gives information about this study which is well worth reading.

Table 11.1 Regular incontinence in the community

Age in years	% Male	% Female
5–14	6.9	5.1
15–64	1.6	8.5
over-65	6.9	11.6

Stated in another way, both reports say that there are probably about 3 million people who are incontinent living in the United Kingdom and no more than 10% of them are receiving any kind of specialist help at all.

Neurogenic bladder

To begin to understand the complexities of incontinence one can examine the term 'neurogenic bladder'. It is used when there is interference with the nerve supply to the bladder, and it can result in various types of incontinence. In one type the desire to pass urine may be appreciated but there is no cerebral inhibition so the bladder contracts resulting in urge incontinence, and evacuation of the full bladder. In another type the full bladder empties reflexly with no sensation. Yet another variation is the atonic bladder which fills so full that the pressure stretches the sphincters and urine dribbles out continuously (overflow incontinence or retention with overflow). Such dribbling incontinence can also occur when the sphincters are incompetent and the bladder no longer acts as a reservoir. The medical diagnosis for people with these different types of incontinence can be as diverse as a stroke (cerebro-vascular accident), spina bifida, paraplegia, peripheral neuropathy in diabetes mellitus, multiple sclerosis, a brain tumour, dementia or a head injury. This list shows clearly that incontinence is a symptom and not a disease; it presents the patient with a problem related to the AL of eliminating and the patient requires nursing help to cope with it (p. 197) since the damage to the nervous system cannot be cured. Norton (1983) discusses various ways to assist voiding; she says that clean intermittent self-catheterisation is probably the single most

significant advance in the management of patients with a neurogenic bladder.

Dribbling incontinence

Dribbling incontinence can come from the non-neurogenic bladder if there is obstruction in or pressure on the urethra from such conditions as an enlarged prostate gland, a full rectum, or a cystocele. There is therefore a mechanical reason for the ensuing retention of urine and when there is sufficient pressure in the bladder it stretches the sphincters and produces dribbling incontinence. The treatment of the cause will theoretically cure the incontinence but in a few instances it is followed by a different type of incontinence.

Urge incontinence

Urge incontinence can also occur in the non-neurogenic bladder. Awareness of the desire to pass urine is immediately followed by passage of urine; this can be a small or large amount while the person is on the way to the toilet. Naturally patients are very distressed about this problem and the more anxious they become the worse the condition gets. If they can find a means of relaxation, perhaps breathing deeply the moment they are aware of the desire to pass urine, micturition will be delayed until the toilet is reached. Such patients may be able to cure the condition by regularly visiting the toilet at perhaps 3 or 4 hourly intervals. It is obvious that confidence is required to cure this distressing problem. In Egan's report (1984) urge incontinence in women increased between the ages of 35 and 64 years.

Stress incontinence

Stress incontinence occurs in people who have an unstable bladder. Should coughing or sneezing or running for a bus — indeed anything which increases intra-abdominal pressure — occur in the presence of a full bladder, the pressure 'squeezes' the bladder wall and stretches the sphincters so that urine escapes against the person's control. Referring to Egan's report (1984), stress incontinence was reported more commonly in those aged 45–64 and the prevalence decreased in the 65–74 age group. Schofield and Schofield (1981) describe how they designed a bodyworn pad in which voided urine is converted into a non-extrudable mass, that is, it is solidified, and in trial this was helpful for patients coping with stress incontinence.

Although the foregoing is a short account of different types of incontinence for the sole purpose of understanding the subject, in reality there can be mixed causes of a person's incontinence. This can be the case for a large group of people who are physically and/or mentally handicapped. Children and adults with physical handicaps which impair their appreciation of the sensation of bladder distension, or render them unable to cope independently with the AL of eliminating, often suffer permanently from incontinence. These people need to be helped to cope with this problem so that they can lead as normal a life as possible. Often the best approach is to utilise special appliances available (p. 199) but sometimes long-term catherisation is necessary.

Incontinence and mental handicap

There is a high incidence of incontinence amongst those who are severely mentally handicapped because there is often damage to the nervous system and this may impair the individual's ability to exercise voluntary control over elimination. Even if there is no physical defect, the mentally handicapped usually have difficulty in coping with the AL of eliminating. However, if they are helped to learn the skills of independent toileting, incontinence often can be overcome. An effective method of toilet training the mentally handicapped is by the use of behaviour modification procedures.

This approach to teaching involves very careful and gradual shaping of new behaviour using reinforcement techniques. Detailed behavioural assessment is carried out first and, from evaluation, changes in behaviour are monitored. The effectiveness of behaviour modification toilet training with severely handicapped patients in a ward environment was evaluated as part of a research project carried out by Tierney (1973). She found that nurses once trained in the techniques involved had considerable success in toilet training patients by this method.

Promoting continence

There is now considerable literature about this subject and if the available knowledge were translated into practice using a positive attitude, many incontinent people would regain continence. An individualised approach is absolutely essential if success is to be achieved and the framework of the nursing process — assessing, planning, implementing and evaluating — can accomplish this. Norton (1984) provides an example of an 'Incontinence assessment checklist' suitable for general purposes. She says that a checklist should not be used as a questionnaire, but as a tool together with accurate information about each incontinence episode to give a picture of the individual person and the incontinence. She also provides a table of symptoms, causes and interventions in incontinence. Rooney (1984) says that accurately defining a patient's incontinence problems is vital for effective treatment and management. Much of what she says will help nurses to assess incontinent patients so that the problems can be identified.

There is undoubtedly an increase in knowledge about promoting continence and the following three references will give readers an idea of up-to-date information. White (1984) gives a table of aids to maintain continence; it includes clothing for both males and females, toilet aids, toilet surround, commodes and hand-held urinals for both males and females: she says that they will give at least some independence to the most handicapped person. Her article includes another table of examples of incontinence aids in each of the following categories — pants with a pouch, stretch pants, pads (waterproof backing), bed protection, bed pads and urosheaths for males. She lists four types of body worn urinals, and a 'bed alarm' and 'night trainer' which can be used in regaining overnight continence.

Robbins (1984) proposes that incontinence is not inevitable in the elderly, mentally infirm. She says that continence relies on the operation of a network of skills both mental and physical and she lists these. She discusses various nursing activities which can be carried out to support the failing systems of continence in this group of people.

Harrison (1984) gives a detailed account of how patients with the problem of stress or urge incontinence can be helped to overcome it. A weak pelvic floor is a contributory factor but she points out that constipation and obesity can also be detrimental to achieving continence. This seems an appropriate place to mention the fact that the efforts of a multidisciplinary team are often necessary to the promotion and maintenance of continence — doctors, nurses, physiotherapists, occupational therapists, dietitians, and supplies officers can all make an important contribution. Indeed chiropodists can be important members of a team since painful feet can prevent people from getting to the toilet quickly.

Nursing the incontinent patient

Although incontinence can be prevented and treated successfully in many instances, there are some patients who need nursing help in order to cope with what has become an intractable problem. For containing urine there are body-worn and bed drainage fabrics so that the skin is no longer in constant contact with urine and they can be used for both ambulant and bedfast patients. However when there is incontinence of faeces the patient does need to be changed immediately. In many ways it is easier for the nurse to manage an episode of faecal incontinence in a bedfast patient. Coping with such an episode in an ambulant patient is a more problematic task: this was highlighted in the research done by Reid (1976). Her observations of the nursing management of incontinence revealed how ill-equipped are many hospital wards for enabling nurses to adequately wash patients and change their day clothes. Either the patient needs to be taken to his bed if this is to be managed properly, or the toilet facilities require to be adapted to provide the nurse with appropriate facilities. Some modern hospitals are equipped with bidets and these permit thorough washing of the perineum and indeed enable many patients to carry out this personal cleansing procedure themselves.

Despite the availability on the market of adequately functioning body-worn pads and pants; bed pads, sheets and waterproof duvet covers, they are not always available to nurses for nursing patients in hospital and in their own homes.

In hospital the use of a drawsheet over a plastic sheet is still common practice as it allows easy replacement of one item of linen with minimum disturbance to the patient in bed. However, drawsheets tend to allow urine to pool under the patient; they also slip and crease readily which is particularly undesirable if pressure sores are to be avoided. The use of incontinence pads is not an ideal solution either because they are seldom effective in containing the urine in one area and frequently cause irritation to the skin and therefore they too may contribute to pressure sore development.

At home, however, protection of the bed is very necessary because most families are without a large resource of linen, and laundering wet and soiled linen becomes a major task for relatives, one which may be impossible if they are elderly or infirm. In the U.K. some areas have a laundry service through which bed linen is loaned and laundered and this is a tremendous help for a family when coping with an ill member at home.

Supporting the patient. The importance of the nurse showing discretion, tact and kindness when helping patients who have problems with the AL of eliminating cannot be overemphasised. It is especially important when nursing incontinent patients. Some nurses do not find it a pleasant activity and it is sometimes difficult for them not to feel annoyed or disgusted at having to deal with another person's excreta. However, such feeling must not be conveyed to the patient who should never be scolded or made to feel like a child. Realising that it is probably equally distasteful to the patient, and communicating an understanding of his feelings by sympathetic and tactful nursing, can make what might otherwise be an unpleasant nursing activity a satisfying and important aspect of nursing.

Because incontinence may make people feel ashamed and cause them to lose dignity it may cause loss of interest in personal appearance which can mean being less attractive to other people including those of the opposite sex. For those who are sexually active there is an even bigger problem and Webb (1984) reminds us that incontinent patients should be helped to continue expressing their sexuality and continue to be sexually active if this is desired.

CHANGE IN MODE OF ELIMINATING

For various reasons it sometimes becomes necessary for urine or faeces to be removed from the body by an alternative or artificial route. For the patient, this causes problems arising from the imposed change in mode of eliminating.

Urinary catheterisation

Urine can be drained to the exterior through a tube — a catheter — inserted into the bladder via the urethra.

Reasons for catheterisation. There are many reasons for catheterising a patient. They include catheterisation to re-establish a flow of urine in urinary retention; to ensure an empty bladder preoperatively; to prevent urinary complications postoperatively; to provide a channel for drainage when micturition is impaired; to maintain a dry environment in urinary incontinence; or to facilitate bladder irrigation procedures.

The procedure of catheterisation. An aseptic technique must be used in order to prevent the introduction of pathogenic microorganisms into the urinary bladder. A Foley catheter (Fig. 11.9) is commonly used. Insertion of

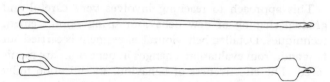

Fig. 11.9 A Foley catheter. Above: catheter before inflation of balloon. Below: self-retaining balloon inflated

a catheter into the female urethra is shown in Figure 11.10 and in Figure 11.11 a male patient with a catheter *in situ* is shown. Infection is a common and potentially dangerous complication of catheterisation. Jenner (1983a) says that urinary tract infection is the commonest hospital-acquired infection. It accounts for approximately 30% of all such infections (Fig. 7.7, p. 103) and at least 500 deaths per year in the U.K. In a second article

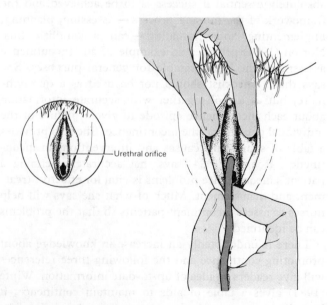

Fig. 11.10 Female catheterisation

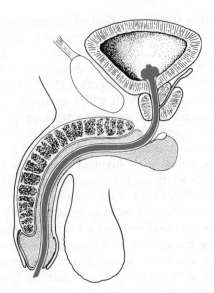

Fig. 11.11 A catheter *in situ* in a male patient

(1983b) Jenner discusses cutting the cost of catheter infections; the causes which can be responsible are:

- inadequate cleaning of the periurethral area prior to catheterisation
- poor technique during catheterisation
- trauma due to ineptitude or by using the wrong size of catheter
- entry of bacteria at the urethral meatus
- breaking the closed system of drainage for collecting specimens or for irrigation procedures
- retrograde flow of urine following contamination of the urine bag

By using a closed system of urinary drainage the likelihood of urinary infection is significantly lessened. The five points at which bacteria can enter a closed urinary drainage system are shown in Figure 11.12.

The patient's problems. The patient who is catheterised has a variety of problems to contend with. He is subjected to the embarrassment of the procedure of catheterisation and then has to put up with the inconvenience of having attached to the body a tube and bag. The patient has to get used to the difficulties this presents when carrying out such activities as bathing, walking or getting in and out of bed. He may also be embarrassed about explaining the appliance to visitors. Not least, the patient is at risk of developing a urinary infection. Helping the patient to come to terms with such varied problems demands sympathetic and skilful nursing.

Urinary diversion

If urethral excretion of urine is not possible at all, as occurs in some diseases affecting the lower urinary tract, a permanent method of urinary diversion becomes necessary. For the patient this involves a drastic change in his mode of eliminating. A cystostomy is the insertion of a

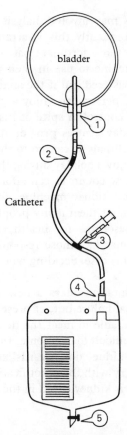

Fig. 11.12 Points at which bacteria can enter a closed urinary drainage system: 1 — the urethral orifice; 2— connection of catheter and drainage tube; 3 — where sample of urine taken; 4 — connection of drainage tube and collecting bag; 5 — drainage bag outlet.

tube directly into the bladder via the abdominal wall. An alternative procedure sometimes carried out is the ileal conduit. In this, the ureters are surgically implanted in the ileum and the distal end of this is brought to the exterior on the abdomen.

Patients with such appliances need to be helped to learn to accept psychologically the change in the mode of eliminating and to cope with the practicalities involved. Lawson (1983) gives the results of a trial which she carried out with urostomy patients to evaluate a new appliance.

Renal dialysis

Renal dialysis is required for acute renal failure but as this is a reversible condition it is usually a short-term life-saving treatment. In end-stage renal failure the kidney damage from disease is so extensive that in order to maintain life, an 'artificial kidney' must be provided. In the process of renal dialysis the patient's blood is continually removed via an artery and in a closed circuit passed through a thin membrane which is bathed in dialysing fluid. This, just like the kidney nephrons, functions to remove urea and other waste products from the blood before it returns through a vein into the circulation. Patients with end-stage renal failure require life-long management. This may involve dialysis once every few days or so, and frequently this is arranged on an out-patient basis. The more fortunate patients are provided with a dialysis machine to use in their home and, once the procedure is mastered and if the anxieties are not too overwhelming, the person can enjoy a greater degree of independence and control in spite of his chronic illness. A few special holiday centres provide dialysis machines and people on renal dialysis can go to these centres, dialyse at night and enjoy a holiday during the day.

Unfortunately, few countries can afford to provide dialysis treatment and kidney machines for all those who require them. Without them many people die each year. When economic resources for health care are limited, many moral dilemmas face those responsible for allocating finance, as in this case, deciding who should have the available machines.

Kidney transplantation offers a new hope for people with end-stage renal failure but, at present, there are not enough organs available to meet the demand and this is a problem that is difficult to overcome. In some countries, such as the U.K., 'kidney donor cards' are distributed so that people can carry with them notification of their willingness to have their kidneys used in the event of sudden death.

Ileostomy/colostomy

When destructive lesions of the colon such as those caused by cancer or severe ulcerative colitis cannot be treated conservatively, surgery may be performed to create an artificial orifice for removal of faeces. An orifice from the small intestine is called an *ileostomy* and one from the large intestine is called a *colostomy*. The faeces are diverted to the opening (the stoma) on the abdominal wall for discharge.

A patient undergoing stoma surgery has a great many problems to contend with. Preparation of the patient both physically and psychologically must be carried out pre-operatively so that he is in the best possible condition for, and understands the implications of, the operation. It is not easy to imagine what a stoma will be like. If the prospect seems unacceptable, the patient may avoid facing up to it by employing various mental mechanisms (p. 38) which the nurse should be alert to recognise.

In the postoperative period the patient will need a lot of support and encouragement and the attitude of the nurses and members of the family must convey their sympathy and respect for his dignity because, more than anything, the patient may feel a loss of self-respect until he regains control over this basic bodily function. People wonder how they can live without a bowel and worry that they may never look normal again to other people; sometimes the visible protrusion of the gut revolts the patient and often the faecal odour is an embarrassment. Reassurance needs to be given that health and normality are com-patible with a stoma; practical advice must be offered on how to look after the stoma and avoid malodour.

A comprehensive nursing assessment is a necessary prerequisite to planning individualised nursing for the stoma patient. Particular attention should be paid to obtaining information which will help the nurse to know how to implement the important teaching component of the nursing plan and, of course, criteria for evaluating effectiveness of nursing must be identified at the outset. Care of the stoma itself involves care of the skin locally and use of an appliance for collection of the faecal matter. Disposable plastic bags of the stick-on variety are usually used and these should be leak-proof, odour-proof, comfortable, non-irritant and easy for the patient to use.

Teaching the patient to cope with the appliance, dispose of excreta, maintain his skin in good condition and experiment with his diet to help establish regular bowel action are important aspects of the nurse's role. Prevention of leakage and quick disposal of excreta will prevent the problem of malodour. Rehabilitation of the patient involves consideration of all activities of living, in particular, those of eating and drinking, working and playing and expressing sexuality.

Stoma care needs a long-term nursing plan, nurses in hospital helping the patient with immediate problems and beginning his rehabilitation, and community nurses carrying out further rehabilitation and teaching. Some nurses in the U.K. specialise in stoma care. In addition to the help available from these specialists and other members of the health care team patients can be greatly helped by the support of a fellow sufferer. The Ileostomy Association and the Colostomy Welfare Group are two self-help groups that operate nationwide in the U.K.; similar groups exist in the U.S.A. and other countries.

CHANGE OF DEPENDENCE/INDEPENDENCE STATUS FOR ELIMINATING

The concept of a dependence/independence continuum is useful when focussed to the AL of eliminating because movement can be in either direction. Many patients are only temporarily dependent on the nurse for example for inserting a suppository or giving an enema and they quickly regain independence. On the other hand when a person succumbs to disease of the urinary or defaecatory system the dependence may be for information and advice about the condition; it may be about short-term changes, for example in diet and fluid intake and how abatement of the condition can be evaluated until the previous state of independence has been regained. For others, the change in dependence/independence status can be caused by limited mobility, confinement to bed or psychological disturbance and these will now be discussed.

Limited mobility

As mentioned earlier (p. 188) several physical skills are involved in the AL of eliminating. Any limitation on mobilising obviously reduces a person's potential for independence. A person who is unable to walk easily, or for any distance, will have difficulty in getting to and from the toilet, especially one which is situated upstairs. Those confined to a wheelchair may have problems when having to rely on public toilets unless there are facilities specially designed with an entrance ramp and the cubicle door wide enough to allow the wheelchair through. Someone with an arm in plaster or with hands badly affected by arthritis has a different problem. That person will be able to get to the toilet but may be unable to undress and dress or use toilet paper.

Any impairment of movement, be it of the arms and/or legs, may render a person incapable of managing to use the toilet without assistance.

Particular problems arise for the patient in hospital whose mobility is completely restricted on account of confinement to bed.

Confinement to bed

When for any reason confinement to bed is prolonged, there may be loss of tone in the gastrointestinal and trunk muscles which may predispose to constipation. Urinary stasis can occur especially if the patient is nursed in the supine position, since urinary flow from the kidneys to the bladder is assisted by the force of gravity. The attendant sluggish flow of urine is conducive to the formation of stones (calculi). In addition, when there is reduced muscular activity, there are fewer acid waste products in the urine so it tends to be alkaline — another condition which favours stone formation.

Nursing activities include supervising an adequate fluid and dietary fibre intake and encouraging the patient to use all muscles as much as possible. Some patients may require help from the physiotherapist in learning to exercise their abdominal and pelvic floor muscles.

Patients confined to bed or the bedside area are totally dependent on the nurse for help with the AL of eliminating. Unless a patient is too ill or incapacitated to move, a commode at the bedside is preferable to a bedpan. In fact, whenever possible, the patient should be transferred to the toilet in a wheelchair or sanichair. In all cases the nurse should anticipate the patient's need to eliminate at regular intervals and be responsive to requests or signals for help with eliminating.

This help may simply involve bringing the receptacle to the bedside or may involve lifting the patient on and off, and assisting with clothing and post-elimination hygiene. Toilet paper should be made available and hand-washing facilities provided. As much privacy as possible should be given. Patients who need this kind of very intimate assistance from the nurse tend to experience worry and embarrassment.

Wright (1974) found that worry and concern about bowel habit was more common among patients who used a sanichair, bedpan or commode than among those who could use the toilets; discomfort and general dislike of the bedpan were reported by almost 40% of those who used it. Having to wait for the receptacle to be brought increased this worry. Of those using bedpans and commodes, 44% experienced constipation compared with only 26% of those who went to the lavatory.

These findings are hardly surprising. Being perched on a bedpan is not very comfortable and, in this position, how does one carry out post-elimination hygiene? And how does the patient feel, knowing that the bedcurtains do not mask either smell or noise, when he passes faeces or flatus? Even if a nurse gives her help sensitively, the patient is likely to find using a bedpan embarrassing and possibly degrading for no-one has helped in this way since he was an incontinent child.

Another disturbing finding of Wright's study was that less than a third of the patients (29%) were provided with handwashing facilities after eliminating. If for any reason it is not possible to provide the patient with a bowl of warm water and soap, disposable 'wipes' should be made available as a substitute. Meticulous handwashing is the single most important method of infection control (p. 102).

Psychological disturbance

Various mental abilities are necessary for the person to appreciate and conform to the various social customs associated with elimination. Knowledge is also needed to understand the importance of disposing of excreta hygienically, to recognise abnormalities of urine and faeces which may indicate the presence of disease, and to prevent the occurrence of problems such as constipation and urinary infection.

Psychological disturbance which results in confusion, depression or disorientation may mean that the person does not remember when he last went to the toilet for example, so he may keep returning absent-mindedly or else forget to go again when necessary. Other patients become incontinent because they fail to recognise the signals of a full bladder or rectum, or recognising them, fail to respond to them. Sometimes patients who are disorientated, particularly at night, cannot find their way to the toilet and others may be so confused that they eliminate indiscriminately in their beds or on the ward floor.

Often the mentally handicapped, and sometimes those with mental illness, may not know how to cope independently with eliminating. Occasionally they engage in unhygienic practices such as handling faeces. If patients who show signs of such psychological disturbance are taken to the toilet regularly and are instructed about elimination skills, it may help them to achieve or retain considerable independence in the many different aspects of this important AL.

Loss of consciousness results in loss of the ability to respond to a full bladder or bowel and the unconscious patient becomes totally dependent on others for ensuring that urine and faeces are removed and disposed of. The nurse should carry this out in a manner that acknowledges the human dignity of the unconscious person.

It is impossible to capture on paper the large variety of patients' problems which necessitate assessing, planning, implementing and evaluating any change in either direction on the dependence/independence continuum related to the AL of eliminating.

DISCOMFORTS ASSOCIATED WITH ELIMINATING

Pain related to eliminating

Here we have to consider pain which can arise in any part of the urinary or defaecatory systems. The discomfort of an overfull bladder or that experienced when trying to expel hard, dry faeces have already been mentioned.

Dysuria is the name given to painful micturition. The problem for the patient is a burning sensation as urine is passed and a constant feeling of an overfull bladder and a frequent urge to pass urine. There may be a constant dull ache in the groin. Some preventive and comforting activities for this condition are mentioned on page 206.

Ureteric colic is usually caused by a stone moving in one of the ureters and the muscular contractions on, and the irritation caused by the stone produces the patient's problems which are excruciating pain, restlessness and sweating. The condition usually constitutes an emergency admission to hospital where muscle relaxant and pain killing drugs will be prescribed by the doctor unless surgery is imminent when the prescription will be for preoperative drugs.

Tenesmus is the medical name for painful, ineffectual straining to empty the bowel. People with this problem should be advised to see the doctor because the cause can be as diverse as proctitis, prolapse of the rectum, rectal tumour or irritable bowel syndrome. Meantime, a warm bath may be comforting.

Colonic flatulence can cause abdominal distension or a colicky sort of pain. Peppermint water is a carminative and is most effective when given in hot water. Sometimes a warm bath can result in the passing of flatus. Or a hollow flatus tube can be passed via which the gas escapes. Flatus with an offensive odour may result from some items of diet, or disease of the bowel, and can cause great embarrassment to the patient.

Haemorrhoidal pain is increased on defaecation. Haemorrhoids ('piles') are dilations of the terminal parts of the veins which lie in the submucosa of the anal canal. The doctor can prescribe medication, which when applied locally reduces the inflammation and discomfort. Constipation predisposes to haemorrhoids: should a nursing assessment reveal this problem then teaching about prevention and ordering a high fibre diet are possible nursing interventions to achieve the goal of a soft bulky stool which is easy to pass.

Postoperative pain on defaecation is feared by many patients after abdominal or urogenital operations and this may predispose to the problem of constipation. Discomfort will be alleviated to some extent by ensuring that faeces are soft and as easy as possible to pass without straining. The patient can also be advised to lean forward while sitting on the toilet, folding the arms against the abdomen to give support to the wound and increase intra-abdominal pressure.

Discomforts associated with investigations/surgery

In the diagnosis of the cause of a problem related to eliminating, the doctor may require to carry out certain medical investigations. For example, sigmoidoscopy may be carried out to assist in the diagnosis of chronic diarrhoea. This procedure involves the insertion of a tube-like instrument into the bowel via the anus through which the rectum and sigmoid flexure of the colon can be viewed. It is not surprising that a patient may find the prospect of such a procedure somewhat anxiety-provoking.

The fact that patients do experience discomfort and anxiety related to investigations is highlighted by Wilson-Barnett (1978). She points out that the level of anxiety is not necessarily related to the seriousness or invasiveness of the particular test and urges nurses to pay attention to the feelings of individual patients. The research also attempted to assess whether information and explanations about scheduled investigations would reduce anxiety. Barium enema was one of the investigations studied and it was found that explanation of the preparation for, and procedure of, a barium enema did help to make the patient feel less anxious. Any invasive procedure constitutes a discomfort.

Whatever the patient's individual bowel habit it is customary to achieve evacuation before investigation of the bowel, before surgery whether or not it is on the bowel, and before childbirth. However readers of the *Daily Telegraph* (1981) were told that after a controlled project in which 125 women in labour were not given an enema and a control group of 149 were given an enema, there was no significant difference in the number of infected babies or the length of labour. Similar results were obtained by Romney in 1982. Many mothers are becoming more voluble about their objections to enemas in labour, and many surgeons are being selective and do not prescribe invasive bowel preparations for patients having minor surgery not on the bowel.

This still leaves a large number of instances in which complete evacuation of the bowel is necessary and Peters (1983) in her article describes some of the current methods which are a discomfort for the patient. The traditional one of aperients, enemas and rectal lavage is still commonly used. Total colonic lavage is a recently introduced method; it is achieved by passing a nasogastric tube, through which a mean volume of 9.5 litres of saline are introduced while the patient sits on a padded commode for a mean duration of 3.5 hours. Non-invasive techniques of producing total colonic lavage include giving oral mannitol or oral polyethylene glycol, or elemental enteral diets. Peters (1983) quotes a study which found that to achieve total colonic lavage there was no advantage in the use of saline given by nasogastric tube over oral mannitol in either efficacy or patient acceptability. As yet it is too early to evaluate the use of oral polyethylene glycol for this purpose. Elemental diets are not particularly palatable and only nine patients were in the study so that more research is needed before they can be accepted as an efficient method of bowel preparation prior to surgery and investigation.

Related to the AL of eliminating, a variety of problems and discomforts which patients can experience have been discussed. This background information will provide nurses with a generalised idea of these; it will be useful in assessing, planning, implementing and evaluating an individualised programme for each patient's AL of eliminating. At all times nurses need to appreciate the intimate nature of this AL and carry out nursing activities in such a way as to provide privacy, prevent embarrassment and preserve the patient's dignity.

This chapter has been concerned with the AL of eliminating. However, as stated previously it is only for the purpose of discussion that any AL can be considered on its own; in reality the various activities are so closely related and do not have distinct boundaries. Figure 11.13 is a reminder that the AL of eliminating is related to the other ALs and also to the various components of the model for nursing.

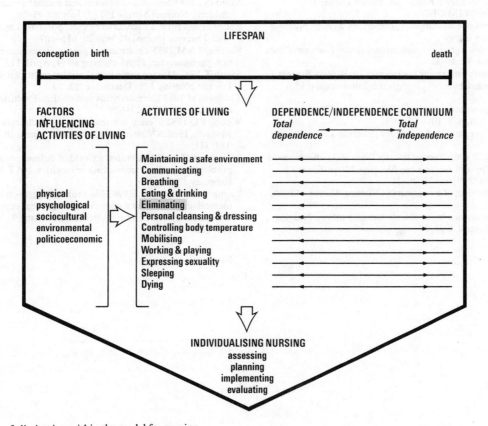

Fig. 11.13 The AL of eliminating within the model for nursing

REFERENCES

Burkitt D 1983 Positive Health Guide. Don't forget fibre in your diet. Martin Dunitz

Chambers T 1981 Fears and tears (Bedwetting). Nursing Mirror 153 (24) December 9: 52–53

Culank L 1979 Detective work in the lab. Nursing Mirror Supplement 149 (4) July 26

Daily Telegraph 1981 Don't need enemas. October 28

Dawson P 1982 Patient's page: as fate would have it: coming to terms with an ileostomy. Nursing Mirror 154 (8) February 24: 24–25

de Mont A 1984 Laxatives. Nursing Times Community Outlook 80 (6): 44–49

Duffin H M, Castleden C M, Chaudhry A Y 1981 Are enemas necessary? Nursing Times 77 (45) November 4: 1940–1941

Egan M 1984 Urinary incontinence quiz. Nursing Times Supplement April 4: 14, 27

Fay J 1979 Colour clues to hidden danger. Nursing Mirror Supplement 149 (4) July 26

Gibson J A, Wilson K M 1976 The diarrhoeas. Nursing Mirror 143 (22) November 25: i–iv (Nursing Care Supplement)

Harrison S 1984 Re-education of the pelvic floor muscles. Nursing Times Supplement April 4: 29–30

Jenner E A 1983a Prevention of catheter-associated urinary tract infections. Nursing Supplement May: 1–3

Jenner E A 1983b Cutting the cost of catheter infections. Nursing Times 59 (61) July 13: 58, 60, 62

King M R 1980 An automatic midstream urine collector. Nursing Times 76 (23) June 5: 1010–1013

Lawson A 1983 A new system for the urostomist. Nursing Times 79 (8) February 23: 37, 39

Lowthian P 1977 Frequent micturition and its significance. Nursing Times 73 (46) November 17: 1809–1813

Meadow R 1981 Help for bedwetting. Churchill Livingstone, Edinburgh

Meers P D, Strong J L 1980 Hospitals should do the sick no harm. Urinary tract infection. Nursing Times 76 (30) Supplement

Metcalf J 1982 Better cookery for diabetics. British Diabetic Association, London WIM 0BD

Mills H 1984 Problems of elimination . . . preserving dignity. Nursing Times 80 (4) January 25: 49

Moore J 1984 Confusion, ignorance and inconsistency. Nursing Times Community Outlook 38: 41–42

Norton C 1983 Training for urinary continence. In: Wilson-Barnett J (ed) Patient teaching. Churchill Livingstone, Edinburgh, p 153, 155–156

Norton C 1984 The promotion of continence. Nursing Times Supplement April 4: 4, 6, 8, 10

Peters D 1983 Bowel preparation for surgery. Nursing Times 79 (28) July 13: 32–34

Ractoo S, Baumber C D 1983 Testing times. (Testing the effectiveness of two Dulcolax suppositories and one Micralax Micro-Enema.) Nursing Mirror 156 (24) June 15: 26–27

Reid E A 1976 The problem of incontinence. Nursing Mirror 142 (14) April 1: 49–52

Robbins S 1984 Incontinence in the elderly mentally infirm. Nursing Times Supplement April 4: 25, 27

Romney M L 1982 Nursing research in obstetrics and gynaecology: research to test value of predelivery shaving and administration of enemas. Internation Journal of Nursing Studies 19 (4): 193–203

Rooney V 1984 Incontinence in the elderly in the community. Nursing Times Supplement April 4: 13–14

Schofield D, Schofield D 1981 Stress incontinence: the solution solidified. Nursing Times 77 (43) October 28: 1885–1886

Swaffied L 1979 Dietary fibre. Any questions. Nursing Times Community Outlook 75 (15) April 12: 94–95

Thomas T M, Plymat K R, Blanning J, Meade T W 1980 Prevalence of urinary incontinence. British Medical Journal 281: 1243–1245

Tierney A J 1973 Toilet training. Nursing Times 69 (51/52) December 20/27: 1740–1745

Webb C 1984 How would you feel? Nursing Times Community Outlook February 8: 45–46

Wilson-Barnett J 1980 Prevention and alleviation of stress in patients. Nursing (Oxford) Part 10 (February): 432–436

Wright L 1974 Bowel function in hospital patients. The study of nursing care project reports. Series 1 Number 4 Royal College of Nursing, London, p 18

ADDITIONAL READING

Cannon J 1982 Urinary incontinence: a disposable flannel and wipe for incontinent patients. Nursing Times 78 (4) January 27: 165–168

Carado-Davis T 1982 Faecal incontinence. Geriatric Medicine 12 (7) July: 65, 66, 68, 69

Freeman R M, Baxby K 1982 Hypnotherapy for incontinence caused by the unstable detrusor. British Medical Journal 284: 1831–1834

Lloyd E E 1983 Bowel stimulator for quadriplegic patients: a follow up survey. Rehabilitation Nursing 8 (3) May/June: 30–31

Mayberry J F 1982 Colostomy management in babies: a survey of parents' difficulties. Practitioner 226 (April): 763–764

Meed D 1983 Chronic constipation and soiling: a training scheme for children. Nursing Mirror 157 (3) July 20: 25–26

Ramsbottom F 1982 Incontinence aids: purchased by post. Health and Social Service Journal 92 May 20: 626–627

Shepherd A M 1983 Treatment of genuine stress incontinence with a new perineometer. Physiotherapy 69 (4) April: 113

Smith T 1982 Moving some bowel myths: constipation. Journal of District Nursing 1 (6) December: 22, 24

Thomson H 1982 Haemorrhoids and all that. Practitioner 226 (April): 619–620, 623–624, 627–628

Welsby P D 1982 Present day management of diarrhoea and vomiting. Midwife, Health Visitor and Community Nurse 18 (8) August: 336, 338, 341

Whitehead M 1982 Ostomists: a world of difference: particular problems of patients from ethnic minorities. NAT News 1962 February 18–20

Younger J B, Hughes L S 1983 No-fault management of encopresis: medical and behavioural approaches to prevent regular soiling of underwear by older children. Pediatric Nursing 9 (3) May/June: 185–187

12

Personal cleansing and dressing

The activity of personal cleansing and dressing

Through the ages man has paid attention to his personal hygiene; there is archeological evidence of the means whereby these activities were performed by members of previous civilisations. In each historical period there was a gradual refinement of the articles used for cleansing the skin, hair, nails and teeth. Today, the ever-increasing budgets of the perfumery and cosmetic industries and hairdressing salons are indicative of an increased sophistication and interest in personal grooming.

Clothing worn by members of previous generations on formal occasions is evident from paintings. Also depicted are the clothes worn for leisure time activities and for different sorts of work. Progress in manufacturing processes has resulted today in a wide variety of 'easy-care' clothes for every conceivable occasion so that people can now enjoy this part of everyday living.

THE NATURE OF PERSONAL CLEANSING AND DRESSING

The objective in most cultures is to socialise children into independent performance of personal cleansing and dressing, usually in privacy and in rooms set aside for these purposes. Even for those children who do not have their own bedroom, the bed and bedside area are symbols of privacy, and they usually dislike other members of the family 'interfering' with this area. For most people the attitude is inculcated from an early age that cleansing and clothing one's body is a personal concern, which if not carried out in privacy is accomplished in the presence of close family members only.

But the end result is observable by others, cleanliness and good grooming being commended in most cultures, while lack of these is deplored, particularly if accompanied by malodour and infestation. As there are several different activities concerned with personal cleansing, they will be discussed separately.

Washing and bathing. Most people clean the skin by washing with soap and water, rinsing and drying. It can be an 'all-over' wash using a basin of water, an immersion bath or a shower. The disadvantage of the immersion bath is that the bather is surrounded by the debris which is washed off the skin, and as the bath empties, some of this 'scum' adheres and has to be removed. The shower, in contrast, is said to be more hygienic and has the advantage that it saves space and water. Children are socialised by membership in the family into a frequency norm for their 'all-over' cleansing, such as daily or weekly, however it is accomplished.

Hand washing. Everyone is now encouraged to wash their hands before preparing or eating food and after visiting the toilet. Notices to this effect are displayed in kitchens where food for large numbers of people is being prepared, and in toilets. This concern for more frequent hand washing resulted from the discovery that hands can act as a vehicle for the microorganisms that cause food poisoning and others that cause diseases of the bowel such as typhoid fever. If hand washing before meals is not feasible as on planes, finger wipes should be provided. Frequent removal of the skin's natural oily secretion (sebum) may produce chafing, and broken skin is a route of entry for microorganisms which can lead to local infection. Dryness can be counteracted by using an emollient hand lotion after washing and adequate drying; when applied before sleeping it has maximum time to act.

Perineal toilet. The moist membranes in the female perineal area require special attention to maintain health and comfort and to avoid malodour. Females are encouraged to cleanse this area from front to back after elimination, especially of faeces. Microbiological data has confirmed that the majority of infections of the female bladder (cystitis) are caused by microorganisms that normally inhabit the bowel and are present in faeces and can therefore be in close proximity to the short urethra. Such organisms do no harm in their natural habitat but are pathogenic (disease-producing) in other organs.

Care of hair. A healthy condition is achieved by at least daily combing and/or brushing with a clean comb and brush; weekly hair washing is the norm for many people. Of all the personal cleansing activities, hair washing over the years has become the least 'private' (witness modern hairdressing salons). To cater for every kind of hair, there are numerous lotions and shampoos many of which help to keep the scalp free from dandruff. Spraying water over

hair is thought to be the best way of completely removing shampoo, but many people still manage with a basin of clean water. Since hair grows daily albeit slowly most people have their hair cut at frequent intervals in a chosen style.

Care of nails. Cleanliness can be achieved by removing any obvious dirt with a blunt instrument before using a nail brush while hand washing. After drying, while the cuticle is still soft it can be gently pushed backward with the towel to prevent it growing down on to the nail. A ragged cuticle can provide an entry point for microorganisms and a whitlow can result. Cuticle cream helps prevent raggedness. For toe nails it is thought that if they are cut in a straight line, any pressure on the middle of the nail from the shoes will slightly raise the two sides and avoid an ingrowing toe nail. Finger nails are usually rounded to the shape of the finger end, although some people wear their nails long and pointed. A few occupations cannot be performed safely for the client by a person with long nails. For instance bakers, hairdressers and nurses are strongly encouraged to have short clean finger nails.

Care of teeth and mouth. Whereas many of the cells in the human body, if damaged, can be replaced the teeth cannot be. The best that can be done for decayed teeth is to remove the careous part by drilling and to fill the space with a metallic substance. To avoid dental caries, people must follow a rigorous routine of teeth and mouth care.

Fluoride protects the teeth; it is present naturally in some drinking water supplies throughout the world and is added artificially (in some countries) to others. Where it is not present or has not been added, fluoride-containing toothpaste should be used by all age groups.

Brushing the teeth with a slightly abrasive alkaline paste or powder helps to remove plaque from the exposed tooth surfaces. Plaque is a sticky film of food and saliva deposits, cells shed from the mucous membrane and microorganisms; it adheres to the surface of the teeth and is not easily removed.

In Figure 12.1 a dye disclosing agent reveals plaque still adhering to the teeth after cleaning. Plaque builds up quickly in the absence of cleaning and starts attacking the teeth shortly after the ingestion of sugars or refined

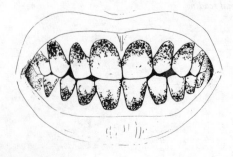

Fig. 12.1 Plaque on teeth

carbohydrates. Therefore it is important that the teeth are cleaned immediately after eating sweet things. A good 3-minute brush at least once a·day is recommended to remove plaque, best carried out before sleeping.

Vigorous up and down movement when brushing teeth is now discouraged and a rotary movement is recommended, not forgetting the backs of the teeth. The gums are also damaged by plaque and gum disease accounts for the loss of more teeth than any other cause in adulthood. Regular dental care, flossing between the teeth and adequate and proper brushing help to prevent gum disease. Recession of the gum, common in older age groups, encourages dental caries; desensitising toothpaste enables brushing to be accomplished without discomfort if the gums are painful.

Ideally food debris should be removed from the teeth after each meal. When tooth brushing is not feasible at these times, the abrasive action from chewing something fibrous like an apple or orange is helpful. A drink of water removes food particles from the mouth but is not so effective in removing them from between the teeth; dental floss (Fig. 12.2) or a tooth-pick can accomplish this.

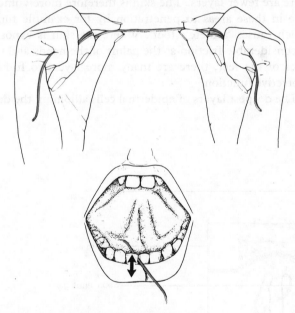

Fig. 12.2 Use of dental floss

In spite of improved knowledge about the causes and prevention of dental caries, many countries are experiencing an increased incidence of dental caries and a lowering of the average age at which people become edentulous and require dentures. The social changes whereby fizzy drinks and ice cream are readily available to children who eat and drink these simple sugar-containing confections between meals contributes to the problem. Sticky sugar adheres to the teeth; it breaks down into acid more readily than starch; acid in contact with tooth enamel for a sufficient time erodes it, and dental caries ensues.

Dressing. Changes in tradition and culture are reflected in clothes and each succeeding generation modifies dress to suit the changing environment and social conditions. Victorian crinolines would be difficult to manage as everyday clothes in today's fast-moving world and would certainly not fit in with the present-day attitude that clothes should be easy to launder and require minimal pressing and ironing.

Clothes are a medium of non-verbal communication. They can signify ethnic origin, level of income and social status, as well as personal preference of colour, style and fashion. They can convey mood: when well, people keep their clothes in good condition; when dejected, they frequently do not mind stained clothes and down-at-heel shoes.

The manual skills required for independence in dressing are achieved by most people, but dressing includes much more than simply learning how to put clothes on. Children usually accept the type of clothing worn by members of the community in which they grow up. They learn that different clothes are worn for different occasions, such as for school and sport, and that a 'uniform' is worn by employees in many occupations.

Clothes which are next to the skin are in contact with sweat, sebum, epithelial scales and microorganisms. The latter have optimal conditions for rapid multiplication, consequently clothes worn during waking hours should not be worn for sleeping and ideally should be changed daily.

THE PURPOSE OF PERSONAL CLEANSING AND DRESSING

Apart from feeling pleasure when relaxing in a bath and experiencing confidence from knowing that one is suitably dressed and groomed, people have a social responsibility to maintain cleanliness of body and clothing. Unnecessary calls on public expenditure arise from infestation, dental caries and spread of some infections, all of which can be prevented by each person accepting this responsibility.

No-one has the right to subject another to malodour from body and clothes. This is an increasing problem because of the extensive use of man-made fibres for clothes: if sweat dries on them, there is an unpleasant odour. Perspiration and sebum are constantly present on the skin, together with dead epithelial cells (scales), fluff from clothing, dust and soot. Removal of these substances at regular intervals before they decompose will prevent unpleasant odour and permit the skin to function optimally.

The skin, mouth and nose each have a natural flora of microorganisms, those on the skin and in the nose being mainly streptococci and staphylococci. Each one can reproduce in 20 minutes and the body by its various defence mechanisms can cope with reasonable numbers, but it can be overwhelmed by larger numbers.

It is to keep the numbers within manageable limits that such activities as mouth care, washing, bathing and manicuring are recommended. As noted above microorganisms attached to the scales shed by the skin collect in clothes, especially those next to the skin. Shedding of these organisms into the atmosphere can be a means of spreading infection. Hill et al. (1974) discuss the effect of clothing on dispersal of microorganisms by males and females.

Sensible selection of clothing can reduce strain on the heat-regulating centre in the brain by the protection afforded against rain, wind, cold, heat and sun. Clothing can also protect from injury, an example being crash helmets. Most people dress for personal adornment and get great satisfaction from so doing. The activity of dressing offers the opportunity for making decisions which help to develop a feeling of self-direction, an important part of self-fulfilment. And last but by no means least clothes are a vehicle of communication.

BODY STRUCTURE AND FUNCTION REQUIRED FOR PERSONAL CLEANSING AND DRESSING

The main body structures which will be outlined in this section, because they are directly related to personal cleansing, are the skin, its appendages, and the teeth. However it has to be remembered that structures cannot function in isolation and the many activities associated with these ALs require an adequately functioning nervous, musculoskeletal and cardiopulmonary system, among others.

The skin: integumentary system

The skin is a remarkable structure; it has the living body in contact with it on one side and the outside world on the other. It gives contour to the body; has erotic zones and manifests a particular complexion so that it is an organ of sexual attractiveness. It is constantly being renewed and it can repair its tissues when injured. It is composed of two layers: the outer one is known as the epidermis and it rests on the inner layer called the dermis (Fig. 12.3).

The epidermis

A variable number of layers of cells make up the epidermis. Where the skin is thin as in the axillae, below the breasts, along the groins and between the fingers and toes there are fewer layers. The skin is therefore more vulnerable in these areas to penetration by for example fungi which causes 'athlete's foot'. Where the skin is exposed to considerable friction as the palms of the hands and the soles of the feet, there are many more layers to fulfil a protective function.

The deepest layers of epidermal cells adjoining the der-

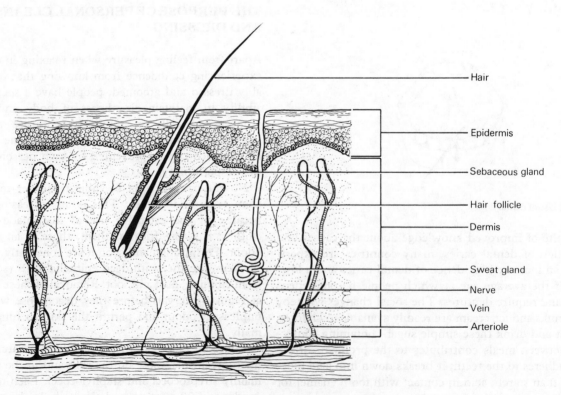

Fig. 12.3 The skin

mis are arranged in a wavy (papillary) line. These cells are very active and are continually dividing and pushing the older cells out to the surface. On their way the cells become hardened by inclusion of keratin, so that they form a layer of scales which are shed from the surface by the million each minute. This hardened, keratinised layer protects the living cells underneath from friction, too much drying and heat loss, and prevents the entry of microorganisms. Although an active tissue, blood vessels are in fact absent and the deeper layers are bathed in lymph, the fluid part of blood.

The papillary line of union between the epidermis and the dermis increases the surface area for distribution of blood vessels in the dermal tissue, from which the lymph for the epidermal tissue is derived. Similarly, there is a greater area for the distribution of sensory nerve endings, thus the skin is an 'information receiver'. Along this line ergosterol is deposited and when it is activated by the sun's rays vitamin D is produced this being part of the skin's nutritional function. Pigment is also deposited determining whether people are fair or dark-skinned; it protects from the sun's rays, and when more is laid down in response to sunshine the skin becomes 'tanned'.

The nails are an appendage of the skin and arise from special infolding of the epidermis. The nail continues to grow from underneath the proximal fold, the nail-bed; the two lateral folds transmit the nail to the finger end. Nails are present on all the digits of the hands and feet and provide protection.

The dermis

The dermis is a layer of loose connective tissue supporting the sebaceous glands, the hair follicles and the small muscles attached to them, the sweat glands, blood vessels and nerves. Below the dermis is a layer of subcutaneous tissue, in the base of which fat is deposited as a food store which also acts as an insulator. The dermis blends with the connective tissue enclosing the muscles.

The hair follicle and sebaceous gland. The hair follicle is a tubular structure, placed obliquely, with a bulb-like projection into its base for the entry of a blood vessel. The follicle rises through the dermis and epidermis and terminates at the surface. Growing from each bulb-like projection and passing through each hair follicle to project beyond the epidermal surface is a hair. A follicle that has a slight curve produces loosely curled hair; the greater the curve, the curlier the hair (Fig. 12.4). Each spiralled hair can easily become entangled with neighbouring ones

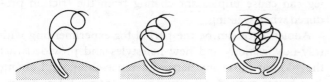

Fig. 12.4 Hair follicle with curly hair

which can cause 'matting'. Surrounding each hair follicle and pouring an oily secretion into it is a sebaceous gland. It is well supplied with blood vessels to enable the secretion of sebum, a nourishing, protective bactericidal substance which coats individual hairs to prevent them from becoming dry, brittle and lustreless. Inserted into the lower portion of the hair follicle and originating from the papillary line of union of dermis with epidermis is a strap of muscle tissue, which on contraction, usually in response to a lowered body temperature, raises the hair and produces 'goose flesh'. The air entrapped by the raised hairs, being a bad conductor, prevents further heat loss.

The sweat gland is a fine tube appearing on the epidermal surface as a 'pore'. The tube descends through the epidermis and the dermis and eventually is coiled around blood vessels so that from the blood it can make its secretion: sweat. Its nerve supply allows it to respond automatically to even slight changes in the temperature of the blood passing through the heat regulating centre in the brain (hypothalamus). With an increased body temperature the blood vessels dilate (vasodilation) and bring more blood to the sweat glands so that more sweat is produced and poured on to the skin surface; heat is taken from the skin to evaporate the sweat with resultant cooling of the skin. The secretion of sweat is a continuous process but when the air is still, warm, humid and cannot absorb sweat as it arrives at the surface, it is visible as beads of perspiration. When the body is making sufficient heat to maintain its normal temperature the skin's vessels contract (vaso-constriction) and less blood flows near the surface, so that there is minimal secretion of sweat thus reducing loss of heat from evaporation. The kidneys deal with the water balance by excreting more urine.

Because of its structure the skin portrays several individual characteristics. It can convey emotion and according to the balance of a person's sympathetic and parasympathetic nervous systems, it can either blush or become pale in response to fear, fright, anger or guilt. Erection of visible hair can be a reaction to either cold or fright. Increased age is revealed by the skin; there is usually a general thinning and increased dryness causing it to lose its turgor and elasticity and become wrinkled. The amount of pigmentation provides information about ethnic groups. Individuality is portrayed by such things as freckles, moles, birthmarks and finger prints.

Knowledge about the complex structure and the wide range of functions of the skin helps people to understand the rationale behind the many everyday activities associated with caring for and clothing it.

The teeth

The teeth are formed in fetal life and by the time that the baby is born there are two sets of teeth embedded in the gums. The milk teeth start erupting at about 6 months and the process is usually complete in 6 years. They are then shed gradually as the permanent teeth appear and the last permanent ones to erupt are the wisdom teeth which appear in the late teens.

The visible part of each tooth (crown) is covered with calcium-containing enamel; the invisible portion (root) is surrounded by cement which also contains calcium. The layer below both of these is made of dentine and encloses the pulp cavity richly supplied with blood, lymphatic vessels and nerves (see Fig. 10.2, p. 162). The vulnerable area is where enamel gives way to cement at gum level and it is here that food particles lodge between the teeth. Microorganisms act on the food producing an acid medium in which calcium is soluble, thus begins the process of dental decay which is preventable.

LIFESPAN: EFFECT ON PERSONAL CLEANSING AND DRESSING

The AL of personal cleansing and dressing is performed throughout the lifespan but, in its various stages, there are some different concerns and preferences, and these are described in this section.

Infancy. An infant's helplessness determines that another person, usually one of his parents, attends daily to his personal hygiene and dressing. For bathing the water is prepared at body temperature as an infant's skin is sensitive to heat. As well as a daily bath babies need to have any milk spillage removed immediately to prevent a sour odour. Because of their incontinent state the perineum and buttocks must be sponged, dried and powdered after elimination of urine and faeces, followed by application of a clean nappy or diaper which is non-irritant and absorbent. Excessive thickness between the legs should be avoided as the bones at this stage are still quite soft, being mainly organic matter. Loose-fitting and cross-over garments are chosen for the very young baby because even momentary confinement and darkening (as when clothes are drawn over the head) are frightening. Also the blinking reflex and tear glands do not work efficiently in early life.

At the crawling stage all-in-one suits are the most suitable day-time wear, for they will not impede the first attempts at standing unaided. As toddling is achieved, dungarees are useful as they afford some protection against the inevitable grazed knees. Gradually clothes characteristic of the culture are introduced. Night clothes should be made of non-inflammable material and pyjamas are safer than gowns which more easily catch fire.

The toddler can progress to the family bath where there is space for him to enjoy sailing his duck and boat so that bathing is associated with pleasure. The cold water is run first to avoid overheating of the bath itself and scalding of the eager child. All clothes for children should fasten at the front and children should be able to dress themselves by the time they go to school. Road safety authorities are presently concerned about small children wearing coats with hoods, which can restrict hearing and vision as the wearer steps out on to the road. A fluorescent garment should be worn when children travel to and from school in inadequate daylight.

Care of the teeth is an extremely important aspect of this AL in the early years of the lifespan. Fluoride increases the resistance of teeth to decay, particularly when given during the developmental period, and it is recommended as a preventive measure by the British Dental Association and the World Health Organisation. It can be administered systematically throughout childhood or topically by use of fluoride toothpaste (Cormack, 1983).

The habit of regular and proper brushing of teeth can be established as soon as a young child is able to hold a toothbrush and, indeed, at that early stage, it is fun rather than a chore. Dental education is increasingly being brought to young children through playgroups and nursery schools, and to their parents through the mass media and child health clinics. The main recommendations are proper brushing; regular dental inspection; and minimum intake of sugar-containing foods (and drinks) and refined carbohydrates. Sweets are better given following a meal and should be avoided altogether for snacks between meals; preferable alternatives include nuts or crisps, and fruit. Started at an early age, it is more likely that habits which avoid harm to the teeth can be established.

Childhood. Increasing development of the neuromuscular system allows the child gradually to master the technique of attending to his own personal hygiene and dressing with supervision. Increasing psychological development permits practice in decision making about these activities resulting in eventual independence and individuality. During these stages he gradually develops a concept of modesty in relation to the AL of personal cleansing and dressing.

Adolescence. As adolescence is reached there are several changes in the skin activity which may require specific attention. There is usually increased under-arm perspiration and most people need to use a deodorant and antiperspirant. Dandruff on the scalp can occur. Many adolescents, particularly males, have to contend with acne sometimes sufficiently severe to warrant medical treatment. Obesity creates a risk of maceration in the skin folds, for example under the breasts and in the groins which can affect care of the skin and choice of garments. Also excessive tissue on the upper inner aspects of each leg can cause unpleasant chafing from the friction produced when walking.

Adolescence can be the period for experimenting with way-out fashions and new hairstyles and provided that they do not cause any harm, tolerance and good humour reap better rewards all round than continual derisory remarks. It can be seen as part of the young person's bid for independence and as much a medium of communication as language.

Adulthood. As adult years are reached the reasons for and time of bathing may vary according to work and recreation. The choice might be an invigorating cold bath on waking or a soothing hot bath before sleeping. A whole lifestyle is reflected in a person's clothes: those for work, for formal social occasions, for informal social occasions, for relaxation, for leisure time activities and for sleeping. Most adults have acquired the ability to dress according to the socially acceptable norm for their culture, whatever the occasion, and to derive pleasure from so doing. Hair styling, grooming and use of cosmetics are ways to express personality and sexuality.

Old age. In the declining years, elderly people may have increasing difficulty getting into and out of the bath. Many gadgets are now available to enable older people to maintain their standards of personal cleanliness. Skin dryness may make moisturising lotions necessary to prevent excessive flaking. Failing eyesight and shaking hands may make it increasingly difficult for older people to retain their independence with conventional clothing. Back fastenings of garments are difficult to reach and front fastenings are therefore preferable; zips and Velcro tapes are easier to manipulate than small buttons or hooks and eyes. Many older people more readily feel the cold and may need to wear extra clothing to keep warm. Two layers of thin material (because of the entrapped air which is a bad conductor of heat) are warmer than one thick layer.

FACTORS INFLUENCING PERSONAL CLEANSING AND DRESSING

The way the AL of personal cleansing and dressing is performed varies among individuals and many different factors are responsible for this. In keeping with the model, this section is sub-divided into physical, psychological, sociocultural, environmental and politicoeconomic factors which influence the AL.

Physical factors

Stage of physical development, and the physical changes which occur in the process of ageing, have a direct as well as an indirect influence on the way the AL of personal cleansing and dressing is carried out. For example, because growth of teeth is a development of infancy and childhood, preventive dental care is an especially important aspect of this AL in these early stages of the lifespan. Similarly, the changes which occur in the physical properties of skin in the course of the lifespan mean that personal cleansing and dressing requirements are different at different stages of the lifespan: acne is a problem of adolescence and dry skin of old age.

Obviously, an individual's level of physical ability will determine the extent to which he is able to carry out the various activities involved in personal cleansing and dressing; and people who are physically disabled may have difficulty in some aspects of this AL.

The physical differences between females and males are relevant to discuss in relation to personal cleansing activities.

Female. Knowledge of the reason for effective perineal toilet (p. 206) will help to motivate girls to carry out this preventive technique. As the breasts develop extra care is needed to avoid maceration in the lower skin fold; daily washing, powdering under large breasts and support in a brassiere usually is sufficient preventive action. Girls require knowledge about the structure of their external genital organs so that they can remove excess secretion from the folds of skin and mucous membrane before it decomposes and causes an unpleasant odour. Psychological preparation for the onset of menstruation will help them to cope with its occurrence; during menstruation all glands are more active and a daily bath or all over wash is even more necessary. Girls acquire the behaviour of their cultural setting related to body hair; it can include removal of unwanted hair from the upper lip and legs, and from the female pubic area before the marriage ceremony.

Male. The bulbous end of the penis is the glans and the foreskin is the prepuce. Between the glans and foreskin at birth there are fine adhesions which prevent retraction of the foreskin and the necessity for cleansing under it. The adhesions dissolve in 6 months to 5 years when retraction of foreskin is easily accomplished. If it is forcibly pulled back before this, the adhesions may be broken down and infection introduced. Boys are then taught to draw the foreskin daily over the glans and cleanse the circular skin fold. Like girls, boys must be taught that this cleansing is a necessary part of their personal hygiene to prevent unpleasant odour and infection. Before puberty boys need to be psychologically prepared for the possibility of wet dreams (ejaculation of semen during sleep); they may wish to bath on waking to remove the characteristic odour of semen. At puberty they acquire the culturally determined behaviour of shaving or having a beard.

It is customary in some cultures for baby boys to have the foreskin removed (circumcision) shortly after birth. In other instances when parents wish to have a son circumcised they are usually advised to wait until he is toilet trained as this reduces the risk of infection. There is some evidence that there is less cervical cancer in women whose husbands have been circumcised.

Psychological factors

Although modern society in general pays less attention to such things as dressing baby boys in blue and girls in pink, and adolescents nowadays tend to favour 'unisex' fashions, there is still a basic difference in psychological outlook between the sexes with regard to the AL of personal cleansing and dressing.

Girls do tend to be more concerned with cleanliness and appearance, and boys may require greater encouragement to carry out personal cleansing activities with sufficient rigour. Adolescents of either sex may deliberately lower their standards of cleanliness as a form of protest against the authority of parents and teachers. On the other hand, their desire to be sexually attractive may result in a somewhat obsessional interest in appearance, make-up, hairstyle and clothes.

In later years, too, standards of cleanliness and dress often reflect personality and emotion; an extrovert is more likely to wear bright colours and the latest fashion than a shy person; and a person who is depressed is likely to lose interest in appearance, sometimes even to the point of neglecting essential, basic hygiene.

Attending properly to the AL of personal cleansing and dressing does require knowledge, for example about the importance of handwashing and the measures involved in preventive dental care. Therefore, lack of knowledge is likely to result in inadequate attention to cleansing and dressing activities which, in turn, may result in problems such as infection, infestation, skin disease and dental caries. People who are mentally handicapped and therefore, by definition slow to learn, require patient and repeated teaching in order to gain confidence and independence in personal cleansing and dressing activities.

Sociocultural factors

Not all cultures place the same value on cleanliness, and the personal cleansing pattern into which a person is socialised becomes deeply ingrained, but probably for an increasing number of people their norm is daily bathing and such people experience discomfort when facilities do not permit them to follow this pattern. There are others who remain healthy while observing their norm of weekly bathing. Some people believe that the 'natural' smell of the body is part of sexual attractiveness.

There are ranges of norms for shampooing the hair (dryness or greasiness often being the deciding factor) and for cleaning the teeth, although many dentists would prefer that everyone accepted as their norm cleaning after meals and before going to bed at night. From a health point of view there is an essential norm for handwashing which is before touching food, and after elimination to prevent food poisoning and diseases spread by ingesting microorganisms from faeces.

There are still instances where culture dictates the type of clothing worn. In the West it has become acceptable for women as well as men to wear trousers; in some cultures it is customary for the men to wear flowing robes and for the women to wear trousers. Religion still influences dress, for instance the clothing worn by monks and nuns. In most countries, not only culture and religion but also the law determine those parts of the body which must be clothed when in public.

Environmental factors

It is easy for those whose homes have a piped supply of hot water and a fixed bath or shower to presume that these facilities are available to all people. Again it is readily presumed that at the turn of the tap, water will be available until the threat or reality of a water shortage reminds people that even such a basic amenity cannot be taken for granted. The AL of personal cleansing and dressing does require the availability of certain amenities in the home environment if the activities involved are to be adequately carried out.

This is true also of the work environment. Some industries expose the skin to risk from such things as coal dust, tar, soot, asbestos and other cancer-producing agents. Showers are considered to be more efficient than baths for removal of these substances and the workers are encouraged to shower before going home. In some countries protective clothing may be obligatory if there is a known health risk to the workers.

The climate of the surrounding environment is another factor which influences the AL of personal cleansing and dressing. For example, in tropical climates there may be the need for more frequent bathing or showering to remove excessive perspiration. Many people in hot climates find that they are more comfortable in clothes made of cotton because it absorbs perspiration and less comfortable in man-made fibres which are less absorbent. Garments made from man-made fibres and wool are useful for providing warmth in colder climates. White and light colours are chosen by people in sunny regions, since they reflect the sun's rays; in contrast dark colours, because they absorb the rays and are therefore warmer, are often the choice of people in cold climates.

Politicoeconomic factors

With the world shortage and consequent high cost of fuel, many people who have the facilities for a hot water supply are experiencing difficulty in affording it. This can apply especially to a nation's disadvantaged groups such as those on a fixed income, be it a pension, social security or unemployment benefit. Some governments consider the amenity of a fixed bath sufficiently important to warrant a financial grant towards its installation in old property.

The importance of preventive dental care and treatment is recognised by those governments which provide a free (or subsidised) service for people unable to afford to pay for it themselves and/or who most need it: such as children, pregnant women, the elderly and the unemployed. Whether or not fluoride should be added to the water supply has been something of a political issue in recent times in some areas.

There is certainly an economic dimension to the AL of personal cleansing and dressing at the individual level. Personal income determines the amount of money which can be spent on articles used for personal cleansing, such basic things as soap, shampoo, comb, hairbrush, toothbrush, toothpaste and manicure tools. When income is limited, emphasis is less on appearance and more on basic health issues — the prevention of infection, skin irritation or disease, dental caries and infestation with lice.

Economics also enters into the number of clothes a person can buy: minimally a person needs to possess enough clothes to wash or dry clean them sufficiently often to prevent odour from dried perspiration or irritation to the skin from dirty fabric. For those who are impoverished, clothes become a matter of basic necessity and the person is denied the pleasure of attractive clothes and variety in dressing.

DEPENDENCE/INDEPENDENCE IN PERSONAL CLEANSING AND DRESSING

The close relationship within the model of the dependence/independence continuum and the lifespan is reflected in almost all of the Activities of Living, and the AL of personal cleansing and dressing is no exception. In infancy there is almost total dependence on others for cleansing and dressing activities; childhood is characterised by ever-increasing independence; and independence is expected in adolescence and throughout adulthood, except for those unable on account of physical or mental handicap, or during a period of illness. Declining physical and mental ability in the final stage of the lifespan may render an old person dependent on help, for example with bathing or cutting nails. A variety of aids are available on the market which can help people to cope independently with cleansing and dressing activities which they would otherwise be unable to manage. Some of the available aids are described later in this chapter (p. 220) within a more detailed discussion of dependence/independence for personal cleansing and dressing in the context of the model for nursing.

INDIVIDUALITY IN PERSONAL CLEANSING AND DRESSING

The purpose of the model of living is to highlight a person's individuality in the Activities of Living. Taking into account all the variables described in the foregoing discussion of the various components of the model (the list below provides a résumé), it should be easy to appre-

ciate that people develop marked individuality in relation to the AL of personal cleansing and dressing.

Lifespan: effect on personal cleansing and dressing

- Infancy
  — skin care (incontinent state)
  — suitable clothing for mobility/safety
  — growth of teeth

- Childhood
  — developing independence and individuality
  — developing concept of modesty
  — importance of care of teeth

- Adolescence
  — increased underarm perspiration
  — dandruff
  — acne
  — expression of feelings/individuality through clothes, make-up, hairstyle
  — puberty (menstruation/ejaculation)

- Adulthood
  — routines related to working and playing
  — reflection of personality in clothes

- Old age
  — skin dryness
  — difficulties with bathing, care of nails and feet
  — difficulties with dressing

Factors influencing personal cleansing and dressing

- Physical
  — stage of physical development
  — physical ability/disability
  — skin state
      colour
      bruising/scars/blemishes
      dry/moist
      turgid/wrinkled
      areas of discontinuity
      cleanliness
  — state of hands and nails
      cleanliness
      handwashing habits
      condition
  — state of mouth and teeth
      moist/dry mouth
      odour of breath
      teeth   (number/condition dentures)
      teeth cleaning routine
  — condition/style of hair
      type (dry/greasy)
      dandruff/lice
      hair washing routine
  — dress
      style/appropriateness

standard of cleanliness/
odour
quality/suitability of footwear
special clothing for work/
play
— sex/biological differences
female: perineal toilet
breast care
menstruation
normal/excess body
hair
male: cleansing under
foreskin
shaving

- Psychological
  — sex differences/sexuality
  — standards related to personal-
  ity/emotional state
  — knowledge (e.g. handwashing,
  dental care)
  — intelligence

- Sociocultural
  — values concerning cleanliness/
  appearance
  — social norms for cleansing/
  dressing routines
  — cultural influences/rules on
  dress
  — religious influences/rules on
  cleansing/dressing

- Environmental
  — bath/shower in the home
  — piped hot/cold water in the
  home
  — exposure at work to substances damaging to the skin
  — availability of bathing/hand-
  washing facilities at work
  — climate

- Politicoeconomic
  — adequacy of necessary facilities for low income groups
  — personal income for articles
  for personal cleansing
  — personal income for essential
  clothing and footwear

Dependence/independence in personal cleansing and dressing

- Dependence in infancy/old age/illness
  — on people
  — on aids and equipment

Personal cleansing and dressing: patients' problems and related nursing activities

Detailed knowledge about a patient's individual habits related to personal cleansing and dressing activities is necessary if this important aspect of everyday living is to be given due emphasis in individualised nursing. In the past, when hospital nursing was highly routinised — with the emphasis on tasks more than on patients — little account was taken of the usual routines and established preferences of the individual. Patients had their faces washed and hair brushed on waking and, as soon as breakfast was over, nurses began on the 'bedbaths' and 'big baths' — in order — strictly according to bed position in the ward!

Such rigid routine completely ignored the fact that in-dividual habits in everyday life are very varied. Some people bathe in the morning, others at night; some never have a bath, always a shower (and vice versa); and while some people bathe only once or twice a week, others like to do so twice a day. Whatever the habits, they often become so ingrained that the person may go to consider-able trouble to ensure that they can be kept up, for ex-ample while staying in a hotel or in lodgings. Nowadays, hospitals are becoming increasingly flexible over the routine of the patients' day and, within reasonable and necessary limits, the continuation of established personal habits in the activities of living is something which is tolerated, if not actively encouraged.

There is another change too. In describing the days of routinised care, words were deliberately chosen which emphasise the idea that, in relation to cleansing and dressing activities, patients had things done *to* them by nurses. This idea that the patient is always a passive re-cipient of nursing care (though, of course, sometimes he is) is fast disappearing. Personal cleansing and dressing activities are normally carried out independently on a daily basis. For any adult, the idea of being washed and dressed by another person — unless help is absolutely in-dispensable — is a very odd one indeed. Most patients who are able to cope with cleansing and dressing activities themselves are likely not only to want to do so, but to obtain pleasure and satisfaction in the process. They may not achieve an end result as clean and tidy as a nurse would wish, but if that causes a problem, it is the nurse's rather than the patient's problem.

If individuality and independence in the AL of personal cleansing and dressing are to be encouraged within the context of individualised nursing, nurses need to have information about the patient's usual routines; what can and cannot be done independently; what previous coping mechanisms have been employed; and what problems exist or may develop. Such information can be obtained at the initial nursing assessment of a patient. Nurses can discuss the AL of personal cleansing and dressing with the patient, using the résumé presented at the end of the preceding section as a guide to relevant topics, and bearing in mind the following questions:

- what are the individual's usual personal cleansing and dressing habits?
- when and how often are the various activities performed?
- what factors influence the individual's personal cleansing and dressing habits?
- what does the individual know about the relationship of personal cleansing and dressing to health?
- what are the individual's attitudes to personal cleansing and dressing?
- does the individual have any longstanding difficulties regarding personal cleansing and dressing activities and, if so, how have these been coped with?
- what problems does the individual have now (or is likely to develop) with the AL of personal cleansing and dressing?

Of course, the nurse may not have to actually *ask* these questions. More often than not the answers are obtained in the course of discussion, or in what the patient chooses to say in response to a general, open-ended question from the nurse. And, of course, all the questions should not come only from the nurse — valuable information can be gleaned from questions the patient asks, and this is something to be encouraged. An assessment, perhaps especially on admission to hospital, has the purpose of *obtaining* information from patients but, equally, it is an opportunity to *give* information to them as well. And, of course, assessment involves much more than use of interview technique alone. Use of all the senses, especially observation, is vital and it may be that some patients' problems are self-evident, requiring discussion only for corroboration.

On the basis of information obtained from assessment, the patient's problems will be identified (as perceived by both nurse and patient) and noted. If relevant, priorities among the problems will be determined and then realistic goals will be set. Some of these will be concerned with alleviating or solving actual problems; others with preventing potential problems from becoming actual ones; and others, perhaps, which aim to help the patient to cope with problems which cannot be solved. Maintaining and encouraging the patient's independence in aspects of this AL is more likely to be achieved if the nursing plan contains details of what the patient is able to do without help, in addition to requirements for nursing assistance. Decisions about appropriate interventions to achieve the set goals must be made within the constraints of prevailing circumstances, existing facilities and available resources. Alongside the written plan of intervention is put the date on which evaluation will be carried out to ascertain whether or not the stated goals have been achieved. All of these activities — the various steps of the process of nursing — are necessary in order to carry out individualised nursing.

The problems which a patient may experience in relation to personal cleansing and dressing are many and varied; recognising and solving them calls for sensitivity, empathy and ingenuity on the part of the nurse. Many of the problems relate to change of environment which increases anxiety and when focused on the many activities related to personal cleansing and dressing, the anxiety is mainly centred on loss of control for such an important part of living and on loss of privacy.

These issues are central to the first section which follows this introduction. Then there is discussion of some circumstances which demand a change in mode of personal cleansing and dressing. The next section considers some causes of dependence in this AL; and patients' dependence on nurses for mouth care, prevention and management of pressure sores and prevention of wound infection. Finally a few discomforts associated with personal cleansing and dressing are discussed.

Neither the problems nor their solutions can be dealt with exhaustively in a book; only guidelines can be given so that nurses can begin to think creatively about nursing activities related to the AL of personal cleansing and dressing.

CHANGE OF ENVIRONMENT AND ROUTINE

Not all patients are nursed in hospital and the discussion later in this section applies to patients regardless of location. However admission to hospital creates particular problems and these will be discussed first.

Unfamiliar ward routine
The newly admitted patient cannot know the ward routine concerning personal cleansing and dressing activities unless information is given. It is usual for patients who are to be admitted from a waiting list to receive general information usually in leaflet form about toilet articles and night attire which they should bring with them, whether or not they can retain their daytime clothes, and if not, the alternative arrangements which they should make.

On arrival, a patient's problem is that he does not know the specific routine of time and place for carrying out personal cleansing and dressing activities. He needs this information on admission and a function of the nurse assigned to admit him is to provide it and to create an atmosphere in which questions can be asked.

Those people who are admitted from the waiting list and who have had a bath before setting off for the hospital will, to say the least, be surprised to be asked to have a bath as part of the admission procedure. Should the patient be admitted for surgery, the explanation that frequent baths in the preoperative period reduce the number of microorganisms on the skin will be useful. Otherwise this part of the admission procedure should be used selectively, that is for those who have not bathed within the preceding 24 hours.

If all patients must have baths on admission then the objective clearly must be for observation of their skin condition including bruising which is important for several reasons. The patient may subsequently have an accident and claim that it resulted in a bruise, which in fact was present on admission; or the patient may have been subjected to ill-treatment, referred to as 'battering' or 'non-accidental injury'. Any evidence of pressure sores must also be carefully noted, together with the patient's ability to perform the ALs of personal cleansing and dressing. Unless nurses explain that the condition of each patient's skin has to be recorded, a patient is likely to feel disquiet at having to have an admission bath and to infer that the nurses think his personal hygiene has been deficient.

For most people clothes are important symbols of their independence and patients can experience distress when their clothes are sent home or to the hospital store cupboard, in which case the nurse makes a detailed list of each item and asks the patient to check the list and sign it. The patient will feel less distressed if it is understood that the staff would prefer possessions to be kept in the ward and that the only reason for their removal is inadequate ward facilities for safe keeping. It is important that nurses understand the patient's problem: being without clothes creates a sense of 'depersonalisation' and also means being deprived of the freedom to decide to leave the hospital immediately, should there be any reason to do so.

Change from the usual routine

For most people the ritual of personal hygiene is an essential part of caring for themselves. These hygiene habits are built into a routine which gives a pattern to the day, an important contribution to a feeling of security and stability. But most patients realise that in hospital the routine will differ from their own. The word routine must accommodate the needs of a group; it must be both expeditious and safe and must not put the patients at any risk. When the nursing workload is heavy, time can be saved by alternative arrangements for personal cleansing and dressing activities; for example, finger wipes before meals; toothpicks and a drink of water after meals; and a dry hair shampoo.

Most people, even those who are housebound, wear daytime clothes and change into night attire. It is most unusual for people to wear night attire during the day. Many newer and upgraded hospitals encourage ambulant patients to wear daytime clothes; this not only improves their self-image but also gives temporal demarcation to being in bed and being 'up', and it also helps to create a sense of normality.

Lessened decision-making

As already noted, most patients have been used to making decisions about the simple activities of personal cleansing and dressing and this is something which should be encouraged as far as possible. There are not many decisions, however, which a bedfast patient can make about personal hygiene. It is therefore important that nurses allow the patients to make the few decisions left available to them — for instance whether or not they want soap on their face, or deodorant applied, what they would like to wear, and so on. It is equally important to recognise when patients are too exhausted or too ill to make decisions, or perhaps unable to make them because of confusion or intellectual impairment.

When all decision-making is removed from patients they cease to make the effort to consider alternatives thereby losing initiative and accepting imposed routine; they become institutionalised. When routine is rigid, members of staff cease to question and to consider alternatives; decision-making becomes unnecessary; they too lose their initiative, become bored and institutionalised thus compounding the patient's problem of lack of stimulation.

Lack of privacy

Most people prefer privacy when carrying out personal cleansing and dressing activities, as has been noted. Curtained washing cubicles or curtains round the bed do not provide the same security as the locked bathroom door, and some patients feel threatened when using such facilities. Shrunken or incompletely drawn curtains can preclude privacy and some patients, particularly women, fail to attend to perineal toilet because of this. Should a nurse become aware of a patient's difficulties in this area she can arrange for use of a private facility or replacement of shrunken curtains; and at all times nurses should be vigilant in making sure that curtains are completely drawn.

CHANGE IN MODE OF PERSONAL CLEANSING AND DRESSING

Habits of personal cleansing and dressing are integral to a person's lifestyle and are important manifestations of self-image and self-esteem. Enforced change in the mode of carrying out any of the activities involved means that a patient has to cope with the change, and nursing activities aim at helping him to do so with minimum discomfort or distress.

Imposed non-bathing

Empathising with patients who are not permitted to bath is easier when one remembers the unpleasant 'grubby' feeling experienced on a long trip. How much worse the feeling must be when for any reason a bath cannot be taken for a long time: for post-radiotherapy patients it can be weeks; for patients with extensive skin destruction it can be many months. Most people's objective when bathing is to feel clean and relaxed and prevent malodour. The nurse can therefore make suggestions as to how these objectives might be achieved during a period of imposed non-bathing. Unless contraindicated, exposed skin areas (e.g. face, neck, hands and feet) and areas where sweat glands are concentrated (e.g. axillae and anogenital area) should be washed frequently. Anti-perspirants/deodorants and perfume/after-shave lotion can help to promote a feeling of freshness and prevent malodour. Frequent changing of clothes and bedlinen would also increase the patient's feeling of cleanliness and comfort.

Some patients, for example those in a plaster cast, though unable to completely immerse themselves in water, might be able to bathe or shower at least some parts of the body if given appropriate help. Other patients, particularly if not mobile and confined to bed, can be bedbathed by the nurse. Provided this procedure is carried out in privacy and adequately (for example, ensuring that the water is warm throughout and that soap is properly rinsed off), it can be both cleansing and soothing for the patient.

Infestation

A change in mode of personal cleansing and dressing is required for treatment of infestation. Lice and scabies are the most common forms of infestation. They have become increasingly common and could be eradicated. Mohylnycky (1983) believes that eradication is hampered by general attitudes towards personal infestation and considers that 'blanket campaigns' directed at the whole community are more effective than orthodox detection and eradication techniques.

Infestation is more common among people who, for any reason, have to be crowded together. Schools are notorious for the spread of head lice and, although previously thought to be more common among children from overcrowded, poorer homes, this may no longer be so. Owen (1982), on the basis of cost-effectiveness, argues the case for abandoning routine head inspections by school nurses and health visitors. She considers that the answer lies in educating parents to inspect and treat the hair of their own children. Priddy (1983) draws attention to the development by his company of a 'hair hygiene kit' which is intended to enable parents to assume this responsibility, emphasising child involvement.

Knowledge of infestation and its treatment can be used by nurses in a wide variety of contexts, hence the following information.

Head lice

The female lays tiny white eggs called 'nits' and cements them to the hairs near the scalp especially behind the ears. These hatch out in 1 week and are fully grown in 3. During a lifetime of 5 weeks they live on human blood. They cause intense irritation with consequent scratching; if this is performed with dirty finger nails infection can result and the resultant dried discharge and matted hair make detection and disinfestation difficult. There is loss of sleep with lowering of vitality; the sores may even give rise to enlarged lymph glands with possible abscess formation.

Head lice are impervious to washing and hair cutting, but a fine comb is effective. Treatment used to be with DDT but lice became resistant to it and, about the same time, its widespread use was banned. Malathion (commercial preparations: Prioderm or Derbac) is currently the most effective chemical for lice. Lotions are preferred to shampoos because they are more effective and help to delay the emergence of resistance. The lotion should be applied to the scalp and the hair.

The hair is then tidied — not combed vigorously which would disturb the lice from the scalp. The nits will be killed but not loosened from the hair. There is substantial protection from re-infestation for some weeks after application because malathion bonds to the hair.

Body lice. The female lays her eggs in the seams of clothing; but in dirty conditions and when day clothes are not changed for night clothes, the eggs can be attached to the body hair. They hatch out in one week, become mature in 2 and live for 4 to 5 weeks. They too live on human blood and their crawling and biting cause intense irritation with consequent scratching and danger of introducing infection.

It is necessary to remove personal clothes into a bag in which they are generously dusted with malathion powder. The bag is securely tied and left for at least 2 hours, after which the clothes are washed or dry-cleaned as appropriate. The infested person takes a cleansing bath, and after drying the skin, sprinkles it with malathion powder. The treatment for pubic (crab) lice is similar but with the addition of shaving the pubic and if necessary the axillary hair.

Scabies. Infestation can become a social problem in overcrowded conditions such as in refugee camps. The itch mite favours those areas where the skin is thin: between the finger knuckles, around the axillae, round the waist, between the thighs, around and especially on the medial aspects of the ankles.

The female burrows under the skin, and at the end of a tunnel, visible to the naked eye as a tiny black line, lays her eggs then dies. The eggs hatch in a few days, the mites crawl out to the skin surface causing irritation; they mate and the cycle starts again, the males remaining on the surface. The scratching and trauma to the skin leaves a route for infection to occur.

After removal of clothes they are washed immediately. A bath is taken after which an emulsion of benzyl benzoate is applied from the neck to cover the whole of the skin. This is left to dry before the afflicted person puts on clean clothes. He is given a bottle of emulsion which he is asked to apply after necessary washing of the hands, but the objective is to leave the first application for 48 hours after which a cleansing bath is taken, clean clothes put on, and removed clothes washed immediately. The condition should be cured. An important part of treatment is to examine, and where necessary treat, people who have been in close contact with the patient.

Whatever type of infestation is concerned, it is important that the nurse relates to the patient in a tactful and sympathetic manner. The person's co-operation is essential if treatment is to be effective, and receptiveness to education with a view to prevention of recurrence, is more likely if the nurse establishes a good rapport.

Modification of clothing

Even with a forearm or ankle in plaster, such things as fitted sleeves or narrow trousers are impossible to put on and clothing has to be modified accordingly. Stretch fabrics, and wide sleeves/trousers — whether or not they are in fashion — are easiest to manage. For a short period this is likely to be accepted by the patient and unlikely to cause undue distress.

However, as was mentioned in an earlier part of the chapter (p. 211) there may be reasons why some elderly people cannot manage to cope with conventional clothing: for example, necessitating wearing front rather than back-opening clothes. Similarly, disabled people may require to modify clothing in order to achieve maximum independence in the activity of dressing. Providing suitable clothing for elderly and disabled people is a basic but often neglected need, as Norton (1983) points out. She recalls how she became aware of this when, as a student nurse some 40 years earlier, she had inflicted pain on a crippled elderly patient when trying to dress her in a hospital issue nightgown. Later, in the course of her research into geriatric nursing problems in hospital (Norton et al, 1962), items of night attire were subjected to systematic study for the first time. Norton acknowledges that since then there has been an increasing awareness of clothing problems and the production of all kinds of gar-

ments for all manner of disabilities. Much of this has been due to the work of the Disabled Living Foundation which has undertaken numerous projects on clothing and dressing problems. However, as Norton says (referring to a recent DLF survey), the practical information which exists does not appear to be widely known. She argues that it is essential for care-givers and administrators to become better informed, '... though knowing of the existence of suitable designs of clothing and footwear to meet the needs of the elderly frail and disabled is only one of a great many factors.' There are problems inherent in the supply of clothing, storage and laundering in hospitals: how to overcome these problems and to introduce successfully a personalised clothing service is the subject of a Disabled Living Foundation publication which Norton commends (Turnbull, 1982).

Nurses, by virtue of their first-hand awareness of the problems, can help in this matter by specifying the clothing needs of individual patients. In addition, empathy is necessary so that any patient who has to wear modified clothing can be helped by the nurse to regain confidence and continue to use dressing as a source of self-esteem and a means of communication.

Wearing a prosthesis

There are various types of prostheses which can be worn, almost all of them resulting in some change in mode of personal cleansing and/or dressing.

An increasing number of people are wearing *dentures* at an earlier age. Some people are very sensitive about being seen without dentures, even for the short time of removal for cleaning. In older people with shrinking gums, dentures can become so loose that they may cause embarrassment in such social activities as eating and speaking. Most dentists now advise that dentures are not removed before sleeping, although many older people still remove them. In contrast, those who have a plate with just one or two teeth attached are strongly advised to remove it before sleeping. In addition to denture cleaning, whole mouth brushing (teeth, gums, palate and tongue) is necessary for oral and dental hygiene to be achieved.

The term 'artificial limb' includes everything from what can reasonably be called a 'wooden leg' to a highly sophisticated powered prosthesis with electrodes placed on opposing muscles that transmit a signal to an electronic device which operates the prosthesis. With the latter device a member of the family is usually taught to help the patient with his personal cleansing and dressing. If the patient has to be admitted to hospital, his anxiety can be reduced if the family member is offered the opportunity to continue his helping role. If this is not possible, he can teach the nurse the method of coping with bathing and so on. There are several grades of sophistication in artificial limbs between these two extremes.

Whatever type is used, one of the patient's problems is the risk of pressure sores on the stump.

People who wear an *artificial eye* become adept at caring for the prosthesis with the necessary apparatus and lotions in a hygienic manner. If for any reason a patient cannot continue to do this, a tissue is placed by the nurse at the outer corner of the eye, the artificial eye is removed on to it using an article with a slight curve and the eye is placed in its container and covered with a suitable lotion such as Optrex. The socket is then wiped with swabs wrung out of water or saline solution. Patients are naturally anxious about the safety of such a precious article, and it is reassuring if the nurse explains exactly what she has done with it and transmits to the patient her mutual desire for its safety.

Various types of *breast prostheses* are available. Mastectomy patients are helped to come to terms with the 'visible' assault on their femininity by discussing and handling these before operation. Indeed in some hospitals a previous mastectomy patient who has learned to cope with her prosthesis talks with a newly admitted patient who is scheduled for mastectomy. It is increasingly recognised that an important nursing activity is the facilitation of such discussions. Another one is helping the patient to realise that hygiene of the prosthesis is important because it is in contact with the skin, at least during waking hours. Clothes do not usually have to be modified.

Although wearing *a wig* is not unusual as a 'fun activity', one's perspective may change if a wig has to be worn for medical reasons. Furthermore one of the most common reasons for having to wear a wig is loss of hair from taking cytotoxic drugs, a treatment for cancer. Such patients may already be debilitated in body and spirit, and loss of hair constitutes an extra problem, often perceived as a major one. Nurses can help by taking an interest in the choice of wig and commending the patient's appearance when it is worn. Help may be needed with shampooing and setting the wig.

CHANGE OF DEPENDENCE/INDEPENDENCE STATUS FOR PERSONAL CLEANSING AND DRESSING

Acquisition of the skills for independent performance of the activities related to personal cleansing and dressing requires an adequately functioning nervous system, not only to control movement in the lower limbs and to facilitate precision movements in the upper limbs, but also to enable learning about the rationale of the skills. Integrity of the musculoskeletal system is simultaneously necessary for carrying out the many manual skills. Inadequacies in these systems at birth may prevent the child from achieving independence for this AL; any dysfunction in the

systems can prevent a person maintaining independence even to the point of rendering him dependent for one or more of the activities which are a part of personal cleansing and dressing.

The nature of the problems in achieving and maintaining independence for this AL varies according to whether the impediment is congenital, immediate, or of gradual onset. Gradual onset permits the patient time to become psychologically adjusted to the changes and to develop physical manoeuvres for coping. Similarly there is a difference in the nature of the problems according to whether the impediment is short or long term. Personal hygiene problems experienced by patients vary according to whether one or more limbs are involved, whether they are upper or lower ones or an upper and lower limb on the same side.

Causes of dependence

There is no easy method of classifying the numerous impediments to independence in carrying out the many skills involved in personal cleansing and dressing. Partly because there are so many skills and partly because such a variety of factors can affect the nervous, musculoskeletal and integumentary systems, there cannot be an exhaustive classification of causes of dependence. The following headings show how causes are categorised for purposes of discussion here:

- limited mobility
- absence of limbs
- involuntary movements
- sensory deficits
- unconsciousness
- psychological disturbance
- illness

Limited mobility

The sites at which a patient experiences limitation of movement determine the particular problems which he experiences in performing some or all of the skills necessary for personal cleansing and dressing. A person with a frozen shoulder should be encouraged to put garments over the arm on the affected side first. Crippled hands cannot hold conventional articles for cleaning teeth, manicuring nails, combing hair; nor can they manage to fasten small buttons or zips. A stiff spine on the other hand interferes with getting into and out of the bath and applying garments to the lower limbs. Immobility of the jaw renders the patient dependent for mouth care but he can usually carry out all the other skills of personal cleansing and dressing.

Absence of limbs

The congenitally deficient child may not feel the absence of limbs to be a problem because for him a limb-deficient body is 'normal'. Should he require admission to hospital there will already be an established regime of managing his personal hygiene. On the other hand a person who loses one or more limbs, is faced with learning alternative techniques according to which limbs are absent. In the early stages there is increased risk of accident should he even momentarily forget the limb deficiency; it is not unusual for him to experience the phenomenon of 'phantom' limb.

Involuntary movements

It is difficult for those who have achieved co-ordination of movement brought about by the smooth, sequential contraction and relaxation of various muscle groups to realise the many difficulties that can be experienced by not being able to control movement. To give an example: exaggerated uncontrollable hand movements make such apparently simple tasks as dressing, shaving, putting paste on a toothbrush and even combing the hair arduous.

Sensory deficits

When for any reason the brain is not receiving warning stimuli from the skin about the temperature of the water being used for bathing, there is increased risk of scalding. Lack of pressure stimuli can mean that tissues are subjected to increased pressure which may result in pressure sores (p. 222). Many blind people achieve the necessary skills to attend to all aspects of their personal cleansing and dressing; others require some help with some of the activities related to this AL.

Unconsciousness

An unconscious patient is totally dependent on the nurse for preserving his dignity and for ensuring the safety and integrity of his body during all aspects of personal cleansing and dressing. The limbs will probably be stiff and spastic and will need to be supported by one nurse without stretching the muscles and tendons, while the other nurse washes and dries the skin. Prevention of pressure sores is very important (p. 222).

Psychological disturbance

Even after healthy habits of personal cleansing and dressing have been established, these can be disrupted during psychological disturbance. There may be a general deterioration in the standard of personal cleansing skills and an apparent disregard for dirty malodorous clothing. Development of a nursing plan for such patients usually requires goal setting in small gradations to achieve the final goal of regaining healthy personal hygiene habits.

Illness

Illness can interfere with independence in several ways. Sometimes it is sheer exhaustion which prevents patients attending to themselves; sometimes it is breathlessness, when the slightest movement causes further respiratory embarrassment. When the illness dictates that patients are attached to various machines or gadgets, this can be yet another reason for dependence in some or all of the activities related to personal cleansing and dressing.

These are but a few examples of circumstances which can impede the many skills necessary for personal cleansing and dressing. There can be no hard and fast rules for activities in this AL and a high degree of professional judgement is required to enable the development of an individual nursing plan and expertise in carrying it out.

It is obvious that on admission an accurate assessment of each patient's manner of performance of this AL is imperative. Many disabled people have become experts at coping with their condition. Nurses should acknowledge this, listen to them and encourage them to continue to cope where this is permissible. In instances of psychological disturbance, and illness, the nurse may well have to take the lead in development of a nursing plan, and for an unconscious patient it would be advisable to discuss previous hygiene habits with the relatives before devising a nursing plan. Unconscious patients, demented patients and some mentally handicapped people are dependent on the nurse for preserving their right to privacy during personal cleansing and dressing activities.

The nursing plan indicates where the patient's personal cleansing and dressing will take place: in bed or in the bathroom; what activities can be carried out independently and what sort of help is required with the other activities. There are many variables to consider when these decisions are made, and the following are some principles which nurses can bear in mind when helping patients:

- Patients are entitled to privacy during the activities of personal cleansing and dressing.
- There is a possibility of lack of congruence between the nurses' and patients' concept of privacy and modesty.
- Activities related to patients' safety, integrity of their body systems, dignity and modesty are a nursing responsibility for which nurses are accountable.
- Most patients are entitled to make some decisions about aspects of their personal cleansing and dressing, and thus make an important contribution to preventing deterioration of self-image, and institutionalisation.
- When patients are experiencing problems in relation to any or all of the activities necessary for personal cleansing and dressing, provision of relevant aids to independence can help both patients and nurses.

Aids to independence

Many types of equipment have been developed as aids to independence for personal cleansing and dressing activities.

For bathing and showering. Although some baths are sufficiently long to accommodate the reclining body it is difficult to lift and lower a person who has to remain in this position into such a bath. Technologists have overcome the problem by providing 'mobile' reclining baths: part of the bath is a 'trolley' on to which the patient is lifted at the bedside, then wheeled over to the bath which is at a comfortable height for the nurse to bath him. Another version allows the patient to be lifted on to a nylon stretcher at the bedside on which he is transported to a bath system and lowered on the stretcher into the water; there is a 'high/low' mechanism whereby the bath can be raised to a comfortable height for the nurse to bath him.

For those who must remain in the sitting position there are fixed baths with a modelled seat. In more sophisticated versions the patient is helped into the 'seat' portion at the bedside then is wheeled into the bath. Hermetic sealing takes place followed by introduction of water at a controlled temperature. After bathing the water is drained away before the 'chair' end of the bath can be removed and wheeled out so that the patient's toilet can be completed.

Another alternative for a patient with mobilising difficulties is to help him at the bedside into a special bath chair in which he is wheeled to the bathroom. Here a hoist fixed near the bath lifts him, in the removable 'chair' that has a lavatory-type seat, above the level of the bath. A swivel movement puts him above the water, then the hoist lowers him into the water. The reverse process takes place after bathing and he can be dried and dressed before being lowered into the mobile chair for return to bed.

Similarly a portable shower has been developed for bed patients who must remain in the supine position. The patient is placed on the shower bed and moved into the shower cabinet, a similar idea to putting a patient in a cabinet-type respirator. His hair can be washed while he is in the cabinet. For those who can maintain the sitting position during showering there are special chairs with shower attachments and a lavatory-type seat so that the perineal area can be attended to.

Bush (1984), examining what the nurse can do to enhance the sense of well-being of residents who are both physically and mentally handicapped, points out that bath aids available to the public can be used to increase independence. For example, 'soap on a rope' can be hung around the neck so that it is not lost in the bath water. Another idea is to put a bar of soap into a towelling bag, thus combining the soap and flannel and making washing easier for residents who lack fine motor movements and co-ordination.

For care of hair. Extra large combs and brushes with modified handles may be helpful for patients who have difficulty in gripping or with above-shoulder movement.

Such a simple measure as positioning a mirror at sitting height may enable some patients to brush and comb hair without help, for example those in a wheelchair or who have difficulty in standing or balancing. The use of dry shampoo is a substitute for wet hairwashing, enabling independence on occasions for patients who require to have their hair washed. Davis (1977) illustrates the type of combs and brushes which are necessary for care of thick curly hair, together with hairgrooming techniques for black patients. Bush (1984) points out that drying of the hair often poses problems for spastic people and suggests use of a towelling hood to make drying easier.

For care of nails. With a total impediment of one hand there is usually no way in which a person can manicure unaided the nails of the other hand, though he may be able to manicure his toe nails. Some patients dislike filing their nails or having them filed; if unable to use nail scissors they may find that they can use nail clippers.

For care of teeth and mouth. Electric tooth brushes may be more effective for handicapped patients' use. However a small baby tooth brush is advisable when brushing the teeth of another person; mouth care procedures are discussed in more detail on page 206. When there is a reduced flow of saliva it is usually thick, and if there is mouth breathing it dries and forms sordes. Lovelock (1973) recommends the use of an electric toothbrush dipped in a solution of bicarbonate of soda, or toothpaste foams. There is also a foam stick applicator (Copperman, 1977) which is proving to be pleasant and efficient when a patient's mouth has to be cleaned by a nurse. For those with dentures who prefer to remove them for sleeping, labelled covered denture baths are provided. It is customary in some hospitals to use denture kits for naming patients' dentures, especially useful where there are confused patients.

For dressing. Velcro and long zip fastenings often help frail elderly and disabled people to continue dressing

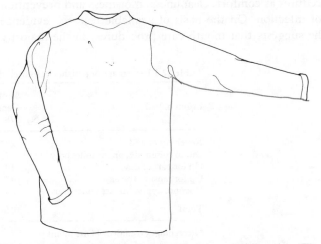

Fig. 12.5 Clothing when both upper limbs are handicapped. (The coloured line indicates zip fastener or velcro in sleeve and side seam.)

themselves or doing so with minimal help from another person (Hinks, 1977). Where there is impediment of one arm or leg, the limb is put into the garment first so that maximum use can be made of the flexibility of the normal limb. When both upper limbs are disabled it may be that one sleeve can be drawn over one limb, the garment arranged over the front and back of the trunk and Velcro or a zip used along the second side (Fig. 12.5). For those with disabled legs it is usually preferable to put on trousers while lying on the bed. There are several gadgets which help them to be independent at this manoeuvre. Similar gadgets help with putting on pants and stockings.

Dependence for mouth care

Howarth (1977), in a short article based on her thesis, reviewed mouth care procedures for the very ill and identified many shortcomings of the procedures as practised. Among suggestions offered, Howarth recommends that small toothbrushes (childsize) should be used because for nurses to clean a dependent patient's teeth with an adult's toothbrush is difficult to accomplish without causing discomfort. She also found that, of substances available, sodium bicarbonate — although unpleasant — was an effective cleansing agent if sores and dry encrusted areas were present. Vaseline was preferred as a lubricant for patients with dry and sore mouths as it lasted longer than other agents, such as glycerine.

Gibbons (1983), a dental officer, refers to Howarth's work in his review of the research into mouth care procedures. Reference is also made to a study which showed that twice-daily use of a chlorhexidine mouthwash inhibited the development of dental plaque and gingivitis, and suggested that it was possible that this agent could remove plaque and treat some cases of gingivitis. Chlorhexidine gels have become available and have been shown to be beneficial in maintaining oral hygiene when applied on a toothbrush.

Gibbons summarises the objectives of mouth care procedures as comfort, cleanliness, moistness and prevention of infection. On the basis of available research evidence he suggests that mouth care procedures, in the majority of instances, can be based on the following recommendations:

- use of a small headed, multi-tufted, childsize toothbrush.
- use of fluoride toothpaste or, where the patient has particular problems, a chlorhexidine gel.
- use of sodium bicarbonate for dry, encrusted mouths.
- use of Vaseline for patients with dry mouth and lips.
- use of chlorhexidine mouth washes for prophylatic purposes.
- whole mouth brushing — which includes gums, palate and tongue as well as teeth. (This requires to be stressed for patients who wear dentures and who normally receive assistance only with denture cleaning.)

It is suggested that a regime based on these recommendations will meet the objectives of mouth care procedures and will also be cheaper than use of prepacked mouth care trays, presently used by nurses in many hospital wards.

It is also the case that patients who receive good mouth care from nurses during a period of dependence might well become aware of ways in which they could improve their own habits, once independence is regained.

Dependence for prevention of pressure sores

Patients who are at risk of developing pressure sores are dependent on nurses either for teaching them how to avoid developing sores and for carrying out the necessary preventive measures. Current use of the term 'pressure sores' in place of the previously used term 'bedsores' or 'decubitus ulcers', is indicative of the recognition of the cause, and acknowledgement that there are surfaces other than the bed which can produce pressure sores. It also acknowledges a changed pattern of nursing care, from most patients being confined to bed for the major portion of their hospital stay, to the majority of patients being up for some part or most of the day (Table 12.1). The changed pattern is referred to as 'early ambulation' and it was instituted as a preventive measure aiming to pre-

Table 12.1 Percentage of patients in four clinical settings related to in/out of bed status

| In/out of bed | % of patients per clinical section | | | |
| | General | Maternity | Psychiatric | Community |
N	378	67	135	194
Never out of bed	23*	2	—	2
Out to commode, up for toilet only	7	—	—	10
Up for part of day	19	13	4	10
Up for most of the day	47	34	95	77
Does not apply, infants under 1 yr	5	51	1†	2
Total	101	100	100	101

*Percentages rounded; †One infant

Source: Roper, N 1976 Clinical experience in nurse education. Churchill Livingstone, Edinburgh

vent pressure sores as well as many other possible complications of bedrest.

The objective of prevention of pressure sores has not however been achieved as shown by a survey carried out in one area of the U.K. (Clark et al, 1978). Of a population of 10751 patients in hospital and in the community, 8.8% had at least one pressure sore, ranging in severity from superficial to a deep cavity, and in number from one to fourteen. There were more sores on the chairfast than on the bedfast patients, the site of the sore in the chairfast not following the theoretically expected change: from over the sacrum to over the ischial tuberosities. In other words the chairfast patients had more sores over the sacrum than over the ischial tuberosities. Another study is needed to investigate this phenomenon but it could be due to patients sliding forward on the chair seat creating a shearing force in the sacral tissues. The survey showed that age-wise it is the over 70s who, whatever the disease, are at special risk and disease-wise it is those of any age with multiple sclerosis, cerebal palsy, spina bifida or paraplegia.

David (1981) points out that it is difficult to be certain about the precise size of the problem of pressure sores because data obtained from various studies are not directly comparable. She reviews the findings of four studies, including that reported above, and illustrates differences which could account for the range of results ound: for example, the type of patients included in the populations studied and the method of grading sores. Nevertheless, it is clear that the prevalence increases in parallel with age; and that chairfast patients require just as much attention as those who are bedfast. Working on the basis of a prevalence of 5%, David estimates that there are some 25–30000 patients in hospitals in this country who have at least one grade 2 pressure sore ('superficial') or worse.

Pressure areas or sites. These are where body prominences, and the tissues overlying them support the body weight when sitting or lying (Fig. 12.6).

Factors contributing to pressure sores
In order to understand the rationale of nursing activities which aim to prevent the development of pressure sores, it is essential to know about the various factors, both direct and indirect, which contribute to their development. Pressure sores result from an interruption of the tissue's blood supply, causing a local ischaemia and, if this continues, necrosis of the affected area. There are many predisposing factors but the main factors in pressure sore formation are continuous direct pressure and shearing force.

The various factors contributing to pressure sores are listed in Table 12.2 and thereafter are discussed in turn.

Table 12.2 Factors contributing to pressure sores

Compression of tissues
Shearing force
Heat
Moisture
Friction
Poor skin hygiene
Poor general nutrition
Lack of oxygen
Lack of spontaneous body movements

Compression of tissues. Compression of tissues between two hard surfaces is the major cause of pressure sores. Compression of the skin and deeper tissues between the hard, bony skeleton and the unyielding surface of a bed is the most common example, but the same effect can result from the chair seat, stretcher, trolley, operating theatre table or X-ray table. The effect of compression is to reduce the blood supply to the cells so that they receive fewer nutrients and less oxygen, and there is less efficient removal of their waste products. Tissue death results from anoxia, not from mechanical damage to cells. It is understood that pressure evenly distributed over a larger area is less injurious than local 'point pressure'. Prolonged low pressure is more hazardous than a short period of high pressure.

On the basis of this knowledge, it is self-evident that relief of pressure is the single most important nursing activity in the prevention of pressure sores. Bearing in mind the particular hazards of localised pressure and prolonged low pressure, it can be deduced that frequent, minor changes of position — which may be accomplished by the patient, if properly instructed — should be incorporated into the nursing plan as well as the more familiar intervention of 'regular turning'. For example, when a patient is bedfast a monkey pole or overhead trapeze is a

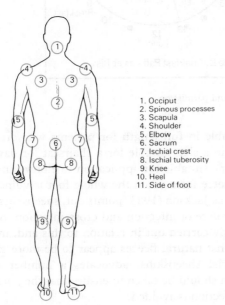

1. Occiput
2. Spinous processes
3. Scapula
4. Shoulder
5. Elbow
6. Sacrum
7. Ischial crest
8. Ischial tuberosity
9. Knee
10. Heel
11. Side of foot

Fig. 12.6 Pressure areas/sites

simple means of achieving frequent relief of pressure by lifting the buttocks off the bed. When they are necessary, turning regimes are usually based on a 2-hourly schedule which to the best of our knowledge is the necessary frequency if those patients particularly at risk are to be adequately protected from developing pressure sores. Lowthian (1979) designed a turning clock (Fig. 12.7) to

possible to accomplish, or indeed as an adjunct to it, pressure-relieving devices can be employed.

Careful positioning and intelligent use of pillows can help to minimise tissue compression. Bed cradles strategically placed relieve the weight of the upper bedclothes from particular parts of the body. Sheepskins and synthetic fleeces also help to reduce compression. They are

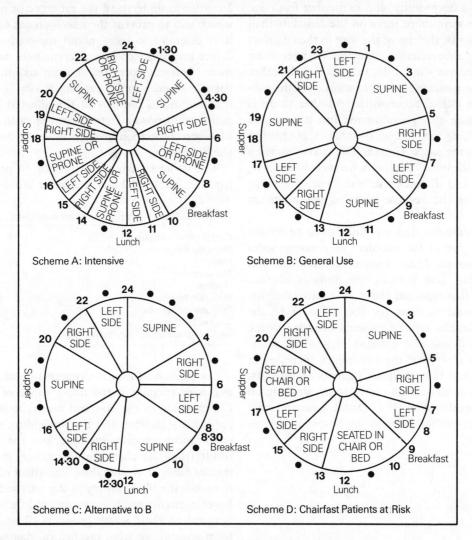

Fig. 12.7 Lowthian's 24-hour turning clock (Lowthian, 1979) (Reproduced by kind permission of the author and *Nursing Mirror*.)

assist nurses in carrying out this preventive measure. The scheme can be adapted to suit each individual's routine and requirements. A list of scheduled times and a signature space accompanies the clock so that there is documentation of the actual implementation of the planned nursing intervention.

Torrance (1983) points out, however, that there are disadvantages in regular turning. First, there is the inconvenience to the patient of regular disturbance, disrupting sleep and perhaps causing pain. Second, it is a time-consuming activity for the nursing staff. In circumstances when regular turning is either undesirable or im-

available in full length for patients who are confined to bed; in a size suitable for a chairseat for daytime use; in a shape suitable for application to elbows and heads; and in bootee form when the whole foot is vulnerable. However, as Jackson (1983) points out, sheepskins are a potential source of infection and cross-infection. She describes a study carried out in relation to this and, in view of the fact that natural fleeces appear to be more effective than artificial sheepskins, advocates a number of measures which should be taken to ensure that the potential hazard of infection is avoided.

Devices are also available which alternate the area of

body under pressure, the most common example being the alternative pressure mattress or ripple bed. The basic system consists of a cellular air mattress connected to an electrical air pump and the air cells are alternately inflated and deflated. Most pump units can be adjusted to an appropriate weight setting, though in practice the heaviest setting is usually best for most patients. The Simpson-Edinburgh low pressure air bed was designed by the bioengineering unit at the Princess Margaret Rose Hospital in Edinburgh in an attempt to produce a relatively low cost but effective patient support system. A study of the bed concluded that it was useful in reducing the frequency of turning, but problems included instability, difficulty in changing the bottom sheet and difficulty in rolling the patient on to one side and when using bedpans (Torrance, 1983).

Although there are many aids of various kinds available, the importance of regular change of position and manual turning where necessary cannot be overemphasised in relation to the prevention of tissue compression, the major cause of pressure sores.

Shearing force. When any part of the supported body is on a gradient, the deeper tissues (mainly muscle) near the bone 'slide' towards the lower gradient while the skin remains at its point of contact with the supporting surface because of friction which is increased in the presence of moisture. The blood vessels in the deeper sheared area are stretched and angulated, thus the deeper tissues become ischaemic with consequent necrosis. Shearing force can be created by badly executed lifting of patients.

Nursing activities to prevent shearing include skilled lifting of patients and positioning which will ensure prevention of sliding in any direction for patients in beds and chairs (Fig. 12.8). Sliding down the bed can be prevented by adjusting the mattress or inserting pillows so that the knees are slightly bent and the thighs supported. A padded footboard is also helpful. The possibility of

shearing in sacral, ischial and heel tissues should not be forgotten when patients spend some part of the day in chairs. The patient is less likely to slump in the chair if his back does not slant too much and if his feet are well supported.

The chair needs to match the patient's physique and be covered with a material which prevents him sliding down. Torrance (1983) identifies a number of factors which contribute to risk of pressure sores in the chairfast patient: slumped posture, badly fitting wheelchairs, or geriatric chairs, and poorly adjusted footrests or footstools. He advocates that patients should be taught to lift free of the chairseat (by hand push-ups) if no pressure-relieving cushions are employed. On the subject of cushions, he emphasises that selection must be individual in relation to size and fit. Air, rubber and foam rings are not recommended.

Heat. Friction and pressure combine to produce a localised increase of temperature. The metabolic rate is raised which increases the demand for oxygen yet its supply is lessened by compression of blood vessels. Two hourly relief of pressure increases the blood supply and reduces the local temperature simultaneously.

Moisture. Excessively moist skin from perspiration, urine or faeces encourages pressure sores which start as maceration of devitalised epithelium. It is therefore important to keep patients' skin as clean and as dry as possible. To this end, retraining for continence is planned and implemented for patients who are incontinent of urine. Immediate washing and changing of patients after incontinence also helps to prevent malodour from decomposing urine and/or faeces.

Friction. The adherence property of friction has already been mentioned. It can also cause injury resulting in the loss of epidermal cells (abrasion). Sometimes the first evidence of a frictional sore is a blister. It can occur on the heels, ankles and knees, especially in restless patients.

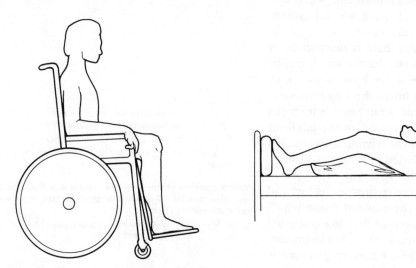

Fig. 12.8 Prevention of shearing force in wheelchair and in bed

Maintaining patients in a non-friction position and comforting them are important nursing activities.

Poor skin hygiene. As noted previously skin has a natural flora of microorganisms which are constantly multiplying so their number is higher if skin is unwashed. Consequently abrasion or maceration of unwashed skin is more likely to become infected.

Poor general nutrition. Poor nutrition results in loss of subcutaneous tissue and muscle bulk, both of which normally act as mechanical padding. Lack of specific nutrients in the blood such as protein and vitamin C render a patient more liable to pressure sores. Particular attention to the dietary intake of patients at risk of developing sores is an important nursing activity.

Lack of oxygen. Localised lack of oxygen due to lessened blood supply caused by compression and shearing has been mentioned. Anaemia is one cause for a generalised reduction in oxygen in the blood (hypoxaemia) and interference with oxygen absorption in the pulmonary membranes is another. Patients with hypoxaemia from any cause are at risk of developing pressure sores. Adequate intake of iron-containing foods such as red meat, egg yolk, green vegetables and salads is useful to maximise the blood's oxygen carrying function.

Lack of spontaneous body movements. People when sitting, lying and sleeping make many small movements in response to sensory stimuli received by the brain. This is a protective physiological phenomenon to avoid excessive pressure on a particular part of the body. In any condition which prevents this protective mechanism, such as frailty, illness, anaesthesia, loss of sensation as in paralysis or being under the influence of alcohol, drugs, and sleeping pills, there is an increased risk of pressure sores.

Types of pressure sores

Various classifications of pressure sores have been suggested but for the purposes of this introductory-level discussion of the subject, types of sores are categorised simply as 'superficial sores' and 'deep sores'.

Superficial sores. In these sores there is destruction of the epidermis with exposure of the dermis which can be caused by such things as creases in the bedclothes and/or personal clothes, crumbs, harsh linen, abrasion from bedpan or commode and persistent scratching. Superficial sores can be precipitated by excessive moisture from fever or incontinence which increases the friction between skin and the surface supporting it. Friction produces blisters, which may be the first sign of damage. Once the epidermis is removed, the skin's protective function is lost and microorganisms can penetrate the exposed tissue which is moist with lymph. A non-adsorbent dressing is applied using aseptic technique and secured in position to prevent entry of microorganisms (p. 228). Relief of pressure is essential until healing has occurred. There can be further

destruction including the dermis and the sore is then classified as a deep one.

Deep sores. In these sores there is destruction of the epidermis and dermis exposing deeper tissues which can include muscle and even bone. Unlike the superficial sore the damage can be established in the deep tissues before tracking out to the surface. Deep sores are usually infected, discharging an exudate which results in protein and fluid loss so that there has to be reciprocal modification of the AL of eating and drinking. Deep sores can take many weeks, indeed months to heal and quite often require surgical closure to prevent further debility. The site, whether or not it is surgically dressed, must not be exposed to pressure and meticulous hourly relief over the other pressure areas is essential.

Identifying patients 'at risk'

Knowledge of the factors which contribute to the development of pressure sores leads to an appreciation of those groups of patients who are particularly at risk. The elderly constitute the single largest section of the patient population at risk of developing pressure sores. However any bedfast or chairfast patient should be considered as vulnerable.

The Norton scoring system for identifying geriatric patients at risk of developing pressure sores is illustrated in Figure 12.9. Although it is now some 20 years since the initial publication of the score (Norton et al, 1962), widespread knowledge of it and its increasing use in nursing is a relatively recent development. The system is dependent on the subjective judgement of the assessor and,

		A	B	C	D	E	
		Physical Condition	Mental Condition	Activity	Mobility	Incontinent	Total score
Name	Date	Good 4 Fair 3 Poor 2 V. bad 1	Alert 4 Apathetic 3 Confused 2 Stuporous 1	Ambulant 4 Walk/help 3 Chairbound 2 Bedfast 1	Full 4 Sl. limited 3 V. limited 2 Immobile 1	Not 4 Occasionally 3 Usually/urine 2 Doubly 1	

Instructions for use

1. Identify the most appropriate description of the patient (4, 3, 2, 1) under each of the five headings (A to E) and total the result.
2. Record the 'score' with its date in the patient's notes or on a chart.
3. Assess weekly and whenever any change in the patient's condition and/or circumstances.

With a 'score' of 14 and below the patient is 'At Risk' denoting need for intensive care, i.e. 1-2 hourly changes of posture and the use of pressure-relieving aids.

Note: When oedema of the sacral area has been present a rise of score above 14 does not indicate less risk of a lesion.

Fig. 12.9 The Norton scoring system

therefore, cannot be considered as a foolproof tool. According to Goldstone & Goldstone (1982) the scores on 'physical condition' and 'incontinence' appear to be the crucial elements and, if so, accurate assessment of these would be especially important. The advantage of the Norton score is that it provides at least some means, which is not time-consuming, of assessing patients' risk of developing pressure sores and providing timely warning of the need to take appropriate preventive nursing activities. Assessments should be repeated regularly (and frequently if the patient's medical condition deteriorates), preferably by the same nurse, and a downward trend in the score is particularly significant.

A more recent development in the diagnosis of incipient and existing pressure injury is in the form of measurement of skin temperature by thermography (measurement of the infra-red energy emitted by the skin). Davis & Newman (1981) describe a study of the use of thermography as a screening technique and conclude that, although it does offer an accurate means of predicting those patients at risk of developing an 'early' sore, further work is needed before its clinical value and cost-effectiveness can be established. They say: 'It is possible that skin temperature measurements made with a simple thermistor or thermocouple probe could detect the presence of inflammation, and thus predict early sores. This could be developed into a very simple procedure requiring little training.'

An instrument is now available, called the Denne pressure gauge (Fig. 12.10), which measures skin pressure. The gauge which is inexpensive, simple in design and easy to use, consists of a small, slim air sac, connected to a mercury column. The air sac is placed under the selected area and the pressure (measured in mmHg) is displayed on the left hand side of the gauge. On the right-hand side, the gauge shows the maximum period of time which may elapse before pressure should be relieved: e.g. a pressure of 100 mmHg requires relief at least every 4 hours. The instrument was invented by Dr Bill Denne at the Oxford Orthopaedic Engineering Centre (U.K.). It had been established that a pressure level on any site of over 40 mmHg will probably, given time and unrelieved, lead to pressure damage. What Dr Denne wanted was a simple instrument to check the pressure as it happens so that appropriate preventive measures can be taken. The result of his efforts is the gauge described. He maintains that it might be of special value to active wheelchair users; that every community nurse should have one; and that there is no reason why patients should not use one themselves (Nursing Times, 1981; Wells, 1983).

A simple pressure gauge which can be used to plan pressure relief, and which can show how pressure is reduced by changes in seating and positioning, would seem to be an instrument of great value to nurses — and to patients. Of course only extensive testing will prove its real value, but it seems an exciting development in the area of pressure sore prevention.

Prevention of pressure sores
As a summary of the foregoing discussion, which has been based on evidence from research as far as possible, there follows a statement of the principles of prevention of pressure sores:

- assessment of risk (based on knowledge of predisposing factors/use of tools, e.g. Norton score)
- relief of pressure to avoid damage by tissue compression — especially point pressure and prolonged low pressure (maximal exposure being 2 hours for those at highest risk or as estimated by pressure gauge instrument)
- avoidance of shearing force (by skilled lifting/positioning in bed or chair to prevent sliding)
- avoidance of heat, moisture and friction
- maintenance of adequate skin hygiene
- maintenance of adequate nutrition
- correction of oxygen lack/anaemia
- avoidance/correction of conditions which decrease spontaneous body movements

The problem of pressure sores is no longer regarded as an indication of poor nursing care. Nevertheless, there is the need for nurses to adopt a more systematic, research-based approach to the prevention of pressure sores. Those patients who are dependent on nurses for

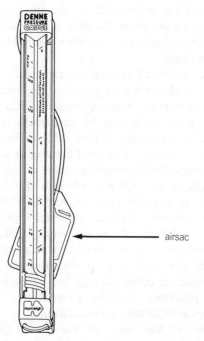

airsac

Fig. 12.10 The Denne pressure gauge (reproduced from Wells 1983 with permission of the editor of *Nursing*)

prevention of pressure sores have every right to expect that the care which is planned for them is based on available up-to-date knowledge, and is tailored to their individual needs.

Dependence for management of pressure sores

If preventive measures are rigorously implemented, many pressure sores can be avoided and those which do occur, if noticed early enough as a result of regular assessment, can usually be treated successfully. When pressure sores do occur, Torrance (1983) suggests that their management can be considered as comprising three aspects:

- removal of pressure (i.e. to keep the ulcerated area free of further pressure)
- treatment of predisposing factors (as described for prevention)
- care of the wound

It is the third aspect—wound care—which remains one of nursing's most controversial issues. Numerous treatments have been invented, advocated, used and later discarded. There seems to be little evidence that any of the many agents which have been used to encourage healing have real proven value. What is needed is rigorous clinical research and that is now only beginning to get underway. Torrance offers the advice that nurses should choose products and treatments which can be demonstrated to aid healing, and avoid those which have no explanation for their mode of action. From his detailed review of pressure sore management (Torrance, 1983), which should be read in full, Torrance draws a number of conclusions about wound care. Certainly, debridement, treating infection and protecting the sore from dehydration and contamination are important, but what the best methods are for achieving these objectives is not clear-cut. Wound cleansing, frequent dressing changes and wound irrigation may also have some value. An adsorption dressing (e.g. Debrisan) which removes bacteria and exudate without drying the wound surface and becoming adherent is effective. Op-Site is appropriate for a clean, superficial wound, if left in place until healing is complete. Torrance emphasises that no single method will suit all patients and, whichever treatment is employed, pressure sores should be given the same meticulous attention which is advocated for any surgical wound.

An article in Nursing Mirror (1983), on the subject of pressure sores, contains extracts from the nursing practice manual which has been developed for staff of London's Royal Marsden Hospital. In tabular form, information is provided on agents and dressings used in the hospital for pressure sores, and both advantages and disadvantages are listed. Readers are recommended to refer to this article, not only for very useful information on pressure sore management (and prevention) but also because it is an excellent example of a resource which provides information but does not remove the need for decision-making by the individual nurse. In addition, the advantages and disadvantages listed take account of patients' likes and dislikes, thus reminding nurses that they are concerned with patients and not just pressure sores! Individualised nursing is a vital aspect of the management of pressure sores.

Dependence for prevention of wound infection

In the preceding section, prevention of infection was mentioned in the context of management of pressure sores. This section discusses the subject in a little more detail, with particular reference to surgical wounds. There is no attempt to go into details of available dressings, wound drains or dressing techniques; rather the aim is to explain the rationale behind some of the routine nursing activities, pre- and postoperative, which have as their objective the prevention of wound infection.

The objective of preoperative skin preparation is to render the skin as free as possible from pathogenic microorganisms. It must be remembered that there is no such thing as 'sterile' skin, even after thorough cleansing. Nursing activities to achieve maximum skin cleanliness traditionally include a 'preoperative bath' for the patient. Some hospitals advocate the addition of a bactericidal agent to the water but the value of this is not proven. Indeed Clarke (1983) states: 'Savlon baths have no affect in reducing skin bacteria'. In the hospital where the study of skin preparation which she reports was carried out, it was routine for all patients to have a Savlon bath on the morning of the operation (and on three mornings preoperatively for major orthopaedic and cardiac surgery). However, swabs from the skin of patients who did not have a Savlon bath grew no more countable bacteria than those who had.

On the subject of bathing before surgery, Stokes (1984) refers to evidence which points to the ineffectiveness of a single antiseptic bath in reducing skin flora. As the surface of the bath may be contaminated, she recommends that showering is preferable to bathing. Specifically, Stokes states: 'Repeated bathing or showering with 4% chlorhexidine detergent solution reduced the number of organisms on the skin' (though this has only been shown to reduce the infection rate in a trial relating to vascular surgery). In fact, thorough application of an alcoholic solution of an antiseptic (chlorhexidine or povidone-iodine) at the time of surgery will give a better reduction of skin flora at the operation site. On the basis of the evidence collected together by Stokes, traditional nursing practices regarding preoperative bathing/showering appear to require reconsideration.

Removal of hair from the skin around the site of incision is another nursing activity routinely carried out in the preoperative period and, again, has prevention of infection as the objective. Customarily this has been achieved by shaving but there is some evidence (Powis et al, 1976) that the use of depilatory creams results in a lower microorganic count. Certainly, this method is increasingly being advocated, and, indeed, whether hair removal with the purpose of infection control serves any purpose at all is being questioned (see Bond 1980 with regard to perineovulval shaving before childbirth).

It is interesting that in the study previously referred to (Clarke, 1983), hair removal was by shaving rather than by use of depilatory cream. In the hospital concerned there was no standard routine regarding time of shaving. However, patients shaved on the morning of operation or in theatre grew more countable bacteria than those who were shaved the day before. On this basis, Clarke states: 'If shaving is to be done it should be the day before surgery.'

However, according to Stokes (1984) there is some evidence that wound infection is higher in patients who are shaved preoperatively than in those who are not. In contradiction to Clarke's statement, Stokes advocates that shaving (if necessary) should be carried out as close to the time of operation as possible because any small abrasions can become colonised with pathogens overnight. For shaving she advocates a disposable razor (or sterilised razor with a clean blade) and foam (rather than soap), or an electric razor (with removable head which can be immersed in 70% alcohol).

Clearly, there is not yet certainty about the most effective method of skin washing and shaving. More extensive clinical trials require to be undertaken before it is clear what precisely is the most effective procedure for skin preparation prior to surgery in relation to prevention of infection.

Most patients are dressed by the nurse in a special 'theatre' gown and cap. Since cotton has a smooth surface to which microorganisms do not readily adhere the patient wears a cotton split-back gown for his visit to the operating theatre. To decrease the possibility of microorganisms being shed from the hair, it is enclosed in a cotton theatre cap. These necessary modifications in the AL of personal cleansing and dressing can add to the normally raised anxiety level of the patient who requires surgery. Adequate explanation of the rationale helps to allay fears.

When the patient returns to the ward after surgery the wound will be protected from invasion by microorganisms with a cellular dressing secured with a bandage or an adhesive strip, or by a transparent adhesive dressing. An adhesive strip or a transparent dressing usually permits bathing or showering when again it may be the practice to add a bactericidal solution to the water. A nursing responsibility when there is a cellular dressing and bandage is to observe that it remains *in situ*, otherwise it cannot fulfil its function as a barrier. Observation is also needed to detect dampness from exudate or blood. A dressing may be covering a wound which is being 'drained' (Hall, 1978) and here there is an additional nursing responsibility to change the dressing before the outer bandage becomes moist, since the minimal requirements for microorganisms to multiply rapidly — nutrients and warmth — exist.

Whenever wounds are exposed, precautions are necessary so that the air contains minimal microorganisms. Sometimes a treatment room with special ventilation is available. If not, the wound is dressed in the ward; domestic and nursing 'dust-producing' activities such as sweeping and bedmaking should have ceased at least one hour previously, during which time the 'dust' will have settled out of the atmosphere. Every hospital has its particular regime of 'aseptic technique' to prevent microorganisms gaining access to wounds, equipment and lotions.

After using aseptic technique for dressing the wound and immediate surrounds, the skin enclosed by the bandage must be washed in the usual way. Cleanliness of the rest of the skin is accomplished by washing which can take place in bed or or in the bathroom. Some patients will be able to do this themselves, others will need help with parts that they cannot reach and some may feel so ill that they are completely dependent on the nurse for keeping them clean and free from odour.

Nursing activities, such as those which have been described, have an important part to play in the prevention of wound infection. There is no doubt that efforts to improve the effectiveness of prevention are required when one remembers the prevalence of hospital-acquired infection, surgical wound infection accounting for over 18% of the total (p. 103). The incidence of wound infection after surgery, according to Westaby (1982), ranges from 1% for 'clean' operations after elective surgery not involving the gastrointestinal or urinary tract to 30% after frank bacteriological contamination of the operative field by faeces or pus. Westaby points out that although bacteria are the basic cause of wound infection, other factors such as host resistance to infection should not be ignored. The fact is that every operation site is contaminated to some extent by airborne or other microorganisms, but not every patient develops a wound infection.

Observation of signs of infection in a wound is an important nursing activity and prompt reporting will enable the doctor to prescribe appropriate treatment. Inflammation, pain and tenderness at the site of the incision, usually accompanied by an increased body temperature, are the classic signs of wound infection. In the absence of other signs, elevated temperature does not necessarily indicate wound infection. Sometimes pus may be produced around the sutures or drain site or along the incision. Bacteriological analysis of a specimen of exudate from the wound will identify the organism responsible and permit appropriate antibiotic therapy to be prescribed.

As will be apparent from this discussion, prevention of wound infection is an excellent example of the interdependence of nurses and doctors in their daily work. Indeed, as was pointed out earlier in the book in a general discussion of this subject (p. 103) infection control can only be accomplished on a teamwork basis. And, of course, although in a position of dependence, the patient must be seen as a member of that team.

DISCOMFORTS ASSOCIATED WITH PERSONAL CLEANSING AND DRESSING

The total surface area covered with skin is extensive and it is therefore not surprising that anything which causes 'difference' can produce discomfort. The minimum areas of the skin which are exposed in most cultures and climates during the day are the face, neck and hands and they are customarily mutually observed when a person is in the company of others. Some people have extensive birthmarks (naevi) and if they are on a part of the body normally covered by clothing during the day, they do not cause discomfort. Yet if they are on the face and neck they are a source of discomfort, usually psychological in

nature. Nurses can help by having a positive not a discriminating attitude toward people with visible birthmarks or other disfigurement of the skin.

Psychological discomfort

Any visible stigma can produce psychological reaction in the person bearing the stigma and in the observer. Either of them can react by being self-conscious, embarrassed, anxious, fearful, shocked and even repulsed if the sight is of extensive skin trauma.

Most children experience self-consciousness and embarrassment in response to loss of the front milk teeth. People react differently to wearing dentures; most suffer initial self-consciousness and embarrassment and thereafter go to great lengths so that they are never seen without their dentures, perhaps even by their spouse. Naturally for such people, admission to hospital presents them with a very special personal problem. Nurses need to be sensitive when caring for patients who have such idiosyncrasies.

Idiopathic loss of hair can sometimes be accepted by cancer patients because they hope that the cytotoxic drugs will improve their condition. Shock and anxiety can be precipitating factors in patchy baldness which the patient finds disconcerting. If the condition can be accepted as a temporary one it will be remedied, but continuing anxiety results in increasing baldness. En-

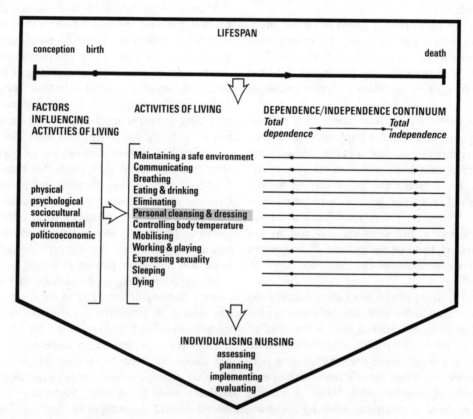

Fig. 12.11 The AL of personal cleansing and dressing within the model for nursing

couraging the patient to talk about his anxiety and help-ing him to identify its cause is an important part of treat-ment.

People with skin disease can become very depressed; indeed some skin diseases are a somatic expression of a psychological disturbance. Attending to the afflicted areas can be time-consuming and healing can be slow. Also in periods of excessive stress the condition can exacerbate which is disappointing to all concerned. If pateints with visible skin disease experience avoiding actions by others, they naturally feel uncomfortable and discriminated against. Nurses can help by positive behaviour towards patients with skin disease.

Excessive sweating

There are changes in a patient's internal environment in response to such states as anxiety and fear. At whatever point they contact the health care system, whether at a doctor's surgery, clinic, health centre or hospital, and on going to such places as the X-ray department and the operating theatre, they will experience some degree of anxiety. One of the body's reactions is increased secretion of sweat. There may be added embarrassment at wet patches on clothing in the axillary region and damp foot-wear. A constant readiness on the nurse's part to give adequate preparatory explanation; to listen to the patient, and to observe non-verbal behaviour for clues as to the cause of anxiety is necessary. Arranging for a daily change of clothing will help to prevent odour which could cause further embarrassment. The patient may benefit from knowledge about stronger antiperspirants and deodor-ants.

Itching (pruritus)

Itching is not a disease *per se* but can be symptomatic of many diseases. The patient's problem is that he is cross, irritable and cannot sleep because of the discomfort. A natural reaction is to scratch an itching part of the body; scratching can induce more itching and more scratching can break the skin so that there is a portal of entry for microorganisms. The sight of the broken skin may make the patient feel guilty and this can add to his misery.

The nurse can help in a general way by offering sugges-tions that short clean nails will lessen trauma and risk of infection. Cotton gloves may help especially if scratching during sleep is a problem. Use of bland non-perfumed talcum powder and soap is helpful; soap should be well rinsed off before drying the skin, and the addition of bath oil to the water is undesirable. Over-spiced food and hot baths are best avoided. Overheating from any cause is undesirable. Loose clothing made of non-irritant material is advisable especially for night clothes. If the patient's mental activity can be diverted so much the better. The objective in all these activities is a cool, calm patient.

Causes of itching
- Allergic reaction to
  topical application
  ingestion of specific drugs or food
- Infectious disease
  german measles
  chicken pox
- Skin disease
  impetigo
  eczema
  dermatitis
- Other disease
  obstructive jaundice
  diabetes
- Infestation
  head lice
  body lice
  scabies
- Discharge
  vaginal

When itching from skin disease is severe, particularly in children, arm constraint is sometimes necessary to prevent further skin damage from scratching, but wherever possible patients are taught the reasons for self-restraint and are praised for compliance.

The many everyday activities associated with personal cleansing and dressing, being of a private and personal nature, are very important parts of each person's self-concept. For conscious and rational patients, discovering their perception of the help which they require in order to cope with problems being experienced in relation to this AL is an important part of nursing. No less impor-tant is the privilege of attending to this AL for uncon-scious, confused and disorientated patients, and those with severe mental handicap, so that their human dignity is preserved.

In the second half of this chapter some of the problems and discomforts which can be experienced by patients in relation to the AL of personal cleansing and dressing have been described. This provides the beginning nurse with a generalised idea of these; it will be useful in assessing, planning, implementing and evaluating an individualised programme for each patient's AL of personal cleansing and dressing.

This chapter has been concerned with the AL of personal cleansing and dressing. However, as stated previously it is only for the purpose of discussion that any AL can be considered on its own; in reality the various activities are so closely related and do not have distinct boundaries. Figure 12.11 is a reminder that the AL of personal cleans-ing and dressing is related to the other ALs and also to the various components of the model for nursing.

REFERENCES

Bond S 1980 Shave it . . . or save it? Nursing Times 76 (9) February 28: 362–363

Bush T 1984 The sense of well-being. Nursing Times 80 (1) January 4: 31–32

Clark M O, Barbanel J C, Jordan M M, Nicol S M 1978 Pressure sores. Nursing Times 74 (9) March 2: 363–366

Clarke J 1983 The effectiveness of surgical skin preparations. Nursing Times Theatre nursing supplement September 28: 8–17

Copperman H 1977 Foam stick applicators. Nursing Times 73 (13) March 31: 459

Cormack J F 1983 Dentistry. Nursing (April) 2nd Series 12: 329

David J 1981 The size of the problem of pressure sores. Journal of the Society for Tissue Viability and the Wessex Special Interest Groups 1 (1) July: 10–13

Davis M 1977 Getting to the root of the problem: hair grooming for black patients. Nursing 77 (7): 60–65

Davis N.H, Newman P 1981 Pressure sores — thermography as a screening technique. Nursing Times Occasional Paper 77 (21) July 15: 81–82

Donaldson R J 1977 Head infestation. Nursing Mirror 144 (3) January 20: 56–57

Gibbons D E 1983 Mouth care procedures. Nursing Times 79 (7) February 16: 30

Goldstone L A, Goldstone J 1982 The Norton score: an early warning of pressure sores? Journal of Advanced Nursing 7: 419–426

Hall S E 1978 Caring for wounds. Nursing Mirror Supplement 146 (10) March 9: ix, xi, xii

Hill J, Howell A, Blowers R 1974 Effect of clothing on dispersal of staphylococcus aureus by males and females. Lancet 2: 7889, 1131–1133

Hinks M D 1977 Clothing and the long-term patient. Nursing Mirror 144 (10) March 10: 39–41

Howarth H 1977 Mouth care procedures for the very ill. Nursing Times 73 (10) March 10: 354–355

Jackson J 1983 Sheepskins — a potential hazard? Nursing Times 79 (18) May 4: 41–45

Lovelock D J 1973 Oral hygiene for patients in hospital. Nursing Mirror 137 (42) October 12: 39

Lowthian P 1979 Turning clocks system to prevent pressure sores. Nursing Mirror 148 (21) May 24: 30–31

Mohylnycky N 1983 Parasitic skin infections. Nursing 2nd series No. 9 (January): 246–248

Norton D 1983 Clothes sense. Nursing Times 79 (44) November 2: 12–14

Norton D, McLaren R, Exton-Smith A 1962 An investigation of geriatric nursing problems in hospital. Churchill Livingstone, Edinburgh (Reissued in 1975)

Nursing Mirror 1983 Pressure sores. (Extracts from Royal Marsden Hospital manual) Clinical Forum 5 156 (23) June 8: i–vii

Nursing Times 1981 Pressure sores: Gauging the problem. (The Denne gauge). Nursing Times Community Outlook 77 (20) May 14: 166

Owen C M 1982 Too much nit-picking? Nursing Times 78 (15) April 14: 632–634

Powis S, Waterworth T, Arkell D 1976 Preoperative skin preparation: clinical evaluation of depilatory cream. British Medical Journal 2: 1166–1168

Priddy M 1983 The death knell of the school head inspection? Nursing Times 79 (44) November 2: 53–54

Stokes E 1984 Showering before surgery. Shaving before surgery. Nursing Times 80 (20) May 16: 71

Torrance C 1983 Pressure sores: aetiology, treatment and prevention. Croom Helm, London

Turnbull P 1982 A guide to the introduction of a personalised clothing service. Disabled Living Foundation, DLF Sales Ltd, Book House, 45 East Hill London SW18 2QZ

Wells R J 1983 Prevention of skin breakdown. (including description of the Denne pressure gauge) Nursing 2 (9) January: 263

Westaby S 1982 Wound care (9): Wound infection-treatment. Nursing Times 78 (20) May 19: Centre supplement.

ADDITIONAL READING

Barton A, Barton M 1981 The management and prevention of pressure sores. Faber and Faber, London

Hadley A, Sheiham A 1984 Smile please! (Promotion of dental health). Nursing Times 80 (27) July 11: 28–31

Hughes J 1983 Footwear and footcare for adults. Disabled Living Foundation, London

Lowthian P 1982 A review of pressure sore pathogenesis. Nursing Times 78 (3) January 20: 117–121

Monk B 1982 Common infestations. Nursing Times 78 (34) August 28: 1431–1433

Ruston R and others 1977 Dressing for disabled people: a manual for nurses and others. Disabled Living Foundation, London

Sidhanee A C 1983 Structure and function of the skin. Nursing 2nd Series 9: 239–242

Swaffield L 1981 Foot care — with older people in mind. Nursing Times Community Outlook 77 (37) September 9: 307–308

Urbanska D A 1977 Care of the mouth and teeth.
  1 Introduction. Nursing Mirror 144 (20) May 19: 13–15
  2 Pregnancy. Nursing Mirror 144 (22) June 2: 29–30
  3 Infancy. Nursing Mirror 144 (24) June 16: 21–23
  4 Childhood and adolescence. Nursing Mirror 144 (26) June 30: 25–27
  5 The elderly. Nursing Mirror 145 (2) July 14: 27–29
  6 The mentally handicapped. Nursing Mirror 145 (4) July 28: 24–26

Westaby S 1981 Wound care series (Nos 3 and 4) — Healing: the normal mechanism (1 and 2) Nursing Times 77 (47/48) November 18, December 16: Centre Supplements.

13

Controlling body temperature

The activity of controlling body temperature

Unlike the cold-blooded animals whose temperature fluctuates according to the changing temperature of their external environment, man is able to maintain his body temperature at a constant level, independent of the degree of heat or cold in the surrounding environment.

THE NATURE OF CONTROLLING BODY TEMPERATURE

For most of the time man is unaware of his body temperature and this is because it remains constantly at a comfortable level. For healthy adults the range of normal body temperature is 36 to 37.5°C. This control is accomplished because a special regulating centre in the brain carefully balances the amount of heat produced and lost by the body.

When the body temperature rises or falls outside this range of normal a person is aware of feeling too hot or too cold. In either circumstance, the individual must perform certain activities to assist the physiological process of body temperature control. If people feel too hot when indoors, they can cease being active if that is the cause; or they can turn down heating appliances, open windows, draw curtains to keep out the sun, remove some clothing, take a cool shower or bath, or have a cold drink. If they are outside doing manual work they can remove an article of clothing or they can rest for a while until they cool down; if they are in direct sunshine they can move into the shade and they can use any suitable article as a fan to move the surrounding air thereby cooling themselves further.

When people feel too cold indoors or outdoors, they can perform various activities which are the converse of those indulged in by the people who are too hot. Physical activity quickly generates body heat and additional items of clothing provide extra warmth and protection from the chill of a wind. Materials made of fibres which entrap air are warmer since air, being a poor conductor, preserves body heat. If the cloth (e.g. wool) has a rough texture, some additional heat is generated by friction between it and the skin. Man also makes use of the fact that dark colours absorb heat from the sun and so help to keep the body warm whereas light colours reflect heat.

Regulating the temperature of the atmosphere in homes and buildings is another activity which must be performed if body temperature is to be controlled satisfactorily. Any householder knows how expensive it is to equip a home so that it is capable of being cool in hot weather and warm in cold weather. Coal, electricity, gas and oil are all expensive commodities and, in addition, many countries are experiencing a shortage of energy resources. Some governments, in an attempt to minimise wastage of these important and scarce resources provide financial aid to householders for double-glazing windows and insulating walls and roofs. Special publicity campaigns are also common to remind the public to save these particular resources. When the temperature outdoors is low it is essential for health and comfort that homes are kept especially warm; this is particularly important for the very young and the elderly.

THE PURPOSE OF CONTROLLING BODY TEMPERATURE

In man, maintenance of a constant body temperature is essential. Most of the numerous chemical processes occurring almost continuously in the body can only take place if the temperature of the body remains at a fairly constant level and within a relatively narrow range. The functioning of the nervous system is easily disturbed by temperatures outwith that narrow range of normal and, at the same time, many other systems of the body are adversely affected. Eventually, if the body temperature rises or falls excessively, there is permanent damage to body cells and the possibility of death.

In addition, the fact that body temperature remains constant within a relatively narrow range of normal, irrespective of the temperature of the external environment, enables man to adapt not only to very different climates but also to daily and seasonal variations in the environmental temperature. If this adaptation was not possible, the scope of human activity would be severely limited and the individual would suffer such discomfort from extremes of heat and cold that everyday living would be disrupted and miserable.

THE BODY STRUCTURE AND FUNCTION REQUIRED FOR CONTROLLING BODY TEMPERATURE

Early in a nursing career an outline of the body structure and function required for controlling body temperature is necessary. However later on, much more detailed knowledge from the biological sciences is essential so that nurses can understand and safely carry out nursing procedures such as inducing and maintaining hypothermia during surgical operations. Here there will be an introduction to the temperature regulating centre, heat production and heat loss.

Temperature-regulating centre. An area of nerve tissue in the anterior part of the hypothalamus of the brain acts as a centre which regulates body temperature. Nerve cells in this area respond to changes in the temperature of circulating blood. It is thought that the centre also responds to impulses from the temperature sensitive receptors in the skin and muscles.

The centre's function is to balance the amount of heat produced by the body and the amount of heat lost by the body. It works just like a thermostat; there is a constant 'set' temperature which is maintained as the centre responds by balancing heat production and heat loss. To achieve this the centre has two control mechanisms: its *heat promoting centre* activates processes which increase heat production and its *heat losing centre* stimulates actions which increase heat loss. These two centres work reciprocally; when one is activated, the other is depressed.

Heat production. All the metabolic processes continuously proceeding in the human body produce heat. At rest and during sleep the body is kept warm enough by the amount of energy produced at the basal metabolic rate. Additional heat production results mainly from skeletal muscle movement and, if this is not sufficient, the body initiates reflex muscular activity — shivering — which greatly increases the rate of heat production. At the same time, stimulation of the sympathetic nervous system speeds up the process of cellular metabolism and raises the hairs on the skin to trap the warm air next to the body, thereby insulating it.

The prevention of unnecessary heat loss is an important way of conserving body heat. Most heat loss occurs through the skin by evaporation, conduction, convection and radiation. Vasoconstriction, the constriction of blood vessels, minimises this heat loss because less warm blood circulates in the subcutaneous tissue. At the same time sweating usually stops, reducing heat loss by evaporation.

Heat loss. A variety of means are used by the human

body to lose heat. Heat is lost from skin which is in direct contact with cooler air by the process called conduction; this is assisted by convection-currents of air circulating around the body. Heat is also lost by evaporation of moisture from the skin surface, naturally increased by sweating. There is some loss of heat by radiation from the body into the cooler atmosphere. Vasodilation enhances loss of heat through the skin by bringing more blood to the surface of the body. Panting, more common in animals though it does occur in man, aids heat loss by speeding up the removal of warmed air from the respiratory tract. At the same time the heat losing centre depresses the mechanisms which result in heat production, metabolism is slowed down and muscular activity is decreased.

It is the balance between heat production and heat loss which must constantly be regulated to keep the body temperature within the limits of the range of normal. This concept of temperature control by balance is illustrated in Figure 13.1.

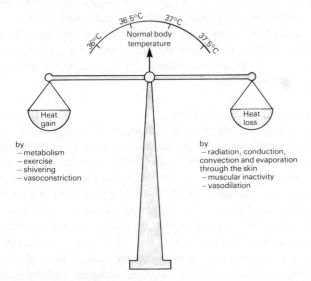

Fig. 13.1 Heat loss/heat gain balance

LIFESPAN: EFFECT ON CONTROLLING BODY TEMPERATURE

The lifespan component of the model of living is especially relevant to the AL of controlling body temperature. As long ago as 1900 a French neonatologist observed that the survival rate in the postnatal period was only 10% for infants whose body temperatures were 32.5 to 34°C and that survival rose to 77% when the infants were kept at 36 to 37°C (Drummond, 1979). Survival rates have improved among preterm and low birth weight babies and this is partly attributable to a better understanding of body temperature control.

The newborn baby requires to have the skin dried immediately to prevent loss of heat by evaporation, and to be wrapped in warm clothing to prevent further loss of heat through conduction, convection and radiation. An infant's body weight comprises 2–6% brown fat (Drummond, 1979). This is richly supplied with blood and has many nerve endings: these provide the stimulus for increased metabolism when the baby is exposed to cold, but prolonged exposure depletes the store of brown fat and this is undesirable. The heat receptors in the face are particularly sensitive and it is especially important that a baby is kept free from draughts. In the first few months and indeed years of life, the heat regulating system continues to be highly sensitive to stimuli which cause heat production, for example, even the exertion of prolonged crying can raise the body temperature above the range of normal. Until the young child learns to associate for instance the discomfort of being hot and sweaty with the relief obtained by taking off a garment and sitting still for a while, parents need to be vigilant on the child's behalf to avoid unpleasant excessive rises in body temperature. The same principle applies to falls in body temperature.

Throughout a woman's fertile life there is a slight rise in temperature just after ovulation and until 2 days before menstruation but many women are not aware of it. Some women have hot flushes as part of the menopause caused by the hormonal imbalance which occurs at this time. They usually manage to cope by wearing a jacket or cardigan which is easily removed when they are too hot.

Towards the end of the lifespan too, body regulation is less efficient and older people can quickly suffer from the ill-effects of extreme heat or extreme cold. At the same time they may be less active and take less food so that it becomes important to provide extra environmental warmth for them, to prevent the potential problem of hypothermia becoming an actual one.

FACTORS INFLUENCING CONTROLLING BODY TEMPERATURE

The factors influencing controlling body temperature will now be considered. The objective of this component of the model is to encourage consideration of how the five factors — physical, psychological, sociocultural, environmental and politicoeconomic — influence the way a person develops individuality in carrying out the AL of controlling body temperature.

Physical factors
There are several factors in this category and they will be discussed as exercise, hormones, food intake and time of day.

Exercise. Body heat production is stimulated by skeletal movement and so the body temperature is related to a person's activity level. It is because heat production increases with activity that, on feeling cold, people spontaneously begin to move about more, rubbing their hands together and stamping their feet. Conversely, the sensible thing to do when feeling too warm is to reduce activity because this reduces heat production. The body temperature is highest during periods of great activity and lowest during periods of sleep.

Hormones. During the female fertility cycle some temperature variations occur due to the influences of the female sex hormones. In the menstrual cycle there is an abrupt slight rise in temperature just after ovulation; a couple of days before menstruation the temperature falls again. This naturally occurring variation of temperature is the basis of the 'rhythm method' of birth control in which abstinence from sexual intercourse is practised during the fertile phase of the monthly cycle, the time of which is ascertained from the temperature variation.

There is a hormonal reason for the slight rise in a woman's temperature during the first trimester of pregnancy; it falls in the second and third trimesters and returns to normal level after delivery.

An excess production of the hormone thyroxine results from over-activity of the thyroid gland and this increases the body's metabolic rate, thus raising the body temperature. Conversely with an underactive thyroid gland less thyroxin is produced and body temperature is lower than normal.

Food intake. Body heat is generated by the metabolism of food and the body's metabolic rate is increased directly as a result of ingestion of food. This is particularly so when the food eaten is high in protein and the stimulatory effect may last as long as 6 hours. Mothers who encourage their children to take a nourishing protein breakfast in order to keep warm in cold weather are therefore, albeit unknowingly, encouraging a practice which is based on sound knowledge of factors which influence body temperature.

Time of day. Variations in body temperature which are related to time of day are obviously influenced by the day and night pattern of activity and sleep. Body temperature is highest in the evening (1700 to 2000 hours GMT) and lowest in the early morning (0200 to 0600 hours GMT). The converse is true for people who work at night and sleep during the day.

Psychological factors

Extremes of emotion sometimes affect the body's metabolic rate causing slight increase or decrease in body temperature. Excitement, excessive anxiety or anger may cause an elevation of temperature and, indeed, this fact is reflected in such phrases as 'flushed with excitement' and 'hot with rage'. On the other hand apathy or depression may cause the body temperature to fall.

Knowledge acquired in the formative years about the sort of precautions to be taken when the outdoor temperature is very high or low will influence how a person carries out this dimension of the AL of controlling body temperature. Similarly the value which a person attaches to making the home capable of being cool in hot weather and warm in cold weather will influence actions to achieve this. A person's temperament and personality traits will have an effect on whether or not a person takes sensible precautions, or risks exposure to the potential problems of heatstroke or frostbite. Current mood will influence how a person carries out this AL, for example when advised to wear a coat, a child may resent this and may react by going outdoors inadequately clad.

Sociocultural factors

The sociocultural customs which can have an effect on the AL of controlling body temperature relate to such things as clothes. For instance many participants withstand feeling uncomfortably hot when in elaborate dress, including head-dress and knee length boots for summer ceremonial parades which are an essential part of their culture. And some with religious impositions wear a characteristic head-dress at all times regardless of the environmental temperature: others might find it uncomfortably hot. Everyone is socialised into acceptance of the areas of skin which can be uncovered in public in that community; this varies widely throughout the world and can vary with the sexes.

Environmental factors

As previously mentioned, changes or extremes of environmental temperature can cause the body temperature to vary and the person to feel warm or cold. In any extreme climate there can be dramatic temperature variations: for example, in parts of North Africa it can be bitterly cold during the night but as hot as 40°C in the mid-afternoon of the same day. Even in the so-called temperate climate of the U.K. there are considerable seasonal variations; the temperature can fall to −10°C or lower in winter and reach 40°C in summer. However, by the process called acclimatisation, the human body is capable of adaptation to very hot, very cold or very extreme climates.

The body's ability to tolerate extremely high temperatures is closely related to the humidity of the atmosphere. A hot day which is dry and breezy, as opposed to one which is humid and still, is less uncomfortable because body heat is readily lost by convection and evaporation of sweat. Similarly, cold, dry weather is less chilling than cold, damp weather.

The availability of hot/cold baths and showers will determine whether or not a person can take advantage of these facilities in controlling body temperature. Likewise, whether or not a house has central heating, air conditioning and double glazing will influence the activities which the occupants need to carry out to help control their body temperature. These are discussed in the next few paragraphs.

Politicoeconomic factors

Many of the activities subsumed in the AL of controlling body temperature need money — to buy clothes, bedding and food; to heat a house and prevent loss of heat from it by excluding draughts, installing double glazing and insulating cavity walls and lofts. Inadequate provisions of this kind may mean that a person cannot prevent the body temperature falling below the range of normal. The two most vulnerable groups are the young and the elderly.

A national survey of hospital admissions carried out by the Royal College of Physicians in 1965 showed that 0.68% of all admissions had temperatures below 35°C. Of these the highest incidence was in children aged 0–1 years which worked out at 82.2 cases per 1000 admissions. It has to be pointed out that hypothermia was not the reason for admission nor did the patients have clinical signs and symptoms of hypothermia; nevertheless they had an unacceptably low body temperature (Millard, 1977). In 1972 the DHSS recommended a temperature of 70°F for a living room when the temperature outside is 30°F. Yet in the early 1980s the Electricity Consumer Council's annual reports stated that some elderly people were attempting to heat their homes on less than £1 per week. The inference was that the homes of those spending so little on heating were inadequately heated. Age Concern, a voluntary organisation, is seeking a better deal for the elderly to prevent the 700 deaths annually from hypothermia recorded on the death certificate (Taylor, 1982), and to reduce the number of cold-related deaths which appear on a death certificate as coronary heart disease, stroke and chest infections. A better deal for the elderly would also help to improve their quality of life.

DEPENDENCE/INDEPENDENCE IN CONTROLLING BODY TEMPERATURE

It is evident from the discussion so far that the concept of a dependent/independent continuum as a component of the model has relevance to the stages of the lifespan when considering the AL of controlling body temperature. As well as children's physiological control being highly sensitive to stimuli, the many behavioural aspects of this AL have to be learned, as well as the perception of when they are necessary. However at any stage a person can have an infection when the body's response is to increase its temperature and make the person dependent on drugs such as aspirin or antibiotics to reduce it, or on people to carry out cooling activities until normal temperature is regained. Conversely the body can respond to inadequate food, clothing, bedding and house warmth by lowering its temperature to the level of hypothermia (35°C) and even in the absence of clinical signs and symptoms such a person is dependent on others for gradually warming the body to restore it to normal temperature.

INDIVIDUALITY IN CONTROLLING BODY TEMPERATURE

From the foregoing discussion it is evident that there are many dimensions of each component of the model which help us to describe how a particular person develops individuality in the AL of controlling body temperature. The following is a résumé of these dimensions:

Lifespan: effect on controlling body temperature
- Infants' body temperature kept at 36–37°C
- Baby kept dry, warmly clad, out of draughts
- Store of brown fat not depleted unnecessarily by exposure to prolonged cold
- Young children, parents vigilant to avoid excessive rise or fall in temperature
- Old people require extra atmospheric warmth, suitable food, clothing, bedding and exercise to avoid hypothermia

Factors influencing controlling body temperature
- Physical
  - exercise
  - hormones
  - food intake
  - time of day
- Psychological
  - knowledge about precautions in high or low outdoor temperature
  - value on making home appropriately warm/cool
  - temperament }
  - personality traits } does/does not take sensible precautions
- Sociocultural
  - clothing
  - socialisation regarding areas of skin which can be uncovered
- Environmental
  - extremes of environmental temperature
  - high/low humidity, velocity
- Politicoeconomic
  - vulnerable people — young, elderly
  - availability of money for clothing, bedding, food
  - heating, excluding draughts, double glazing and insulating.

Controlling body temperature: patients' problems and related nursing activities

Knowledge about the person's individual habits in carrying out the AL of controlling body temperature is absolutely crucial for planning individualised nursing. The foregoing discussion will give nurses an idea of what they should keep in mind when carrying out the initial assessment. The following questions will help the nurse to focus on the sort of information being sought:

- does the individual perceive the body temperature to be comfortable, too high or too low?
- what factors influence the way the individual carries out the AL of controlling body temperature?
- what does the individual know about controlling body temperature?
- are sensible precautions taken to avoid excessive rise or fall in body temperature, or does the individual take risks relating to, for example, the potential problems of hyperthermia (hyperpyrexia/heatstroke), hypothermia and frostbite?
- what value does the individual put on adequate food, clothing, bedding, heating, excluding draughts, double glazing and insulating as part of the AL of controlling body temperature?
- are there any financial reasons for the above-named accessories being absent from the home?
- has the individual any longstanding problems with the AL of controlling body temperature and, if so, how have these been coped with?
- what problems if any does the individual have at present with controlling body temperature and are any likely to develop?

The information will be examined to identify, in collaboration with the patient whenever possible, any actual or potential problems. The nurse may recognise from the information that the ward temperature is higher than the one to which the patient is accustomed and can verify this, and make suggestions about how it can be coped with. Many patients in hospital and in the community do not have a changed body temperature and merely need help and guidance when for example anxiety has increased body temperature and produced extra perspiration. If the newly-admitted patient does have an increased or decreased body temperature then the goal will be a return to that person's normal body temperature. The nursing interventions to achieve the set goals will be selected according to local circumstances and available resources. The interventions will be written on the nursing plan together with the date on which the evaluation will be carried out to discern whether or not they are achieving the set goals. All these activities are necessary in order to carry out individualised nursing related to the AL of controlling body temperature.

However, before nurses can begin to think in terms of individualised nursing they need to have a generalised idea of the kind of problems which patients can experience in carrying out the AL of controlling body temperature. These will be discussed together with relevant nursing activities which are likely to be encountered early in a nursing career. They will be grouped together under three headings:

- change of environment
- change in controlling body temperature
- change of dependence/independence status for controlling body temperature

CHANGE OF ENVIRONMENT

When people are confined to bed at home, whether it is for a short or long time the problem may well be that they exchange the atmosphere of the living room for the distinctly chill atmosphere of most bedrooms, unless of course bedrooms have been included in the central heating system and the members of the household can afford to use it.

Those patients who are admitted to hospital, almost invariably find the atmosphere warmer than that at home and this can be a problem. When people are ill, they become less tolerant of minor discomforts and are more quickly prone to feel miserable if the environment is too cold or too hot, draughty or stuffy, or changeable. Some people like to wear a lot of clothing and have the room well ventilated; others prefer to have the room well heated and wear less. In an open hospital ward, it is impossible to cater for each patient's particular preference.

However, it is essential for the nurse to find out from assessment, each patient's usual habits. If any patient is feeling very uncomfortable the nurse can help by adjusting the heating and ventilation for the majority, and advising extra or less clothing for individuals according to their needs and wishes. Elderly and immobile patients feel the cold more readily and may appreciate the extra warmth of a blanket around the shoulders or over the knees.

Body temperature falls during the night and patients should be encouraged to express their preference as to the amount of bedclothes they require in order to keep warm during sleep. In helping to maintain a comfortable environmental temperature, nurses should always give first consideration to the patients' needs and remember that, being active in their work, they are less likely to appreciate that it may be cold for the patients when it seems warm to them.

CHANGE IN CONTROLLING BODY TEMPERATURE

For healthy adults the range of normal body temperature is 36 to 37.5°C. Therefore, if a person's temperature goes higher than 37.5°C or lower than 36°C it can be regarded as abnormal, suggesting a problem has arisen with the AL of controlling body temperature. An abnormally high body temperature is referred to as *pyrexia*; the name given to describe the condition of an abnormally low temperature is *hypothermia*. The upper and lower limits of survival are not known exactly but are thought to be at body temperatures of 45°C and 25°C respectively (Fig. 13.2).

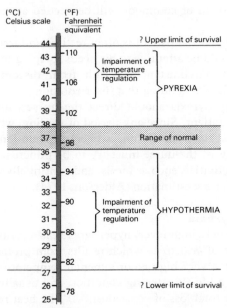

Fig. 13.2 Range of normal/abnormal body temperature

Pyrexia

The condition of pyrexia exists when the body temperature rises above the upper limit of the range of normal, that is above 37.5°C. It is one of the cardinal signs of physical illness, often the first indication that there is some disturbance of body function. Most commonly, pyrexia is a manifestation of infections, neoplasms, diseases of the nervous system, and metabolic disorders. There is reason to believe that pyrexia actually helps the body to combat infection because bacteria survive less readily, and production of immune bodies increases, when body temperature is raised above normal.

Pyrexia itself is a very debilitating condition and a

dangerous one for young children, even if the associated disease condition is not particularly serious. The abnormally high body temperature is a source of discomfort and anxiety for the patient and it places considerable strain on the body. These consequences are particularly undesirable in some instances, for example postoperatively when the excessive demands on body systems may impede recovery and wound healing. (Postoperative pyrexia is often the result of temporary inefficiency of heat loss mechanisms but it may be a warning sign of such diverse complications as infection of the wound, respiratory tract or urinary tract; or of formation of a blood clot in a vein, a deep venous thrombosis.)

Onset of pyrexia. Although the onset of pyrexia is sometimes sudden, more often it is gradual and the problem is a feeling of unwellness. The person may complain of a headache, loss of appetite, lethargy and tiredness and, usually fairly quickly begins to feel cold and shivery. This is what is referred to as *chill* and it can last for a few minutes or even an hour, depending on the speed of onset of the pyrexia.

Chill can be explained — the infection or causative factor raises the 'set' point of the body temperature and to cope with this, heat production increases due to shivering, the skin hairs stand on end (piloerection), the metabolic rate increases, there is a vasoconstriction and reduced sweating. The patient feels cold and often lies curled up, a position which prevents excess heat loss by radiation. Once the body temperature is raised, the balancing mechanism keeps it at the new 'set' level.

Features of pyrexia. Once the temperature stabilises at the higher than normal level, the patient has the problem of feeling uncomfortably hot. In an attempt to lower the temperature again, heat loss mechanisms are activated; vasodilation makes the skin warm and flushed and sweating increases which creates another problem. At this stage the hot patient desperately tries to get cool by removing clothing, fanning himself and keeping as still as possible. Usually he will feel thirsty due to excess fluid loss through the skin and dehydration can result quite quickly. Loss of appetite turns into loss of weight, contributing to the person's overall feeling of lethargy and weakness which are further problems.

There are also mental changes associated with pyrexia. The person becomes irritable and restless and this is very obvious in a child as he cries, refuses to be comforted and tosses and turns in bed. Sometimes severe headache, photophobia (sensitivity to light) and drowsiness may add to the patient's problems: sometimes he becomes disorientated and it is known, for example that 'speeded time' perception can be caused by a high body temperature. The problem for the patient is that time seems to drag because his 'internal clock' runs more quickly than his watch. Sometimes mental processes are upset to such an extent that hallucinations may occur and delirium may result. Not infrequently convulsions (p. 328) occur in young children.

During the course of a fever, body temperature may fluctuate quite dramatically as there is continual adjustment to reduce the raised temperature. Alternating episodes of fever and chill are characteristic of pyrexia until the reduction of the 'set' level is permanently achieved. Usually the return of the body temperature to normal occurs gradually. A typical temperature chart of a pyrexial patient is shown in Figure 13.3.

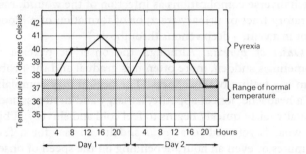

Fig. 13.3 Example of a typical temperature chart of a pyrexial patient

Nursing a pyrexial patient. If a raised body temperature is not lowered, it tends to get higher and higher; eventually the regulating mechanisms become impaired, damage to cells occurs and death ensues. The aims of nursing intervention are threefold:

● to prevent any further increase of body temperature
● to reduce body temperature to the patient's normal level
● to alleviate the discomforts associated with pyrexia

The nursing activities that are carried out are based on the principles involved in the body's heat production and heat loss mechanisms. Which activities are appropriate depend on the stage and severity of the pyrexia and are selected on the basis of the nursing assessment. Regular assessment of the patient is necessary as his condition changes and as the outcome of nursing intervention is ascertained by evaluation. Measurement of body temperature (p. 242) is an important part of evaluation and it is essential that accuracy is ensured so that the progress of the fever is recorded and effectiveness of treatment ascertained.

Promotion of heat loss by radiation is encouraged by removing excess clothing. Heat loss by convection is encouraged by using fans to circulate air. Body heat can be dispersed utilising the principles of conduction and evaporation as when tepid sponging or applying cold wet sheets or ice packs. Although it seems radical, and in contradiction to a mother's instinct, a cold immersion bath may be the most effective way of quickly reducing severe pyrexia in a child.

Additional heat gain can be prevented by limiting the patient's activity and encouraging as much relaxation, rest and sleep as possible. For this reason, patients with pyrexia are usually nursed in bed; body temperature is lowest during periods of inactivity and sleep.

Alleviating discomforts associated with pyrexia, involves a variety of nursing activities. Special help may be required with personal cleansing and dressing because with excessive sweating, the patient will want to wash more frequently than usual. It is important to pay special attention to the skin folds and the genitalia, and to change the nightclothes and bedclothes when they are damp with perspiration.

To prevent dehydration, and the discomfort of a dry mouth, frequent drinks should be encouraged and opportunities made for the patient to clean his teeth and rinse out his mouth. Although unlikely to have a good appetite, the patient should continue to eat because while the temperature remains high, the metabolic rate is also high. An appetising well-balanced diet containing protein and carbohydrate foods should be provided. Being confined to bed, the patient will be unable to use the toilet facilities and a bedpan or commode will be needed at regular intervals.

As the pyrexial patient is often restless and irritable the nurse should be attentive to his needs, helping him to feel as free as circumstances permit from discomfort and anxiety. Understanding that disorientation to time can be caused by pyrexia should direct the nurse's interaction with the patient. Since any period of waiting, when there is speeded time perception, is likely to seem longer than it actually is, the nurse must try to be punctual in time-related activities, such as meals, and continually assist the patient in time estimation (Alderson, 1974).

Hyperpyrexia

An extremely high fever, hyperpyrexia, is a feature of the condition of *heatstroke* which results from prolonged exposure to a very high environmental temperature. Heatstroke is a life-threatening condition and usually there is partial or total loss of consciousness. The heat regulating centre loses control and as a result of the physical effect of heat on brain tissue and that of other large organs, various injurious processes are triggered off. The most important of these is clotting of blood in the capillaries which, in turn, reduces oxygenation of vital organs, such as the heart and liver. Without immediate treatment to cool the body and maintain functioning of the large organs the person affected by heatstroke will die (Davies, 1977).

Illness or death from heatstroke are not unusual in parts of the world where the temperature is very high during the hot season. But even in temperate climates a heatwave may cause some people (particularly the very young and the elderly) to succumb to heat exhaustion. The affected person becomes pale, complains of nausea and headache and shows signs of shock. Usually moving the individual to a cool place and providing a cold drink are sufficient to relieve the discomfort.

When heat exhaustion turns to heatstroke there are signs of very high temperature: the skin is flushed, hot and dry, and there is impaired consciousness. Sometimes if the person has been exposed to excessive direct sunlight, there is accompanying sunburn which is extremely painful as well as hazardous. As a result of excessive loss of body fluid in perspiration, causing salt depletion, heat cramps may occur. These are severe muscle cramps and they are often accompanied by extreme thirst, nausea and dizziness. A long salt-containing drink usually gives relief.

Lack of acclimatisation plays a major role in people's intolerance of heat, and illness due to heat is most likely to occur when there is excessive physical activity while working or playing in exceptionally hot or humid conditions. The nurse concerned with industrial health services, or with health education for the young and the elderly, can contribute to the prevention of illness due to heat by advising those at risk to limit activity, keep as cool as possible and maintain hydration when exposed to heat for any length of time.

Hypothermia

In 1966 the Royal College of Physicians defined hypothermia as a 'deep body' or 'core' temperature of 35°C or under measured either rectally or in freshly passed urine (Taylor, 1982). The most common cause is prolonged exposure to a cold and damp environment.

It is well-known that exposure in cold water or winter blizzard conditions can cause hypothermia to develop rapidly. Fishermen, sailors, farmers, skiers, climbers, yachtsmen and motorists are a few of the many people who, in the course of working or playing, are exposed to cold, wet and windy conditions. Without wearing special clothing and taking safety precautions they have little chance of staying alive when the weather conditions are severe.

However, within the walls of a house people can succumb to the dangerous effects of cold and dampness and recently it has been recognised that the elderly constitute a group at risk of hypothermia. On low income they are often forced to live without adequate heating or warm clothing; in addition, they are less active physically and tend to eat less well so that body heat production is lowered. Sometimes an elderly person who lives alone falls or suffers a stroke and, having lain on a cold floor all night, when discovered, is found to be hypothermic.

The risk is also great for those at the opposite end of the lifespan. Without stability of body temperature or the ability to increase heat production voluntarily very young babies are susceptible to hypothermia unless at all times they are kept warm, dry and out of draughts. Premature babies, or others considered to be at risk, may be nursed in an incubator so that a constant warm environment can be provided, thus preventing hypothermia.

Features of hypothermia. The most significant feature of hypothermia is that even parts of the body well covered with clothing feel extremely cold to the touch. As the body temperature falls the whole of the body becomes cold to the touch, looks waxy and the face appears swollen. As the metabolic rate lowers, breathing becomes slower and more shallow and there is a progressive fall in heart rate, cardiac output and blood pressure. The onset is often insidious; this is why people affected often have failed to recognise the serious cause of their feeling of lethargy and extreme tiredness. All they want to do is to lie down and go to sleep which is the worst possible course of action. Quickly their drowsiness increases and eventually coma results. Then the body temperature falls even more rapidly and, if the condition remains untreated, death will occur.

If, in addition to exposure to a cold atmosphere, parts of the person's body actually come directly into contact with extreme cold, hypothermia is likely to be accompanied by frostbite. This is often the case when an inadequately clothed person is caught in a snow storm.

Nursing a hypothermic patient. The primary aim of nursing intervention is slow re-warming of the body to return it to its usual temperature. Rapid re-warming, although it may seem appropriate, is dangerous because it may cause circulatory collapse. Direct heat is inadvisable too, as this causes peripheral vasodilation which draws heat away from the vital organs in the core of the body. Slow rewarming, a rise of 0.5°C/hour, can best be achieved by putting the patient to bed, covering him with lightweight blankets and warming the room temperature to 26–29°C (79–84°F). Regular measurement of body temperature using a special low-reading thermometer (p. 242) is the method of evaluating the effectiveness of intervention.

As the body temperature gradually rises (Fig. 13.4) and

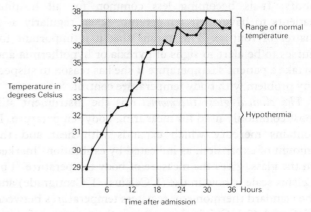

Fig. 13.4 Example of a typical temperature chart of a patient with hypothermia

consciousness is regained, the patient can be encouraged to increase mobilising and, by taking warm drinks and nourishing food, increase heat production further until the temperature reaches normal levels.

Preventing hypothermia. There is scope for all nurses, in their role as health educators, to attempt to prevent hypothermia and to detect those at risk. The elderly in the community must be helped to understand and implement the principles involved in prevention. Cold seriously affects the elderly and many old people do live in surroundings which are too cold. A room temperature of 21°C (70°F) is recommended; it may be most economical if one room of a house is kept warm and used throughout the day and night. It must be remembered that the coldest time is just before daybreak. The amount and type of clothing worn is also important. Several layers of light but warm material provide more warmth and protection from cold than one heavy garment; heat is conducted away from the body when clothing is damp and so dryness of material is essential as well as warmth.

MEASURING BODY TEMPERATURE

It is clear that being able to measure body temperature objectively is extremely helpful in the identification of an abnormal body temperature and in the evaluation of the outcomes of related nursing intervention. Body temperature measurement provides the nurse with an objective assessment and evaluative tool.

The aim of measuring body temperature is to identify deviations from the range of normal (and, in particular, from the individual's usual body temperature) or to monitor changes over time and those resulting from specific nursing activities. It is usual to take a patient's temperature on admission to hospital although, because many factors influence temperature control, this single measurement may not be representative. However, if a deviation from normal is found, or is anticipated, the procedure is repeated at regular intervals of 2, 4 or 12 hours. It is becoming less common for all hospital patients to have their temperature taken regularly as a matter of routine. This means that it is important for nurses to be alert to signs of pyrexia or hypothermia and to take a patient's temperature if she has reason to suspect any problem with body temperature control.

The clinical glass thermometer is the instrument still most commonly used for measuring body temperature. It contains mercury which expands with heat and the amount of expansion, as indicated by calibrations marked on the glass, gives the measure of body temperature. The Celsius scale is now in use (1°Celsius = 1°Centigrade) and the standard thermometer registers temperatures between 35°C and 43.5°C. The low-reading thermometer, for use with patients at risk of or suffering from hypothermia, registers down to 21°C. All clinical thermometers have a constriction above the bulb so that when the mercury has risen it remains at the level reached until forcibly shaken down. The special thermometer for use in the anal site only has a short, blunt bulb to prevent injury to the anal mucous membrane; it is coloured to distinguish it from those used in the oral or axillary sites (Fig. 13.5).

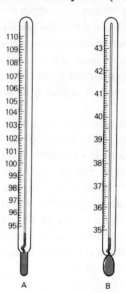

Fig. 13.5 Clinical glass thermometer A. oral F
B. anal C

Accurate measurement of body temperature is essential if the exercise is to be useful. To achieve this the nurse must use a reliable instrument, select an appropriate site, leave the instrument *in situ* for the necessary length of time and, finally, read the thermometer accurately.

Most nurses consider taking temperatures to be a simple basic procedure requiring little skill or knowledge, but the findings of some recent research projects suggest that traditional practice is far from accurate and is being continued in ignorance of the facts. An excellent review of the relevant literature is provided by Sims-Williams (1976) and, on the basis of evidence, she gives guidance on the procedure which should be followed.

The oral site is most commonly selected because it is convenient and is considered to be the most sensitive to changes in the temperature of the blood in the arteries. It is certainly the most appropriate site in the case of the fully conscious adult.

The exact placement of the bulb of the thermometer is important. This should not go just anywhere in the sublingual cavity (under the tongue); the exact place where the maximum mouth temperature is ascertained is at the junction of the base of the tongue and the floor of the mouth either to the left or to the right of the frenulum. Areas of the mouth other than these two 'heat pockets' (Fig. 13.6) are lower in temperature and, therefore, are not an accurate reflection of the actual body temperature.

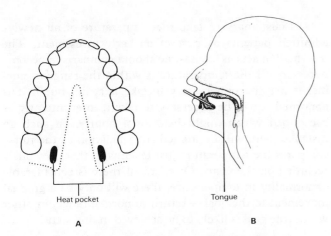

Fig. 13.6 The oral site A. position of heat pockets on mouth floor
B. thermometer in position in a heat pocket

Still further precautions must be taken to ensure an accurate measurement. If the patient has taken a hot drink, a time lapse of 6 minutes is needed prior to inserting the thermometer and 15 minutes if the drink is an iced one. A hot bath may raise body temperature and the effect can last up to 45 minutes; strenuous exercise has a similar effect. People who wear lower dentures require relatively longer to return to a stable oral temperature after such activities. Contrary to most people's expectations, smoking does not appear to affect recordings.

To ensure a reliable recording, the optimum placement time is 8 minutes for men, and 9 minutes for women in room temperatures of 18–24°C (65–75°F) and 7 minutes for both men and women in room temperatures of 24.5–30°C (76–86°F).

The axillary site is useful for babies, children or patients who are confused, breathless or unconscious. The thermometer must be maintained in a secure underarm position for about 9 minutes in adults and 4 to 8 minutes in babies and children. Variations have been found between the temperature recorded in the left and right axilla and so the same side should be used for consecutive recordings of a patient's temperature and the side used should be recorded on the patient's temperature chart.

The anal site is more usually referred to as the 'rectal' site but, in fact, the thermometer is placed into the anus and does not reach the rectum. This site is traditionally reserved for babies and those adults, particularly the elderly, whose temperature is highly variable, or suspected of being abnormally low. It is considered to be the site best able to provide a recording which is an accurate reflection of the temperature of the core of the body. However, the procedure does subject the patient to considerable embarrassment and so should not be used unless essential. There is, in addition, the hazard of cross-infection when a thermometer is coming in contact with faeces.

The reason for using this site with babies is that en-

vironmental temperatures alter axillary temperatures more than anal temperatures. However, as Eoff et al (1974) are able to point out, the environmental temperature of the nursery is usually kept stable and, in fact, the very small differences between recordings taken in the two sites do not pose any risk to the baby. Given this, use of the axillary site avoids two risks associated with the anal site; firstly, reflex defaecation and secondly, there is no chance of accidental injury to the mucous membrane of the anus.

Measuring body temperature is an important aspect of nursing assessment, and of evaluation of the effectiveness of nursing activities related to the AL of controlling body temperature. It is clear that traditional practice which does not take account of all relevant knowledge and which adopts a 2 or 3 minute placement time is unsatisfactory. It is essential that nurses apply research findings about this particular nursing activity to their practice.

Alternative temperature-recording instruments are becoming increasingly popular. This is not surprising as entrepreneurs in business are aware that many queries still remain about the satisfactory use of glass thermometers. The electronic thermometer (Fig. 13.7) is an ex-

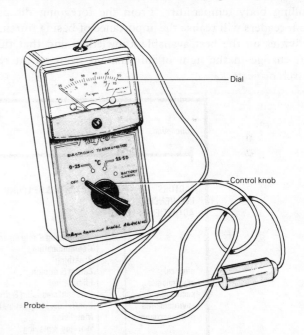

Fig. 13.7 One type of electronic thermometer

ample. It is the most expensive but it is in the main accurate, registers the temperature in 25–35 seconds when the lever comes to rest at the appropriate point on the scale. Another version is the Philips electronic digital thermometer HP 5310; it works from a battery and the probe fits into a neat case after use. It takes 60 seconds to register and there is a digital display on the handling end.

Stronge & Newton (1980) carried out a clinical trial to

compare another electronic thermometer, the IVAC 821 with the current system of glass thermometers in performance and cost. They concluded that the time saved using an electronic thermometer on the surgical ward equalled one extra nurse a week.

Campbell (1983) states that of 100 comparative readings between glass thermometers and the electronic thermometer, only 18% registered the same temperature recording. Higher readings were made on the electronic thermometer in 58%, and lower readings in 24% of the recordings. She concluded that the glass thermometer does not accurately reflect body temperature.

Fever Scan is a development of liquid crystal technology. It is robust and can be re-used. It is like a band and is gently pressed against the forehead: within 15 seconds an accurate temperature reading is displayed. It is said to be especially useful for babies, children and the elderly. The Optrex digital thermometer is a circular liquid crystal display system which can be used repeatedly: when it is pressed to the forehead it gives a clear accurate reading within seconds.

Measuring body temperature is the most frequently carried out nursing activity in relation to the AL of controlling body temperature. From the foregoing discussion, readers will realise the importance of basing nursing activities on the best available knowledge; and that this can change in the light of information from recent research projects.

It is customary to take the temperature of all newly-admitted patients as part of an early assessment. The information acts as a base-line should comparison become necessary. If the temperature is within the range of normal it may be unnecessary to take it again, but if it is abnormal it will be necessary to take it intermittently as prescribed which might be 2 or 4 hourly. In such an instance there will be immediate evaluation as the nurse compares the temperature just taken with that previously recorded on the chart. Of course if there is considerable abnormality in temperature, there will only be a gradual movement to the goal — return to normal range, in other words, the goal is likely to be achieved in tiny steps.

CHANGE OF DEPENDENCE/INDEPENDENCE STATUS FOR CONTROLLING BODY TEMPERATURE

In the model of living the dependence/independence continuum for the AL of controlling body temperature is closely related to the lifespan, a varying level of dependence being a characteristic of those people at either end of it. This is also the case in a nursing context; many of the patients who have problems which change their dependence/independence status are children or are elderly. But people can have a change in status when they are at any stage on the lifespan, and the sort of change in status

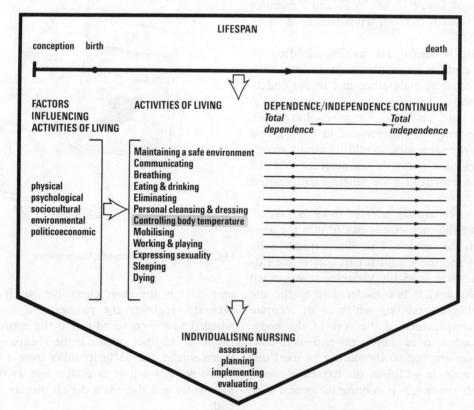

Fig. 13.8 The AL of controlling body temperature within the model for nursing

will be different according to the problem causing the change. Some of these will now be discussed.

As already mentioned many adult patients do not have an abnormal body temperature. The minority who do have problems associated with an increase/decrease of body temperature, may well be dependent on the nurse for measuring and monitoring the increase/decrease: for administering the prescribed drugs, in the prescribed dose, at the prescribed time, by the prescribed route; and monitoring the effect not only on the temperature but also the general effect, for example the extent of sweating and restlessness, return of appetite and a moist mouth. Should the prescribed treatment be tepid/warm sponging, exposure of the body to air currents produced by a fan, or to ice packs, or to cold/warm immersion baths, or whatever, then the patient is dependent on the nurse's knowledge and efficient method of carrying out these intimate procedures in such a way that the anxiety level is not increased, and hopefully is decreased. When the stated goal of return to that particular patient's normal body temperature has been achieved, the patient is dependent on the nurse for encouraging return to the previous status of independence with (when appropriate) adequate knowledge to prevent recurrence of the condition, for example hypothermia, which caused a change in status.

In the second half of this chapter some of the problems and discomforts which can be experienced by patients in relation to the AL of controlling body temperature have been described. This provides the beginning nurse with a generalised idea of these; it will be useful in assessing, planning, implementing and evaluating an individualised programme for each patient's AL of controlling body temperature.

This chapter has been concerned with the AL of controlling body temperature. However, as stated previously it is only for the purpose of discussion that any AL can be considered on its own; in reality the various activities are so closely related and do not have distinct boundaries. Figure 13.8 is a reminder that the AL of controlling body temperature is related to the other ALs and also to the various components of the model for nursing.

REFERENCES

Alderson MJ 1974 The effect of increased body temperature on the perception of time. Nursing Research 23(1) January/February:42–49
Campbell K 1983 Taking temperatures. Nursing Times 79(32) August 10: 63–65
Collins KJ, Dore C, Exton-Smith AN 1977 Acidental hypothermia and impaired temperature homeostasis in the elderly. British Medical Journal 1:353–356
Davies AG 1977 Illness due to heat. Nursing Mirror 144(25) June 23:13–14
DHSS 1972 Keeping warm in winter. Simple guidance notes for those engaged in helping old people. DHSS, London
Drummond G 1979 Hypothermia: its causes, effects and treatment in the very young and the very old. Nursing Times 75(49) December 6:2115–2116
Eoff MJ Meier RS, Miller C 1974 Temperature measurement in infants. Nursing Research 23(6) November/December: 457–460
Millard PH 1977 Hypothermia in the elderly. Nursing Mirror 145 (18) November 3:23–25
Sims-Williams AJ 1976 Temperature taking with glass thermometers; a review. Journal of Advanced Nursing 1 November: 481–493
Stronge JL, Newton G 1980 Electronic thermometers. A costly rise in efficiency? Nursing Mirror 151(8) August 21:29
Taylor G 1982 Cold comfort. Nursing Times 78(5) February 3:181

ADDITIONAL READING

Barrus DH 1983 A comparison of rectal and axillary temperatures by electronic thermometer measurement in preschool children. Pediatric Nursing 9(6) November/December:424–425
Roper N 1982 Principles of nursing, 3rd edn. Churchill Livingstone, Edinburgh, ch 16
Takacs KM, Valenti WM 1982 Temperature measurement in a clinical setting. Nursing Research 31(6) November/December:368–370
Yorkman CA 1982 Cool and heated aerosol and the measurement of oral temperature. Nursing Research 31(6) November/December:354–357

14

Mobilising

The activity of mobilising

The reason for selecting the word 'mobilising' for this AL has already been discussed (p. 21). By its very nature it is closely associated with most of the other Activities of Living. The ability to move the body freely is taken for granted by the majority of people. To push, to pull and lift; to walk, run, jog or indeed just to maintain posture, various groups of large voluntary muscles surrounding the trunk and limbs are used. Other groups of smaller muscles are constantly in use to bring about movement of the hands and feet. It is well known that muscles which are used regularly are kept at a desirable tension which makes them firm to touch, and this usually results in a feeling of well-being which can be recognised in the person's appearance. Conversely, muscles which are used infrequently lose tone, become soft and flabby and are inadequate at maintaining the body in a desirable posture so that the person looks dejected, and this is not conducive to a feeling of well-being.

THE NATURE OF MOBILISING

Physical activity is a basic human drive and is important throughout life, even into old age. When awake, healthy children are constantly on the move; most adolescents seem to have boundless energy; for adults, work and recreational activities involve overt movement; the cherished independence of the older person is impossible without some degree of mobility.

The acquisition of motor skills is, however, a very complicated process. At birth the nervous system is not sufficiently developed to permit co-ordinated movement and even when the nervous system is in a state of readiness for learning to take place, human infants, if compared to young animals and birds, are relatively slow to adopt independent co-ordinated movement. Observation of a baby trying to walk will indicate how many failures there are before he eventually manages to stand and walk unsupported and even then, the sense of balance is unpredictable.

Good walking, standing and sitting positions (Fig. 14.1), as well as being aesthetically pleasing to the on-

have opposing functions; as one muscle (the flexor) contracts and flexes, the other (the extensor) relaxes and extends to allow movement in the desired direction. When, for example, the flexor muscles on the anterior aspect of the upper arm contract to bring the forearm up towards the shoulder, the extensors on the posterior aspect relax to allow movement in the desired direction (Fig. 14.2). This diagram is a simplification of the highly sophisticated muscle activity in the human body, indeed muscles

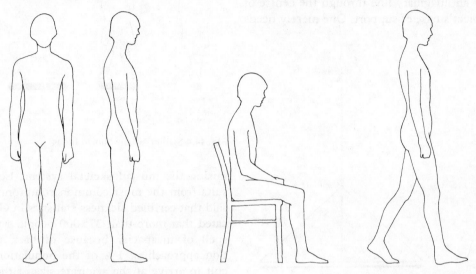

Fig. 14.1 Effective standing, sitting and walking positions

looker, conserve energy and are cultivated for everyday activities at home, at work and at play; and many recreational activities such as gymnastics, ice-skating and dancing encourage good posture. To achieve some understanding about the nature of mobilising there are several physical principles which are helpful, for example, those of contraction and relaxation, leverage and gravity.

Contraction and relaxation (extension). In health, all muscle fibres are in a state of what is called muscle tone, ready for instant, smooth movement. Muscles contract to produce action and are often arranged in pairs associated with two or more bones and a joint, such that the pair

usually work not only in pairs but in groups and Figure 14.2 merely demonstrates one of the principles of muscle action.

Leverage. The principle of leverage is also useful in understanding the nature of mobilising. A lever is a rigid bar which revolves around a fixed axis or fulcrum and a simple example of a lever is a see-saw. Two children of equal weight and equidistant from the middle will balance the see-saw but if one child moves further back, that end of the see-saw will move towards the ground assisted by the pull of gravity, and to elevate his end the child must push upwards against the force of gravity. By

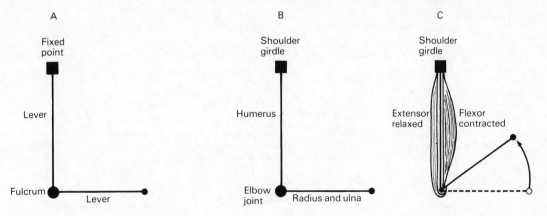

Fig. 14.2 Principles of muscle movement at the elbow joint

using the board as a lever it is possible for one child to lift the other quite some height off the ground, which would probably be impossible using only the arms. Utilising the principle of leverage increases an individual's lifting power.

Law of gravity. Knowledge about the law of gravity is also important in understanding the nature of mobilising. Every object has a centre of gravity (in the human it is around the level of the second sacral vertebra) and it is possible to draw an imaginary line through the centre of gravity to the object's base of support. One merely needs

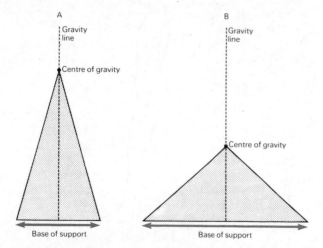

Fig. 14.3 Stability in objects: base of support and centre of gravity

to visualise a tall slender object and a low squat one to appreciate that the broader the base of support and the lower the centre of gravity, the more stable is the object (Fig. 14.3).

Similarly the baby who is starting to crawl has a low centre of gravity and wide base, and when he first stands, somewhat unsteadily, he places his feet wide apart.

Likewise, patients out of bed after an illness hold on to furniture or lean on someone's arm or use a walking stick in an attempt to increase their base of support (Fig. 14.4).

A knowledge of body mechanics and its application can help people to acquire techniques of mobilising: and lifting bulky heavy equipment (Fig. 14.5) without compro-

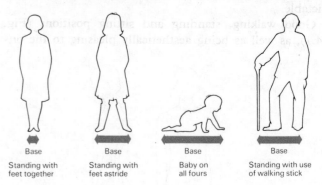

Fig. 14.4 Stability in the human frame

mising the musculoskeletal system. Low back pain results from the most common compromise. Evans (1981) said that certified sickness statistics in Great Britain indicated that more than 375 000 people a year experience a spell of incapacity because of back pain — a proportion approaching 1% of the population. But it is difficult to arrive at the accurate size of the problem in the population, because some people continue at work and statistics are not even available on all those who are off work.

A pilot study in 1979 indicated that of 430 000 nurses in the National Health Service (England & Wales) 40 000 were affected by back pain which caused them to take sick leave (Rogers 1983). Compared with the rest of the working population, nurses had twice the amount of sick leave as a result of back pain. Ways and means of minimising the risk will be discussed later in this chapter.

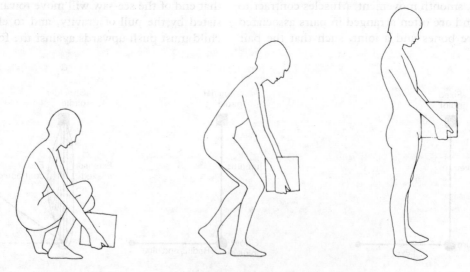

Fig. 14.5 Desirable body positions when lifting a heavy object from the floor

THE PURPOSE OF MOBILISING

With an AL which has as many dimensions as mobilising it is difficult to encapsulate the wide range of purpose, as can be seen from the headings under which it will be discussed — exploring the environment, enjoying rhythmic movement, channelling emotional energy, promoting well-being, and transferring man and goods.

Exploring the environment. It is the capacity for movement which first allows the infant to explore himself and his environment. If the child's movement is restricted or if he is deprived of opportunities to respond to stimuli in his surroundings, his physical and psychosocial growth may be impeded. Intellectual development too may be curtailed if the growing child is denied exposure to new experiences beyond the home environment, with people other than the immediate family. This capacity for physical movement to explore the environment is critical to many aspects of the individual's development, and lack of or loss of mobility, or reduced mobility, can have a devastating effect on the person's image of himself, perhaps ultimately affecting his capacity to take his place effectively in society.

Enjoying rhythmic movement. Young children seem intuitively and uninhibitedly to engage in body movement as a response to music and in time with the rhythm. Many adults too seem to enjoy rhythmic body movement, almost subconsciously, and when sitting alone or in company can be observed tapping a foot or a hand, or swinging a leg. Recreations such as dancing, ice-skating and even gymnastics are frequently performed to the accompaniment of music, probably enhancing the pleasure derived by both performers and spectators. At work too, long before the advent of piped music, artisans were known to sing while busy with the weaving frame, or hauling in the fishing nets, and many well-known songs reflect this rhythmic association.

Channelling emotional energy. Some people use physical activity as an outlet for emotions, for reasons as diverse as boredom and aggression. Many 'normal' teenagers and young adults who engage in strenuous activities say that they do so to 'let off steam' and, many admit that by so doing they experience relaxation and recreation. In a similar vein, physical activities are deliberately encouraged in social clubs for young offenders, so that energies may be expended in a way which is pleasurable to the individual, rather than in uncontrolled, and sometimes violent, types of behaviour.

Promoting well-being. It is well known that not only the musculoskeletal system benefits from regular exercise but the function of all the other systems is enhanced. Currently the media extol the benefits, both physiological and psychological, of exercise for all age groups and deplore the sedentary lifestyle of people in most industrialised countries; a lifestyle which is considered to be a major contributing factor to conditions such as hypertension, coronary heart disease and obesity. All of these have increased in incidence in the last few decades, indeed coronary heart disease is a major cause of death in most countries of the Western world.

Transferring man and goods. In industrialised countries the capacity for personal physical movement from place to place is greatly enhanced by machines. In the initial stages of man's existence on this planet he had to rely on his own body energy to move himself and his goods from place to place, but as he learned to domesticate animals, he came to conserve his own energy by riding a horse or a bullock or an elephant. With the advent of the wheel, he was able to construct a carrier of sorts which could be drawn by animals. Making an immense chronological leap down to the industrial and technological revolutions, he was able to harness other forms of energy in devising fuel-powered vehicles such as cars, trains, ships and planes for rapid transit of people and vast quantities of goods.

It is interesting that man is now showing concern about the dwindling natural energy sources in the world and there is a drive to conserve existing supplies. There is also considerable activity in the development of nuclear power, and exploration of the possibilities for utilising solar and wave energy to man's advantage so that he can continue to augment his own capacity for physical mobility. Hopefully man will find the appropriate balance between exploiting the mobilising power of machines, and maintaining a personal exercise level which is conducive to health and the enjoyment of everyday living.

BODY STRUCTURE AND FUNCTION REQUIRED FOR MOBILISING

Normal motor function is a very complex activity involving many body systems which are inextricably linked, but overt physical movement most obviously involves bones, joints and muscles, and these are the structures which in the model for nursing, are related to the AL of mobilising. Of course the muscular and nervous systems function co-operatively to produce body movement. However, in the model for nursing the nervous system is part of the body structure and function required for communicating which is discussed in Chapter 8. What follows is an introduction to the skeletal and muscular systems; later in the programme nurses will need to know more about these systems to understand the diseases, infections and traumas which can occur in them and produce the patient's problems with mobilising.

The skeletal system
To allow physical movement, a system of rigid braces, attachments, levers and joints activated by muscles is re-

quired and in the human, the basic arrangement is provided by the skeletal system.

The adult height is genetically determined but achievement of height potential requires an adequate diet, particularly of protein, calcium, phosphorus and vitamin D which are needed for bone formation. The deposition of new bone which increases height is controlled from birth to adolescence mainly by the growth hormone secreted by an endocrine gland situated at the base of the brain: the pituitary gland. But growth is also affected by the hormones secreted by the thyroid gland which lies in front of the larynx and by the androgens and oestrogens secreted by the ovaries and testes to influence, among other functions, the male/female skeletal characteristics.

The bony skeleton is made up of four main types of bones:

- *long bones* form the limbs and have a shaft and two extremities
- *short bones* are found in groups at the ankles and wrists and permit intricate movement, yet can support considerable weight
- *flat bones* are found in the skull, ribs and pelvis providing protection for vital organs in the head, chest and abdomen respectively
- *irregular bones* as the name suggests are irregular in shape, for example, the bones of the face and of the spinal column

All bones where they form joint surfaces are smooth in texture to allow easy movement, and conversely they present a roughened appearance where muscles are attached.

Before describing individual bones of the skeleton it is necessary to define some terms which identify their position in relation to the anatomical position:

- *anatomical position:* this phrase is used to describe the body in the upright position, the head facing forward, the feet together and the arms by the sides with the palms of the hands facing forward (Fig. 14.6)
- *midline:* if the body in the anatomical position were divided longitudinally into two equal parts, this imaginary line would be the midline
- *medial:* indicates that a structure is nearest to the midline
- *lateral:* indicates that a structure is farthest from the midline
- *anterior:* indicates that a structure is nearest to the front of the body
- *posterior:* indicates that a structure is nearest to the back of the body
- *superior:* indicates that a structure is nearest to the head
- *inferior:* indicates that a structure is farthest from the head

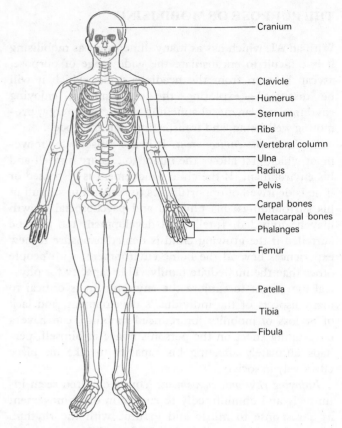

Fig. 14.6 The skeleton: anterior view

Labels: Cranium, Clavicle, Humerus, Sternum, Ribs, Vertebral column, Ulna, Radius, Pelvis, Carpal bones, Metacarpal bones, Phalanges, Femur, Patella, Tibia, Fibula

- *proximal and distal:* these terms are used in relation to the limbs. The proximal end of the bone is nearest to the point of attachment of the limb to the trunk, and the distal end is farthest from the point of attachment
- *foramen (plural foramina):* a hole in a bone usually allowing the passage of blood vessels and nerves

Vertebral column

The human being has a spine or backbone which forms a central support yet allows considerable flexibility. This spinal column is made up of 33 irregular bones called vertebrae, hence the vertebral column. Some of the bones are quite separate, others are fused together and they are named according to their position (Fig. 14.7):

- 7 cervical vertebrae
- 12 thoracic vertebrae
- 5 lumbar vertebrae
- 5 sacral vertebrae — fused to form the sacrum
- 4 coccygeal vertebrae — fused to form the coccyx.

Most of the bones are similar in shape but they vary in size. The smallest are nearest the head, then they become progressively larger down to the lumbar region, then reduce in size down to the level of the coccyx.

Most of the vertebrae have a body which lies anteriorly.

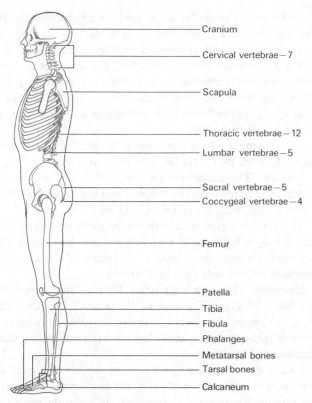

Fig. 14.7 The skeleton: lateral view

Projecting back from it is an arch enclosing the neural canal through which passes the spinal cord. From the arch, three processes project for the attachment of muscles which move the vertebral column, and the most prominent, the spinous process, can be felt easily under the skin of the back (Fig. 14.8).

The vertebral column, though firmly held together by

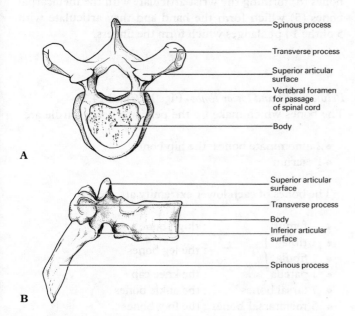

Fig. 14.8 A vertebra: A. superior view B. lateral view

ligaments and muscles, is capable of a range of movement because of the slightly movable joints between most vertebrae and because of the presence of cartilagenous discs between each vertebra — intervertebral discs — which act as cushions and shock absorbers (Fig. 14.9). When the

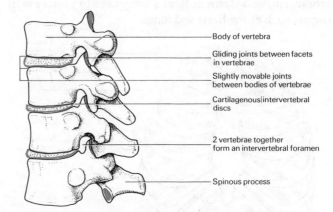

Fig. 14.9 Vertebrae and intervertebral discs

spine bends forwards, the area of pressure on the disc is at the front, and similarly at the back when bending backwards and at the side when bending laterally. Should the disc become displaced, however, there can be pressure on the spinal nerves causing severe pain. At the level of each vertebra, pairs of spinal nerves branch off from the spinal cord and pass through intervertebral foramina to be distributed to every part of the body (see Ch. 8).

In summary, the vertebral column has three main functions:

1. Protection. The strong bony column with its neural canal is a protective framework for the delicate tissue of the spinal cord. The cells of the brain and spinal cord unlike most others, cannot regenerate and it is critical to protect them because once damaged, they are irreplaceable.
2. Movement. Because of the presence of slightly movable joints in the vertebral column and the disc-like cushions between the bodies, a limited amount of movement is possible.

   - flexion   : bending forward
   - extension   : bending backward
   - lateral flexion: bending to the side
   - rotation   : turning round

3. Support. The spine supports the skull which encloses the brain tissue. The vertebral column also provides attachment for the ribs, shoulder girdle and upper limbs; and the pelvic girdle and lower limbs. In addition, it provides attachment for the many muscles which allow intricate and powerful movements of the human frame.

Thorax (Fig. 14.10)

The thorax is the upper cavity of the trunk. Posteriorly are the 12 thoracic vertebrae, articulating with them are the 12 pairs of ribs, and these in turn are joined by cartilage to the sternum or breast bone. Together, the vertebrae, ribs and sternum form a bony cage to protect vital organs such as the heart and lungs.

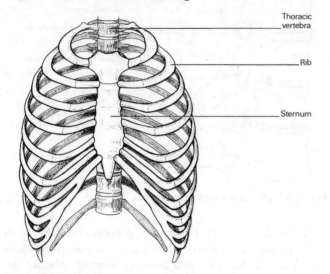

Thoracic vertebra

Rib

Sternum

Fig. 14.10 The thorax

Sternum. This is a flat bone shaped, it is said, like a dagger and can be felt easily under the skin. Beneath the sternum lies the heart and when, in an emergency, external massage is required to stimulate heart action, pressure is rhythmically applied over the sternal area.

Ribs. These 12 pairs of flat curved bones form the lateral walls of the thoracic cage. With the exception of the last two pairs, they are attached by cartilage to the sternum. Cartilage helps to give resilience to the thoracic cage should excessive pressure be applied thus helping to prevent fracture of the ribs.

Shoulder girdle and upper limbs (Figs 14.6 and 14.7)

The shoulder girdle, attached by strong muscles to the upper rib cage, consists of:

- 2 scapulae: the shoulder blades
- 2 clavicles: the collar bones

The bones of each upper extremity are:

- 1 humerus : the arm
- 1 radius ⎱
- 1 ulna ⎰ : the forearm
- 8 carpal bones : the wrist
- 5 metacarpal bones : the hand
- 14 phalanges : the fingers

Scapula. This triangular bone curves to fit the contour of the upper ribs and the lateral border forms one of the boundaries of the axilla, the space under the shoulder. At the top of this axillary border is a shallow socket, the glenoid cavity which is covered with hyaline cartilage and receives the head of the humerus, the arm bone. This makes the freely moving, ball and socket shoulder joint. Projecting from the back of the bone is the spine and it ends in a prominence which articulates with the clavicle forming a gliding joint.

Each scapula gives attachment to muscles and ligaments and the two scapulae help to protect the two lungs.

Clavicle. The clavicle is an S-shaped bone, one end of which articulates with the scapula and the other end with the sternum. Both are synovial, gliding joints.

The clavicles give attachment to muscles and ligaments and act as a brace to the shoulder; they hold back the scapulae. When the clavicle is fractured, the entire shoulder on that side falls forward.

Humerus. This is a long bone. Its proximal extremity fits into the glenoid cavity of the scapula to form the shoulder joint. The distal extremity broadens to form two smooth surfaces which articulate with the radius and ulna forming a hinge joint.

Radius and ulna. The radius is on the lateral aspect of the forearm (when the body is in the anatomical position). Its proximal extremity is rounded, articulating with the humerus to form part of the elbow joint, and also with the ulna to allow the very important pivoting movement in the forearm. The distal extremity articulates with the wrist bones.

Near the wrist, on the lateral border, the radial artery passes over the bone and because it is near to the skin surface, this artery can be felt easily. It is the site where the pulse rate is most commonly counted.

Carpal bones, metacarpals and phalanges. The carpal bones (8) forming the wrist articulate with the metacarpal bones (5) which form the hand and they articulate with 5 of the 14 phalanges which form the fingers.

Pelvic girdle and lower limbs (Figs 14.6 and 14.7)

The bones which make up the pelvis or pelvic girdle are:

- 2 innominate bones: the hip bones
- 1 sacrum

The bones of each lower extremity are:

- 1 femur : thigh bone
- 1 tibia ⎱
- 1 fibula ⎰ : the leg bones
- 1 patella : the knee cap
- 7 tarsal bones : the ankle bones
- 5 metatarsal bones : the foot bones
- 14 phalanges : the toes

Innominate bone (hip bone). Each hip bone is made up of the fusion of three bones:

- the ilium
- the ischium
- the pubis

The upper flattened part of the ilium is called the iliac crest. The ischium lies posteriorly and takes the body weight in the sitting position. The pubis is the anterior part of the bone and articulates with the pubis of the other innominate bone to form what is called the symphysis pubis. All three parts unite in a deep depression called the acetabulum which acts as a socket for the head of the femur and forms the ball and socket hip joint (Fig. 14.11).

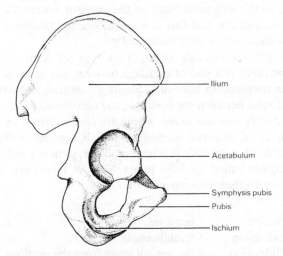

Fig. 14.11 The innominate or hip bone

The pelvis is formed by the two hip bones which articulate anteriorly at the symphysis pubis and posteriorly with the sacrum (Fig. 14.12). It contains the organs of reproduction and the shape in the male differs from that of the female. The male pelvis is larger but narrow and funnel-shaped; the female has a lighter, shallower pelvis to allow room for the passage of the baby at the end of pregnancy.

Sacrum. It consists of the five fused sacral vertebrae.

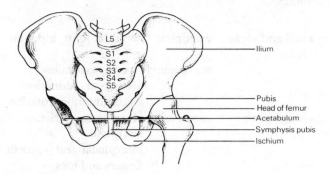

Fig. 14.12 The pelvis

Femur. The thigh bone is the longest and strongest in the body. The upper extremity has a rounded head which forms the ball and socket hip joint with the acetabulum. The distal extremity presents two articular surfaces which take part in the formation of the knee joint.

Patella. This triangular shaped bone forms the knee cap and articulates with the femur. It takes the weight of the body when kneeling.

Tibia and fibula. The tibia, situated on the medial aspect of the leg, is commonly known as the shin bone. It is a long bone whose thick, flat upper extremity has two smooth surfaces which articulate with the distal end of the femur to form the knee joint. The fibula is on the lateral aspect of the leg. It, too, is a leg bone and at the proximal end its rounded head can be felt on the lateral aspect of the knee. The distal extremity along with the tibia and tarsal bones form the ankle joint.

Tarsal bones, metatarsals and phalanges. The structure is similar to the hand: 7 tarsal bones, 5 metatarsals and 14 phalanges. When walking, it is important to have some spring in the foot and this is achieved by the arches. The foot bones are maintained by ligaments and tendons in such a way that they form three resilient arches, two lengthwise and one across the foot. When, for some reason, these bridge-like structures fall (the condition is called flat foot) there is a varying degree of pain and an ungainly gait.

Skull
The skull is made up of 22 bones and has two main parts (Figs 14.13 and 14.14):

- the cranium: 8 bones
- the face   : 14 bones

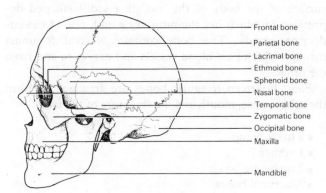

Fig. 14.13 The bones of the skull: lateral view

Cranium. The cranium consists of eight flat bones arranged to form maximum protection for the brain tissue.

The frontal bone, as its name implies, is at the front of the cranium and forms the forehead and the roof of the orbits (eye sockets).

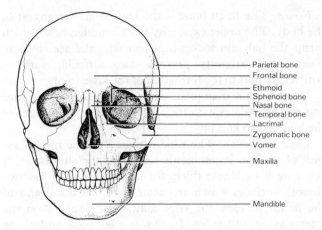

Fig. 14.14 The bones of the skull: anterior view

Parietal bone
Frontal bone
Ethmoid
Sphenoid bone
Nasal bone
Temporal bone
Lacrimal
Zygomatic bone
Vomer
Maxilla
Mandible

The 2 parietal bones meet in the midline and form the dome of the cranium. The 2 temporal bones form the sides of the head. Each has a triangular portion which juts inwards to form part of the structure of the ear. The occipital bone lies at the back of the cranium and contains the foramen magnum through which the spinal cord passes as it leaves the brain. On each side of the foramen are surfaces for articulation with the atlas, the first bone of the vertebral column.

The ethmoid bone forms the anterior part of the base of the skull, part of the orbital cavities and the bony framework of the nose. The portion forming the roof of the nasal cavities has numerous small foramina through which pass the nerves of smell conveying stimuli from the nose to the brain for interpretation.

The sphenoid bone is an irregular bone shaped somewhat like a bat with wings outstretched and occupies the middle portion of the base of the skull. On the superior surface of the body of the 'bat' is a saddle-shaped depression in which lies the pituitary gland, one of the endocrine glands. The bone contains several foramina through which pass blood vessels and nerves to and from the brain.

Face. Fourteen irregular bones are arranged to form the orbits, nose, mouth and the structure of the face:

- 2 nasal bones
- 1 vomer
- 2 turbinate bones
- 2 lacrimal bones
- 2 malar bones
- 2 maxillary bones
- 2 palatal bones
- 1 mandible (jaw bone)

Joints

A rigid, bony framework would not be of much use for mobilising. Movement is dependent on the presence of joints and these are found where two or more bones come together or articulate. Some joints have no movement, some have slight movement and some are freely movable.

1. *Immovable joints.* Sometimes these are called fibrous joints because of the presence of fibrous tissue which fixes the joints firmly together. Examples of this type include the innominate bone, the teeth in their sockets, and the joints of the skull.

Apart from the mandibular joint, all the joints of the skull are immovable. The bone edges are serrated and fit together closely from an early age. In the newborn child, however, there is a space at the junction of the frontal and two parietal bones — the anterior fontanelle — and at the junction of the occipital and parietal bones, the posterior fontanelle. These spaces allow moulding of the skull during the baby's descent in the birth canal but ossify soon after birth. Blood vessels can be felt easily beneath the soft membrane of the anterior fontanelle before ossification and this is a useful site for assessing the pulse count of the very young infant.

2. *Slightly movable joints.* This type of joint occurs where there is a pad of cartilage between the ends of the bones involved in the joint. Slight movement is possible as is found between the bodies of the vertebrae.

3. *Freely movable joints.* These are characterised by the presence of synovial membrane which secretes a thick, sticky fluid to provide lubrication, indeed, these joints are sometimes called synovial joints. Various terms are used to describe their movements:

• flexion	:	bending
• extension	:	straightening
• abduction	:	movement away from the midline
• adduction	:	movement toward the midline
• circumduction:		the combination of the 4 above
• rotation	:	turning
• pronation	:	turning the palm of the hand down
• supination	:	turning the palm of the hand up
• inversion	:	turning the sole of the foot towards the midline
• eversion	:	turning the sole of the foot outwards

The synovial joints are classified according to their movement:

• ball and socket joint	examples:	shoulder joint, hip joint
	movement:	flexion, extension, abduction, adduction, circumduction, rotation
• hinge joint	examples:	elbow, knee, wrist, ankle and interphalangeal joints in fingers and toes
	movement:	flexion and extension

- pivot joint   examples: atlas/axis joint, radius/ ulnar joint

  movement: rotation

- gliding joint   examples: sternoclavicular joint, carpal joints, tarsal joints

  movement: surfaces slide easily over each other

Synovial joints have certain common characteristics (Fig. 14.15):

a. the bones forming the joint are covered by hyaline cartilage

b. the joint is surrounded and enclosed by fibrous tissue which though binding the bones together is sufficiently loose to allow a range of movement in the joint capsule

c. synovial membrane lines the capsule and covers the part of the bones not covered by hyaline cartilage. It secretes synovial fluid to lubricate the joint

d. outside the capsule are extracapsular ligaments which strengthen it and lend stability to the joint

e. muscles, by contracting and expanding, control the movements of the joint

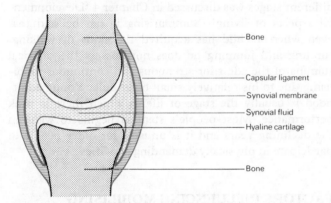

Fig 14.15 The main structures in a synovial joint

The muscular system

The bony skeleton with its joints requires the presence of muscles to provide movement. These are termed voluntary or skeletal muscles. Each passes over one or more joints and by contracting, it pulls on the bone and causes movement, for example, flexion, extension, circumduction. Each muscle fibre contracts in response to a stimulus delivered by a nerve which initiates complicated enzyme and chemical reactions resulting in the production of heat, energy and waste products which are transported in the blood. Much of the heat needed to keep all body tissue 'warm' is generated in the muscles in the process of movement.

The human body is capable of powerful but intricate movement and the muscles each have a name but only

those making up the main groups of muscles will be given in this section (Figs 14.16 and 14.17).

Upper limb muscle groups

Deltoid. This is the muscle lying over the shoulder joint assisting with movement of the shoulder and raising the arm.

Biceps/triceps group. The biceps lies anteriorly on the upper arm and on contraction it flexes the elbow. The triceps lies posteriorly and extends the elbow.

The lower arm, hand and fingers have numerous smaller muscles capable of intricate movement.

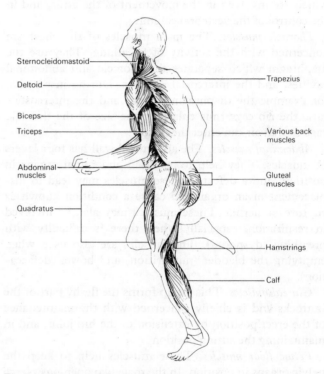

Fig. 14.16 Muscles of the trunk and limb

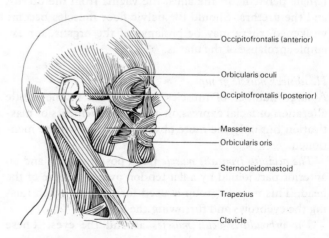

Fig. 14.17 Muscles of the face

Lower limb muscle groups

Quadratus/hamstrings group. The quadratus muscle to the front of the thigh extends the knee joint and plays a part in moving the hip joint. The hamstrings lie posteriorly and are essentially concerned with flexion of the knee joint.

The lower leg muscles form the calf of the leg, and along with smaller foot and toe muscles are extensively used in activities such as walking, running and jumping, and with maintaining the body in the upright position.

Trunk muscle groups

Back muscles. There are many strong back muscles which are involved in the movement of the arms, and in the control of the vertebral column.

Thoracic muscles. The main muscles of the chest are concerned with the activity of breathing. They are the diaphragm which separates the thoracic and abdominal cavities, and the intercostal muscles. During inspiration for example the diaphragm flattens and the intercostals raise the rib cage thus enlarging the size of the thoracic cage so that air can enter the lungs.

Abdominal muscles. The abdominal wall has four layers of muscles. They help to maintain abdominal organs in position, and a defect in these muscles may lead to displacement of an organ and cause a condition known as rupture or hernia. These muscles may also be involved in respiration, especially when there is difficulty with breathing (dyspnoea). The muscles are also used when emptying the bladder (micturition) and bowel (defaecation).

Gluteal muscles. This group forms the fleshy part of the buttocks and is chiefly concerned with the maintenance of the erect position by extension of the hip joint, and in maintaining the sitting position.

Pelvic floor muscles. These muscles help to keep the pelvic organs in position. In the male two openings pierce the pelvic floor: the anus from the rectum, and the urethra from the bladder. There are three openings in the female pelvic floor: the anus, the vagina from the uterus, and the urethra. Should the pelvic floor muscles become weakened, there may be prolapse of the organs, for example, prolapse of the uterus.

Head/neck muscle groups

A large number of muscles are involved in the subtle alteration of facial expression and the movements of mastication but only the more obvious muscles will be mentioned.

The occipito frontalis muscle has a posterior part and an anterior part joined by a flat tendon over the dome of the head. This muscle group is used for example when raising the eyebrows and furrowing the brow.

The orbicularis oculi muscles around the eyes. These muscles are used when closing and 'screwing up' the eyes.

The orbicularis oris muscle surrounds the mouth. It is used to close the lips, and when pouting and whistling.

The masseter muscles extend from the cheek bones to the angle of the jaw. They are used in the process of chewing and for example when blowing musical wind instruments.

The sternocleidomastoid muscles stretch from the sternum and clavicle to the mastoid process of the temporal bone. The head is drawn down to the shoulder when the muscle on one side contracts.

The trapezius muscles cover the neck, shoulder and upper part of the back. These muscles are used when putting the head backwards, squaring the shoulders and controlling the action of the scapulae.

It can be seen that all these structures are necessary to enable a person to carry out the AL of mobilising which as said earlier, includes all the movement of which the human body is capable.

LIFESPAN: EFFECT ON MOBILISING

It is evident that the lifespan component of the model has an effect on mobilising. The range of norm for the development, maintenance, and decline of this AL for the different stages was discussed in Chapter 4 'Developmental aspects of living'. Summarising it can be said that even when a child has acquired the skills of walking, running and jumping he does not possess the physical stamina of the adult for strenuous and continuous mobilising due to his relatively small body bulk. Young adulthood is usually the stage of life in which there is peak performance. Most people's stamina begins to wane in the declining years and it is unusual for older people to participate in physically demanding activities.

FACTORS INFLUENCING MOBILISING

An important part of the model of living is how five factors — physical, psychological, sociocultural, environmental and politicoeconomic — influence the way in which individuality in mobilising develops, and they will now be discussed in turn.

Physical factors

A fully functioning musculoskeletal system is essential for acquisition of the skills related to mobilising. The capacity for unaided physical mobility is therefore affected by any circumstance which interferes with any part of the musculoskeletal system and its associated nerve pathways. The adverse circumstance may be congenital in origin but good obstetric care aims at prevention of birth injuries and disabling conditions occurring in the neonatal period.

Fractured or diseased bones can interfere with mobilising in many different ways. Joints too may become diseased and so painful that movement is impeded. Should the hips, knees or ankles be affected, walking becomes difficult; when the small joints of the hands are involved there can be interference with many aspects of mobilising for example those used in domestic activities, personal cleansing and dressing and working and playing. A muscle sprain may cause swelling and thereby reduce movement. Any form of paralysis such as hemiplegia caused by a stroke, or paraplegia caused by accident, severely restricts mobilising.

For those who have a permanent physical impairment which reduces mobility, the aim is to help them to enjoy everyday living to the optimum level. If physically impaired from birth, the goal will be the achievement of a lifestyle where they will have the maximum possible mobility. For those who succumb to an immobilising disease or injury, it may mean adapting to a lifestyle which is less physically active but just as personally fulfilling, and the adaptation may be merely temporary or it may require to be a lifelong adjustment.

Psychological factors

A minimum level of intelligence is necessary to learn the skills necessary for safe mobilising. Temperament also influences this AL; there are people who are constantly curious and characteristically active; their mobilising is often of an adventurous nature. There are others whose curiosity relates to acquiring knowledge; they are usually less active in mobilising and may be described as 'thinkers rather than doers'. A person's values and beliefs may provide the motivation to exercise in order to keep fit, and indeed they may provide a driving ambition so that daily practice for many hours can be sustained. People also display different attitudes to safety while mobilising, for example complying with speed regulations and the wearing of seat belts.

Sociocultural factors

Some sociocultural factors were mentioned on page 249 — artisans' songs to bring rhythm to the movements involved in weaving and fishing. Most countries of the world have national dances which are a much valued expression of national pride and patriotic fervour, and have been handed down from generation to generation. On the other hand members of some religious and cultural groups exclude, for example, dancing as a form of pleasurable exercise. Social class may well determine how this AL is carried out, for example whether a person travels on foot or public transport, by car or in private plane or yacht. There are also sports and other leisure activities which are characteristic of the higher and lower social classes; children from the former may go skiing abroad while those from the latter play football on a piece of waste ground near their home. Of course social class undoubtedly dictates the mobilising component of the working day; the majority of people in the higher classes have sedentary jobs while many in the lower group are manual workers.

Cultural factors make their contribution to the sort of sport which is characteristic of countries. The names of many famous tennis and cricket clubs, and rugby leagues are indicative of the strong tradition attached to the sport in that part of the world. At international gatherings too, the influence of culture can be observed in for example the style of dress and the music chosen to accompany the movement, as in gymnastics and ice skating.

Environmental factors

The type of residence is an important determinant of optimal achievement in mobilising.

High rise flats are not conducive to children's optimal development of the AL of mobilising. A third-floor flat which is not serviced by a lift may deter a frail elderly person from taking a daily walk. Available space within the home is another influencing factor; the type of furniture for toddlers and frail people to use as a support while walking is also important. Ergonomists pay special attention to the design of furniture, particularly chairs so that for example a desirable sitting posture is maintained. There are many other environmental factors which influence the AL of mobilising particularly for those with impaired vision, hearing or agility. These include having to cross busy streets, having to climb a gradient when setting out from or returning to the house, or lack of parks and open spaces in which to take exercise in an unhurried manner.

One should not forget that local climate and terrain can affect mobilising. The majority of people do not exercise strenuously in a hot and humid atmosphere, and where facilities are available are much more likely to go swimming for example. People who have a tendency to breathlessness fare badly in a windy climate and may not get sufficient outdoor exercise. Those brought up in hilly districts may be influenced to take up fell walking as a hobby and the adventurous ones may be attracted to mountaineering.

Politicoeconomic factors

It is said that every city has its slums and areas of substandard housing and these are usually owned by the local council, or administrative body. The environs of such areas are often in bad repair and poorly lit, so that there are restrictions on young children in terms of possibilities for physically active pursuits. Councils vary in the provision of parks and open spaces, children's playgrounds, playing fields, swimming baths, sports arenas and leisure centres and all these can directly influence the mobilising habits of the population.

The local council is of course responsible for the state schools in which physical education is available. The range of sports can vary from one city to another, but if for instance the school does not have facilities for swimming, tuition arrangements can usually be made with the city swimming pool so that pupils are not deprived of this sport which is such a healthy form of mobilising.

The council is also responsible for the state of city pavements so that pedestrians can walk safely. There is usually a kerb of several inches between pavement and street and these can be hazardous for both adult and child when a pushchair is being used. Such kerbs also present problems to those of all ages whose form of transport is a wheelchair whether it is manually wheeled by another person, or is self-propelled or battery driven. Some people feel sufficiently strongly about this restriction that they campaign for the council to provide ramps between the street and pavement to cater for the special needs of these groups of people.

The central government in the UK encourages local councils to provide wheelchair access to public buildings and shops so that the users of this form of mobilising are not deprived of entry. A transport allowance is available to disabled people and if their cars display the necessary sticker, they can park in areas which are normally forbidden to private vehicles, or restricted in some way.

Pedestrian crossings are usually sited at traffic lights but where these are absent on a long straight street or road, many campaigners have succeeded in getting the council to instal a pedestrian-controlled crossing so that particularly those with some impediment in walking can take time to cross safely.

DEPENDENCE/INDEPENDENCE IN MOBILISING

It is relevant here to point out that with regard to the AL of mobilising, the dependence/independence component of the model is closely related to the lifespan component. For the majority of people, after a period of dependence in infancy, there is increasing independence in childhood. At the other end of the lifespan, the majority of old people experience a gradual decrease in the level of independence until many of them become dependent on some type of aid, often a walking stick, to broaden the base and take some of the body weight when walking.

However there are some people who at birth do not have adequate body structure and function to achieve independence in mobilising, as they progress through the stages of the lifespan. There are others, who having achieved independence, are deprived of it at a further stage on the lifespan, perhaps due to accident or disease. Aided independence may be a possibility by learning to use such external aids as walking frames, crutches, leg calipers, and artificial limbs which may be body worn

aids. There may be dependence on another person for help with applying the aid. For those who cannot stand, mobilising has to be achieved by dependence on a wheelchair and possibly another person to push it; some are able to use a self-propelled or a battery operated wheelchair. Some can also manage to drive a modified car and indeed become independent as they use a hoist to transfer from wheelchair to car.

INDIVIDUALITY IN MOBILISING

The purpose of the model of living is description of a person's individuality in mobilising. With so many facets influencing the AL of mobilising, it is not surprising that by the time a person reaches adulthood, he has developed highly individualised mobilising habits. Sometimes the person who has a physically active work pattern also chooses to have strenuous play activities. On the other hand he may deliberately engage in more sedentary recreation in order to balance his daily energy output. There are many variations on the theme and they provide an interesting diversity in the life of a community. When describing a particular person's individuality in mobilising the nurse will find the foregoing description of this AL in the context of the model useful, and the following résumé helpful:

Lifespan: effect on mobilising

- Infancy and childhood — increasing skills in mobilising
- Adolescence and young adulthood — peak performance in mobilising
- Later years — decreasing agility

Factors influencing mobilising

- Physical
  - fully functioning musculoskeletal system
  - congenital interference with function
  - trauma, disease
- Psychological
  - intelligence; temperament; values, beliefs, motivation, ambition; attitudes
- Sociocultural
  - rhythm of mobilising; dancing; religious constraints; social class; tradition
- Environmental
  - type and place of residence; local climate and terrain; influence on hobbies
- Politicoeconomic
  - substandard housing
  - kerbs and pavements
  - access to buildings ⎫
  - safe street crossings ⎬ in home area
  - exercise facilities

Dependence/independence in mobilising
- Increasing independence in childhood
- Dependence on another person
- Body worn aids ⎫
- External aids   ⎬ for aided independence
- Transport   ⎭

Mobilising: patient's problems and related nursing activities

For the majority of people, an episode of illness which requires a spell in hospital will involve some change in mobilising habits. To minimise problems nurses need to know about the patient's previous habits and at least some of this information will be gained at the initial assessment. The following questions will help the nurse to collect the required information:

- how much exercise does the individual take daily/weekly?
- when does the individual exercise?
- what factors influence the way the individual mobilises?
- what does the individual know about mobilising, particularly with regard to health?
- what is the individual's attitude to mobilising?
- has the individual any longstanding problems with mobilising and if so, how have these been coped with?
- what problems, if any, does the individual have at present with mobilising, and are any likely to develop?

It will probably be unnecessary to ask all the questions; answers to some of them may be evident from observation of the patient. There may be relevant information in the medical records and some might be revealed when the patient talks about his occupation; the nurse could ask for example, how far the workplace is from the home, and what form of transport is used and so on. Indeed the ALs of working and playing, and mobilising are so closely related that it may be advisable to collect information about them simultaneously. The collected information will then be examined, in collaboration with the patient whenever possible, to discover what the patient can/cannot do independently and to identify any actual problems with the AL of mobilising. There may be potential problems and these too will be discussed with the patient. For each actual and potential problem a realistic and achievable goal will be set, again in discussion with the patient.

The goals may well be to prevent potential problems becoming actual ones; or to alleviate or solve the actual problems; or help the patient to cope with those which cannot be alleviated or solved. The nursing interventions to achieve the goals will take into account the local circumstances and the available resources: they will be written on the nursing plan together with any activities which the patient has agreed to carry out, for example foot exercises to prevent the potential problem of foot drop. A date for evaluation will also be written on the nursing plan to discover whether or not the interventions are achieving or have achieved the stated goals. These activities incorporate the four phases of the process of nursing and they are necessary to carry out *individualised nursing* related to the AL of mobilising.

However before nurses can begin to think in terms of individualised nursing they need to have some idea of the kinds of problems which patients can experience in carrying out the AL of mobilising. They will be discussed under the following four headings:

- change of environment and routine
- change in mobilising habit
- change of dependence/independence status for mobilising
- discomforts associated with mobilising

CHANGE OF ENVIRONMENT AND ROUTINE

Any change of environment is likely to change a person's routine related to the AL of mobilising and this is certainly true of admission to hospital. This will be discussed as change in mobilising routine, and lack of specific knowledge about mobilising routine.

Change in mobilising routine
In order to prepare an individualised plan related to the patient's AL of mobilising it is important to collect information about previous routines at the initial assessment. As mentioned previously, this AL is, for many people, so closely related to working and playing that it may be advisable to seek information about them, either together or in sequence. Knowledge about the previous pattern of the patient's day will help the nurse to help the patient to adjust accordingly. The help, of course, will be different according to whether the patient is mobile, bedfast or chairfast.

Mobile patients. Inevitably there is a degree of restriction in activities, even for mobile patients although some hospitals have amenities which permit them to exercise in the attractive grounds. Nowadays an increasing number of hospitals, particularly those providing long stay treatment for psychiatric and geriatric patients, acknowledge the important part mobilising plays in daily living and make arrangements to ensure that patients continue this AL.

Admission to hospital almost always causes a patient distress and anxiety of some sort. The anxiety may be exacerbated however for the person with a long-standing mobility impairment which has been present perhaps from birth and who may have learned to cope adequately in his home surroundings. Admission to hospital may be for some quite unrelated reason and disrupts his daily mobilising routine. Activities which he managed at home perhaps independently, perhaps with family help in the privacy of his bedroom or bathroom, may become a problem in an unfamiliar setting which does not have his accustomed aids and fixtures. In these circumstances, the nurse must be sensitive to his need for privacy and appreciate that, for example, he may require a longer time for dressing/undressing or for feeding. Help from the nurse may be interpreted as an intrusion and a threat to personal dignity and independence, so it is of paramount importance to assess the patient's capacity for self-help, leaving him to control the situation yet without leaving him to struggle unnecessarily.

Bedfast and chairfast patients. Those patients who are confined to bed are deprived of many of their mobilising routines and may well feel angry and distressed at their predicament. On the other hand they may be so ill that they are glad to regress and hand over control to the nursing staff. They may have difficulty maintaining the sitting position which (unless contra-indicated) is desirable for eating purposes and to facilitate breathing, and is usually preferred by the patient during waking hours.

Bedfast patients may require assistance to maintain the sitting position and there are specific techniques for lifting patients which are effective, cause minimum upset to the patient, and are crucial for the nurse to know and perfect if she is to avoid back injury (Figs 14.18 and 14.19). The same lifting principles are used to help patients out of bed into a chair and vice versa (Figs 14.20 and 14.21) and to help a seated patient into the standing position (Fig. 14.22).

Those patients who are chairfast for most of the day are frequently adapting to change in their mobilising routines. They usually require the help of a nurse to rise from the chair and to walk whatever distance they are capable of walking, supported by another person; and usually the walking exercise is organised to include a visit to the toilet.

Whether in bed or seated in a chair, the patient with reduced capacity for movement must be assisted to feel as independent as possible and it is the nurse's responsibility to ensure that a glass of water, the call-bell, and articles such as spectacles, paper tissues, books and newspapers are within reach; that an immobilised arm or leg is adequately supported by pads and pillows in a desirable position; that the patient is not exposed to chill; that the patient is not left in one position for too long a period (this maxim is just as important when the patient is sitting in a chair). When a conscious patient with reduced capacity for mobility is left in one position for too long a period, he will almost certainly experience discomfort; even if there is loss of sensation in the impaired part, other parts of the body may be strained in maintaining that position.

Lack of specific knowledge about mobilising routine

It is important for the patient to know what he can, and what he should not do in relation to mobilising. Newly admitted but mobile patients may feel insecure about continuing the AL of mobilising unless they are told where it is permissible for them to walk; whether or not there are specific times when they require to be in bed or at the bedside; whether it is customary for patients to leave the ward, for example, to go to the hospital shop, the public telephone booths or for a walk in the grounds.

Patients who are on 'early ambulation' programmes need to understand exactly how much and what type of activity they may carry out each day; and the increasing activity should be clearly described in the patient's nursing plan. It is interesting to note that Lelean (1973) found eight different interpretations among nurses of the phrase 'up and about' written in the nursing kardex.

All patients are exposed to potential problems because of their reduction in mobilising. However they can, whether they are ambulant, chairfast or bedfast help to prevent the potential problems becoming overt, if they are given adequate information, encouragement and supervision.

One important purpose in exercising is to assist return of blood against gravity to the heart by the 'massage' action of active muscle on blood vessels, particularly in the legs. This is further assisted when the increased 'suction' from deep breathing draws blood along the large vessels back to the heart. Both these actions help to prevent stagnation of blood in the leg vessels. With reduction in mobilising there is a danger of stagnant blood clotting (thrombosis). A portion of the clot can become detached (embolus) and flow in the blood until it impacts in a vessel too narrow to permit its passage, usually in the lungs. This condition, called pulmonary embolism, may be fatal and it was to help to prevent this condition that 'early ambulation' was introduced in the 1950s. Patients should therefore be taught to do deep breathing exercises and instructed about moving their feet and toes in a circular direction at regular times throughout waking hours.

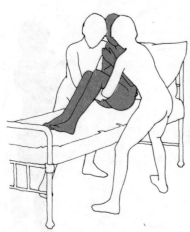

The nurses stand close to the bed.

The patient is asked to cross his arms across his chest and bend his head forward.

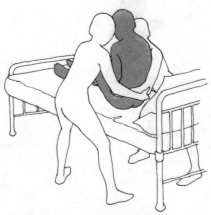

The nurses clasp each other's arms and have their feet wide apart to give the greatest possible support. The weight is then taken by the nurses' thigh muscles and as they lift the patient, they transfer the weight from the leg nearest the foot of the bed to the other leg.

Fig. 14.18 Two nurses lifting a patient in bed: orthodox lift

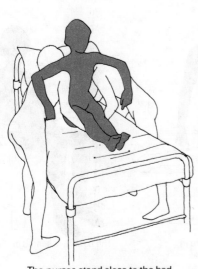

The nurses stand close to the bed with their 'inner' shoulders under the patient's axillae. The patient's weight is taken by the nurses' shoulder muscles and by straightening the flexed hips, the nurses lift the patient.

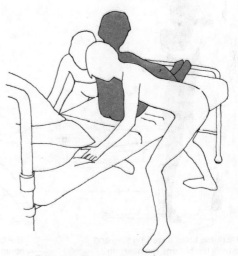

The nurses' outer arms are free either for support on the bed while lifting or to adjust the pillows and bottom sheet. The nurses' feet are wide apart, to give the greatest possible base of support.

Fig. 14.19 Two nurses lifting a patient in bed: Australian lift

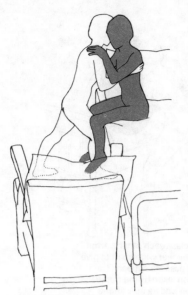

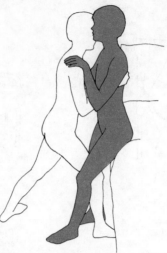

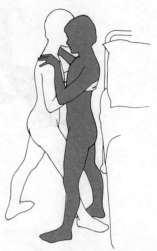

The nurse is standing with her weight over her front foot and keeps close to the patient; her arms are under the patient's arms.

The nurse's weight is transferred to the back foot as she thrusts upwards with her arms.

The patient slides his feet on to the floor, wide apart (the chair has been removed from the diagram to show the position of the feet).

The patient and nurse stand upright, each with their weight central over their own base of support.

The nurse continues upthrust with her arms (the chair has been removed from the diagram to show the position of the feet).

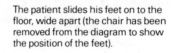

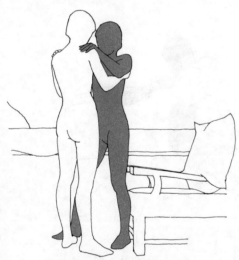

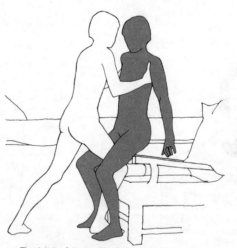

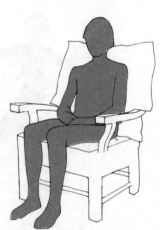

The nurse takes a walking step and swivels the patient, maintaining upthrust with her arms.

The back of the patient's legs are in contact with the chair. The nurse, maintaining a straight back, takes her weight forward and starts to lower the patient by bending her front knee.
The patient bends his knees and stretches the hands backwards to hold the chair.

The patient is seated on the chair.

Fig. 14.20 One nurse helping the patient from the bed to a chair

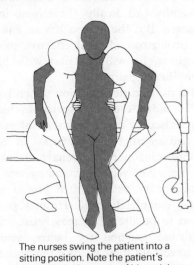

The nurses swing the patient into a sitting position. Note the patient's arms which place most of his weight across the nurses' shoulders and the right nurse's right instep against the patient's right foot.

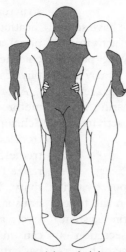

The nurses straighten their legs and transfer the patient on to the edge of the bed.

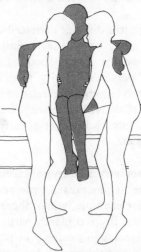

The nurses help the patient to the middle of the bed. Note the position of the nurses' legs.

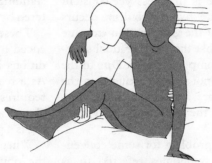

One of the nurses helps the patient to swing his legs into the bed.

Fig. 14.21 Two nurses helping a standing patient into bed

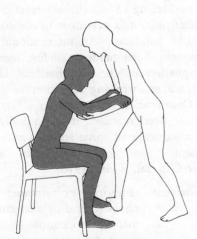

The patient's feet are placed well apart; he is leaning forward and is supported on the nurse's arms. The nurse's knees are bent so that the thighs take the weight. The instep of the nurse's right foot is against the patient's left foot.

Fig. 14.22 One nurse helping a seated patient to stand

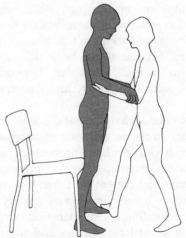

The patient has achieved the standing position by using his anti-gravity muscles and the upthrust of the nurse's support.

Both patient and nurse have their feet wide apart to give the greatest possible base of support and the nurse still has her right foot against the patient's left foot.

CHANGE IN MOBILISING HABIT

Although it is difficult to describe, most people have some idea of what constitutes normal or average activity in relation to the human body. Comment may be passed when a person's activity level changes from busy and bustling to lethargy and relative inactivity. There are gradations of activity/inactivity, but when appearing in an extreme form both over-activity and under-activity are pathological.

Hyperactivity and hypoactivity

A change to generalised hyperactivity and hypoactivity is found, for example, where there are defects in the function of the thyroid gland, part of the endocrine system. Hyperthyroidism occurs when there is oversecretion of the gland and the person has problems because of hyperactivity, breathlessness on exertion, increased pulse rate, and may be palpitations; there is tiredness yet constant restlessness. On the other hand hypothyroidism occurs when there is undersecretion of the gland and in extreme cases the patient's problem is that there is a gradual slowing down to a state of almost complete inertia. Due to the hormone deficiency, energy is not being produced in the body. Usually drugs can be prescribed to achieve hormonal balance and counteract the hyperactivity/hypoactivity.

Muscular hyperactivity is a problem for some congenitally brain-damaged people, sometimes referred to as 'spastics'. The sinuous, writhing, purposeless movements interfere with manual dexterity and if the muscles in the lower limbs are affected, they dictate the strange and unco-ordinated movement of the legs, while walking. Writhing, purposeless movement along with a shuffling gait is characteristic also of Parkinson's disease, currently of particular interest because it can be a side-effect of some antidepressant drugs. Muscular hyperactivity occurs too, though usually transiently, during an epileptic fit (p. 328).

Some psychiatric illnesses have physical manifestations which include change in the normal level of activity. The patient with a neurotic disorder has a problem because of difficulty with emotional adaptation to circumstances. In a florid anxiety state the patient is acutely distressed because he experiences intense feelings of anxiety. One manifestation of the condition is an increased output of energy indicated by general restlessness and sometimes uncontrollable tremors. Some patients reduce the anxiety level by the use of a mechanism called a conversion reaction. The mechanism is always unconscious and it produces physical impairment in a part of the body which would normally be under voluntary control. Motor symptoms include paralysis of the limbs, twitchings, tics and fits and there may also be sensory symptoms including numbness and pain. A description of the symptoms is often a reflection of the person's own idea of anatomical structure and when examined medically, there is no indication of organic disease. But the person has an emotional and a physical problem, and until effective psychiatric treatment is given, he will not part with his physical mobility/immobility impairment.

Another example of a psychiatric condition which has motor manifestations is called catatonic schizophrenia. Schizophrenia is characterised by a withdrawal of interest from everyday affairs and an emotional coldness. In extreme forms of catatonic schizophrenia, behaviour may range from stupor to excessive excitement and hyperactivity. In complete stupor, the patient often lies in an unusual position in bed, completely rigid. He may passively allow his position to be altered or may resist and can maintain the unusual position for hours; some patients are known to have held their heads a few inches above the pillow for many hours or to have remained standing on one leg until their position is physically altered by one of the staff.

These are examples of mobilising problems experienced by patients who have neurotic and psychotic conditions involving physical hyperactivity or hypoactivity. As a result, apart from their emotional imbalance which requires expert psychiatric care, problems arise related to almost all the activities of everyday living, since mobilising is a part of all the ALs.

When considering changes in mobilising habit, some of the obvious examples however are related to physical handicap.

Physical handicap

Before considering an individual's reaction to a change in mobilising habit, it is pertinent to consider the meaning of physical handicap. At international level, several attempts have been made to define handicap, such as the compilation of the International Classification of Diseases, and as a working definition for the International Labour Organisation (ILO). Although no conclusive definition has been reached, it is generally accepted that there is a sequence of three stages which can be termed impairment, functional limitation and disability (Director-General, WHO, 1976):

- impairment: temporary or permanent psychological, physiological or anatomical loss/abnormality; for example, loss of a limb, paralysis following poliomyelitis, mental handicap
- functional limitation: due to impairment, and consists of partial or total inability to perform those activities necessary for normal motor, sensory or mental function; for example, walking, speaking, reading
- disability: difficulty in performing one or more

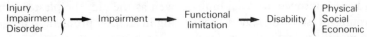

Fig. 14.23 Disability: the sequence of stages

functions that are generally accepted as normal and essential in daily life; for example, self-care, social relationships, earning a living

The sequence is illustrated in Figure 14.23.

This form of definition highlights the nurse's responsibility as one of the health team in relation to prevention or intervention which can diminish the impact of disability. It can be said to operate at three levels:

- first level prevention: action to reduce the occurrence of impairment; for example, immunisation against conditions such as poliomyelitis; health control of workers; provision of a safe environment in the home and at places of employment
- second level prevention: when impairment has occurred, emphasis is placed on prevention of long-term functional limitations and this depends on:

a. speedy diagnosis such as immediate detection of a fracture
b. care in the acute stage such as intelligent first aid, effective care in the intensive care unit, the early use of exercise to assist in the return of muscle function
c. care in the chronic stage such as establishment of a suitable regime in the activities of living for that individual

- third level prevention: the mobilisation of available services — medical, social, vocational, educational — to prevent dependence, or in other words to encourage self-care and economic independence

Useful though this concept of physical handicap is, nurses need further information about how they can help a patient who is experiencing a reaction to the initial change in mobilising routines then how to help those who have to cope with long-term change.

Reaction to initial change. Physical handicap, especially after sudden trauma, is a shattering experience for the patient and the rehabilitation process may take many months. During the initial dramatic change and the attendant personal confusion and disorganisation, the patient is aware only of deprivation. There may be loss of a limb and a sequence of painstaking stages may have to be worked through — grief for loss of the part, shock, denial, depression, aggression, regression — only then can the individual explore the reality of the situation and be helped to identify possibilities for social and emotional reorganisation of his life. It requires time and courage to adapt to a disfigured body image, an altered role image, loss of security, loss of self-esteem and loss of freedom.

Reaction to long-term change. Loss of even part of a limb to a young person can be worrying in terms of career and economic prospects, recreation choice and social acceptance. Much more so is the total limb and trunk paralysis (tetraplegia), a not uncommon result of diving accidents. But it must not be forgotten that impaired mobility is equally disrupting to an elderly person who is slower at re-learning to use injured muscles and slower at adapting to changed circumstances especially when other faculties such as sight and hearing may also be failing.

Even in the protective environment of the hospital, the patient keeps on discovering just how much his mobilising impairment affects his other activities of living. After all, one can do very little without moving some part of the body. But if it is a long-term disability he requires further adaptation to the harsh realities of twentieth century living when he is discharged and coping in the outside world. Sometimes a patient will progress through a rehabilitation unit to ease the transition, but whether or not, a team of health and social service professionals is usually involved in the patient's care and adaptation — doctors, nurses, physiotherapists, occupational therapists, social workers, rehabilitation officers, educationists, employment officers, employers, housing officials — and the chaplain and voluntary agencies may also make an invaluable contribution.

The most important members of the team however are the patient and his family. The patient's motivation to help himself is critical to successful rehabilitation, so it is imperative to include him in the planning process and the decision making about his future mode of living. Rehabilitation implies restoration to the fullest physical, mental and social capability for that individual. The family, too, must be convinced that their efforts are worthwhile and be helped to understand that it is not always in the patient's interests if they continue to do for him things he finds difficult to do for himself. For the nurse and the family, it is important to learn when to give assistance and when to withdraw.

CHANGE OF DEPENDENCE/INDEPENDENCE STATUS FOR MOBILISING

It is important to remember that change of dependence/independence status for mobilising can be in either direction along the continuum. For example after amputation of a lower limb there is dependence for a varying period, but technological advances have improved artificial limbs to such an extent that a young person can regain independence for such intricate mobilising activities as dancing. This is of course an instance of aided independence. There are other people who have become dependent for their mobilising on walking aids to relieve for example weight bearing on painful hips. Hip replacement surgery is now so successful that many such people are able to mobilise independently without aids. But for a variety of reasons these facilities are not available to all the people who have limb defects, so a few of the difficulties which such people encounter will now be discussed, together with some strategies for overcoming the problems.

Upper limb defects. Many actions carried out by the two hands can be performed by one hand. Often the second hand is merely used to hold an object steady. In principle therefore, if some other means can be used for 'steadying', for example securing vegetables on a spiked board, the good hand can be used to carry out the activity of peeling the vegetable. Similarly bread can be steadied ready for buttering; a grater can be fixed to the wall in a suitable position; a hot water bottle can be placed securely in a specially adapted wall fixture and the kettle held in the good hand; clothes can be washed using one hand then wrung out by twisting them round the tap. When eating, a rubber pad under the plate will hold it securely, a plate guard on the plate will prevent food sliding on to the table and a fork with a cutting edge allows manipulation of food by one hand.

It is possible to surmount the problem of upper limb mobility at work too, and also for leisure activities. A paper-weight can secure writing paper and allow handwritten correspondence; a typewriter can be manipulated with one hand; various aids have been devised to facilitate, for example, manual skills at the place of employment and for hobbies such as knitting, sewing and gardening.

Lower limb defects. If the mobilising problem is associated with one of the lower limbs, a walking stick with a rubber tip or a quadrupod (light metal stick with four small feet) can increase the base of support and help to maintain balance. It is crucial that the stick is of the correct length for that person and it is useful to have a loop of elastic attached to the handle so that the person is free to grasp door knobs and open doors himself without dropping the stick.

On stairs there should be rails on both sides to assist ascending and descending and until the patient gains confidence, the helper should always stand below the patient, that is behind him when going up, and in front of him when he is coming down. When ascending, the patient should use his good leg first and when coming down, his affected leg first. Manipulation of stairways may be particularly difficult for an elderly person who has a plaster of Paris bandage on a lower limb. For the young as well as the old, the plaster is heavy and unwieldy resulting in another problem — fatigue.

At home in the kitchen, a re-arrangement of storage space and adjustment of working heights can help to increase the patient's independence, and articles such as long-handled dustpans can make floor cleaning relatively simple. A trolley can be used for transporting articles from one place to another.

Some people have a lower limb incapacity which necessitates use of a wheelchair. In the U.K. a wheelchair can be provided free, under the national health service arrangements, indeed more than one may be supplied if medically recommended: a transit chair to take in a car and another for use in the house. It is almost impossible to get all the desired features in one model and it is important to assess individual needs: width (important in relation to size of doorways, corridors, lifts, public toilets), depth, seat height, position of foot support, angle of back, wheel diameter, type of tyre, weight, fixed or detachable arm rests and so on. When choosing a wheelchair for long-term use it is imperative to see the home surroundings. It will almost certainly be necessary to rearrange furniture and carpets, and it may be necessary to widen doorways or provide ramps, modifications which may qualify for a local authority grant in the U.K.

Problems related to dependence in the AL of eliminating were discussed in Chapter 11, those related to personal cleansing and dressing in Chapter 12, and those related to incapacity because of body paralysis were discussed in Chapter 8. They are all associated with mobilising, yet another instance of the relatedness of the ALs.

Attitudes to dependence

For many people, their concept of 'dependence' in a health context is of physical and/or mental handicap. And in the not too distant past, many such dependent people were segregated from the general public and were cared for in large, old fashioned institutions. Ordinary people therefore did not have opportunity to develop a positive attitude to dependent people. In an attempt to encourage a positive attitude to people with a handicap, the World Health Organization designated 1981 as 'The Year of the Disabled Person'. Many of the year's events were reported by the media, and because disabled people took part in some of the programmes, people were made more aware of the many hobbies and sports in which disabled people can take part. The best organised, but possibly the least well known of these is the 'Paralympics' which includes shooting, bowling, archery, fencing, field and track events, snooker and weightlifting. Ball (1984) gives an account of the 7th World Wheelchair Games which were held at Stoke Mandeville in the U.K., where there is an Olympic village which was built to mark the Year of the Disabled Person. The change of title of the wheelchair games to 'Paralympics' is to put these games on an equal footing with the 'Olympics' and this surely is a measure of the success of the games.

The Year of the Disabled Person also drew ordinary people's attention to the types of work which can be accomplished by disabled people. In the work context, disabled people have fared less well, but some of the opportunities open to them are mentioned in the chapter on working and playing under the headings 'Physical disability' (p. 286), 'Mental handicap' (p. 286), 'Mental illness' (p. 287) and 'Sensory loss/impairment' (p. 287).

Dependent people can be distressed by the public's attitude to their dependence. Some members of the public show their discomfort by using 'distancing' techniques which make the disabled person feel uncomfort-

able from health and social services, from housing agencies, from education and employment departments and from voluntary organisations (Figure 14.24). Indeed in one study Blaxter (1976) found that 59 different organisations were offering help of various kinds related to disability within one city in the U.K. It is obvious that coordination of the services is needed if the disabled person is to have maximum benefit, and the Snowdon Working Party (1976) considered, among other things, that in the U.K., the health visitor was a suitable health care worker to undertake this role.

In an ideal world no one would be dependent, but in the real world there will always be a reservoir of dependent people and perhaps the most helpful way of develop-

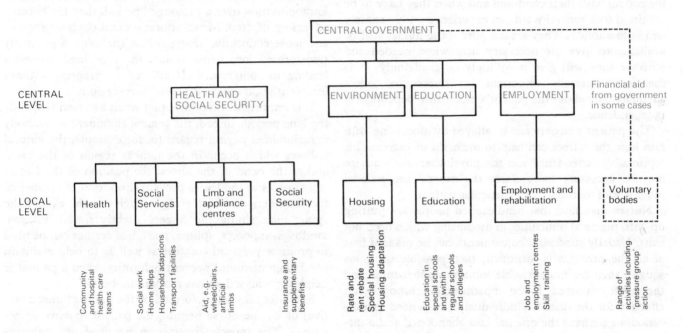

Fig. 14.24 Some services available to handicapped people

able; some may be embarrassingly over-solicitous; yet others manage a mature interaction, conveying that the patient is valued as a person and yet acknowledging, probably by non-verbal communication, the reality that he is dependent.

It is desirable that ordinary people should become more aware of the ways in which handicapped people can be helped to achieve a satisfactory life-style in work, leisure, recreation and family situations. Adequate provision for their needs will overcome their disadvantages to some extent and help them to make a positive contribution to the life of the community in which they live.

The idea still persists that disabled people should be protected from the rigours of everyday living. It is becoming more accepted, however, that instead of a passive role, it is preferable to assist them to face the stress of active participation in the life of the community. To help them to do this, a wide range of facilities must be avail-

ing a positive attitude to dependence is given by Waldron (1983). She wrote a detailed account of co-operation between the multidisciplinary staff at a special school and a comprehensive school so that three dependent children from the special school were integrated into the comprehensive school. Waldron writes 'Sixth-form debates on "The place of the physically handicapped in our community" take on a new dimension when personal experiences can be used.' She ends her article by saying 'The best way to learn is through experience. Perhaps the children now in daily contact with their handicapped peers will grow up with a healthy attitude to handicap.' However here it is necessary to discuss professional attitudes to dependence.

Professional attitudes to dependence. Nurses, like members of any other professional group, have a variety of attitudes to dependence, fashioned by their previous experience and current knowledge. In the acute hospital wards they gain considerable experience with patients who are temporarily dependent for some aspects of the AL of mobilising. However, they must be on their guard against expecting patients to be independent for mobilising before they can comfortably be so. For example, when can a patient after extensive abdominal surgery reasonably be expected to get in and out of bed independently? Nurses need to develop professional judgment of patients' individuality in readiness for regaining independence for this AL. Roper (1982) discusses the reasons for and the meaning of 'early ambulation' which is not a licence for patients to be up and about all day in the early postoperative days.

Dependent people have usually developed mechanisms for coping with their condition and when they have to be admitted to a general ward can experience undue anxiety and vulnerability. They are not sure if the nurses will be available to give the necessary help when needed and whether they will give it willingly or grudgingly. It is therefore especially important for nurses to collect adequate data about the patient's mobilising dependence/independence.

The patient's anxiety can be allayed by discussing with him how the nurses can help to maintain or increase his 'optimal' independence and the physiotherapist's advice may be necessary to reinforce the nurses' professional judgment of 'optimal' for a particular patient.

Nurses may find that handicapped people are putting up with practical difficulties in mobilising which need not exist. Usually successful adjustments can be made if first of all the problem is identified, then possible solutions sought, then the most feasible solution implemented and the result evaluated. If the implemented solution is not effective for the disabled individual, it may need modification, or perhaps the original idea abandoned and a different solution sought.

Thinking through this type of problem requires the same logical thought sequence as is used for the process of nursing. Probably the nurse will not seek to solve this kind of patient's problem alone, however. All members of the health team should combine their knowledge and expertise to provide what is best for the individual patient and help to achieve his optimal level of mobilising.

DISCOMFORTS ASSOCIATED WITH MOBILISING

The body structures associated with mobilising are extensive and it is understandable that patients can experience a wide variety of discomforts related to this AL which involve many of the other ALs. Prolonged bedrest in the home or in hospital, for example, causes reduced activity in all the body systems and can create discomfort related to almost any facet of daily life.

The discomforts mentioned in this section, however, will refer essentially to the musculoskeletal system itself.

Musculoskeletal discomforts
When muscles are inactive, atrophy (wasting) commences and this muscle degeneration in turn depletes the capacity for movement and leads to further impairment and so the cycle continues.

In the bones too, lack of muscle action leads to degenerative changes. A process of decalcification or release of calcium from the bones (osteoporosis) begins and even if halted, it may take months for the bone to return to normal.

Understandably, if joints are left in one position due to immobilisation over a prolonged period, they too become adversely affected. Muscle fibres around the joint shorten and loose connective tissue within the joint is gradually transformed into dense tissue, the combined processes leading to contracture. If allowed to progress without intervention, these processes are irreversible.

It is important, therefore, that when a person is spending long periods in bed, the general alignment of the body is maintained paying regard to, for example, the natural hollows which occur in the lumbar region of the back, and at the bend of the knees; the position of the feet at right angles to the leg to prevent drop foot; the planes of the shoulders and hips at right angles to the axis of the spine; maintaining the fingers slightly flexed. Pillows, sandbags, supports, splints, pads, bed cradles can be used to promote personal comfort as well as to help maintain good alignment and prevent deformity when a patient is helpless/paralysed, or has reduced mobility.

Exercises may be performed by the patient himself (active) or by the nurse helping the patient (passive or assisted). The muscle contraction involved not only increases muscle strength, it improves circulation and the movement preserves muscle tone and helps to prevent contracture (Fig. 14.25).

Therapeutic immobilising procedures
Local discomforts may arise because of certain therapeutic procedures related to the musculoskeletal system. After certain injuries such as those involving a break in the skeletal framework, action may be taken deliberately to immobilise the affected part. There are two main methods of immobilising broken bones in the limbs: the use of plaster of Paris bandages and the use of a technique called traction. The principle behind both methods is the same. The broken fragments are aligned and the limb is immobilised until the bone has an opportunity to heal. Then the immobilising agent is removed. Some of the general problems experienced by the patient due to immobility/reduced mobility of the upper or lower limbs have already been discussed in this chapter (p. 266). The

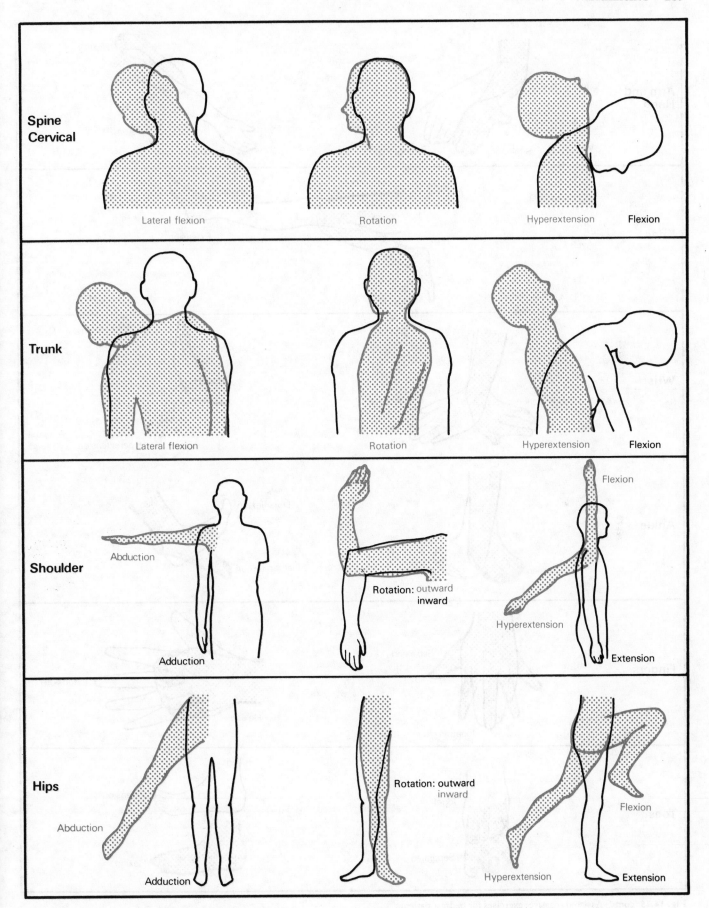

Fig. 14.25 Assisted (passive) exercises for bedfast patients

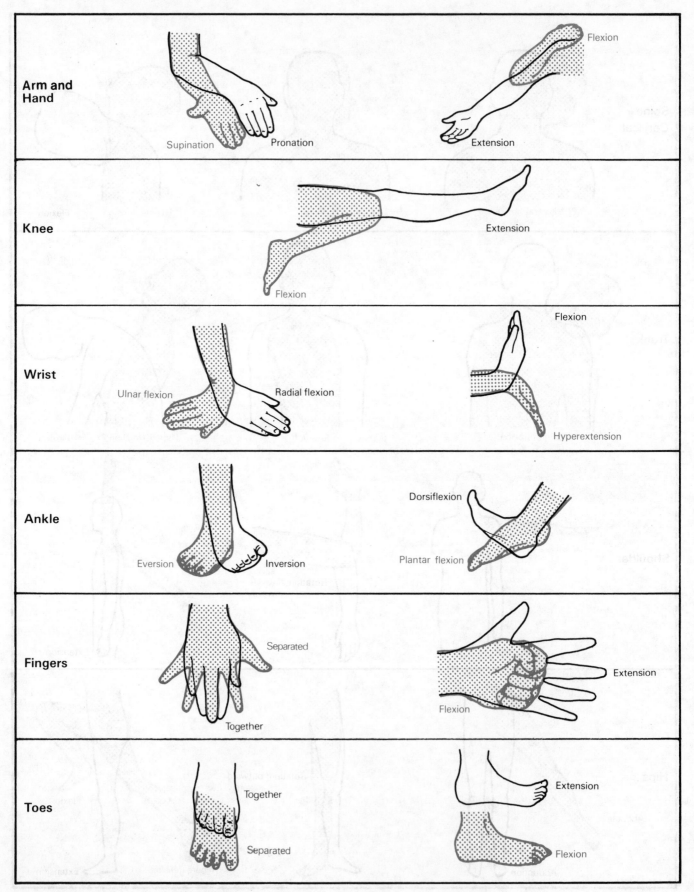

Fig. 14.25 (contd) Assisted (passive) exercises for bedfast patients

immobilising agents themselves, however, may create specific local discomforts.

Discomforts may arise even in the first few hours if a plaster has been applied too tightly. It is most important for the nurse to observe the limb for any sign of discolouration in the relevant fingers/toes as this is indicative of excessive pressure, causing occlusion of the blood vessels to the part. When this occurs, the patient will comment on excessive discomfort, pain and loss of sensation. If the pressure caused by the tight plaster is not relieved, the limb would become gangrenous, so the plaster may have to be removed and re-applied.

The plaster cast itself causes discomfort. Even after it dries it is still heavy and unwieldy, and older people or those who are already physically handicapped often find its weight very fatiguing. Everything possible should be done, therefore, to assist the person to retain his independence in everyday living activities without allowing him to become excessively exhausted.

Even when the plaster is removed, the patient may have problems. In relation to the lower limb, there is often initial discomfort in rising and exercising the joints and muscles which have been relatively immobile during the time when the plaster was in position. In addition the affected limb may look discoloured and it may be covered with scales of dead skin. These discomforts are usually rectified within a few days, however, as the limb is exercised and the circulation is improved. The scales of skin, too, gradually become detached if gently bathed. They should not be removed forcibly and sometimes an emollient is helpful.

The technique called skeletal traction involves passing a specially-designed, sterile pin through a fragment of the bone distal to the fracture, and maintaining the bone's position once it has been aligned, by a system of pulleys and weights attached to a special bed-frame. Countertraction (a force in the opposite direction) is necessary and is provided, in the case of a lower limb, by elevating the foot of the bed.

The same effect is achieved by applying adhesive tape to the skin in the area of the fracture (skin traction) and attaching the adhesive bandaging to a similar system of pulleys and weights. In both instances, there may be discomfort due to irritation of the skin and in the former, the small wounds where the pin protrudes may cause discomfort unless carefully tended.

After an initial period of awkwardness in manipulation, people who have a plaster of Paris bandage applied to a limb are usually ambulant and can carry out the AL of mobilising without too much discomfort; when the traction methods are used, however, bedrest is needed, with all the attendant discomforts of restriction on freedom and independence. The patient in traction usually has to remain in the supine position, and ingenuity is needed to help the patient to be as comfortable as possible, to make activities such as eating, drinking and eliminating as easy as possible, to prevent the formation of pressure sores and to reduce boredom and frustration. Another problem which requires thought is the positioning of bedclothes such that the traction ropes are unimpeded yet the patient is protected from draughts and loss of modesty. Small blankets can be strategically placed to provide warmth and adequate cover and the patient will usually wish to wear bedsocks. Especially for the older patient on traction, it is important to be on the alert for indications of hypostatic pneumonia and encouragement of regular, deep breathing exercises will help to prevent this distressing complication.

Pain

Because the prime purpose of the musculoskeletal system is to produce movement, it is not unnatural to expect that many of the dysfunctions produce pain on movement. And different kinds of pain can be experienced in relation to mobilising.

Sudden severe pain. The pain experienced by a person when a limb is fractured is certainly sudden and usually severe. It results from muscle spasm and tissue damage; it produces deformity and shortening of the limb, impaired mobility and loss of function. The immobility continues until the person can have specialist treatment usually in hospital, to align the bone ends and immobilise the limb. The person needs an analgesic but as in all probability he will require an anaesthetic to undertake the bone alignment, the drug is not given orally but by injection. It is important that a written note of the drug, dose, time and route is sent with the person to the hospital.

Chronic pain. Many people experience chronic pain associated with the musculoskeletal system variously referred to as muscular rheumatism (fibrositis), low-back pain (lumbago) and joint pain (arthritis). These dysfunctions are responsible for much temporary and permanent disablement and are the cause of much absenteeism from work.

As pain is the main reason for seeking medical aid, much of the treatment is aimed at relieving this distressing symptom. The measures used involve, for example, rest of the involved joints, physiotherapy, use of anti-inflammatory drugs, analgesics and corticosteroids, surgery to restructure affected joints with prostheses and rehabilitation programmes to restore maximum function.

District nurses, particularly those 'attached' to a family doctor's surgery, can help these patients by assessing whether or not they protect themselves from chill, take reasonable exercise outdoors according to their disability, get the best advantage from their drug regime and so on. As excessive weight usually exacerbates the pain, those who are overweight can be encouraged to reduce their kilojoule intake.

Some patients obtain relief by the application of dry or moist heat to the painful area and they can be taught to do this safely. Others find the application of liniment useful.

Sharp shooting pain. When there is injury to an intervertebral disc, the person usually finds that a particular movement causes a sharp shooting pain which is experienced along the pathway of the sciatic nerve: through the buttock and down the back of the leg. Since it is a mechanically induced pain — a tiny fragment of the disc pressing against the nerve — control by oral analgesics is necessary until the fragment shrinks. The patient may or may not be on bedrest, but most people with an acute attack of sciatica find rest in bed helpful.

The nurse should discover whether or not these patients do heavy lifting at work or at home and what knowledge they have about safe lifting methods. Again overweight is not advisable for people with a disc lesion and the nurse can advise accordingly.

Deep boring pain. Pain in bone is often described as excruciating. Since bone is a relatively dense structure it has little space to accommodate the swelling caused by inflammation or the extra tissue from a new growth like a cancer. The nurse can help by careful positioning and supporting of the part relative to the rest of the body and by giving analgesics, anti-inflammatory and any other prescribed drugs promptly and safely.

Phantom pain. A discomfort which is particularly dis-turbing to the patient who has had an amputation is 'phantom limb pain' (p. 40); he has the sensation of pain in the amputated part of the limb. The mechanism of this type of 'referred' pain is not clearly understood but it is probably related to his previously established body image. Pain is a subjective experience and as such it is a psychological event, not a physical one. The concept of pain must involve location in the body for the experience, even when there is not a physical cause. So phantom limb pain is peculiarly distressing to the patient, because he can see that, physically, the amputated part is no longer there. Usually the experience is transient but while it lasts, the person requires special care and attention from the nurse, to help him with this manifestation of pain which is very real to him.

Social and emotional discomforts

When there is interference with mobilising there is emotional discomfort and upset because of loss of freedom, loss of independence and loss of personal dignity. In addition there is anxiety about the state of immobility and its cause. There may also be a change in social role related to family, and to work and leisure activities which can be destructive to the individual's self-image. Together these assaults on personal identity may manifest themselves as aggressive behaviour or as apathy, or frustration or regression.

The nurse must therefore learn to listen to the patient

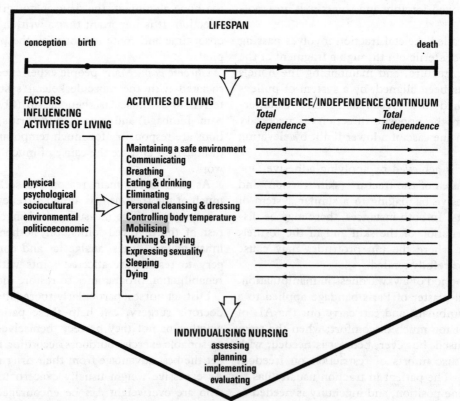

Fig. 14.26 The AL of mobilising within the model for nursing

and help him to work through these stages so that he can restore his image of his personal worth and dignity. In these circumstances, it is necessary to support the relatives by, among other things, allowing them to express their feelings in response to behaviour of this type. Aggression or apathy may be quite atypical of the person's usual behaviour and can cause extreme discomfort, distress and bewilderment to the family.

Related to the AL of mobilising, a variety of problems and discomforts which patients can experience have been discussed. This background information will provide nurses with a generalised idea of these; it will be useful in assessing, planning, implementing and evaluating an individualised plan for each patient's AL of mobilising.

This chapter has been concerned with the AL of mobilising. However, as stated previously it is only for the purpose of discussion that any AL can be considered on its own; in reality the various activities are so closely related and do not have distinct boundaries. Figure 14.26 is a reminder that the AL of mobilising is related to the other ALs and also to the various components of the model for nursing.

REFERENCES

Ball D 1984 News Focus: Paralympics. Nursing Times 80 (34) August 22: 16–18

Blaxter M 1976 The meaning of disability. Heinemann, London

Director-General WHO 1976 Disability, prevention and rehabilitation. WHO Chronicle 30(8) 324–328

Evans D 1981 Lean back and exercise. Nursing Mirror 152 (24) June 10: 16–19

Harris AI, Cox E, Smith RW 1971 Handicapped and impaired in Great Britain Part 1. HMSO, London

Lelean SR Ready for report nurse? Royal College of Nursing, London, p 61

Rogers P 1983 Sharing the load. Nursing Mirror 156 (26) June 29: 28–29

Roper N 1982 Principles of nursing, 3rd edn. Churchill Livingstone, Edinburgh, p 170

Waldron S 1983 Integration of handicapped pupils. Nursing Times 79 (15) April 13: 54–56

ADDITIONAL READING

Dardier EL 1981 The early stroke patient. Positioning and movement. Bailliere Tindall, London

Downie PA, Kennedy P 1981 Lifting, handling and helping patients. Faber, London

Mansell CA 1981 Partage — not just another course. Nursing Times 77 (42) October 14: 40:43

Nursing Times 1982 The seven ages of disability. Nursing Times Supplement August 4

Royal College of Nursing 1979 Avoiding low back injury among nurses. Royal College of Nursing, London

Scholey M 1982 The shoulder lift. Nursing Times 78 (12) March 24: 506–507

Stubbs DA, Rivers PM, Hudson MP, Worringham CJ 1981 Back pain research. Nursing Times 77 (20) May 14: 857–858

Tarking C 1981 A choice of hoists. Health and Social Service Journal May 15: 577, 579–580

Vasey J, Crozier L 1982 A neuromuscular approach.
   1. A move in the right direction. Nursing Mirror 154 (17) April 28: 42–47
   2. Get into condition. Nursing Mirror 154 (18) May 5: 22–28
   3. At ease. Nursing Mirror 154 (19) May 12: 28–31
   4. Handle with care. Nursing Mirror 154 (20) May 19: 30–32
   5. Easy on the base. Nursing Mirror 154 (21) May 26: 36–42
   6. Safety first. Nursing Mirror 154 (22) June 2: 44–48

Wright B 1981 Lifting and moving patients. 1. An investigation and commentary. Nursing Times 77 (46) November 11: 1962–1965.
   2. Training and management. Nursing Times 77 (47) November 18: 2025–2028

15

Working and playing

The activities of working and playing

What do people do during the hours of the day when they are not sleeping? Broadly speaking, people spend the major portion of their day 'working' and what free time they have left over is available for 'playing'. Work and play are complementary to each other, and both are fundamental aspects of living. As the following discussion shows, the activities of working and playing have many dimensions and, according to the different stages of the lifespan, their nature and purpose are open to various interpretations.

THE NATURE OF WORKING AND PLAYING

Working is the word most commonly used to describe an individual's main daily activity and tends to be thought of first in terms of gainful employment. People work to earn an income in order to provide for the necessities of living, for themselves and their dependants. Because work is necessary, it is often thought of in a rather negative way. However, it is worth remembering that a job not only provides an income: it is also an important part of a person's identity and it provides a sense of purpose and accomplishment, a structure to each day and the year, a source of company and a certain status in the family and in society. In these times of high unemployment, it is vital to recognise that many people are being deprived of these benefits as well as being denied the right to earn their living. Nevertheless, they — like others, such as schoolchildren, students, mothers at home, housewives, voluntary workers and retired people — would still describe much of their daily activity as 'work'. So, although discussion of the nature of the activity of 'working' inevitably focuses on gainful employment, the broader interpretation of the term should not be forgotten.

Playing is the term being used to describe what a person does in 'non-work' time. It is a convenient term because it emphasises that, by nature, 'playing' is the opposite of 'working' and it is an all-inclusive term which covers many other words such as leisure, relaxation, recreation, hobby, exercise, sport and holiday. In recent years as unemployment has grown, retirement has come at an earlier age and working hours have become shorter, so there has been increased interest in the use of leisure. Enjoyment and occupation are prime objectives in all forms of playing. However, for children, playing is also essentially a means of learning and development: this is also true of many non-work activities which adults pursue. For some people, play becomes work: for example, there are sportsmen and women who earn their income as 'professionals'. Indeed, there are many examples of activities which can be one man's work and another man's play, illustrating that work and play are relative terms.

THE PURPOSE OF WORKING AND PLAYING

The purpose of these activities is hardly separable from their essential nature. Since its main purpose is to earn an income, there is an element of compulsion about *working*. However, as has already been pointed out, not all work is paid and, even if it is, it fulfils a variety of other purposes and so the remuneration is not the only consideration when choosing a job or career. For example, nursing is frequently chosen by those who describe their main purpose as finding a job which allows them 'to work with people'. Others pursue their jobs with the purpose of finding an opportunity to use their hands or their intellect or particular qualifications; to be able to go to sea or to travel; or to become famous. People who choose to do voluntary work see their purpose as giving service to the community. Women who choose to stay at home to look after children would describe their purpose in terms of their children's well-being. Whatever the job, be it paid or unpaid, prevention of boredom and meaningful use of time are basic purposes of working.

Playing, the main occupation in childhood, has the purpose of enabling learning and development to take place. Through play the child learns about the surrounding physical and social environment and acquires many of the physical, psychological and social skills which are necessary to cope with independent, adult life. Adults pursue different types of leisure activities with different purposes — outdoor activities to get fresh air; sporting activities for exercise, slimming or competition; group activities for company; reading, theatre or musical activities for relaxation and enlightenment. Whatever the choice, enjoyment and prevention of boredom are the basic purposes of playing.

LIFESPAN: EFFECTS ON WORKING AND PLAYING

The inclusion of the lifespan in the model serves as a reminder that the way an individual carries out any Activity of Living varies throughout the stages of life. This is certainly true of the AL of working and playing and there is a change in the balance between the two activities at different stages of the lifespan.

In infancy and early childhood it is the activity of playing which assumes priority. The importance of purposeful playing in the development of physical, intellectual, interpersonal and social skills is undisputed. Play begins spontaneously and there is general agreement that its satisfactory development depends on continuing adult encouragement and the provision of suitable toys and play equipment. Four provisions are of primary importance — playthings, playspace, playtime and play fellows. There are many different types of play — ranging from the exploratory finger play of the young infant to imitative play, constructive play, make-believe play, games with rules, and hobbies. These different types of play emerge in sequence as the child first learns to use the senses and body movement and then, later, the ability to communicate, interact with others and use creativity and imagination (Sheridan, 1977).

Recognition of the importance of playing in early life has resulted in widespread provision of playgroups and nurseries for children of pre-school age. In primary school, there is little distinction nowadays between working and playing, for much of what is traditionally described as school 'work' is accomplished nowadays through 'play' activities. However, most people's perception of secondary school would include a clearer differentiation between 'working' and 'playing' activities. In the past, the emphasis was very much on preparation for work and acquiring qualifications for employment. However, in the context of high unemployment and with an increasing awareness of the need for preparation for all aspects of adult life, school education has taken on a broader perspective.

Nevertheless, the choice of, and establishment in, an occupation must be regarded as a central task of young adulthood. As Barnard (1981) points out:

The process of choosing a career and the period of adaptation to work or vocational training can be stressful. For many young people the transition from school to work is extremely uncomfortable. Their general education, at home and at school, may have been inadequate to prepare them for the world of work.

In both the activities of working and playing, peak performance is usually reached in the years of adulthood. However, whereas young athletes may be past their peak by their 30s, at the other extreme there are people, such as judges and politicians, who do not reach their peak until an age when many people are retiring from their work. The effects of the process of ageing on working and playing vary greatly according to the nature of the work and play, and the person's health and psychological outlook. Hammond (1981) highlights some of the different effects in relation to unskilled, semi-skilled, skilled and professional workers.

With retirement from work, which comes around the time of entry into the 'old age' stage of the lifespan (p. 51), there is more time for activities which fall into the category of 'playing'. Society now recognises the importance of providing suitable and varied leisure activities for older people so that mental and physical health is maintained. *Preparation for a healthy retirement* is now regarded as extremely important in view of the increased life expectancy. Ferguson (1984) emphasises the need for people to be educated about measures which can be taken to maintain health and prevent illness in retirement. Psychological readiness for retirement is also important and, increasingly, employers see it as a responsibility to provide pre-retirement courses so that people can prepare themselves to cope with the changes involved.

Garrett (1983) observes that withdrawal from gainful employment is a relatively new phenomenon. Although there is now an almost universal acceptance of the principle of retirement, in pre-industrial society the worker was expected to continue at his job just as long as he remained physically able. Garrett says that for working class men, retirement is often associated with four 'losses' — the loss of social status and role; of companionship; of income; and of a meaningful lifestyle. Seen this way, it is not surprising that retirement is viewed as a negative event.

As Homewood (1981) points out, though, all 'work' is not necessarily linked to paid employment and she argues that the many non-financial benefits of work could be obtained in other ways in the post-retirement period. She asks, 'Can individuals be helped to disengage from work and re-engage in other rewarding activities?'

So, it can be seen that the AL of working and playing undergoes considerable change as a person progresses through the stages of the lifespan. For most people, the lifespan is punctuated by significant work-related events — starting school, leaving school, starting work, changing jobs, gaining promotion and, ultimately, retiring. Though 'working' predominates in the adult years and 'playing' in the early years, both activities are an integral and important aspect at every stage of the lifespan.

FACTORS INFLUENCING WORKING AND PLAYING

The nature of the AL of working and playing is multifaceted and, as just described, there is variation in both of these activities in the course of the human lifespan. However, there is great variation in working and playing even among individuals of similar age because many factors can influence this AL. In keeping with the relevant component of the model, this section is subdivided into physical, psychological, sociocultural, environmental and politicoeconomic factors. The last of these is discussed in some detail in view of its importance to the subject of this chapter.

Physical factors
In infancy and childhood, the development of increasingly complex and varied play is closely related to physical growth and the maturation of the neuromuscular system.

Physique enters into the suitability of a person for some occupations, examples being a minimum height for policemen and a maximum weight for jockeys. Some jobs — such as those in heavy industry, those which are concerned with sport and others like nursing — require considerable physical fitness and energy. Others, most notably sedentary jobs such as working in a bank, do not require this. People who work in the physically demanding occupations may experience considerable tiredness towards the end of their working lives, when physical fitness and energy decline in the process of ageing.

The capacity for both working and playing, at any stage of the lifespan, is obviously influenced by a person's state of physical health. Obesity, heart disease, respiratory problems, musculoskeletal disorders and certain specific conditions, such as diabetes mellitus, may dictate that certain types of work and play are impossible or undesirable or necessary to regulate within certain limits.

Any physical disability or impairment of the senses are important factors which influence this AL. A physically disabled person may need to be retrained for work within his physical capacity. Similarly the blind and the deaf need to choose work which is compatible with their disability. What disabled people choose to do in non-work time is influenced by what special facilities are available to them. In recent years the scope of playing activities for the physically and visually disabled have increased, though deaf people have fared less well and many are frustrated by inadequate leisure time activities.

Psychological factors
As described in the section on the lifespan, both purposeful playing in childhood and productive work in adulthood contribute to an individual's intellectual and emotional development and, indeed, to the development

of their total personality. There are many different kinds of psychological factors which can influence a person's working and playing habits and preferences.

A person's level of intelligence is usually one factor in the type of occupation which he can satisfactorily follow, as are temperament and personality traits. These traits range from patience to impatience, from gregariousness to being a loner. No one is patient all the time but an impatient person is unlikely to enjoy working at intricate tasks or with ill people. Similarly a gregarious person usually enjoys being alone sometimes and a loner sometimes seeks the company of others, but a loner is unlikely to enjoy working with a lot of people in the same room or constantly meeting new people as in nursing. It is hoped that career counselling will help people choose occupations suited to their particular attributes. Some occupations devise and use entrance tests in an attempt to reduce misplacement.

Level of intelligence, temperament and personality traits also play an important part in choosing leisure time activities. There is now a wide range of activities available, catering for most skills and tastes. If the desired ones are not available in the locality in which a person lives, he can usually travel to a nearby centre at weekends and in holiday periods.

Those people who have not learned to be punctual, reliable and honest and who have little appreciation of a team concept will from the beginning have difficulties at work. Personnel officers are usually alert to these problems and try to help. Lateness, uncertificated absence, lessened concentration and deterioration in personal relationships in a person with a previously good work record can be due to a number of factors such as a family crisis, alcoholism, drug taking and incipient disease. The occupational health nurse is aware of these possibilities, and if the help which she can offer proves inadequate she can encourage such a person to visit his own doctor.

Lack of development in self-discipline can result in difficulties at work. Workers may fail to take adequate precautions in hazardous occupations, for instance miners not wearing safety helmets and nurses not using well-defined lifting skills and not taking adequate preventive measures in relation to infection.

So far, discussion of psychological factors has concentrated on people in work, but the absence of work has equally important psychological considerations. Redundancy (even the fear of it) and unemployment can have severe consequences for the individual and his family. Not only is there the loss of financial independence, but also the loss of self-esteem and self-confidence. The person is denied the opportunity to use his skills and to develop new ones; and there is too the loss of social contacts. These losses can lead to feelings of frustration and anger, or to depression and a feeling of worthlessness, even to the point of contemplating suicide. Although a

different situation, for similar reasons, retirement from work may also cause these kinds of reactions. Coming to terms with the absence of work requires considerable psychological adjustment and, in turn, a new attitude towards playing.

Sociocultural factors

In earlier, simpler times both working and playing were centred round small, self-sufficient communities of families. For all members there was no differentiation between those people comprising the work, play and family groups. As society grew more complex, communities began to exchange different commodities and goods by the bartering method. Later money was used as the mode of exchange. The realisation that the commodities produced by one community were 'desired' by another created supply and demand which encouraged more organised trading systems resulting in intercommunity dependence.

These changes had significant effects on the activity of working. It became necessary to leave the community to pursue one's work, thus the work group was differentiated from the family and play groups. The long process of industrialisation brought the gradual changeover from handmade to mass-produced goods, and from intercommunity to international trading systems, resulting in even further differentiation of the play, work and family groups, the basic groups from which a person obtains support and recognition. In most cultures the sex of an individual affects his choice of work. There are preconceived ideas about the kind of work which only men and only women can do, not just as an occupation but also in the home. However, these attitudes are changing rapidly in many countries, and in the U.S.A. and the U.K., it is illegal for advertisements to state the sex of the person required for the work. Also the current trend for both wife and husband to follow their occupations and the gradual acceptance of an equalisation of the parental role is changing the expectations of a man's 'work' in the home.

Similarly in many cultures there are games which are usually played by boys and others which are usually played by girls. However, it is likely that the currently changing attitudes toward adult work will have their effect on the games children (as opposed to boys and girls) will play in the future. Play is often an imitation of adult life and as the distinctions break down for adults so will they for children.

Religious factors can influence work and play; beliefs may preclude some activities in both. There are religions which do not permit drinking or gambling and adherents would not choose to work in industries associated with them. Followers of some religions do not countenance abortion and would not therefore work in any areas connected with it. Some communities will not permit local factories to function on a Sunday. There are still some religious sects which forbid their members to dance, to visit cinemas and theatres, to listen to radio, to watch television and to read any book other than the Bible on Sundays.

The nature of the work contributed by each person is used by many governments to define social class. An example of this, as used in the U.K., is given in Table 15.1.

Table 15.1 Social class by occupation

Social class	
I	Professional occupations
II	Intermediate occupations
III (N)	Skilled occupations: non-manual
III (M)	Skilled occupations: manual
IV	Partly skilled occupations
V	Unskilled occupations

Source: Registrar General's classification

Environmental factors

An infinite variety of climatic and environmental factors affect working; there are conditions which employers have to provide and ones which they are advised to provide for both indoor and outdoor workers. Examples are protective clothing for dirty work; pads for kneeling; gloves for handling hot objects; goggles to prevent not only strain from glare but also injury from sparks, hot metals and corrosive liquids; filters and masks in dusty industries and for prevention of spread of infection.

Excessive heat, climatic or environmental, increases sweating; salted fruit drinks may be needed to maintain the body's fluid balance. Although all workers are entitled to a morning and an afternoon break, a more frequent rest period helps to offset excessive fatigue and stress due to heat, both of which can increase the risk of an accident. Wherever it is important for workers to be easily visible, for example on highways, they are provided with a fluorescent garment.

Outdoor weather conditions can from time to time adversely affect indoor working conditions. For example large expanses of windows can cause excessive cold in winter and excessive heat in summer as well as glare from the sun, resulting in a slower pace of working and frayed tempers. Icy roads increase risk of accident and injury for many, in particular transport drivers.

Leisure time activities necessarily reflect a region's climate and environment, sailing and hill walking being examples. Swimming is associated with hot weather and the sea, but technology has resulted in swimming facilities being available in all weather conditions even thousands of miles from the sea. Similarly ski-ing was once dependent on the availability of snow-covered slopes but there are now artificial ski slopes in many large cities.

The importance of maintaining a safe environment for the activities of working and playing is discussed in some detail in Chapter 7, particularly in the section on 'preventing accidents at work' (p. 86) and 'preventing accidents at play' (p. 86).

Politicoeconomic factors

This section concentrates almost entirely on the 'working' aspect of this AL, with only a comparatively brief discussion of 'playing' at the end.

Work is the means by which an individual earns an income and the level of that income is a very important factor which influences many aspects of living. A person's social class is determined by the nature of his occupation (Table 15.1, opposite) and this, in turn, determines his economic status.

On a larger scale, work is the basis of a nation's wealth. The process of industrialisation, described in an earlier section (p. 277), was essentially a means of increasing wealth and the highly complex national and international economic systems which exist today are a result of industrialisation. Industrialisation may have brought about economic improvement but it also created poor working conditions, and created numerous social problems. Low wages and long hours at work meant that for the majority of the population, now dependent on a monetary income, life was 'work dominated'. Gradually, health and social systems were developed in most industrialised countries to combat these social ills and employment legislation was introduced to establish protective measures, such as:

- the minimum age at which a person can be gainfully employed
- the maximum number of hours to be worked per week
- alternative remuneration during unemployment or absence from work due to illness, injury or maternity leave
- the number of weeks of paid holiday
- the age at which there can be retirement from work on a pension

In any national economy which provides employment, health and social services, the relative numbers of the following population groups are of critical importance: children, workers, unemployed, workers absent because of illness/pregnancy and pensioners.

For work a person receives official remuneration in the form of a wage or salary, exceptions being voluntary work and the occupation of housewife/mother. In the U.K., national insurance paid by the workers, and income tax paid by those with an income above a stipulated amount contribute to the total national income, part of which is used to finance the National Health Service, unemployment and sickness benefit, and the old age pension. There is great disparity, some would say inequity, in the level of income accorded to different occupations. The way in which income is determined is largely historical and any changes in pay structure, and pay increases, are introduced by agreement of the employers, government and trade unions.

Contrary to the impression which may be created by the media, trade unions are not only interested in pay negotiations but, in various ways, act to safeguard the rights of employees. From a health and safety point of view unions are particularly interested in:

- identification of health hazards
- provision of a safe work environment
- provision of education for workers in an attempt to prevent accident and minimise risk
- surveillance of the workers' health
- collection of data to monitor the effect of health on work and vice versa

In the U.K., the Health and Safety at Work Act (1974) is an important piece of legislation which aims to secure the health and safety of workers. Some mention of this Act was made in Chapter 7 (p. 86) and its application to the National Health Service is discussed by Holgate (1980), with particular reference to nursing.

In many countries there is an occupational health service and this also plays a vital part in the promotion of health and safety at work. Nurses as well as doctors are employed in this service and the nurse's contribution to the health of the worker is the subject of ongoing study by the Permanent Commission and International Association on Occupational Health (Rcn, 1983). The nurses' role is essentially preventive and educational, though they deal with any accidents which occur and with certain treatment regimes; and they are also concerned with rehabilitation and resettlement at work after an extended absence due to injury or illness.

Resettlement of physically disabled people in work is a subject discussed in more detail later in this chapter (p. 286) but it is appropriate here to mention the role of government in relation to this matter. There is a wide range of facilities provided to help the disabled to find and keep suitable work and, in the U.K., these are mainly provided under the Disabled Persons Employment Acts of 1944 and 1958. Hall (1979) relates how employment matters in this country have passed in turn from the Ministry of Labour to the Department of Employment and, since 1974, have rested with the independent Manpower Services Commission; and she outlines the Commission's services for the disabled in particular. From the individual's point of view, the disablement resettlement officer is a key figure in the complex system and he works closely with members of the health care professions. Another aspect of the Acts is the provision of a quota scheme whereby firms of a certain size (20 or more employees) are required to employ a percentage (presently 3%) of disabled people. In 1977, the MSC launched a campaign to encourage the integration of disabled people into the workforce and, in particular, to educate the employers. As Swaffield (1980), who describes this campaign and many aspects of the employment of the disabled, says: the message to employers was 'that disabled people are worthwhile employees and need not be taken on as an act of charity'. Six guidelines on employing disabled people were formulated:

- consideration of disabled people for all vacancies
- retention of newly disabled employees
- equality of opportunity at work for disabled people
- modification of equipment or jobs if needed
- adaptation of premises where needed
- co-operation with the disablement resettlement officer.

Employers can apply for financial help, for example grants for adaptations to the workplace, and an award scheme was launched for 'good' employers.

Help with deployment and re-employment is, of course, available too to the nonhandicapped and in many countries advice on employment is offered by guidance units sponsored by the government. Technological advances may mean that some workers in future will need to be trained for a second and possibly a third type of employment in a lifetime. High unemployment in certain occupations, and mid-career redundancy, are other reasons why more people nowadays may need to retrain in the course of their working lives. New attitudes towards working are becoming essential in these times. The age of retirement is becoming earlier; the working week is shorter; more women are working outside the home than before; part-time work is becoming increasingly common; and the concept of job-sharing is gaining ground. Part-time work and job-sharing are ways of spreading the increasingly limited work available more equitably. Tierney (1983) argues that nursing is one profession which appears to have tremendous potential for the widescale introduction of job-sharing, especially in the more senior grades where part-time work is practically non-existent. A substantial proportion of practising nurses work part-time, a fact not surprising because the majority are married women. Tierney draws attention to reactions which indicate that the growth of part-time employment in nursing has been viewed as undesirable, but she argues that it could be viewed as a desirable trend and writes:

One of the major problems of our society today is unemployment. Some 3¼ million people in the U.K. are now unemployed. Facing up to this fact demands a widespread change in personal values and institutional attitudes towards the nature of employment. The strategy of sharing work more equitably is a social necessity. We are faced with the stark choice between a society in which a minority of the population work full-time and are highly paid (and highly taxed in order to support the rest) or a society in which work and its rewards are more equitably shared.

Although this was written in the context of nursing, the statement is generally applicable. There is absolutely no doubt that high unemployment is the greatest single politicoeconomic issue of our time. In the U.K. the number of unemployed people represents over 13% of the population of working age, and many other Western countries have equally high levels of unemployment. The way in which governments attempt to deal with the problem, and the way societies react to it and cope with it, will determine the nature of the activity of working for future generations.

High unemployment and, for others, reduced working hours and longer retirement, means too that people increasingly have more time for the activity which complements working — playing.

All schools encourage physical education and the foundation for enjoying leisure-time activities in adult life is also laid in various school classes, such as needlework, woodwork and music. Social reforms have resulted in provision by local government for community recreation. This includes adventure playgrounds for children and a range of sports and arts facilities to cater for people of all ages.

Although in relative terms more people nowadays have more time for leisure and more money, many recreational pursuits are expensive and this can be a problem for the lowest paid workers, parents with several children, single-parent families, students, the unemployed and pensioners. This fact is recognised for these groups who are often offered reduced rates for travelling, theatres and cinemas.

There is no doubt that, with less work, there will be greater emphasis on play. Education for leisure and the provision of adequate recreation facilities will therefore assume even greater political importance in the future since a bored society can so easily become a troubled society.

DEPENDENCE/INDEPENDENCE IN WORKING AND PLAYING

The inclusion of the dependence/independence continuum in the model draws attention to the fact that there are periods in life when 'dependence' is to be expected and, at other times, 'independence' is the expectation. From what has been written thus far about working and playing, it is clear that the principle applies to this AL. Children are dependent on adults for the development of skills in playing and the provision of playthings and, at a later stage, they are dependent on the education system

for the acquisition of skills to equip them for working.

The so-called 'independence' of adulthood is largely due to the adult's ability to be financially independent, a state which is possible through income from working. By definition, a 'dependant' is a person who is not financially self-sufficient: a child is dependent on parents and an unemployed person on state aid. Independence in playing allows the adult to make choices about leisure activities, including the choice to give up previously compulsory sport and thus to jeopardise health through lack of exercise!

To a great extent, independent control of working and playing activities continues throughout the rest of the lifespan. Whereas some people would say that there is a loss of independence on retirement from work, others might argue that independence is actually increased. However, frailty and ill-health in old age may cause some loss of independence and necessitate dependence on others or on aids.

There are a number of reasons why people, at any stage of the lifespan, might be unable to achieve or maintain independence in the activities of working and playing. The main reasons — physical disability, mental handicap, mental illness and sensory loss/impairment — are discussed later in this chapter.

INDIVIDUALITY IN WORKING AND PLAYING

The model of living places great emphasis on the idea of *individuality*. A person's individuality in the AL of working and playing is the result of many different circumstances and influences. In attempting to draw up a profile of one individual's working and playing habits, consideration would have to be given to a vast array of topics. The list below draws together the range of topics which have entered into the discussion of the various components of the model and which are relevant in considering the idea of individuality in the AL of working and playing.

Lifespan: effect on working and playing
- Infancy — type of play/playthings
- Childhood — play and work in school/out of school
- Adolescence — preparation for work
- Adulthood — type of occupation and recreation
- Old age — retirement

Factors influencing working and playing
- Physical — physique
  - physical fitness/energy level
  - state of health/ill-health
  - physical/sensory disability
- Psychological — intelligence
  - temperament and personality

— self-discipline and attitude to safety
— punctuality, reliability, honesty
— fulfilment/boredom/motivation
— balanced attitude to work/play
— reaction to unemployment/retirement

- Sociocultural
  — sex differences
  — cultural factors
  — religious factors
  — social class by occupation

- Environmental
  — climate and terrain
  — hazards to safety at work/play

- Politicoeconomic
  — personal economic status
  — health and safety at work
  — employment of disabled people
  — unemployment

Dependence/independence in working and playing
- Dependence on others (e.g. children, disabled)
- Dependence on aids (e.g. disabled)
- Financial dependence (e.g. unemployed)

Working and playing: patients' problems and related nursing activities

The time at which the day's work — whatever kind of work it is — begins and ends, are the two points around which the rest of the day is organised. During waking hours, when people are not 'working', they are 'playing'. These two activities then are an integral part of people's lives. However, the nature of the activities and their relation to one another varies at different stages of the lifespan and each person develops individuality in the AL of working and playing.

If individualised nursing is to take account of this aspect of a patient's lifestyle, nurses need information about individual working and playing habits. Such information can be obtained in the course of nursing assessment by discussing with the patient, in the detail and manner appropriate to the circumstances, topics along the lines summarised in the preceding section. While discussing

relevant topics with the patient, the nurse might bear in mind the following questions:

- what kind of working/playing activities does the individual usually engage in?
- how much time does the individual spend working/playing, and when?
- where does the individual work/play, and with whom?
- what factors influence the individual's working/playing?
- what does the individual know about the relationship of working/playing to health?
- what is the individual's attitude to working/playing?
- has the individual any longstanding problems with working/playing and, if so, how have these been coped with?
- what problems, if any, does the individual have at present with working/playing or seem likely to develop?

The objective in collecting this information is to discover the patient's usual working and playing routines; what can and cannot be done independently; previous coping mechanisms; and current problems.

To the extent relevant in the circumstances, the information obtained about the person's working and playing habits is then recorded on the nursing assessment form. The information is examined to identify, in collaboration with the patient whenever possible, any problems with the AL of working and playing. The nurse may well recognise potential problems and these too will be discussed with the patient. Some patients' problems with this AL, although identified from nursing assessment, may well lie outwith the scope of nursing intervention. In such cases, after discussion with the patient, those problems may be referred to other members of the health care team, such as the doctor or social worker.

For those actual and potential problems with which nurses can assist, realistic goals will be set and nursing interventions to achieve these will be decided upon. The problems, goals and interventions are written on the patient's nursing plan, together with the date on which evaluation will be carried out. The steps which have been described are those of the process of nursing, and all of the activities mentioned are necessary if effective *individualised nursing* is to be achieved.

Readers will be familiar by now with how this systematic approach to nursing can be applied to the Activities of Living. But how important is this with respect to the AL of working and playing? Clearly there are circumstances, such as acute illness, when this AL assumes a low priority compared to others, such as the ALs of breathing, eating and drinking, and eliminating. However, in other circumstances, the AL of working and playing assumes considerable importance. Nurses who work in the fields of psychiatry and mental handicap do seem to have developed an understanding of the significance of the AL of working and playing, both in terms of the structure of the patients' day and in terms of the therapeutic value of work and play activities as an integral part of treatment and rehabilitation. And, certainly, the importance of play is now widely recognised by nurses who work with children, whether in the hospital setting or in the community.

Yet in most general hospitals, the AL of working and playing is generally accorded a very low priority and it would seem to merit more attention than sometimes it appears to receive from nurses.

It is usual for nurses to know something about a patient's job and leisure interests. This knowledge is frequently used to initiate social conversation, thus indicating to patients an interest in them as individuals. The perceptive nurse is likely to realise too that events such as starting work, being made redundant and retiring from work constitute significant life crises. Patients who have recently experienced these crises may well be anxious or depressed and welcome additional emotional support from the nursing staff.

What may be less widely recognised is that enforced absence from usual working and playing routines can simply in itself be distressing for patients. This point is made by Wilson-Barnett (1978) in a report of her study of the feelings and opinions of a group of patients in hospital. Many of the patients expressed negative comments on being away from their family and work, ranging from 'wondering what was going on without me' to 'being very bored without work' and 'missing my friends'. A reduction in income affected many self-employed men and fear of actually losing their jobs affected many, especially men over 40 years of age. Research findings like this are not really any revelation but, nevertheless, should help to remind nurses that patients do worry about work, and do feel sadness because of separation from family and friends.

There is also the problem of boredom. In most general hospitals there are few special facilities for patients to occupy that part of the day when they are not undergoing treatment. Gooch (1984) writing about anxiety and stress in surgical care, comments:

The anxiety of how to fill the time when one is denied the normal work or leisure activities can be very real. Boredom and frustration result in greater problems . . . A day-room with books, games and television can provide diversion for a short stay but more needs to be done for the long-stay patients.

It would seem to be important for all nurses to try to understand what absence from work and separation from friends mean to patients, and to use ingenuity in helping them to avoid feeling unduly bored and lonely.

Further discussion along these lines is developed in the section below which, as in previous chapters, considers some patients' problems which arise from the change of environment and routine imposed by the hospital setting. Following that, there is a section which considers some of the main causes of change of dependence/independence status in relation to the AL of working and playing. The final section of the chapter looks at the change in working and playing habit which results from drug taking and unemployment.

These three sections by no means cover the entire range of patients' problems with working and playing, but should go some way towards helping readers to see how an understanding of these activities of everyday living can be applied in the context of nursing.

CHANGE OF ENVIRONMENT AND ROUTINE

A hospital is a very different environment from the surroundings in which people normally spend their day, working and playing. People do not normally spend all day in one place and seldom sleep in the same place as they spend the day. So, it is not surprising that patients who are confined to a hospital ward for days, and sometimes weeks on end, may become tired by the monotony of their surroundings and bored by lack of the stimulation of variety. It is no wonder that patients often take an intense interest in the goings on around them, for they have little else by way of distraction. Another problem for patients in hospital, or indeed for people who are ill in bed at home, is that they are confined indoors.

Confinement to indoor environment
Most children are accustomed to playing out of doors for at least part of the time, and for them it is unnatural to be indoors all day long in a confined space. Similarly those adults whose working and playing activities take them outside for much of the time are likely to find confinement to a hospital ward particularly irksome. Whatever their occupation, there are few people who do not go out for some part of each day, even if it is just travelling to and from work or going to the local shops or collecting children from school. Even though such outings have a specific purpose, they also provide diversion, fresh air, physical exercise and the opportunity to meet and talk to people.

If nurses are to help patients to cope with the change of environment which results from hospitalisation, then they must have information about the patients' usual working and playing habits in order to appreciate the results of deprivation and to plan appropriate alternatives. The day room is intended to provide an alternative and a more relaxing environment than the bedside area and is often equipped with television, books and games.

In some wards, nurses and/or physiotherapists organise daily exercise sessions to compensate to some extent for the sedentary lifestyle which patients lead. Sometimes patients are given freedom to walk about the hospital and if there are facilities for patients, such as a canteen or library, nurses should make sure that patients know about these and where they are. Some hospitals have attractive grounds in which, health and weather permitting, patients can walk and sit at leisure and enjoy a change from the environment of the ward.

Altered daily routine
It has already been mentioned that the activities of working and playing are important in that they provide a structure to each person's day. According to a person's occupation, the time at which work begins and ends each day determines the time of rising and going to bed, and the amount of time left for pursuing leisure interests. Hospital routine has become more flexible in recent years, but nevertheless, there are good practical reasons for patients being expected to conform to set times for rising, going to bed, having meals and undergoing tests and treatments. For the majority of patients this routine, even though different from their normal one, is unlikely to cause undue upset. However, night shift workers will require special consideration, at least until their sleeping pattern has adapted to enable them to cope with the demands of the daytime hospital routine.

Nevertheless, everyone becomes anxious with uncertainty and so nurses should inform patients and relatives about the ward routine — other patients will doubtless inform newcomers about the flexibility or otherwise of the 'official' routine! On the subject of information-giving, Gooch (1984) writes:

To feel secure in their environment people must understand it and the part they themselves are expected to play in it. Patients are unlikely to ask directly for information about the ward environment so should be told what is to happen and when it is to happen, what they will be expected to do and when to do it. If they can discuss these things, they may feel more in command of the new situation.

Being encouraged and enabled to exercise control over their own lives is important to patients. In their everyday lives, adults make decisions and exercise choice as an integral part of working and playing. How difficult then, if as patients, they are treated by nurses as though incapable of making decisions and taking initiatives. Nurses who have been patients may well have experienced the loss of self-esteem which results from such insensitivity. Male patients, especially those whose job gives them authority over others, may resent being dominated by young female nurses. Female patients who, as mothers, are accustomed to running a home and attending to the ceaseless demands of a family, might equally well be demoralised by being made to feel incapable of continuing to do as much as possible for themselves. Nurses not only create unnecessary distress by failing to recognise that patients have a need to cling to their accustomed roles and routines, but they do patients a disservice. After all, their established working and playing routines will hopefully be resumed and so, the least disruption there is to these, the easier rehabilitation will be and the more confident the patient.

How can patients be helped to incorporate their work and play interests into the daily routine of the hospital ward? For many people, having a daily newspaper, reading, watching the news or a favourite programme on television, listening to the radio or making telephone calls are regular daily activities. In hospital, the sale of daily papers, a trolley library service, television facilities, radio earphones and portable telephones are provided to help patients to continue with these activities.

There is no reason either, providing it is not detrimental to health or interferes with treatment, why patients should not continue with work activities if that is possible. Students might keep up with reading and writing essays; teachers might do marking; businessmen and women might be able to keep abreast with correspondence; and mothers might want to make shopping lists and menus, catch up on mending or continue to help with homework when children visit. Not all patients would be able to continue with work in this way, either because of the nature of their job or the severity of their illness. Some patients may need to be convinced that doing work or even worrying about it may jeopardise their recovery, and others may welcome the opportunity of 'doing nothing' for a change. Encouraging patients to do something to occupy the time may not always be in their best interest. However, skilled judgement is needed to assess when a patient is ready and indeed should be encouraged to start occupying his time. Thoughtful yet simple acts can be helpful, like introducing those patients with similar interests. Patients do appreciate the nurse who conveys a concern to prevent their day from being long and boring.

Absence from work and play groups
It is not only the loss of a familiar working and playing *routine* which patients find difficult but, equally, their absence from the *people* with whom they work and play. Apart from the family group (which is discussed separately below), work and play groups make up a major part of an adult's network of social relationships (p. 57). Absence from work and play groups may cause emotional problems for a patient in that he is no longer receiving the day-to-day feedback which is so important as a source of feelings of acceptance and belonging. Since membership of one's play groups is from choice, they are probably chosen by most people to enhance self-esteem and self-confidence. Membership of the work group may re-

sult less from choice than necessity, and may be more or less rewarding. Furthermore when things are going badly in the work group, a person may rely more on the play group for reinforcement of self-esteem, and vice versa. The patient in hospital is thus denied the usual sources of company and emotional support and has to rely on staff and fellow patients instead. It is important that new patients are helped to feel a part of the ward group so that feelings of insecurity and isolation are decreased, and those of acceptance and support are increased.

The importance of the patient group as a source of mutual support is highlighted by Rowden & Jones (1983) in an article describing a nurse-initiated programme of diversional activities for patients with cancer. They wrote:

Patients in hospital are often bombarded with information by doctors, nurses and other clinical staff. On many occasions, we have seen interactions between patients which have eased anxieties about treatment, prognosis, investigations and a host of other subjects. However hard staff try to break down barriers between them and their patients, there will always be an intrinsic value in patient-to-patient contact. We believe our programme allows us to maximise the benefits of that contact in a positive and controlled environment.

The programme itself, for patients with cancer who are no longer receiving active treatment for their disease, was designed to divert the patients' attention in a positive way, and to provide entertainment and relaxation.

The variety of activities — video, concerts, sport, games and relaxation techniques — enables both individual and collective needs to be taken into account, as does the flexible timing of the programme. The more traditional activities, such as basket weaving and carpentry, are also available to the patients and the occupational therapy department and other service departments within the hospital collaborate with the nurses on a team-work basis. Concluding their article, the authors comment:

Through our programme ... we believe we can begin to offer choices which reinforce the importance of individuality as a hospital in-patient. That process is as important as every investigation or drug that we give our patients in determining the quality of his return to a healthy life outside hospital, independent of others.

This example shows that the effects of absence from work and play groups can, to some extent at least, be lessened if the patient group is seen as a means of providing companionship, occupation and support during the period of hospitalisation.

So far in this section discussion has concentrated on adult patients, but children in hospital are also affected by absence from work and play groups. For children of school age, arrangements can be made for homework to be brought in to minimise the effects of absence from school and to provide purposeful occupation. During a long stay in hospital, regular teaching is made available to the child. So important is play in a child's life, particularly in the pre-school age group, that many children's hospitals employ what are variously described as play leaders, play workers or play therapists. This does not mean that nurses have abdicated that part of their role; indeed experience has shown that they become more skilled at helping children to play purposefully when there is a therapist available. The role of nurses, play-workers, voluntary workers and parents complement each other, as Latimer (1978) emphasises in her article which is aptly titled 'Play is everybody's business in the children's ward.' She quotes from the DHSS Report of the Expert Group on Play for Children in Hospitals as follows:

Play is not a purposeless activity seeming only to pass the childhood hours; it is a vital factor in intellectual, social, and emotional development. In hospital, play has special significance as an opportunity for the child to express physically the tension and dissatisfaction generated in a stressful and often otherwise inhibiting situation. For some years, therefore, there has been growing, but still far from widespread, recognition of the value of skilled encouragement of play when children are admitted to the strange environment of hospital.

Absence from family group

Play is certainly important in the child's life, but even more so is the family. An understanding of the adverse effects of separation of children from their parents has resulted in allowing *parents to have liberal access to their sick child*. Increasingly, hospitals have 'rooming in' facilities so that at least one parent can be with the child continuously, if that is possible and desirable, taking into account the wishes of the parents and the needs of the other family members. Lewer & Robertson (1983) indicate that all paediatric wards should have accommodation for families to be resident, and further, that:

The accommodation should not just be available to parents whose child is very ill, but to parents of all children in hospital. *Visiting times should be unrestricted* so that all family members and friends can visit.

Children can be very distressed when an adult member of the family is being taken to hospital. This is now recognised and it is government policy in the U.K. that children should be allowed to visit adults and relieve the nagging fear that the person has gone away and left them. In 1859 Florence Nightingale wrote:

There is no better society than babies and sick people for one another. Of course you must manage this so that neither shall suffer from it which is perfectly possible. If you think the 'air of the sick room' bad for baby, why it is bad for the invalid too, and therefore, you will of course correct it for both. It freshens up a sick person's whole mind to see 'the baby'. And a very young child, if unspoiled, will generally adapt itself wonderfully to the ways of the sick person, if the time they spend together is not too long.

Notes on Nursing

Visiting, and being visited, is very important in the case of children and so it is too for adults. For any patient who belongs to a family, absence from it on account of being in hospital can be a distressing and traumatic experience. Though using the term 'family' here, it needs to be remembered that not all patients have a family and, even if they have, it should not be assumed that members of the family are necessarily the most important people to the patient.

For these reasons, the nurses should find out who are the 'significant others' for each individual patient. It is also important for nurses to appreciate that the separation not only affects the patient, but equally those who have been left at home. Sometimes they may experience considerable difficulties while the patient is in hospital: for example, the young husband who has to take over running the house and looking after the children when his wife is admitted; or the elderly lady who is left to cope alone, deprived of her husband's help on which she has relied heavily due to failing sight and poor health. These are just two examples but serve to illustrate the general point that absence from the family group during hospitalisation does affect the patient, but also affects the rest of the family. Hospital visiting is, therefore, a facility which is important to both parties — the patient being visited and the family members and others who are the visitors.

At home the person had control over who visited, when and for how long. When a patient is in hospital, this control is usually forfeited. Furthermore, patients are in the unusual situation of wearing nightclothes and, even though 'ambulant', may be in bed when visitors arrive. 'Being visited' in hospital is a rather strange experience! The visitors might also find the experience somewhat strange because, after all, a hospital ward does not afford either privacy or comfort; it is busy and often noisy; and to some people it is an intimidating, even frightening environment. For both parties then, hospital visiting may be somewhat stressful but it is an important means of minimising the effects of the patient's absence from the family group.

The norm was for hospitals to have specific daily visiting hours and often a rule that there may be only two visitors per patient at any given time, but the trend now favours more liberal and more flexible visiting hours.

For a flexible policy to succeed there has to be adequate extensive preparation of the staff and the public. It was never intended that visitors (even near relatives) should visit continuously from first thing in the morning to last thing at night. Some relatives who interpreted 'free visiting' in this way felt guilty if they did not stay, and if they did, they found it a marathon task. It was merely intended that patients and their relatives could have mutual choice about the time and duration of visits, subject to staff approval. It was hoped that this would spread the number of visitors in a ward at any one time and the staff could continue their ministrations to those patients who were not being visited at that time.

Also with visitors spread over a longer period it could afford both visitors and staff a much better opportunity to communicate with each other. For each ill person there are anxious relatives and friends who need information, not only to keep their anxiety within reasonable limits, but also to teach them how they can help their ill relative to recover or to die peacefully. Each dying patient has special visiting needs; if he is conscious his wishes should be granted; if he is unconscious it is his relatives who need information and consideration about whether or not to stay with him.

Some hospitals have tried and then abandoned the more flexible visiting policies. Sadler (1981) compares the two systems and concludes that:

old-fashioned though it may seem, I feel that restricted visiting, regulated and adapted humanely, is more conducive to a patients' recovery than 'open visiting'. A patient needs to see his friends and relatives, but have we not reacted too strongly to the former discipline by letting rules become too relaxed? Rules were made not for the convenience of the staff, but to protect the patient.

Though acknowledging that there are problems associated with liberal hospital visiting Gooch (1984), however, argues in favour of this system. She writes:

Why are families considered to be 'visitors' merely because one of their number has become a patient ...? Relatives are part of the patient's care and therefore *belong* in the ward whenever they wish to be there.

Gooch considers that nurses on adult wards should emulate the family-centred care which is now an integral part of sick children's nursing and, therefore, there would be new expectations of the purpose of visiting.

There are of course some patients whose family may not be able to visit and for them, communication by phone and letter may help to compensate for lack of visiting. Other patients, for instance the elderly, may no longer have a family group and nurses can help by discussing with them whether they would like to take advantage of any of the voluntary visitors' schemes, should these be available in the area.

In conclusion, the objectives of hospital visiting are to enable contact to be maintained between members of the family group; to make the patient's day more meaningful; and to provide mutual benefit and pleasure for both patients and their visitors. Nurses are in a strategic position to help in the achievement of these objectives, whatever visiting policy is adopted by the institution.

CHANGE OF DEPENDENCE/INDEPENDENCE STATUS

Independence in the activities of working and playing is regarded as the desirable norm for adults. Clearly, then, those who are unable to achieve or retain independence are disadvantaged members of society. In any country there are some people who are unable to work and, therefore, are financially dependent on their families and/or the state. There are many different reasons for lack or loss of independence and here these are categorised as physical disability, mental handicap, mental illness and sensory loss/impairment. An understanding of the causes and effects of dependence in the activities of working and playing is a relevant part of nursing knowledge. There are many different circumstances in which nurses can contribute to helping people to achieve their optimal level of independence in work and play activities.

Physical disability

Obviously there will be a difference in the difficulties experienced in gaining or maintaining independence for working and playing depending on the nature of the disability and the body systems affected. Disease of the cardiopulmonary system can render a person so breathless and short of oxygen that 'work' is impossible and entertainment only of the passive variety is possible. Many of the chronic disabling diseases affect the nervous system and the musculosketal system, and the patient's work and play problems are in fact mobilising problems. Depending on the person's previous working and playing activities, the degree of dependence caused by the disability will vary and there will need to be more or less adaptation. The outdoor worker and the active sports enthusiast may well find it difficult to settle for sedentary work and more passive leisure time activities. If the sedentary workers can be rehabilitated to an 'independent' wheelchair life, they are likely to be able to resume their previous work.

The importance of helping the disabled patient back to employment as soon as possible is emphasised by Hall (1979), who writes:

Work is habit-forming as well as therapeutic: a newly disabled person can become demoralised almost beyond hope of resuscitation if he is allowed to remain in unproductive idleness for too long. Apart from the physical damage of a disability, it can result in psychological and social ill-effects. The natural confidence of the individual is damaged, and, furthermore, the loss of earnings can cause domestic problems.

Hall describes the role of health care professionals and the Manpower Services Commission (p. 279) in the process of resettlement in work, and ends her article by saying:

The needs of the disabled person differ according to the nature and the severity of the disability, but all should be helped to lead as near normal a life as possible. Although re-introduction to the working force is the final stage in the rehabilitation programme it is, nevertheless, a most important stage for it enables the disabled person to feel he is part of, and is contributing towards, the community.

Physical disablement not only changes a person's independence status for working, but also affects playing.

Increasing awareness of the needs of the disabled in this respect has led to the development of special sports facilities and international sports events are now organised in just the same way as they are for able-bodied sportsmen and women. Cotton (1983), in his book *Outdoor Adventure for Handicapped People*, makes the point that the only difference between the handicapped and the normal person is their degree of ability, and that 'adventure' does not need to involve climbing mountains. Swimming, sailing, canoeing, fishing, riding, camping, and snow sports such as tobogganing, are all possible and all offer the excitement and stimulation which result from the challenge of adventure. Other handicapped people, again no different from normal people, may prefer to choose more passive, indoor leisure pursuits. Nowadays, theatres, cinemas, art galleries, restaurants and hotels are becoming better equipped — and in new buildings, intentionally designed — to enable physically disabled people to make use of and enjoy these facilities.

Mental handicap

By definition, the mentally handicapped are a highly dependent group within society but, nevertheless, they too have the need for the satisfaction and occupation of time which are obtained from working and playing. In industralised societies, 'work' has become so complex that there has been an almost unquestioned assumption that someone who is mentally handicapped is incapable of working. However, this can be seen to be a false notion if a broader view of work is taken. All but the most severely handicapped are quite capable of work which does not necessarily demand a high level of intellectual capacity. Domestic work, work with animals, gardening and horticulture, farming and repetitive industrial jobs are examples of the kind of work which many mentally handicapped people are perfectly capable of doing.

Working is part of normal adult life and those who adopt the principle of 'normalisation' for the mentally handicapped argue that they too have the right and the need to work. To cope with the demands of work in contemporary society, this means that they require education and training for work. In the U.K., where the emphasis has shifted from institutional care to community care, there has been an increase in the provision for the mentally handicapped of what are called 'adult training centres', and also of 'sheltered workshops'. Opportunities for mildly mentally handicapped people to be employed under normal working conditions are still few and far between, but are being actively pursued. However, even if employers adopted a more enlightened attitude, the mentally handicapped are unlikely to fare well in the competitiveness which high unemployment has created.

For people who are so severely mentally handicapped as to be unable to achieve sufficient independence to live in the community, countries vary as to the type of residential provision which is made for them. Some utilise the model of a village with a group of houses, a workshop, shops and a village hall for sports and entertainment. Other countries care for the mentally handicapped in hospitals, the system which has operated in the U.K. Nowadays, in mental handicap hospitals there is considerable emphasis being placed on the residents' need for productive occupation. Hence, there are occupational therapy and industrial therapy units in most hospitals with the aim of giving a sense of purpose and satisfaction, and providing a small monetary income. Much attention has always been paid to the social side of life, and sports and entertainment of increasing diversity provide the opportunity for regular playing. However, more recently there has developed an awareness that play can be exploited to therapeutic advantage too.

Darbyshire (1980) describes the ways in which nurses, teachers and physiotherapists have worked together in a hospital unit for profoundly handicapped children to use play as a means of maintaining or improving the child's level of functioning and quality of life. Water play, hydrotherapy, painting, sand play, music, rough and tumble play and social play are some of the types of play described. In addition, a variety of suitable, sometimes ingenious, toys are mentioned and in that hospital a toy library was established. This is described in another article (Benicki & Cull, 1980) and again, though nurses are heavily involved, this has been a multidisciplinary effort. Toys are important, but only as an aid to play. Benicki & Leslie (1983) write:

> Surrounding the child or handicapped adult with play equipment is not sufficient; the impetus must come from the staff to encourage and demonstrate the use of the toy, and reward must be given when interest is shown. Play ... fosters communication, intellectual development and social interaction. Toys can be said to be tools to aid this development; the right toys at the correct moment can improve and extend these skills.

In relation to adult mentally handicapped patients, Benicki & Leslie comment that nurses often seem to be uncertain as to the appropriateness of play as an activity and again they emphasise:

> Toys alone are insufficient; to offer them to a mentally handicapped adult who has no concept of play will only cause frustration and subsequent rejection of the equipment. Staff must be willing to show interest, understanding, and patience to motivate and develop play skills. ... Play can help to overcome many of the secondary handicaps or problem areas projected by the residents; lack of motivation, poor concentration, difficulties in hand-eye co-ordination, balance and movement difficulties, or general lack of physical co-ordination.

Playing, then, is a means of increasing independence and it, like working, is an important dimension of the lives of people who are mentally handicapped.

Mental illness

Some people experience difficulty in gaining or maintaining independence for working and playing because of mental illness. Some of the common features of mental illness are excessive anxiety, depression, phobias, obsessional thoughts or behaviour, delusions, confusion, overactivity or apathy, aggression, loss of confidence, forgetfulness, dependence on alcohol and disturbed personal relationships. It is not difficult to appreciate that these kinds of psychological difficulties can diminish a person's independence for the activities of working and playing. Mental illness is likely to lessen an individual's ability to secure a job and, if employed, to continue to function satisfactorily at work.

However, the treatment and care of the mentally ill person has changed considerably over the years. The availability of treatment by tranquilliser drugs and antidepressants has meant that many people can be cured, or at least the symptoms sufficiently controlled, without the necessity for admission to a psychiatric hospital or even much time off work. Behaviour therapy too can be provided on an out-patient basis, as can psychotherapy and counselling, and being encouraged to continue with regular working and playing activities may in itself be therapeutic. Certainly these activities are exploited as part of the treatment of psychiatric in-patients, somewhat similar to the situation described earlier in relation to hospital care of the mentally handicapped.

For people who have suffered a severe, perhaps prolonged, form of mental illness there may be the need for resettlement in work, a subject discussed earlier in the context of physically disabled people. Burns (1979) is of the opinion that ex-psychiatric patients do not fare as well when it comes to placement in work, whether in open or sheltered employment. He makes the point that the disability of mentally ill people is not as well understood, citing the example of an employer who considered that all people who have been in a psychiatric hospital are potentially dangerous. This may seem rather ignorant but it is the case that mental illness is a poorly understood subject and, for the sufferer, is still a social stigma. It seems that the mentally ill do need a better planned scheme for resettlement and employment, and Burns, a qualified psychiatric nurse, describes such a scheme for both day patients and in-patients at a psychiatric hospital.

Sensory loss/impairment

Most people who become *blind* are faced with changing their work. Those who have the necessary ability and aptitude can be encouraged to take the special training courses in typing, machine sewing and physiotherapy. There are also various craft courses which can be undertaken in the workshops for the blind. Most people with acquired blindness will be able to continue independently some of their playing habits, and with help from the various organisations for the blind, they can continue others in a modified form, for example reading journals in braille, listening to tape recordings of books and using braille playing cards.

Gradual onset of *deafness* may permit a person to learn to lip read and to make preparation for future working. Some can continue with their previous employment, but there are many types of work which require a person with adequate hearing: serving in a shop, waiting at table, banking and manning a switchboard are but a few examples. There has to be preparation for enjoying leisure time when eventually all hearing is lost. Nurses can encourage patients to develop suitable physical activities in which they are interested and help them to decide about visual activities which can be pursued by deaf people.

Impairment of *speech* will cause considerable problems since for most people verbal communication is an essential part of working and playing. The problem of aphasia commonly results, in addition to paralysis, from a cerebrovascular accident. Whether it is mainly expressive or receptive (p. 129), or a mixture of the two, it will interfere with their ability to communicate. Nurses are guided by speech therapists as to the ways in which they can help these patients to improve or regain their ability to communicate while working and playing.

CHANGE IN WORKING AND PLAYING HABIT

A change in dependence/independence status for the activities of working and playing, often results, as is apparent in the foregoing section in a change in habit. For example, chronic disabling disease which causes physical disability is very likely to necessitate a change in both working and playing habits. In this section, the two problems discussed — drug taking and unemployment — do have links with the concept of dependence/independence. However, primarily they result in change of working and playing *habit* and for that reason are placed here.

Change due to drug taking
Experimentation with drugs usually starts in relation to leisure time activities. In many countries it seems to be part of present day culture and indeed some people look on it as part of growing up. Adolescents claim that the selected 'drug' makes them feel excited and allows them to experience heightened awareness. It could be argued that no one has the right to deprive another of such experience which is a precious part of living, but many people experience the full impact of their emotions in heightened awareness without taking a drug.

However, if adolescents start taking drugs as leisure time experimentation it can, perhaps insidiously, have an effect on working habits. The person finds that he cannot

discipline himself to arrive on time, to take the necessary precautions while at work and to complete the scheduled amount of work before leaving. So he continues taking drugs.

Yet another group who start taking drugs do so as a reaction to stress at work. For some reason, perhaps too heavy a work load, members of this group are not managing and work piles up to the extent that it is unmanageable. One way of tackling the problem would be by adjusting the work load and by informing the authority that it is too heavy. But conscientious people often find it difficult to admit that they are not managing. To gain some respite they indulge in drug taking, only to find it does not solve the problem but brings others in its wake.

The problem of drug taking is something about which nurses should have knowledge as they, along with other health care professionals, have a part to play in prevention through health education of the public, especially youngsters. The main types of drugs involved are described below, starting with one kind of drug taking which has recently become an issue of much publicity — solvent abuse.

Solvent abuse. The term solvent abuse has come to be used in place of 'glue sniffing' or 'fume sniffing'. Morton (1983) describes solvent abuse as 'the practice of inhaling volatile organic substances in order to obtain euphoric effects or to later psychological states.' There are many methods in use: for example, putting glue into an empty crisp bag and inhaling and exhaling into it; or saturating a rag with solvents, such as turpentine, and inhaling; or spraying an aerosol, such as hair lacquer into a polythene bag over the head. As Morton emphasises, solvent abuse is not only harmful but it can be fatal. In the U.K. there has been mounting pressure on the government to make abuse of solvents illegal and, indeed, the Solvent Abuse (Scotland) Act of 1983 was introduced as a response to increasing concern. Enforcing restrictions on retailers, for example prohibiting the sale of 'glue kits' (glue and crisp bags) will not solve this problem but may help to deter some youngsters.

Educating young people, and their parents and teachers, about the danger of this form of drug taking is something positive in which nurses can become involved. The danger of solvent abuse is the immediacy of its effects, and brain damage and asphyxiation can occur. Bizarre and dangerous behaviour, such as jumping out of windows or climbing high walls, have been known to follow intoxication. A severe reaction can cause sudden death and many countries have recorded instances of death from solvent abuse. Pointers to solvent abuse include a lingering smell of solvent on hair and clothes and possession of glue and bags. Staggering walk, slurred speech, violent behaviour, dilated pupils, and spots around the mouth and nose are other signs of solvent abuse. Many cities now have treatment centres which offer guidance and counselling, and involvement of the child's parents is considered to be vital to the success of treatment of habitual solvent abusers.

Marijuana/pot/cannabis. Those adolescents who smoke pot in the hope of alleviating their 'adolescent problems' are the ones who are likely to become continuous users, that is they develop dependence which may interfere with their working and playing habits. The long-term effects of smoking pot are not known for certain. Two nurses have written an informative article about their survey of evidence and they ask 'Why is the literature so contradictory?' (Dell & Snyder, 1977).

There is a possibility that the use of cannabis (a soft drug) can lead to a *life of dependence* on hard drugs which mitigates against health. It is for this reason that society is divided into those who are for, and those who are against the legal use of cannabis. Currently there are many countries in which the use of cannabis is illegal and possession of the drug is a punishable offence.

Amphetamines. These are the much talked about 'pep' pills; they are in tablet or capsule form called 'black bombers', 'French blues' or 'purple hearts'. Another type — methedrine — is called 'speed'. After ingestion the pupils dilate and behaviour can be described as boisterous. When the effects wear off, there is usually lethargy, irritability and unsociability. This psychological see-saw is an indication to members of the family, work and play groups that an individual might be using amphetamines for other than medicinal purposes. Loss of appetite with consequent loss of weight and sleeplessness can also result from taking this drug.

As with other drugs, desire for the next dose can become compulsive, and money is spent acquiring it to the exclusion of food and clothing and this state can lead to stealing. Chronic amphetamine users can become mentally ill and require psychiatric treatment. In many countries amphetamines are only obtainable on a doctor's prescription and doctors are discouraged from prescribing them.

Barbiturates. There is a considerable range of barbiturates previously prescribed as sleeping tablets. After taking them some people experience a 'hangover' which makes them sullen and this can disrupt personal relationships at home, at work and at play. There can be increasing incidents of being late for work and evidence of increased accident-proneness. Continued use can result in psychological dependence.

A more serious development is taking the tablets mixed with water as an injection. The barbiturates may not dissolve properly causing inflammation of the veins and clotting of the blood when death may ensue. Also it is not uncommon for ulcers to occur at the injection sites and the area can become gangrenous. As they are still used for medical reasons in many countries, barbiturates are not illegal but they are only obtainable on a doctor's prescription and doctors are discouraged from prescribing them.

LSD/Lysergic acid. Lysergic acid is a transparent liquid, effective in minute quantities so it can be dropped on sugar cubes or the back of postage stamps which are common means of distribution. It can also be made in tablet form and it is usually taken orally and only rarely by injection. It has the effect of raising the blood pressure and increasing the heart rate; it produces hallucinations which are false perceptions occurring without any sensory stimulus. Coping with the torrent of psychological experience released by the drug can be difficult and dangerous without medical supervision. In most countries lysergic acid is not legally for sale, and to possess it is an offence.

Heroin, cocaine and morphine. Each of these drugs has a useful though small part to play in medical therapy. 'Hard drugs' is the term used when they are peddled for illicit purposes. Introduction to them occurs in a social setting when the uninitiated are invited to experiment with 'just one injection'. The social setting and the personal introduction lead some people to liken the spread of drug-taking to that of the spread of a 'contagious' disease. But for some personalities, even after just one injection, abstinence is not possible. Such people find themselves on the slow road of decline, to a dependence that rules their lives. They become 'drop-outs' from work because obtaining the next dose ('fix') takes precedence over any other activity. Eventually they may have to be injected up to six times daily, the dose getting higher and higher to satisfy the craving. In addition there is always the danger that infected syringes will cause jaundice, local sepsis or even fatal septicaemia. Other common accompaniments of drug taking are loss of interest in personal appearance and lack of appetite to the extent of causing malnutrition with a consequent lowered resistance to infection.

Change due to unemployment

It is not difficult to appreciate that becoming unemployed necessitates tremendous change in a person's established working and playing habits. Loss of work is a problem in its own right, denying the person a whole range of benefits: personal, social and financial. But having no job to go to also obviates the purpose of many daily living habits which are primarily work-related: for example, habitual time of rising; usual daily dress; regular exercise obtained getting to and from work; and the type and timing of meals. Being without work means that there is unlimited time for playing. For some resourceful people this may not pose a problem but for most it does. Almost all leisure activities cost money. Deprived of income from work, established playing habits may be impossible to continue. Apart from that, the person's motivation to seek enjoyment and diversion may be lost and the inevitable stress and gloom which unemployment brings may cause such apathy and depression of mood that there is no enthusiasm or energy for playing. There is little incentive to get up in the morning and sleeping longer is one way of passing the time and obliterating worries. Watching television, smoking and drinking are other ways of coping with boredom and anxiety. None of these habits in excess is conducive to health and some can lead to further financial difficulties.

There is increasing concern that unemployment has deleterious effects on health and it seems reasonable to conjecture that the change in working and playing habits which occurs plays some part in this. Stress-related health problems, such as high blood pressure and heart disease, have been cited in discussion linking ill-health and unemployment, as have psychiatric illness, alcohol-related problems and parasuicide. There is increasing knowledge about the links between ill-health and unemployment but, as yet, no really precise and indisputable findings. It is of course a problem which is very difficult to investigate because there are so many factors involved. Two frequently cited studies, one British and one American, are discussed in an article by Brown (1981) on the subject of unemployment. The British research was undertaken by Fagin, a psychiatrist, and involved an in-depth study of 22 families. The aim was to assess the effects of unemployment on the health of the families. Health changes were not restricted to the unem-

ployed 'male breadwinner' but often affected the wife and children. The men experienced various psychological changes; including depression, loss of self-esteem, suicidal thoughts, violence and increased reliance on tobacco or alcohol. Physical changes included lack of energy and loss or gain of weight; and backaches and headaches were also reported. The younger children of men who were out of work for longer periods commonly had disturbances in feeding and sleeping habits and were more prone to accidents and various ailments. In some cases, there was marital disharmony to the extent of violence, and in three of the families the parents separated.

The American study, done by Brenner of James Hopkins University (U.S.A.) was much larger and involved an epidemiological approach rather than a study of individual cases. The claim is made that a 1% increase in unemployment in the U.S.A. has been associated with a 2% increase in deaths. Suicide, homicide and neonatal mortality rates have risen in association with increased unemployment and, during recessions, so too have admission to psychiatric hospitals and alcohol consumption. Both of these studies have been criticised, both in terms of their method and the conclusions drawn. Nevertheless, they have helped to draw attention to the potentially serious health consequences of unemployment and increasing numbers of health care professionals are now expressing concern about this major contemporary problem.

Governments, while tending to be reluctant to accept

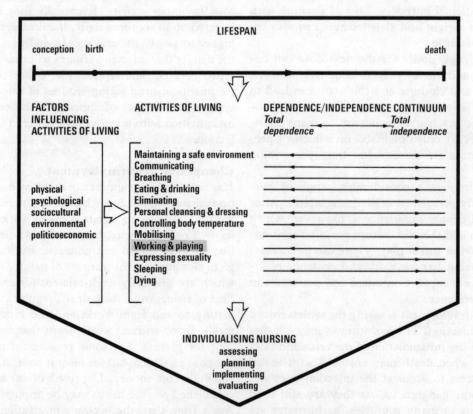

Fig. 15.1 The AL of working and playing within the model for nursing

the evidence which links ill-health and unemployment, nevertheless have begun to make some provisions to ameliorate the effects of the change in working and playing habits which arise. For example, in the U.K. there are schemes which provide productive occupation for unemployed school leavers, and people who are unemployed are allowed free and subsidised entry to some educational sports and leisure facilities. Thus, recognition is being given to the importance of working and playing habits in the lives of people who have the misfortune to be unemployed.

Like many aspects of the AL of working and playing, it is not easy to be precise about the nature of nursing activities which are directly related to the problem of unemployment. After all, the problem of a person's joblessness cannot be solved by nurses. On the other hand, an understanding of this problem — especially its links with ill-health — is relevant in nursing. So too is a sympathetic attitude to those who have the misfortune to be unemployed, for many suffer from feelings of shame and desolation.

Thinking in more specific terms, the knowledge that unemployment can affect the health of the whole family is obviously of relevance to those nurses who are concerned with health surveillance and health promotion in the community. Families in which there are young children, and one or both parents are unemployed, might be visited more frequently, thus allowing them an opportunity to discuss their problems and feelings. Assessment of what changes have been made to compensate for lack of working, and to fill the unlimited time available for playing, might reveal some actual and potential health problems. The member of the family might welcome the opportunity to review their changed lifestyle in this way and to be helped to plan activities which would maintain, rather than endanger, their health.

This might also be very relevant in the context of hospital nursing and, indeed in that setting, the patient might be highly receptive to education about health problems to which he may be vulnerable because he is unemployed. Actual and potential problems might be indentified from nursing assessment on admission and the fact that the patient is unemployed should be borne in mind when assessing all the Activities of Living. When finding out about usual habits and routines, it might be revealing to find out whether these have changed since unemployment. If problems identified, such as excessive alcohol intake or insomnia, do appear to have resulted from unemployment then planning to deal with them would have to take that into account. Indeed, the fact of a person's joblessness is relevant to much of the nursing plan which, after all, is geared towards rehabilitation and discharge. The needs of a patient who is returning to work are different from those of the person who has no job to go back to. This would certainly be a major preoccupation of

treatment and rehabilitation of patients in the context of psychiatric nursing.

There are, therefore, implications of unemployment for individualised nursing, both in hospital and in the community. In direct contact with families and sick people, the nurse may be able to help constructively with some of the adverse consequences of joblessness.

Some would say that nurses have another responsibility too — to become involved politically in the matter of unemployment. Seabrook (1982) writing about suffering of the unemployed says:

the consequences of unemployment in the eighties remain essentially secret: part of an individual burden, contained within families for the most part … This means that those, including health visitors, who actually penetrate the outer defences, those who have access to people's homes, carry a heavy responsibility in that it is up to them to assess the extent of the harm that is done inside the privacy of those despairing and demoralised homes, and to make sure that the rest of us understand exactly what it is we are asking of people.

He ends the article:

The caring professions are uniquely placed, in their privileged access to people's lives, to make sense of some of the remorseless pressures and to raise their voice against them. If they don't, nobody else will.

In the second half of this chapter some of the problems and discomforts which can be experienced by patients in relation to the AL of working and playing have been described. This provides the beginning nurse with a generalised idea of these; it will be useful in assessing, planning, implementing and evaluating an individualised programme for each patient's AL of working and playing.

This chapter has been concerned with the AL of working and playing. However, as stated previously it is only for the purpose of discussion that any AL can be considered on its own; in reality the various activities are so closely related and do not have distinct boundaries. Figure 15.1 is a reminder that the AL of working and playing is related to the other ALs and also to the various components of the model for nursing.

REFERENCES

Barnard J M 1971 The young adult and work. Nursing 1 (25) May: 1076–1078

Benicki A, Cull A 1980 The toy library. Nursing Times, Occasional Paper 76 (7) March 6: 29–32

Benicki A, Leslie FA 1983 The mental handicap nurse's special role. In: Tierney AJ (ed) Nurses and the mentally handicapped. Bristol, ch 5

Brown A 1981 The road to despair. Nursing Mirror 153 (9) August 26: 8–9

Burns DB 1979 Resettlement and employment of psychiatric patients. Nursing Times 75 (19) May 10: 799–801

Cotton 1983 Outdoor adventure for handicapped people. Souvenir Press, London

Darbyshire P 1980 Play and profoundly handicapped children. Nursing Times 76 (35) August 28: 1538–1543

Dell DD, Snyder J 1977 Marijuana: pro and con. American Journal of Nursing April 4: 630–635

Ferguson V 1984 Preparation for a healthy retirement. Nursing Mirror 158 (12) March 21: 28–29

Garrett G 1983 Health needs of the elderly. (The essentials of nursing series.) Macmillan, London p 15

Gooch J 1984 The other side of surgery. Macmillan, London, p 3, 21, 60

Hall EM 1979 Helping the patient with work or productive occupation. Nursing Times June 21: 1061–1062

Hammond G 1981 Effects of ageing on work performance. Nursing 1 (25) May: 1079–1080

Holgate P 1980 Safety in the N.H.S. Nursing 1 (14) June: 602–605

Homewood JV 1981 When you retire. Nursing 1 (25) May: 1081–1082

Latimer E 1978 Play is everybody's business in the children's ward. Nursing Mirror 147 (11) September 14: 21–23

Lewer H, Robertson L 1983 Care of the child. (The essentials of nursing series.) Macmillan, London, p 71

Morton A 1983 Solvent abuse. Nursing Mirror Supplement Community Forum 10 (December 14): i–viii

Rcn 1983 The nurse's contribution to the health of the worker. Report of the Nursing Commission. Permanent Commission and International Association on Occupational Health. Royal College of Nursing, London

Rowden R, Jones L 1983 A diversional programme for patients with cancer. Nursing Times 79 (11) March 16: 25–27

Sadler C 1981 Some thoughts on ward visiting. Nursing Mirror 153 (11) September 9: 14

Seabrook J 1982 The human cost of unemployment. Nursing Mirror 155 (18) November 3: 30–31

Sheridan MD 1977 Spontaneous play in early childhood: from birth to six years. NFER Publishing Co.

Swaffield L 1980 Work — the current state of play. Nursing Times Community Outlook 76 (7): 37–43

Tierney AJ 1983 Married women in nursing. Nursing Times Occasional Paper 79 (24) September 7: 30–33

Wilson-Barnett J 1978 In hospital: patients' feelings and opinions. Nursing Times Occasional Paper 74 (8) March 16: 29–32

ADDITIONAL READING

Melhuish A 1982 Work and health. Penguin, Harmondsworth

Newson J, Newson E 1979 Toys and playthings in development and remediation. Allen and Unwin, London and Penguin, Harmondsworth

Weller BF 1980 Helping sick children play. Bailliere Tindall, London

16

Expressing sexuality

The activity of expressing sexuality

'It's a boy' or 'It's a girl' is almost always the very first thing a midwife tells the mother about her newborn baby. As the basic body structure of males and females is distinctly different even at birth, the midwife's identification of the baby's sex is almost instantaneous. A person's sex is determined at conception and, throughout the entire lifespan, sexuality is a significant dimension of personality and behaviour.

Each human being is a 'sexual' human being and for health, each person requires to have a sexual identity, that is, to perceive 'self' as a boy/girl, then as a man/woman. Aspects of sexuality include enjoying the accessories which, in a given society, characterise man/woman such as the style of dress, wearing personal adornments, perfumes and cosmetics; all are ways in which the individual concept of being man/woman is announced to others.

In many parts of the world social mores are moving away from a rigid interpretation of activities, attitudes, beliefs and values associated with expressing sexuality as 'good' or 'bad', 'normal' or 'abnormal'. The subject is increasingly being aired by the media so that more people are becoming aware of a wide range of practices related to the many dimensions of the AL of expressing sexuality.

THE NATURE OF EXPRESSING SEXUALITY

Human beings have an innate sensuality; being cuddled, rocked and stroked are pleasurable experiences for even the very young infant. It is not long before the child discovers how to create enjoyable sensations himself by,

293

for example, mouthing objects, body rocking and touching particular parts of his body, including the genitals. From the child's point of view there is nothing explicitly sexual about these activities.

However, a little later on, the child's increasing curiosity about body structure and function manifests itself in constant questioning of the parents, not least of all, the age-old questions about sex and reproduction. All of this is quite natural and normal; the child is expressing an interest in sex in general and, in particular, about his/her sexuality.

Children experiment with the concept of sexuality in their everyday play and in their private fantasy world. They act out the ways in which masculinity and femininity can be conveyed in gait, mode of dress, make-up and choice of working and playing activities. Children's play characters can be the stereotype of the strong, aggressive male or the seductive, submissive female. Inevitably families feature prominently in children's play and this allows them to act out their view of the roles of men and women as fathers and mothers.

From these learning opportunities, the growing child becomes increasingly aware of the complexities of human sexuality and the ways in which men and women express their masculinity and femininity. This growing awareness helps the adolescent at puberty to understand his/her own sexual feelings and how he/she is expected to behave as a sexually mature person. There is a great deal of experimentation going on in the adolescent's ways of expressing sexuality. In private, masturbation enables the youngster to learn to enjoy the physical pleasure of sex; in friendships with members of their own and the opposite sex, adolescents begin to learn how human sexuality influences at a fundamental level how adult men and women relate to each other.

Relating to each other in an explicitly sexual way is central to the husband–wife relationship of marriage. Many different ways of expressing sexuality are involved in this adult sexual relationship in addition to the behaviour of sexual intercourse.

THE PURPOSE OF EXPRESSING SEXUALITY

It is clear that at different stages of the lifespan forms of sexual expression vary and so too does the purpose of expressing sexuality. The various forms of sexual behaviour described can enable the individual to express his or her personality, or reflect society's expectations of sex differences, or provide physical pleasure, or attract a mate, or bring about the conception of a child.

It is interesting that in most lower mammals, sexual behaviour tends to occur only when fertilisation can take place and courting and mating activities are inextricably linked to reproduction. In contrast, human sexual behaviour serves both reproductive and non-reproductive functions and, indeed is much more frequently performed for non-reproductive reasons than for the purpose of procreation.

BODY STRUCTURE AND FUNCTION REQUIRED FOR SEX AND REPRODUCTION

The male sex organs

In the model of living the body structure and function related to the AL of expressing sexuality are the male sex organs, the female sex organs, the female fertility cycle and control of fertility. As study of the reproductive system may be arranged later in a nursing curriculum, an outline of the body structure and function required for sex and reproduction is given here. Only the physical aspects are discussed because the psychological and sociocultural aspects are considered later in the chapter. The male and female reproductive systems are described separately. The organs which comprise the male reproductive system are shown in Figure 16.1. The *testes*, equivalent to the ovaries in the female, are glands which produce the spermatozoa capable of fertilising the female ova. The testes are covered by the scrotum which is a pouch-like structure, its skin continuous with that of the trunk. It is thought that the testes require this exposure to external atmospheric temperature for optimum functioning. The male sex hormone — testosterone — is increased in the testes from puberty, and is responsible for initiating and maintaining the secondary sex characteristics of the male.

Semen, the fluid containing spermatozoa, is ejaculated from the penis through the urethra (which also conveys urine to the exterior from the urinary bladder, though not simultaneously). Spermatozoa leave the testes by the *epididymis*, a series of convoluted tubes arranged as an oval body on the surface of each testis. Continuing from the epididymis is the *vas deferens*. This tube enters the pelvic cavity, passes over the top of the bladder and descends behind it. Here it enters the base of the *seminal vesicle* which lies behind the bladder and is a hollow organ acting as a reservoir for semen. It contracts to force semen along the *ejaculatory duct* which passes through the *prostate gland* to join the urethra.

The urethra passes through *the penis*. This is a tubular organ of spongy, erectile tissue. Erection of the penis, caused by sexual excitement, occurs because the spaces in the sponge-like tissue become engorged with blood. After ejaculation has taken place the penis returns to its normal size and flaccid state. The most sensitive part of the penis is *the glans*, an enlargement at the tip of the organ. Certain areas of this contain many nerve endings highly sensitive to touch and pressure. A loose fold of skin, the *foreskin or prepuce*, covers the glans penis. This is not present if the man has been circumcised; in some

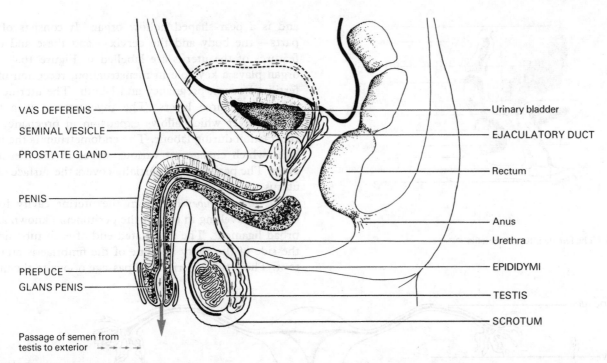

VAS DEFERENS — — Urinary bladder

SEMINAL VESICLE — — EJACULATORY DUCT

PROSTATE GLAND — — Rectum

PENIS — — Anus

— Urethra

— EPIDIDYMI

PREPUCE — — TESTIS

GLANS PENIS — — SCROTUM

Passage of semen from
testis to exterior → → → →

Fig. 16.1 The male reproductive system

religious sects this is performed soon after birth and circumcision may also be carried out during boyhood.

The female sex organs

The female sex organs consist of the external genitalia, the internal genitalia and the breasts.

The external genitalia are shown in Figure 16.2. The *mons veneris* is a pad of fatty tissue overlying the symphysis pubis and, from puberty, is covered with hair. The *labia majora* are two thick 'lips' of adipose tissue extending backwards from the mons veneris to the perineum. Together these two structures form the immediately visible parts of the external genitalia. When the labia are parted, the other structures can be seen.

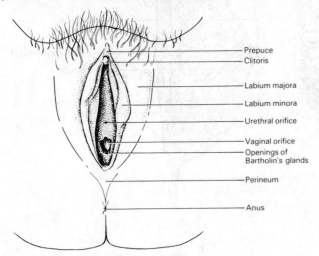

Prepuce
Clitoris

Labium majora

Labium minora

Urethral orifice

Vaginal orifice
Openings of
Bartholin's glands

Perineum

Anus

Fig. 16.2 The female external genitalia

The *labia minora* are two thinner, highly vascular folds of smooth skin within the labia majora. Anteriorly the labia minora join into the hood-like prepuce which surrounds and protects the *clitoris*: a small highly sensitive erectile structure. The *vestibule* is enclosed by the labia minora and clitoris and, posteriorly, by the opening of the vagina. The urethra opens into the vestibule and lubricating glands (Skene's glands) open at its base. The *vaginal orifice* is situated behind the urethra and is covered (before its perforation) by a fold of skin, the *hymen*. Bartholins glands lie on either side of the vaginal orifice and secrete a lubricating fluid which facilitates intercourse. The external genitalia protect the inner organs from trauma and infection and provide the route of entry into the vagina for the penis during sexual intercourse.

The internal genitalia are contained within the pelvic cavity and consist of the vagina, uterus, uterine tubes and ovaries. The position of these organs is shown in Figure 16.3.

The vagina is a muscular canal which opens upwards and backwards from the vulva to the cervix of the uterus. The bladder and urethra lie in front and behind lie the perineal body, rectum and anus. The vagina is the passage to the exterior for menstrual blood and for the baby at childbirth. The vagina is kept moistened by secretions from the cervical glands and vaginal fluid, being acid, inhibits the growth of microorganisms. However, before puberty and after the menopause this mechanism is not so effective and the vagina is more susceptible to infection at these stages of the lifespan.

The uterus is set almost at right angles to the vagina

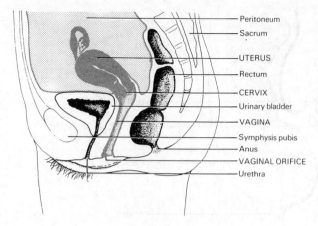

Fig. 16.3 The female internal genitalia

and is a pear-shaped hollow organ. It consists of two parts — the body and the cervix — and these and other features of the uterus are labelled in Figure 16.4. This organ plays a key role in menstruation, reception of the fertilised ovum, pregnancy and labour. The uterine wall consists of three layers. The myometrium is a thick muscle layer which allows expansion in pregnancy and contraction during labour. The endometrium is the inner layer which changes at various stages in the menstrual cycle. The perimetrium partially covers the surface of the uterus.

The uterine tubes run from the uterine cavity to the ovaries, travelling in part of the peritoneum known as the broad ligament. The fimbriated end of each tube lies on the side of the ovary and one of the fimbriae is attached to it. These tubes permit the passage of ova to the uterus

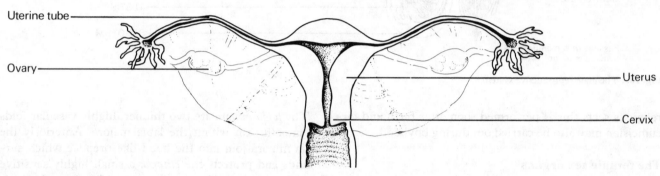

Fig. 16.4 Uterus and appendages

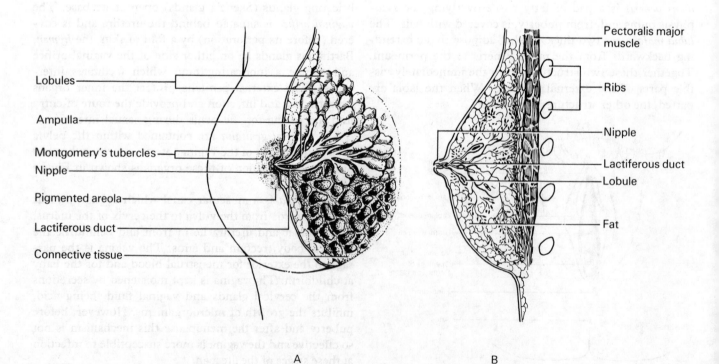

Fig. 16.5 Structure of the female breast A. Front B. Side

from the ovary after ovulation and allow spermatozoa to enter the ampulla of the tube for fertilisation to take place. If fertilised, the ovum embeds in the lining of the uterus and, if not, is discharged in the menstrual flow.

The ovaries themselves are small almond-shaped structures lying in the fold of the broad ligament, attached to the uterine tube and the uterus. The ovaries have two main functions: to produce ova and to manufacture the female sex hormones, oestrogen and progesterone.

The breasts (Fig. 16.5) are accessory organs to the female reproductive system and their function is to produce milk after childbirth. The breasts lie on the anterior chest wall between the second and sixth ribs and are circular in outline, ending in a central prominence called the nipple. This is a highly sensitive erectile structure, surrounded by an area of loose pigmented skin called the areola. The size of the breasts vary, enlarging at puberty and in pregnancy and often atrophying in old age. They are formed of glandular tissue surrounded by fat, each breast consisting of 15 to 20 lobes divided into smaller lobules. These consist of numerous alveoli connected by ducts. Milk is secreted from the alveoli into the ducts and these join to form the lactiferous tubules which open on the surface of the nipple. The process of lactation (milk production) is under the control of the hormone prolactin. This is released after labour, causing first the secretion of colostrum and then of milk. Lactation is sustained by the stimulus of the baby's sucking at the breast.

Sexual intercourse

Sexual intercourse is of course the ultimate function of both male and female reproductive systems. As already pointed out, it deliberately need not result in conception. It involves penetration of the penis into the vagina and, because of friction between the penis and the wall of the vagina, the male ejaculates seminal fluid into the vagina. Ejaculation occurs because of a spinal reflex; it results from contraction of the smooth muscle of the epididymis, vas deferens, seminal vesicles and prostate which causes discharge of seminal fluid into the urethra. A couple of million sperms enter the woman's vagina with each ejaculation and they pass through the cervix to enter the uterus. Despite the very large numbers of sperms, usually only one fertilises the female ovum.

In order for penetration to be achieved the penis must be erect and the vagina must be accessible and lubricated. Erection is the male's response to sexual arousal; it results from a spinal reflex, but is also influenced by impulses from higher centres in the brain. When a female is sexually aroused there are increased vaginal secretions. For both partners to reach this state of readiness for intercourse, there is usually a period of foreplay.

This involves certain types of stimulation which arouse the man and woman to a state of excitement with the result that coitus is more likely to be successful and enjoyable. Kissing, touching of the body's erogenous zones, stimulation of the breasts by the man and handling of the sexual organs of the partner are common components of foreplay. Face-to-face intercourse (the man on top of the woman) is the position most commonly adopted. This allows easy insertion of the erect penis into the vagina and permits stimulation of the sensitive areas (the glans penis and clitoris) with the man's thrusting movements while the penis is in the vagina. The most popular alternative position used is face to face with the woman sitting or lying above the man. Other possible positions include lying side by side and various forms of rear entry.

The duration of intercourse is dictated by the speed with which the male achieves orgasm ('climax'). For most men, ejaculation is reached within a couple of minutes after penetration (although it can be voluntarily delayed). Ejaculation is followed by loss of erection and temporary impotence.

In women the cause and effect of orgasm are less obvious but it is thought that clitoral stimulation and distension of the vagina by the penis are the important factors. Female orgasm tends to be a less defined and less inevitable event than the male sexual climax and it often takes couples considerable practice and patience to achieve mutually satisfying intercourse.

As sexual intercourse is an energetic activity, demands are placed on the cardiopulmonary system; there is an increase in heart rate and rate of breathing, and there may be increased sweating.

The female fertility cycle

The main events in this cycle during the fertile years are menstruation, pregnancy and the menopause.

Menstruation occurs periodically from the time of the menarche which in the U.K. occurs around 13 years of age until the menopause at 45 to 55 years, usually ceasing only during pregnancy. The menstrual cycle ensures the regular release of a ripe ovum and the preparation of the uterus to receive this should fertilisation take place.

The normal menstrual cycle is described as a 28-day cycle, from the first day of one period to the first day of the next. Although the length of the cycle varies between individuals, ovulation always occurs at a fixed point, namely, 14 days before the next period. The menstrual cycle is controlled by the ovarian hormones which are secreted under the influence of the gonadotrophic hormones (the follicle stimulating hormone, FSH; and the luteinising hormone, LH) from the anterior lobe of the pituitary gland of the endocrine system.

At the beginning of the cycle, the FSH is secreted, it activates the Graafian follicles (in the ovarian cortex) to produce oestrogen to ripen the ova. The LH causes the follicle to rupture and the ovum to be released. This is the event of ovulation. At this time, oestrogens stimulate the cervical glands to produce extra mucus which aids fertilisation by protecting the spermatozoa from the acidity of vaginal secretions and by helping their passage through the cervix.

The remaining cells of the Graafian follicle proliferate to form the structure called the corpus luteum. In addition to continuing to secrete oestrogen, this produces progesterone which thickens the endometrium of the uterus ready for the ovum to be received if fertilisation takes place. If this does not happen, the corpus luteum shrinks and the endometrium is shed.

The menstrual cycle therefore comprises a series of events and is often described as having four phases:

1. The *menstrual phase* lasts from 3 to 7 days and involves the endometrium disintegrating, and being shed, accompanied by bleeding from the proliferation of supplying blood vessels.
2. The *proliferative phase* occurs after a brief resting time following menstruation, the level of oestrogens rises again due to the action of FSH and the endometrium begins to proliferate. Ovulation takes place at the end of this phase.
3. The *secretory phase* is when the corpus luteum develops and progesterone is secreted to cause further endometrial growth.
4. The *regressive phase* involves a further increase in the vascularity of the endometrium and a reduction in the levels of oestrogen and progesterone. This is the 'premenstrual phase'.

These phases and the main events of the menstrual cycle are illustrated in Figure 16.6.

Pregnancy is most often suspected on the basis of a missed menstrual period. Although some 350 ripened ova are produced during a woman's fertile years, only two or three on average are allowed to be fertilised to result in pregnancy. Pregnancy lasts about 40 weeks and the expected date of delivery is calculated as 9 calendar months and 1 week from the first day of the last normal menstrual period.

In the early weeks of pregnancy breast tenderness and enlargement, nausea and vomiting, and fatigue are commonly experienced by the woman. Pregnancy tests can be done to confirm the diagnosis of pregnancy. These are based on the fact that human chorionic gonadotrophin (HCG) is produced by the placenta and excreted in the mother's urine.

Later, positive signs of pregnancy become established. Fetal heart sounds can be heard on auscultation and fetal parts felt by examination from about the 24th week.

After the 12th week the enlarging uterus becomes palpable abdominally. The growth of the uterus is the most overt sign of pregnancy, along with changes which occur in the breasts. The nipples and areolae darken in colour and the sebaceous glands (called Montgomery's tubules) become more noticeable. From the 16th week or so, small amounts of colostrum sometimes can be expressed from the breasts.

In addition to changes within the reproductive organs, many other systems of the body alter in adaptation to pregnancy. The cardiovascular system increases its capacity, a 30% increase in blood volume occurring by the 30th week. With this the haemoglobin concentration may fall and iron and folic acid supplements to prevent anaemia may be prescribed. Due to the action of progesterone the veins become relaxed and varicose veins and haemorrhoids may develop. Extra oxygen is needed for the fetus and pregnant women breathe more deeply to obtain this. It is now established that cigarette smoking can diminish the oxygen supply to the fetus via the placenta and so smoking is strongly discouraged (p. 144). Black (1984) in her report of a small study said that individual support was essential to help pregnant women to stop smoking. From other research she reports that the risk of spontaneous abortion was doubled in smokers, but the most common consequence was a lower birth weight of the babies compared to those of non-smokers. The urinary system has to cope with the increased volume of fluid and so the rate of glomerular filtration rises. Increased frequency of micturition is common in the first and last trimester of pregnancy. Progesterone acts on the digestive tract to relax smooth muscle and this can cause the discomforts of heartburn, indigestion, nausea and constipation.

There is no need to increase greatly the amount of food taken but a balanced diet is essential for the health of the mother and the growth of the fetus. Protein, calcium and vitamins are important constituents of the diet at this time. Alcohol is discouraged and the fetal alcohol syndrome is mentioned on page 178. As the body shape alters during pregnancy, posture and gait change and the tendency to exaggerate the lumbar curve often results in

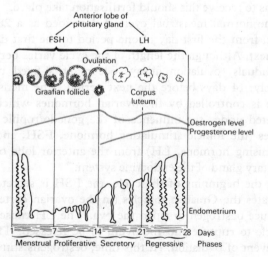

Fig. 16.6 The menstrual cycle

backache. The skin also shows changes with pigmentation occurring on the areola of the breasts, the linea nigra (midline of the lower abdomen) and sometimes the face (called chloasma, 'the mask of pregnancy'). The skin of the abdomen and breasts becomes stretched and marks (striae gravidarum) appear on these areas.

All pregnant women are advised to have regular pre-natal care to help them maintain good health and to enable the early detection and treatment of complications. This care is provided by the family doctor or a midwife and obstetrician at a maternity hospital and includes preparation of the mother and her husband for the birth and the postnatal period. Increasingly husbands are being encouraged to participate throughout pregnancy and most hospitals allow fathers to be present at the birth if the couple wish this.

After pregnancy the reproductive organs gradually return to their non-pregnant state and regular menstruation recommences within 3 months or so of delivery. Because the time of the first ovulation cannot be predicted, contraception should be practised whenever sexual relations are resumed as a further early pregnancy is undesirable.

The menopause most commonly happens around the 50th year of life, but can occur at any time between the ages of 45 and 55. The menopause marks the cessation of ovarian function and the loss of the capability to conceive and reproduce. Discontinuation of the monthly periods is sometimes sudden but more often is gradual with a lengthening of the intervals between periods.

Like puberty, this is a time of hormonal change and imbalance and there are often temporary emotional and physical disturbances. Symptoms can be experienced such as hot flushes, insomnia, palpitations, sweating, vertigo, headache, depression, irritability and fatigue. These result from the decrease in the levels of the sex hormones and can be exacerbated by the woman's distress, albeit at a subconscious level, that she has reached the end of her reproductive life. Loss of libido at the menopause is not uncommon but the physical changes which occur do not in fact reduce a woman's potential to experience normal sexual feelings and to achieve orgasm and sexual satisfaction.

Control of fertility

The availability of contraceptive techniques means that it is possible to control fertility and this allows couples to plan the timing and number of pregnancies as they wish. Advice about contraception and contraceptive supplies is widely available in the U.K. within the N.H.S. Alternative facilities also exist, for example the Brook Advisory Centres which cater particularly for unmarried men and women.

In countries where overpopulation is a problem, for example in India, the governments are active in promoting family planning services and educating people about the importance of birth control.

A wide variety of contraceptive methods is available and some of the most commonly used are described below.

The pill is a hormonal method of contraception. The 'combined pill' (oestrogen and progesterone) works by inhibiting ovulation. It is taken orally and is the most reliable method of contraception available today. There is a small risk of thrombosis associated with prolonged use, and it is now thought that the degree of risk increases with age and in women who smoke. Hamilton & Hamilton (1980) describe the risks in detail.

An injectable long-term contraceptive. Depo-provera, has been the cause of much controversy about its safeness. In response to this, Wigington (1981) reviewed the research findings on its action, side-effects, and use in 65 countries — many of them in the third world. Some governments have reconsidered their ban on this contraceptive and the current position in the U.K. is that as from May 1984 it can be used as a 'last resort contraceptive' (Sadler, 1984), as long as the laid-down precautions, which are given in the article, are observed. Nurses in other countries will need to check the current regulations regarding Depo-provera.

A morning-after pill can be used by those who have had unprotected sexual intercourse but this form of contraception must be supervised by a doctor or a family planning clinic. One pill is taken as soon as possible and the other 12 hours later and they must be taken within 72 hours of the intercourse before the fertilised ovum has had a chance to implant in the uterus. Such treatment is useful in cases of rape.

The diaphragm is a barrier method used by the woman and is a rubber cap which covers the cervix and thereby creates a mechanical barrier between ova and spermatozoa. It is inserted into the vagina before intercourse and removed not less than 6 hours afterwards. There are no harmful side-effects to consider, although some women find the diaphragm a distasteful and bothersome method. It is reliable if used correctly with a spermicidal cream.

The sheath is a male barrier method and is a cover fitted over the penis to prevent the semen entering the vagina. It is a reliable method if the sheath is put on prior to any genital contact and if care is taken to prevent leakage on removal. Reliability can be improved if used in conjunction with a spermicide and the sheath may give some protection to the partner if one of them suffers from a sexually transmitted disease.

The intra-uterine device (IUD) is a device inserted (by a doctor) into the uterine cavity through the cervix. *In situ* it prevents the successful implantation of a fertilised ovum in the endometrium. It is a reliable method and requires no special preparation by either partner prior to intercourse, although for a variety of reasons it may not be the most suitable method for some women to use. Hawkes (1981) confirms this; she reports the surgical removal of an IUD which had perforated the wall of the uterus. Her experience in a gynaecology unit leads her to say that more care should be used in considering the suitability of women for having an IUD fitted.

The 'rhythm' method also called the calendar method involves abstinence from intercourse during the female's fertile time of the menstrual cycle. The time of ovulation is estimated from records of the woman's menstrual cycle or, more accurately, from recordings of body temperature. The temperature rises after ovulation and there should be abstention from intercourse for 7 days prior to the earliest recorded temperature rise and for 5 days afterwards. The method requires high motivation on the part of both partners and is not reliable because the time of ovulation can vary unpredictably.

Sterilisation is a permanent method of contraception, completely reliable in the majority of cases, and often the ideal method after a couple have completed their family or do not wish to have any children. Male sterilisation is called *vasectomy* and involves the division of the vas deferens to prevent spermatozoa reaching the urethra. The operation is performed under local anaesthetic and has no adverse effects on the production of semen or on sexual sensation and performance. It takes some time for the semen to become completely void of spermatozoa and another contraceptive method must always be used until tests of the ejaculate indicate that it is clear. Female sterilisation, *tubal ligation*, is usually performed under general anaesthetic and is effective immediately. It involves the division of the uterine tubes to prevent ova reaching the uterus.

The effectiveness of a particular method, apart from the IUD and sterilisation, depends largely on the correctness of its use. Choice of method must be based not only on the degree of reliability ensured but also on the couple's preference about which method is most appropriate to them and their needs. People's feelings about contraception can be very complex indeed. Their decision to use contraception and which method to choose is influenced by the nature of their relationship, attitude to sex, desire to have or not to have children, knowledge about sex and contraception, family upbringing and religion.

Abortion is the termination of a pregnancy and it can be accidental or induced. Many pregnancies terminate spontaneously during the first trimester, most of these due to fetal malformation or some abnormality in the mother. Vaginal bleeding during pregnancy is the cardinal sign of a threatened abortion.

In the U.K. the 1967 Abortion Act permits termination of pregnancy up to the time (the 28th week) when the fetus becomes viable. Due to improved neonatal intensive care, some infants born before this date have survived so

if possible induced abortion is carried out before the 12th week of pregnancy. As well as medical reasons for carrying out abortion, there may be social and psychological reasons. The politicoeconomic aspects of abortion are discussed on page 303.

LIFESPAN: EFFECT ON EXPRESSING SEXUALITY

The lifespan component of the model of living is intimately connected with the AL of expressing sexuality. Already several aspects of this AL relating to infancy and childhood have been mentioned and a summary of the development of sexuality throughout the lifespan is given in Table 16.1. Adolescence can be a period of experimentation in expressing sexuality. Both male and female adolescents may well have more knowledge of biology than of human relationships and this can lead to unhappy sexual relations. Shy adolescents may believe the extroverts who brag about their sexual conquests, and develop feelings of inadequacy and constant anxiety, which may cause them to experiment simply to be like their peers. The relatedness of the ALs is demonstrated by mention of adolescent clothes and hairstyles at the AL of personal cleansing and dressing (p. 210), and choice of work at the AL of working and playing (p. 277), but they are also aspects of expressing sexuality. Late adulthood, that is from 45 to 64 years can be another turbulent period on the lifespan. Coping with hot flushes at the menopause (p. 299) may have an effect on how a woman expresses sexuality, for example she may need to wear lighter clothes, or a jacket which can be easily removed. The familiar term 'middle age spread' may have some basis in fact because some people's weight does increase and this probably results in a negative feeling about sexual attractiveness. Those who feel dissatisfied about expressing sexuality may begin to fantasise about sexual gratification and this can lead to behaviour resulting in separation, divorce or termination of a longstanding relationship.

FACTORS INFLUENCING EXPRESSING SEXUALITY

In the model of living, factors which influence each AL were considered and they are particularly applicable to expressing sexuality. The five factors — physical, psychological, sociocultural, environmental and politicoeconomic — will now be considered.

Physical factors
The stage on the lifespan is obviously an important physical factor in the AL of expressing sexuality and it was mentioned previously (p. 293). The discussion of normal

Stages in the life-span

	Pre-natal	INFANCY (0-5 years)	CHILDHOOD (6-12 years)	ADOLESCENCE (13-18 years)	YOUNG ADULTHOOD (19-30 years)	MIDDLE YEARS (31-44 years)	LATE ADULTHOOD (45-64 years)	OLD AGE (65+)
PHYSICAL SEXUAL DEVELOPMENT	DETERMIN-ATION OF SEX	Growth of sex organs. Sex differences in body build, appearance and rate of growth		♂ PUBERTY ♀ MENARCHE	Continuing sex differences in body build and strength. Completion of development of secondary sex characteristics	Changes of pregnancy ♀	MENOPAUSE ♀	Physical and hormonal changes may cause decline in libido and potency
PSYCHO-SEXUAL DEVELOPMENT		Establishment of sexual orientation (masculine/feminine)		Consolidation of sexual self-image	Development and modification of sexual self-image and attitudes towards sex, sexual relationships, sexual behaviour and sex-related roles and functions			
SEXUALITY and SOCIAL ROLES		Sex differences in roles and functions within family, school and community settings.			Sex differences in family roles: ♂ as FATHER ♀ as MOTHER Sex differences in social roles Sex differences in occupational roles			Decreasing differentiation of role and function according to sex
INTERPERSONAL/ SEXUAL RELATIONSHIPS		Mainly confined to FAMILY relationships	Friendships with same and opposite sex	Homosexual liaisons Heterosexual friendship and partnerships	ESTABLISHMENT AND DEVELOPMENT OF ADULT SEXUAL PARTNERSHIPS — Temporary liaisons or long-term mateship/marriage (heterosexual or homosexual)			Possible loss of sexual partner through death
SEXUAL BEHAVIOUR		EARLY SELF-STIMULATORY SEX PLAY		MASTURBATION Various forms of non-coital behaviour with same and opposite sex	ADULT SEXUAL BEHAVIOUR PATTERNS Attracting/courting behaviours Self-stimulatory activities Sexual intercourse			Possible decline in sexual behaviour and in libido
SEXUAL REPRODUCTION				CAPABILITY FOR EJACULATION AND FERTILISATION ♂ CAPABILITY TO CONCEIVE ♀	♂ CAPABILITY FOR EJACULATION AND FERTILISATION OF FEMALE ♀ CAPABILITY FOR CONCEPTION AND REPRODUCTION (i.e. FERTILE)			♀ incapable of conception after menopause

Table 16.1 Summary of aspects of the development of sexuality throughout the lifespan

development during each stage of the lifespan in Chapter 4 is also relevant here.

The body structure and function most usually associated with this AL is the reproductive system but equally important is a fully functioning nervous system, sensory system and musculoskeletal system because they are so closely associated with many of the activities which are included in the AL of expressing sexuality.

Overt expressions of sexuality can be seen in the patterns of physical contact which occur in interpersonal communication and interaction. The extent to which bodily contact occurs between individuals depends very much on the nature of their relationship. The mother-infant relationship involves very close physical contact, perhaps the closest being in breast feeding. However as the child grows, the mother engages in less and less direct bodily contact especially towards adolescence when the child's awareness of sexuality is developing. There is a certain amount of physical contact between children of the same sex, but little between adults of the same sex. It is extensive in the husband-wife relationship but, in contrast very limited between adults of the opposite sex who are not in any close relationship.

Jourard (1966) studied patterns of physical contact occurring between people in different kinds of relationships. He showed that the amount of bodily contact is closely related to the degree to which the relationship involves sexual affiliation. Clearly there is a taboo on touching areas of the body which have a sexual connotation when the individuals concerned are not in a sexual relationship.

As so many systems are involved in the AL of expressing sexuality, it is not surprising that some people do not have the necessary physical attributes required for expressing sexuality in the usual ways, whether the condition is congenital or acquired. More is said in the second part of this chapter about how these people can be helped to express sexuality — which, it must be stressed again, is much more than sexual intercourse.

Psychological factors

The intellectual and emotional development as discussed in Chapter 4 in relation to the various stages of the lifespan is clearly relevant to the AL of expressing sexuality. A minimum level of intelligence is necessary for learning about the body and how it functions; the changes that can be expected at puberty and how to cope with them; human relationships; close relationships with people of the same and opposite sex; the social norms concerning courting; contraception; pregnancy; childbirth and rearing a family.

Attitudes to expressing sexuality are developed during early years. Children who are reprimanded for example for touching the genital area or masturbating may develop a negative attitude to this part of expressing sexuality.

Beliefs are also important and those who believe that expressing this AL is pleasurable and natural, will behave accordingly. At the other end of the spectrum of beliefs are people who believe that sexual intercourse is only for procreation and they will only indulge in it when a child is wanted.

Although modes of sexual behaviour are shaped as well as restricted by particular customs, individuals can still exercise considerable control over the ways in which they wish to express their sexuality.

Heterosexuality. Preference for heterosexuality is the norm for the majority of adults. For those who are involved in a heterosexual relationship, various factors influence how the partners express their sexual drives and achieve a mutually satisfying sexual relationship. There is now much greater understanding of the nature of sexual relationships as a result of research investigation, notably the work of Masters and Johnson (1966, 1970). Such work has helped to clarify what constitutes 'normal' sexual behaviour.

In Western societies, married couples engage in intercourse about two or three times a week on average, although individual variation is great. The age of the husband tends to influence the frequency, a decrease being common from several times a week in the early 20s to once a week in the 60s. With advancing age there is a progressive increase in the length of time and amount of stimulation necessary to produce an erection, a decrease in the duration of complete erection and in the capacity for multiple orgasms. Sexual responsiveness varies with changes in physiological condition and, for example, extreme physical tiredness inhibits libido and potency.

Many women experience cycles of increased sexual desire according to their pattern of menstruation. There may be decreased libido during the menopause and in later life. Some societies prohibit sexual intercourse during menstruation, pregnancy and lactation.

Homosexuality. Sexual attraction to a person of the same sex has existed through the ages and is found in all societies. It has been treated in different ways at different times, ranging from acceptance and understanding to hostility, ignorance and sometimes imprisonment. In Western countries today there is a trend towards a greater enlightenment and acceptance of the right of consenting adults to have a homosexual relationship if that is their wish. Preference for homosexuality is much more common than many people imagine. Fong (1978) notes that the Kinsey Report indicated that as many as 37% of men and 13% of women had had a homosexual experience leading to orgasm by the age of 45, that probably up to 10% of the adult population remain exclusively homosexual and that about half of all unmarried men over the age of 35 are homosexual. Many homosexuals are also married and have children; homosexuality is not an absolute state but a sexual orientation on the continuum which ranges from exclusively heterosexual to exclusively homosexual.

Transsexuality. There are a few people who, even in childhood feel that they have been mysteriously born into the sex opposite their actual body structure (Bradshaw & Issa, 1981). Transsexualism has as its central feature disturbed gender identity and the transsexual not only dresses and acts like a person of the opposite sex but usually wants to have surgery and treatment to make the body like that of the opposite sex; although this may not be possible. Transvestites on the other hand, although they dress in clothes of the opposite sex for sexual gratification, do not generally wish to belong to the opposite sex.

Sociocultural factors

Throughout the world similar forms of expressing sexuality are used to attract a sexual partner. Physical appearance plays a role of considerable importance in this, although there are no universal standards of sexual attractiveness. Clothes and hair styles, perfumes, make-up and adornments are also used to enhance sexuality. Elaborate rituals and symbolism usually accompany courtship, and romantic love is displayed by songs, love letters and presents.

Individuals learn to adopt the norms and mores of their society through the process of socialisation. Parents influence the child's sexual development from an early age; femininity or masculinity can be encouraged by the particular choice of clothes and games, and demonstrated by the sexual behaviour of the parents themselves. School education further shapes the child's developing concept of sexuality by reinforcing the attitudes of society towards sex and the respective roles and functions of men and women. Gradually the child begins to learn society's expectations of how men and women should behave and what overt expressions of sexuality are permissible.

Each society has its own code of sexual behaviour based on cultural values, norms, attitudes, morals and laws. While universal regulations prohibit some particularly undesirable sexual relationships such as incest and adult sexual intercourse with children, most societies have their own laws delineating the forms of sexual partnerships which are acceptable. In Western civilisation the monogamous marriage is the norm whereas in other parts of the world, polygamy (two or more females married to one male) is practised.

Some religious rites and some cultural customs result in members having a positive perception of themselves as man/woman. To give but a few examples, all orthodox male Jews are circumcised shortly after birth; female circumcision is still practised in some parts of the world (p. 309), and some cultures have a rite-de-passage to demarcate childhood from adulthood this usually coinciding with the time when the individual becomes physically capable of reproduction.

Environmental factors

Perhaps the only specific aspect of this AL which is influenced by environmental factors is related to physical sex. In the West people in their own homes most commonly associate the bedroom with the central act of expressing sexuality. When the parents and children have separate bedrooms, children can become curious on hearing sounds, coming from the parent's bedroom. Whether or not they voice this curiosity, and if they do, how the parents deal with it may well influence developing attitudes to expressing sexuality. Separate bedrooms for the children, or at least separate beds can influence masturbating habits. However, sometimes from choice and sometimes because there is no alternative, all members of the family may sleep in one room, either separately or huddled together. It is thought that the huddling together can predispose to incest (Young, 1981).

Politicoeconomic factors

It is evident that economic factors influence expressing sexuality. Take for example the money spent on clothes, make-up, shaving requisites and sanitary protection. Contraceptives are subsidised in many countries, and in some are provided free, and in some of those countries where overpopulation is a problem, surgical sterilisation is offered free.

The term 'legal abortion' is acceptable in many countries and its opposite 'illegal abortion' is a punishable offence. Acts of Parliament usually define these terms. Currently in the U.K. there is controversy about the upper time limit for a legal abortion: although the period of 28 weeks is on statute, so also is the term 'child capable of being born alive'. With improved prenatal and obstetric care a few babies born at 22 weeks have survived. Finch (1984) says that the alarming conclusion is that neonates are being treated differently according to whether or not they are 'wanted'. The article gives a clear account of the complicated law as it relates to abortion in the U.K.

Another politicoeconomic factor pertains to abortions — whether termination is easy or difficult to procure in a particular area; whether or not it is free at the time of termination, that is, provided by a national health service, or only available on payment of a fee.

In many countries there are laws regarding permissible sexual relations. Homosexuality was mentioned and in this context it is fair to say that in many countries it is no longer a criminal offence to have a sexual relationship with a consenting adult of the same sex. Incest on the other hand is usually a criminal offence which may well be a reason for under-reporting its occurrence (deChesnay, 1983). The most usual form is between father and daughter but it can be between an adult male family member and a boy, and more rarely between a mother and son. Rape also comes into this category, but the number of victims who report the occurrence to the police is thought to be many less than the number of offenders. Some local authorities contribute financially to special centres organised by women to give help to rape victims.

As part of the model of living, the factors influencing expressing sexuality can be seen to have many dimensions and they show very clearly the complexity of this activity.

DEPENDENCE/INDEPENDENCE IN EXPRESSING SEXUALITY

In the context of the AL of expressing sexuality, the dependence/independence component of the model of living has relevance to the lifespan, another component of the model. Children's dependence is for guidance in development; for knowledge — not only to understand their current individual development but also to anticipate what they can expect will happen in their development at later stages of the lifespan. They are dependent on protection from sexual assault and need to understand the undesirability of going with strangers without impeding the development of friendliness. It has to be borne in mind that when incest does come to light it is often a shock because the offender was above suspicion. Independence can only be achieved by having adequate knowledge and experience; only then can adults trust young people to behave independently according to the attitudes and beliefs acquired in the early years.

By definition, the mentally handicapped are slow to learn and therefore may not be able to achieve independence in some aspects of this AL, as one would expect of people with greater intellectual ability. For example, adolescent girls who are mentally handicapped may not be able to be independent in relation to coping with menstruation, and young adults may be unable to make independent decisions about the appropriateness of a marriage or about the need for, and type of, contraception.

For different reasons, some people who are physically handicapped may not achieve independence for all aspects of this AL. They have the intellectual ability to understand their situation, but lack the physical ability to carry out what they wish to do: for example, to manage a date or accomplish sexual relations or use contraceptives in the way able-bodied people can.

INDIVIDUALITY IN EXPRESSING SEXUALITY

It can be seen from the discussion so far that there are several dimensions to each of the components of the model of living which can influence the acquisition of individuality in expressing sexuality. Since the purpose of the model is to describe how a particular person develops individuality in relation to expressing sexuality, what follows is a résumé using its components.

Lifespan: effect on expressing sexuality
— development of masculinity/femininity in childhood
— puberty in adolescence
— menopause in middle years

Factors influencing expressing sexuality
- Physical   — physical contact in relationships
       — physical disability
- Psychological   — intelligence
       — attitudes negative/positive
       — beliefs
       — sexual preference
- Sociocultural   — permissible expressions of sexuality behaviour to attract sexual partner
       — monogamy/polygamy
       — male/female circumcision
       — rite de passage
- Environmental   — parental bedroom
       — children: own bedrooms, own beds
       — family sleeping in one room
- Politicoeconomic   — money for toilet articles clothes sanitary protection
       — law relating to contraception abortion incest rape

Dependence/independence status in expressing sexuality
- Children need guidance/knowledge
- Mentally, physically handicapped may be dependent for some aspects of this AL

Expressing sexuality: patients' problems and related nursing activities

In the field of health care the subject of human sexuality is being included in the curriculum and sex is no longer the taboo subject which once it was. But even though doctors and nurses are beginning to acknowledge that illness and hospitalisation may cause sex-related problems, some are still reticent about discussing them openly with patients. Talking with patients about sexual problems is not easy; it requires tact, sensitivity, tolerance and knowledge. Perhaps most important, it requires a nurse to be comfortable about his/her own sexuality and at ease when discussing sex-related topics with others.

Those nurses who do experience anxiety and embarrassment when discussing explicit sexual matters such as homosexuality, masturbation and sexual deviance, can be helped to overcome these difficulties. Two articles describe the sexual attitude restructuring (SAR) process, which can be used to accomplish change from a negative to a positive attitude towards sex and sexuality (Linken et al, 1980; Llewelyn & Fielding, 1983).

Most Activities of Living continue to be performed even if in a modified way after admission to hospital. The patient continues breathing, and eating and drinking; and perhaps with more emphasis than usual he performs personal cleansing activities. Communicating, a two-way process between nurse and patient, becomes a most important activity in orientation to the new and unfamiliar environment; the AL of maintaining a safe environment becomes crucial. But what happens to the AL of expressing sexuality? A patient does not cease to be 'male' or 'female' but the significance of this characteristic is not always acknowledged in the context of a hospital ward and this may result in problems for the patient.

The purpose of the process, an integral part of our model for nursing is to provide a method whereby nurses can carry out an individualised nursing plan of those activities which are nurse-initiated and related to the patient's AL of expressing sexuality. Of course there are nursing activities derived from the doctor's prescription and possibly the physiotherapist's, and the radiographer's if the patient is to have radiotherapy to the sex organs, and maybe the dietitian's if the appetite is severely affected; and the carrying out of any of these delegated nursing activities is also influenced by the patient's individuality.

The initial assessment is the means by which the patient's individuality is identified. It involves collecting certain biographical and health details as well as information about the patient's ALs; by observing the patient, family and friends and asking relevant questions. This is supplemented by appropriate information already written on health records, and when applicable, from other members of the health team. From all this information the nurse will become aware of the patient's previous routines in the many activities which make up the AL of expressing sexuality; what can and cannot be done independently in expressing sexuality, and if there is a longstanding problem such as paraplegia, how expressing sexuality has been coped with.

While collecting this information nurses will find the résumé under the heading 'Individuality in expressing sexuality' (p. 304) useful, and it will be helpful to bear in mind the following questions:

- what factors influence the way in which the individual expresses sexuality?
- what does the individual know about expressing sexuality?
- what is the individual's attitude to expressing sexuality?
- has the individual any longstanding problems with expressing sexuality and if so, how have these been coped with?
- what current problems (if any) does the individual have with expressing sexuality, and are any likely to develop?

When the reason for admission directly concerns the reproductive system, explicit information about several intimate aspects of this AL will need to be collected at the initial assessment. After this the nurse will, in discussion with the patient (and partner where appropriate), identify and agree about the current problems and their priority (if any) for which realistic and achievable short- and long-term goals will be set. A date will also be written for evaluating whether or not the goals are being or have been achieved.

There then has to be discussion about the necessary nursing interventions and any activities which the patient agrees to do to achieve the goals and these are written on the nursing plan in sufficient detail for a nurse reading them to be able to carry out the planned nursing. A large part of daily nursing consists of implementing the plan, together with further assessing and evaluating of the patient. Evaluating can only be as good as the goal setting, so it is imperative that the goals are set out clearly and in unambiguous terms. All these activities take into account the patient's individuality which is the basis for individualised nursing.

Before nurses can begin to think about individualised nursing they need to have a generalised idea of the sort of problems which can be experienced by patients with regard to the AL of expressing sexuality. These, as already mentioned, are likely to be different when the patient's reason for admission is directly related to this AL. The problems will be discussed under the following headings:

- change of environment
- change in mode of expressing sexuality
- change of dependent/independent status for expressing sexuality
- discomforts associated with expressing sexuality

CHANGE OF ENVIRONMENT

In normal life people have developed individual ways of expressing sexuality and it is only when faced with change that they might realise the inappropriateness of continuing some of these in a hospital ward. For example, a person may enjoy sleeping in the nude and even changing such a simple habit adds yet another difficulty in getting off to sleep. But by far the biggest problem for most patients is embarrassment and there are many ways in which, if the patient's individuality is appreciated, nurses can help to prevent or minimise embarrassment.

Embarrassment

In doctor–patient and nurse–patient interactions there is violation of the normal social taboos on touching which are closely associated with patterns of sexual affiliation (p. 302). The intimate nature of many medical and nursing procedures can consequently cause much embarrassment and confusion for both patients and staff.

In helping patients with the ALs of personal cleansing and dressing, and eliminating, nurses see patients' bodies exposed, and they handle body parts normally kept discreetly covered. If, for example, a young female nurse is bedbathing a middle-aged man both parties may experience a sense of embarrassment. Understanding that embarrassment is a natural reaction to being in a relationship which disregards normal social taboos can help to ease the uncomfortable feelings experienced. The patient will be reassured if the nurse deals with such situations tactfully and sensibly, acknowledging the mutual embarrassment and helping the patient to maintain dignity and privacy. Nurses soon become accustomed to this aspect of their professional role, but should never forget that patients find intimate procedures disarming and embarrassing.

The vaginal examination is an example of an intimate medical procedure which few women manage to undergo without some anxiety and embarrassment. The woman's genitals are exposed and handled in a way which totally violates the usual codes of allowed physical contact. She may be confused by the sexual overtones of the examination and Moyes (1977), in an article discussing women's reactions to the internal examination given at the prenatal booking clinic, emphasises that such confusion need not arise if the encounter is not seen in sexual terms. However, as she points out, this means that the medical reason for the procedure must be explained clearly to the patient.

Sometimes the anxiety is caused because the woman is afraid she may be unable to allow entry of the speculum (the instrument used to open the vagina) or that the procedure may be painful or damaging. Recognising these natural fears should help the doctor and nurse to prevent undue embarrassment. In preparation for the procedure nurses should appreciate the importance of their explicit explanation concerning its nature and the reason for it being done. During the procedure nurses can convey their empathy by such acts as keeping the patient covered as much as possible.

Lack of opportunity

The restriction which hospitalisation places on normal sexual expression must be seriously considered when long-term care is necessary. A child in hospital for a considerable length of time will be less able to master sexual development if not given opportunities to express normal sexual feelings of childhood and to engage in the usual sex-related games and roles. An adolescent may experience frustration at being cut off from his peers and unable to satisfy sexual desires by normal self-stimulatory activities such as masturbation, unless given opportunities for privacy.

Long-term hospitalisation for an adult can seriously disrupt the continuity of a sexual relationship. The patient and partner may suffer from loneliness and, if abstinence from sexual intercourse is prolonged, loss of libido and even severe dysfunction may result. If appropriate, such patients should be given opportunities to go home from time to time so that social and sexual relationships can be resumed and sustained.

Attitudes towards the sexual needs of the mentally ill and the mentally handicapped in the past have been most restrictive and, in institutions for those people, the practice has been to deny patients any opportunity for expressing sexuality. Somehow it was thought that 'madness' and 'imbecility' rendered a person 'sexless' or sexually dangerous. Gradually it is being realised that it is desirable to allow sexual expression and that mental impairment does not preclude achieving enjoyment from sexuality.

Helping patients to cope with their sexuality and behave in a socially acceptable way is an important aspect of care of the mentally handicapped. These people, like all others, need to be helped to understand how their bodies work and that changes in their bodies and emotions are a normal part of sexual development. For example, instead of being punitive towards patients who masturbate openly in the ward, the nurse can teach them that this is a normal form of sexual behaviour, but should be done in private.

Like all human beings the mentally handicapped are capable of forming and maintaining relationships with others. More and more hospitals now encourage male and female patients to mix together in occupational and recreational activities. This requires nurses to help them to learn about normal social patterns of interaction and it is obvious that the patients enjoy opportunities to behave as adult males and females do in everyday life. It is becoming common practice in hospitals for the mentally handicapped to ensure that female patients are protected from unwanted pregnancy by teaching them about sex and by employing contraception. This removes the anxiety that social integration of patients may have undesirable consequences and encourages the patients themselves to appreciate that adult sexual behaviour carries with it serious responsibilities.

CHANGES IN MODE OF EXPRESSING SEXUALITY

A person may encounter difficulties associated with expressing sexuality at any stage of the lifespan and for a great variety of reasons. However, the majority of disabled people and many of those who suffer certain kinds of physical disease or disfigurement are particularly prone to experience sexual difficulty.

Physical disability

People can be disabled in many different ways. It is probably true to say that most people's perception of disability is associated with musculoskeletal conditions, or people who are chairfast from whatever cause. Here, disability will be discussed under the headings, Sexuality and disablement; Attitudes to sexuality and disablement; and Helping the disabled who have sexual difficulties.

Sexuality and disablement

Wells (1982) gives an extended review of a book by Bullard & Knight (see Additional suggested reading) in which several disabled people express their views on their sexuality needs, the problems which they have in satisfying these because of disability, and how they have achieved satisfaction by physical and psychological adaptation. Contributors include a blind person, a deaf person, an arthritic person, a young nurse of 22 who had a radical vaginectomy; and people with spinal cord injuries, cerebral palsy, head injuries, stoma formation and many other conditions. This list is a useful introduction to the wide range of disabling conditions.

All the contributors to the book viewed themselves not only as human beings but as sexual human beings with the same needs as those who are not disabled. They describe their struggle to maintain or achieve a sexual identity; and emphasise that the issue of a normal sex life is much more complex than erection, penetration and orgasm. These aspects of sexuality assume secondary importance to touch, closeness, alternative methods of satisfying a partner and establishing a lasting relationship thus making it clear that sexual intercourse is only a small part of the whole AL of expressing sexuality. The book states emphatically that society has no right to 'de-sexualise' an individual just because he is disabled, and that it has a duty to think in terms of 'sexualisation' for those with

disabilities from birth, and of 're-sexualisation' for those whose disabilities occur after satisfactory sexualisation has been achieved. There is advice on how to make sexual intimacy a meaningful part of the love-making ritual, for example removal of a leg caliper, or the clothes of a paraplegic person, by the partner.

With such a wealth of information about first-hand experience of problems encountered by people with very diverse physical disabilities, nurses will be challenged to be creative in helping patients to achieve alternative ways of participating in relationships so that they not only express their love, but also feel loved.

Campling (1980) thinks that female sexuality as such is less well attended to in the literature. She says that sexuality exists for everyone and cannot be dismissed because of crutches, wheelchairs, scars or spasms. She quotes Anna Freud: 'Sex is something we do, sexuality is something we are', and an unnamed woman as saying 'Sex may end in the penis, but it starts in the mind.' Campling thinks that the need to be more open and experimental can lead disabled couples to discover a range of touching, positions and pleasures which ablebodied couples might never discover. Disability can have the effect of forcing a couple to be completely honest with themselves and with each other, leading to that 'exchange of mutual vulnerabilities' which Masters & Johnson saw as central in loving relationships.

Attitudes to sexuality and disablement

Sometimes, however, able-bodied people feel repulsed by the idea of the physically handicapped wanting to have sexual relations and even wishing to have children, or by the notion that unconventional modes of sexual activity may need to be used for sexual satisfaction. Anyone with such thoughts would do well to read the book so aptly called *Entitled to Love* (Greengross, 1976) in which the sexual needs and problems of the disabled are discussed with frankness and sympathy, making it clear that many of the problems would be alleviated by a more humane and informed attitude of society.

Helping the disabled who have sexual difficulties

Difficulties of children. A child disabled from birth needs the help of his parents and the encouragement of others to allow sexuality to develop as naturally as possible and to find ways of sexual expression compatible with the handicap. Difficulties will almost certainly arise if the child's sexuality is ignored and, in the course of answering questions and giving information about sex and reproduction, it may be helpful for the special difficulties and needs of the child to be acknowledged and openly discussed. A girl who has to wear an artificial limb may be helped to feel feminine despite this if special attention is paid to her personal appearance and once she begins to menstruate, she may need advice to help her cope realistically with anxieties about the effect of her disability on relationships and reproductive function.

For an adolescent boy confined to a wheelchair, masturbation will provide an outlet for sexual frustration and he should be reassured, if anxious, that this is an absolutely normal activity. Throughout adolescence it is essential for girls and boys who are physically disabled to have opportunities to mix with able-bodied people of the opposite sex and as far as possible, like them, learn to enjoy and come to terms with their own sexuality.

Difficulties of adults. A person who becomes physically disabled in adulthood may have major readjustments to make in the sphere of sexuality depending on his previous level of sexual activity and his feelings about how physical disability may affect sexual function. The disability may be the result of a sudden event, such as a road traffic accident causing the loss of a leg, or the result of a stroke causing paralysis or it may signify the onset of a chronic disabling illness such as multiple sclerosis or rheumatoid arthritis.

The person's sexual difficulty may be the direct result of the physical disablement, perhaps difficulty in coping physically with sexual intercourse, or it may be predominantly psychological, for example a feeling of worthlessness or fear of rejection by the partner. The disability does affect both the person and the partner, sometimes drastically altering their relationship if, for example, the person affected is forced to give up work. Many people too find it difficult to be both nurse and lover to a disabled spouse. A man may, as a result of direct damage to the central nervous system, have difficulties associated with erection or ejaculation (p. 297) or both. If the disability is accompanied by recurring or persistent pain this can cause loss of libido for a person of either sex.

If pain is a cause of difficulty, as for example the pain affecting joints in rheumatoid arthritis, the person could be advised to take analgesics prior to attempting intercourse. Sometimes too, a warm bath in advance may add to relief of pain. Adopting a comfortable position is essential. For full sexual satisfaction the glans penis and the clitoris must rub against each other (p. 297). The conventional 'man-on-top' position may not be the most comfortable or effective and very practical help can be given to couples about alternative positions for intercourse. A complete erection and full penetration of the penis are not essential for ejaculation and a great deal of exertion is not necessary for the achievement of an orgasm. If erection is impossible, a man may wish to try using a penile prosthesis, one of the many available sex aids. There is nothing weird or wrong about people trying out any of these possibilities. The important thing is that the solution to difficulties must be acceptable to both partners.

Physical disease

For those people leading a sexually active life, any one of the wide variety of physical diseases is likely to be accompanied by a temporary loss of interest in sex. Should the disease be acute and temporary in nature it is highly likely that libido will be restored as the illness subsides and the patient's previous sex life will be able to continue at its previous level.

But there are diseases, like those affecting the heart, which are associated in patients' minds with sexual difficulties even although this is frequently unjustified and due simply to lack of knowledge. Other diseases, for example diabetes, can affect body function in such a way that sexual function becomes impaired. And, understandably, patients undergoing surgery or treatment related to the sex organs may anticipate encountering sexual difficulties. These are some examples of perceived and actual difficulty associated with physical disease and they have been selected for discussion here.

Difficulties associated with heart disease

Most people are aware that intercourse makes considerable demands on the cardiopulmonary system and so patients who have suffered a heart attack or have a chronic cardiac condition such as hypertension (high blood pressure), not surprisingly are fearful about the possible harmful effects of resuming normal sexual relations. It is true that sexual intercourse involves considerable activity and exertion. The pulse rate may rise from around 70 to as high as 180 beats per minute, the blood pressure from 120 to over 250, and the respiratory rate from 16 to more than 40 per minute.

However, there is general agreement among cardiologists that sexual activity is compatible with heart disease as long as the patients know how to assess their ability and identify warning signs of heart strain. Roper, Logan & Tierney (1981) provide guidelines about the kind of advice which nurses could give to a male postcoronary patient. Intercourse can usually be resumed within a few weeks, readiness for this assessed on the patient's ability to perform exercises of comparable physical exertion. For example, the 'stair-climbing test' (two flights of stairs at a brisk rate) is a good form of assessment. The patient needs to be advised of warning signs of heart strain: a rapid pulse and respiration rate persisting 30 minutes after intercourse; palpitations 15 minutes after; chest pain during or after; exhaustion following intercourse or extreme fatigue on the next day. Advice on when to avoid sexual relations can also be given and abstinence recommended: soon after a large meal or drinking alcohol; in extremely hot or cold environments; in an anxiety-provoking situation; and if strenuous activity is anticipated after intercourse.

Nurses and doctors see fit to give heart patients every sort of advice — from dietary needs to whether gardening will be too strenuous for a while — but advice about sex is given less frequently. This is probably thought to be the least of the patient's many concerns; and the patient probably feels too embarrassed to ask, thinking it trivial if the subject has not been raised for him. Much of this misunderstanding and anxiety could be avoided if advice and discussion about sexual activity were given to patients as routinely as other subjects concerning rehabilitation and this is becoming more common particularly in coronary care units.

Difficulties associated with chronic respiratory disease
A person suffering from a chronic respiratory disease such as emphysema (alveolar distension resulting in oxygen insufficiency) is likely to experience difficulty with sexual intercourse due to dyspnoea (p. 150). It is not easy to alleviate this problem due to destruction of the lung tissue and the person may be advised to consider finding alternative ways of obtaining sexual satisfaction which do not involve physical exertion with which the cardiopulmonary system cannot cope. The discussion on page 308 is relevant to these patients.

Difficulties arising from diabetes
Men who have had diabetes for a number of years, particularly those whose condition has not been kept well stabilised, may experience difficulty with erection and ejaculation. Erection is particularly affected because the diabetic condition affects the autonomic nerves, especially the parasympathetic supply (Felstein, 1979).

Sometimes female diabetics experience a loss of sexual interest or strength of orgasm. Achieving better control of the diabetic condition may overcome these difficulties.

Difficulties anticipated after surgery/treatment to sex organs
Not uncommonly men in the middle and older age groups require to have a *prostatectomy* (removal of the prostate gland) and it is not surprising that many of them have anxieties about the effect on sexual functioning. Patients can be reassured that impotence is rare in men who were previously sexually active.

Savage (1982) brings together some of the little information that is available on the effects of gynaecological treatments on female sexuality. In the article there is a good description of females' sexuality in general, and the possible conveyance of nurses' non-verbal messages which discourage patients from raising problems concerning sexuality.

Sexual self-image can be influenced in a negative way by post-radiation changes. Fear of damage to skin which is red and scaling may lead to avoidance of sexual intercourse. Savage points out that because gastrointestinal mucosa is especially sensitive to radiation there may be limitation on oral-genital or oral-anal sexual activity.

Loss of vaginal elasticity can shorten and narrow the vagina, and together with pelvic fibrosis make male penetration painful. Patients can be helped to avoid this by being advised to either resume sexual activity or mechanically dilate the vagina and insert oestrogen cream.

Research quoted by Savage (1982) should remove any doubt about women needing help, advice and information regarding what to expect after surgery/radiation to sex organs. In one study 22 out of 28 patients presented major vaginal alterations and impairment of sexual function after treatment with deep X-ray for cervical cancer. Fear of recurrence was given by four women as a reason for sexual abstinence. Three male partners reported that they had stopped having intercourse because they no longer found it satisfying, while 10 spoke of changes, although they were unable to describe them. In preparation for allocation to a gynaecology ward, nurses would benefit from reading the article.

Currently in the U.K. the Prohibition of Female Circumcision Bill is going through Parliament. Female circumcision is practised in over 20 countries mainly in Africa and the Middle East. There is usually excision of the clitoris, the labia minora and majora but the extent of cutting varies from country to country. In Sudan the resulting wound is stitched up and only a small opening is left for the passage of urine and menstrual fluid — so-called 'infibulation'. It prevents male penetration, but the woman is 'opened up' ready for the wedding night and traditionally friends do this.

In Britain there are ethnic groups who practise female circumcision. Midwives, in particular, meet circumcised women who need extensive episiotomies before delivery — sometimes laterally as well as horizontally — and afterwards some wish to be re-stitched as they would not feel 'feminine' if this were not done. Circumcised women can also be admitted to the wards suffering from urinary tract infections, urinary retention, vaginal infections, bleeding, labial cysts and vaginal calculi (Graham, 1984), all of which can cause difficulties with the AL of expressing sexuality.

For many women, *hysterectomy* (removal of the uterus) may mark a positive turning point in sexual function with relief from problems such as heavy bleeding and the final removal of fear of pregnancy. Some women however experience symptoms known as the 'posthysterectomy syndrome' even when the ovaries have been conserved. The ovaries have an endocrine function and among other substances secrete androgen which is thought to be the basic hormone of libido (Savage, 1982). The symptoms are similar to those of the menopause and they can cause difficulty with some aspects of expressing sexuality. Nurses should be especially observant for any signs of undue fatigue and depression. If the patient reports loss of libido and dyspareunia it should be reported to the doctor.

Physical disfigurement

Being and feeling physically attractive is a fundamental feature of any person's sexuality and an important aspect of sexual relationships. Western society places great emphasis on beauty and physical perfection. Any disfigurement such as a facial birth mark, burn, operation scar, physical malformation or loss of a limb, alters a person's sexual self-image. This may cause a man or woman to fear that they may be unable to attract a partner, be regarded by others as sexually unattractive or even be rejected by their spouse.

Difficulties after stoma surgery

Stoma surgery (p. 200) results in a form of permanent physical disfigurement. There is usually no physical reason to cause a loss of interest in sex or in the capacity to enjoy sexual intercourse. However, difficulty in accepting the stoma may lead to psychological difficulties about sex and even to impotence. Couples may simply need reassurance that sexual relations can be resumed without harming the stoma or they may need very practical advice on how to conceal the bag, prevent leakage and odour, and perhaps an alternative position for intercourse. Conception, pregnancy and childbirth are all possible for women who have had stoma surgery.

Difficulties after breast removal

The removal of a breast (mastectomy) is an example of a physical disfigurement which causes tremendous anxiety to a woman. The procedure is usually performed as treatment for cancer and fear about this adds to the patient's anxieties.

Breast cancer manifests as a lump in the breast; if found in its early stages it may be cured. For this reason women are encouraged to examine the breasts routinely. Self-examination of the breasts (Fig. 16.7) should be carried out once a month immediately after menstruation. Any lump, change in shape, puckering of the skin or change of skin colour should be reported to the doctor immediately.

Harwood (1983) reports an evaluation of teaching 50 female staff in a hospital and 50 nurses to examine the breasts monthly. During the course of one year 10 women returned to the occupational health department having detected a change in the breast, and of these, two were confirmed as cancer. At the end of the year 50% of the non-nursing staff continued to examine the breasts monthly whereas only 20% of the nurses did so. There is obviously room for improvement related to nurses examining their breasts each month — Figure 16.7 illustrates how this can be done.

In the Southampton breast study (Nichols 1983), 2% of those who developed cancer were under 45 years of age; 22% were 45 to 64 and 61% were in the 65 + group. Based on this information it is evident that monthly ex-amination of the breasts needs to be a lifelong preventive activity. The earlier breast cancer is treated, the better the outlook.

Radical mastectomy, involving removal of the whole breast and the axillary lymph nodes, is a mutilating operation sometimes followed by gross lymphoedema of the arm. It is thought that this might deter women from seeking help in the early stages of any change in the breast. Currently there is increasing interest in local removal of the tumour (lumpectomy) followed 2 to 3 weeks later by irradiation then by iridium wires threaded into the base of the breast for 2 to 3 days. It is hoped that this less mutilating operation which leaves the majority of breast tissue intact will encourage women to report any change in the breast immediately (Ellis, 1981).

The chairman of the Mastectomy Association (West-gate, 1981) gives excellent advice about what mastecto-mees can do to help patients come to terms with loss of a breast and what can be done in the way of expressing sexuality. For example, mastectomy does not preclude wearing pretty nightdresses and attractive swim suits and nurses should encourage patients to seek satisfaction by these apparently simple activities.

Although being without a breast does not have a direct effect on the mode of sexual functioning, it alters the woman's feelings about her sexuality. The breasts are a recognised sexual characteristic of the female body and after a mastectomy a woman may feel she has lost some of her sexual attractiveness and, indeed, may fear that her husband will be repulsed by the ugly scar. Wearing a breast prosthesis helps to restore the woman's appearance and confidence in public and, coming to terms with her new body image, helps her to cope with her sexual anxieties. In a stable and loving relationship the operation is unlikely to cause any long lasting impediment to shared sexual enjoyment.

CHANGE OF DEPENDENCE/INDEPENDENCE STATUS FOR EXPRESSING SEXUALITY

With an AL which has as many dimensions as expressing sexuality there are many different ways in which there can be a change in a person's dependence/independence status, and it is important to remember that the change can be in either direction. For those born disabled the objective is for them to achieve their optimum 'independence' in each of the activities subsumed in the AL of expressing sexuality. For example McCarthy (1980) after collecting largely anecdotal data from disabled women, reveals that facilitating maximal independence for managing menstruation is a very complex procedure and requires an individual approach to each woman.

Then there are those who, after satisfactory 'sexualis-ation' (p. 307) become disabled as a result of injury or

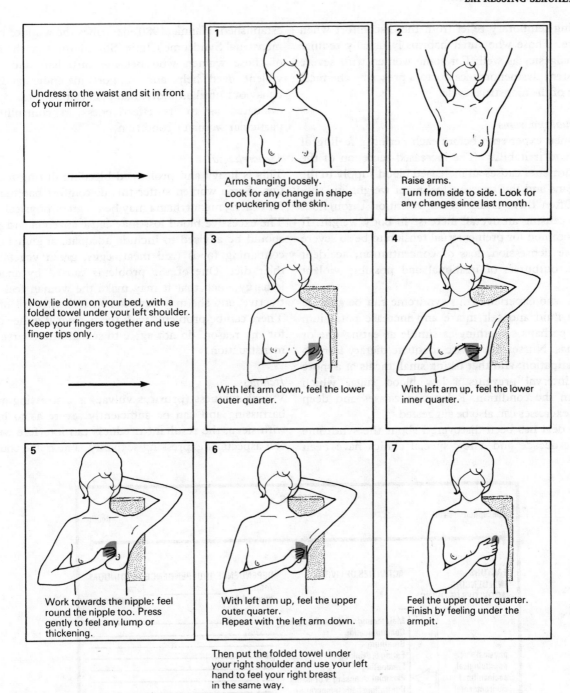

Undress to the waist and sit in front of your mirror.

1 Arms hanging loosely.
Look for any change in shape or puckering of the skin.

2 Raise arms.
Turn from side to side. Look for any changes since last month.

Now lie down on your bed, with a folded towel under your left shoulder. Keep your fingers together and use finger tips only.

3 With left arm down, feel the lower outer quarter.

4 With left arm up, feel the lower inner quarter.

5 Work towards the nipple: feel round the nipple too. Press gently to feel any lump or thickening.

6 With left arm up, feel the upper outer quarter.
Repeat with the left arm down.

7 Feel the upper outer quarter. Finish by feeling under the armpit.

Then put the folded towel under your right shoulder and use your left hand to feel your right breast in the same way.

Fig. 16.7 Self-examination of the breasts (based on an illustration kindly supplied by the Family Planning Association, 27/35 Mortimer Street, London WIA 4QW)

disease so their dependence/independence status for many of the activities in the AL of expressing sexuality changes. These changes can take many forms, some of which are mentioned at 'Helping the disabled who have sexual difficulties' (p. 307), and those who have 'Physical disease' (p. 308), and those who suffer 'Physical disfigurement' (p. 310), together with what nurses can do to help such people.

DISCOMFORTS ASSOCIATED WITH EXPRESSING SEXUALITY

Dysmenorrhoea

This is pain associated with menstruation, either coinciding with the onset of a period or persisting throughout it. Some women find that the pain is relieved by resting, others prefer to remain active. A hot bath is a good way of obtaining temporary relief from the discomfort when it is severe. Those who suffer habitually usually require to take analgesics as well. For some women with severe and persistent dysmenorrhoea doctors prescribe chemical regulation of the menstrual cycle.

Premenstrual syndrome

Some women experience before each period a feeling of tiredness and irritability. The increased secretion of the ovarian hormones causes an increased blood supply to the pelvic organs and this causes a feeling of weight and distension. Often there is also water retention throughout the body, causing an overall increase in body weight. It is not uncommon for premenstrual tension to be so severe as to cause depression, loss of concentration, accident proneness, outbursts of irrational and possibly violent behaviour.

Women who experience this syndrome can be advised to restrict fluid and salt intake and increase potassium intake by perhaps something as simple as eating one or two bananas. Nurses can advise adequate dietary fibre to avoid constipation; and that taking small meals at a more frequent interval prevents a low blood sugar which can worsen the condition. Relaxation classes and deep breathing exercises can also be suggested.

A great deal has been discovered about the syndrome in the last decade and a few special clinics have been established. Hanna (1980) describes the work of one Premenstrual Syndrome Clinic. She advises that the relatives of those women who become turbulent and possibly violent need help and support in understanding the behaviour until an individual plan can be worked out and evaluated as to its effectiveness in controlling that particular woman's condition.

Menorrhagia

This is heavy and prolonged bleeding during menstruation. Some women suffer this discomfort habitually but, for others, menorrhagia may be a sign of physical disease. The excessive blood loss may cause anaemia and patients should be advised to include adequate amounts of iron-containing foods (red meat, eggs, green vegetables) in their diet. One of the problems caused by anaemia is lethargy, such that it may make the woman feel less attractive, and she may have to contend with loss of libido. There can be problems with the partner if either or both, for any reason, do not agree to sexual intercourse during menstruation.

Itchiness

Vulval itchiness (pruritus vulvae) is distressing and embarrassing and can be sufficiently severe as to interfere with sleep: the resultant tiredness can interfere with several aspects of expressing sexuality. The nurse could sug-

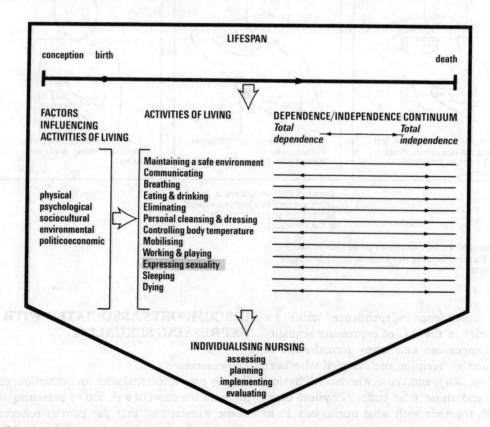

Fig. 16.8 The AL of expressing sexuality within the model for nursing

gest to the patient avoiding tight clothing such as tight trousers, and wearing stockings instead of tights. Frequent washing of the genital area is necessary and only bland soap and talcum powder should be used. Itching can be associated with diabetes, genital herpes or an abnormal urethral or vaginal discharge and the discomfort should always be medically investigated.

Abnormal discharges

Normally there is a discharge of clear or white mucus from the vagina and this thickens and increases in amount just before and after a period and throughout pregnancy. However, there may develop an excessive discharge which causes the woman's underclothes to be permanently wet or one which, when it dries, leaves a green or brown stain. Sometimes the discharge may have an offensive smell. An abnormal discharge may result from infection or perhaps from the presence of a foreign body, such as an unremoved tampon. A discharge which contains blood may indicate a more serious condition, such as cancer in the reproductive tract.

A discharge from the penis may indicate infection and the possibility of venereal disease must be considered. As these are usually contracted during intercourse with an already infected person, they are referred to nowadays as 'sexually transmitted diseases'. Gonorrhoea is common in the U.K. but syphilis is relatively rare. A white or yellow discharge from the urethra, accompanied by an increased frequency of micturition and dysuria, is characteristic of gonorrhoea in the male. Immediate treatment is essential and it is necessary for contacts to be traced and treated in order to prevent spread of the infection.

Dysuria

Sexual intercourse may aggravate dysuria associated with recurrent urinary tract infection (p. 202) and, in addition, the woman's persistent discomfort may be worsened by the act of intercourse. Either reason may mean she is unable to maintain an enjoyable sexual relationship and, indeed, the discomfort may be sufficiently severe as to cause her to abstain from sexual activity altogether.

In addition to advice mentioned previously, the woman should be advised that she and her partner should both wash the genital area prior to intercourse and apply a lubricant jelly before penetration. After intercourse the woman should empty her bladder and take a drink.

Dyspareunia

This is pain actually during sexual intercourse, felt either on penetration or during subsequent movement of the penis in the vagina. The former problem may occur at first intercourse because the hymen has to be completely ruptured to permit entry of the penis or it may be due to soreness from tissue scarring following an episiotomy performed at childbirth, or from tightness of the vagina resulting from inadequate relaxation or dryness due to insufficient lubrication.

Pain felt during intercourse usually means that nearby tissue is receiving pressure, directly or indirectly, and this may occur if the uterus is misplaced (retroverted uterus), or an ovary is enlarged or the rectum distended.

People suffering from dyspareunia should seek medical advice because most of its causes are amenable to medical or psychological treatment, thus enabling the person to resume enjoyable intercourse.

In the second half of this chapter some of the problems and discomforts which can be experienced by patients in relation to the AL of expressing sexuality have been described. This provides the beginning nurse with a generalised idea of these; it will be useful in assessing, planning, implementing and evaluating an individualised programme for each patient's AL of expressing sexuality.

This chapter has been concerned with the AL of expressing sexuality. However, as stated previously it is only for the purpose of discussion that any AL can be considered on its own; in reality the various activities are so closely related and do not have distinct boundaries. Figure 16.8 is a reminder that the AL of expressing sexuality is related to the other ALs and also to the various components of the model for nursing.

REFERENCES

Black P 1984 Who stops smoking in pregnancy? Nursing Times 80(19) May 9:59–61
Bradshaw PL, Issa M 1981 Gender surgery. Nursing Times 77(37) September 9:1595–1597
Campling J 1980 Sexuality and the disabled woman. Nursing Times Supplement August 28:14
deChesnay M 1983 Incest: a family triangle. Nursing Times 79(8) February 23:64–65
Ellis H 1981 Time is of the essence. Nursing Mirror 152(26) June 24: 43–44
Felstein I 1979 When the music goes off key . . . Nursing Mirror 148(8) February 22:16–18
Finch J 1984 The fallacy of time limits. Nursing Mirror 158(20) May 16:24–25
Fong R 1978 Sexual abnormalities 1. Harmless variations. Nursing Times 74(24) June 15:1015–1016
Graham S 1984 The unkindest cut. Nursing Times 80(3) January 18:8–10
Greengross W 1976 Entitled to love: the sexual and emotional needs of the handicapped. Malaby Press, London
Hanna J 1980 Defeating the curse of the calendar. Nursing Mirror 151(14) October 2:36–37
Hamilton D, Hamilton C 1980 Candidates for the pill. Nursing Mirror 150(9) February 28:43–45
Harwood D 1983 Breast self-examination by NHS staff. Nursing Times 79(50) December 14:27–29
Hawkes E 1981 Piercing pain. Nursing Mirror 152(14) April 2:41
Jourard S M 1966 An exploratory study of body accessibility. British Journal of Social and Clinical Psychology 5:221–231
Linken A, Marshall P, Thorpe D 1980 Sexual attitudes factor. Nursing Focus 1(9) May:358–360

Llewelyn S, Fielding G 1983 Sex: more than the facts. Nursing
Mirror 156(11) March 16: 38–39

Masters WH, JohnsonVE 1966 Human sexual response. Little Brown,
Boston

Masters WH, Johnson VE 1970 Human sexual inadequacy. Little
Brown, Boston

McCarthy BP 1980 The management of menstrual flow in disabled
women. Nursing Times 76(10) March 6:409–411

Moyes B 1977 A doctor is a doctor. New Society November 10:289–
291

Nichols S 1983 The Southampton breast study — implications for
nurses. Nursing Times 79(50) December 14:24–27

Power D 1981 Children in danger. Nursing Mirror 152(5) January 29:
29–32

Roper N, Logan W, Tierney A 1981 Learning to use the process of
nursing. Churchill Livingstone, Edinburgh, p. 105

Sadler C 1984 Last resort contraceptive. Nursing Mirror 158(20) May
16:14

Savage J 1982 No sex please, Mrs Smith. Nursing Mirror 154(7)
February 17:28–32

Wells R 1982 The lover. Nursing Times Supplement August 4:8–9

Westgate B 1981 Facts and figures. Nursing Mirror 152(1) January
1:30–32

Wigington S 1981 Depo-Provera: an injectable contraceptive. Nursing
Times 77(42) October 14:1794–1798

Young M 1981 Incest victims and offenders: myths and realities.
Journal of Psychosocial Nursing 9(10) October:37–39

ADDITIONAL READING

Bullard DG, Knight SE (eds) 1982 Sexuality and physical disability,
personal perspectives. Mosby, St Louis

Connell H 1983 More than a physical illness. Multiple sclerosis
management. Nursing Mirror 79(24) June 15:40–41

Hogan RM 1980 Human sexuality in nursing process perspective.
Appleton Century Crofts, New York

Irish AC 1983 Straight talk about gay patients. American Journal of
Nursing 83(8) August: 1168–1170

Lion EM 1982 (ed) Human sexuality in nursing process. Wiley, New
York

Oates JK 1983 Herpes, the facts. Penguin, Harmondsworth

17

Sleeping

The activity of sleeping

All parents can testify to their children asking endlessly 'Why have we to go to bed'? Most parents believe that because children are growing, they need relatively more sleep than adults. Scientists have now confirmed this and have unravelled many other mysteries about sleep, although some still remain. Adults spend about one-quarter to one-third of their lives sleeping so in terms of time alone, it is for everyone an important Activity of Living.

It appears that all living creatures have periods of activity alternating with periods of inactivity and these are governed by the sleep-wakefulness cycle controlled by the hypothalamus. Human beings do not seem to be born with a 24-hour rhythm of sleeping and waking. The recurrence of sleep every 24 hours constitutes a rhythm which the human body has 'learned' through experience. The word circadian describes this learned rhythm, and the term 'biological clock' refers to the mechanism which produces the rhythm. The previous idea that all babies slept for most of the 24 hours is now refuted; each baby is different. In acquiring their rhythm most babies sleep for about 16 hours, at first spread round the clock but by the time they are 3 months old the amount of night sleep has usually doubled.

To include sleeping as an 'activity' is not paradoxical, for although sleep provides the greatest degree of rest, the body systems are still functioning albeit at a reduced level. Sleep has been described as a recurrent state of inertia and unresponsiveness; a state in which a person does not respond overtly to what is going on around him. Although consciousness is lost temporarily, a sufficient new stimulus as from an alarm clock will rouse him. In this respect sleeping differs from the states of coma and anaesthesia which are also discussed in this chapter.

THE NATURE OF SLEEPING

How does one know that a person is asleep? Most people sleep with closed eyes; they lie still for part of the time but they move at intervals throughout the sleep periods; sometimes there is relaxation in the muscles of the face and neck so that the jaw is unsupported and the mouth open; breathing is slower and usually deeper; flaccid muscles in the upper respiratory tract are thought to be responsible for snoring. But what is the nature of this phenomenon called sleep? In recent years, this very question has been exercising the minds of experts in various parts of the world who are conducting research on sleep, and some of the mystery still remains. The writings of a number of researchers are mentioned in this chapter, but most of the references are based on findings from the Sleep Research Laboratory at the University of Edinburgh headed by Professor Ian Oswald who is renowned in this field of enquiry. Although complete answers cannot yet be given to all the queries about sleep, a great deal of information has been collected by recording tracings of the electrical waves from the brains of people who are sleeping — electroencephalograms (EEGs). The information revealed, particularly about sleep occurring in cycles, has helped in understanding the nature of sleeping.

The sleep cycle

Each sleep cycle is approximately 90–100 minutes in duration and there are usually four to six cycles in a person's normal sleep period (Oswald & Adam, 1983). Each sleep cycle can be described as having five stages which are now generally recognised (Fig. 17.1).

Stage 1. The sleeper has just 'dropped off'. There is a general relaxation; there are fleeting thoughts, and the sleeper can be wakened by any slight stimulus. If awakened, the state is remembered merely as one of drowsiness; it is not described as sleep. But if not interrupted, the next stage is entered after about 15 minutes.

Stage 2. There is greater relaxation, and thoughts have a dream-like quality. The sleeper is unmistakedly asleep but can be wakened easily.

Stage 3. This stage usually occurs after 30 minutes of sleep. There is complete relaxation and the pulse rate slows as do most other bodily functions. Familiar noises such as a flushing cistern do not usually waken the sleeper. If undisturbed, the next stage follows.

Stage 4. The sleeper is relaxed, rarely moves, is difficult to waken, and is in a 'deep sleep'. If sleep-walking occurs, or if there is enuresis, it occurs at this stage. (Sometimes Stages 3 and 4 are referred to as slow wave sleep or SWS because of the large, slow waves seen on the EEG tracing.)

Stage 5. This is a period of light sleep during which dreaming occurs and the eyes move rapidly back and forth giving the name Rapid Eye Movement (REM) sleep to this stage. Stages 1 to 4 for obvious reasons are called Non Rapid Eye Movement (NREM) sleep. A baby's sleep has more REM than NREM stages; with increasing age there is less REM sleep. If awakened during the

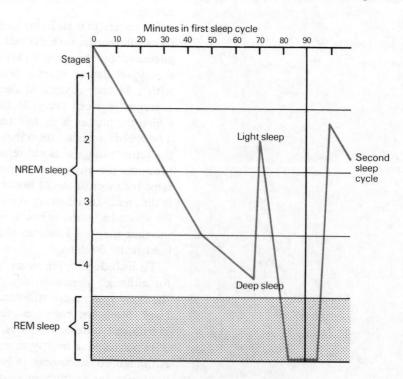

Fig. 17.1 A sleep cycle

REM stages people may report vivid dreams full of action. It is thought that dreams promote psychological integration; it is as if they update memory and integrate emotionally meaningful experiences with those of the past. The REM stages are relatively longer in the later cycles of any one sleep period and the duration of stages 3 and 4 relatively longer in the early cycles.

Although everyone has those sleep cycles, there is considerable variation in the length of time which people will spend sleeping and in what is considered sufficient sleep.

The sufficiency of sleep

It is difficult to say what constitutes sufficient sleep although it is known that adults have an average sleep time of 7–8 hours per night. It would seem however that a sleep debt can be built up over time which can be compensated by a longer than usual sleep period. After deprivation, stages 3 and 4 deficit is made up before REM sleep deficit, and for this reason some writers refer to NREM sleep as 'obligatory'. In one study, in an attempt to discover the effects of sleep loss, experimental volunteers were kept awake for over a week at a time. As well as having difficulty in performing certain tasks it was found that they had a strong tendency to fall asleep yet seemed to be able to maintain semi-automatic activity such as walking while they slept; a point which highlights the danger of continuing to work while short of sleep at jobs which carry risk for the worker and for others. In some instances bizarre hallucinations also occurred after extreme sleep deprivation. It would seem however that the 'effects of sleep loss are not only evident after extreme deficits; fine effects can be detected after as little as 2 hours deprivation' (Wedderburn & Smith, 1980).

To go to the other extreme, 'extra' sleep has not been shown to improve performance. A researcher, quoted by Wedderburn & Smith, gave people extra sleep after they already had a long night's sleep, and found that their performance on some tasks was worse after 'excessive' sleep.

It is difficult to say what 'lack of sleep' and 'extra sleep' mean because a small group of people have been identified who require only about 2 hours of sleep each night and these healthy non-somniacs appear to enjoy a happy and constructive lifestyle (Meddis, 1977). It would seem that each person learns a circadian rhythm of sleep which thereafter is governed by an inbuilt 'biological clock'. During the day however there is a related cycle — the ultradian cycle — which appears to be related to restlessness.

Restlessness and resting

Even in non-sleep time, alertness and drowsiness can come and go according to a 100-minute ultradian rhythm. Generally people are so involved in what they are doing or the people they are with that they are unaware of the rhythm but on their own, in a dull or boring situation, research has shown that individuals 'become more restless and less restless about every 100 minutes' (Oswald & Adam, 1983). It is interesting to ponder on the states of restlessness and resting.

The state of resting incorporates the art of relaxation, both physical and mental, although it is now a common belief that as the pace of living has greatly increased, there is less time for relaxation, and man has become less skilled in the art. In recent years, a growing interest in, for example, yoga and transcendental meditation may be indicative of a renewed public awareness of the value of relaxation and rest. Often the term relaxation is used to describe pleasurable activities such as sport or reading or art usually as a change from the daily work routine but sometimes involving a great deal of activity. The relaxation of yoga however is claimed to be not a change but a resting period, a cessation of activity, a complete 'letting go' permitting refreshment of body and mind. Authorities on yoga believe that 20 minutes of yoga can bring greater benefits than hours of sleep (Lathlean, 1980). By whatever means it is achieved, it would seem that there is a link between the 100-minute rhythms of resting and sleeping.

THE PURPOSE OF SLEEPING

Sleep researchers are by no means in agreement about the purpose of sleeping. Oswald (1983) supports the restorative theory, that sleep promotes the restoration and growth of all body cells. REM sleep seems to be particularly associated with brain cell renewal and maintenance; and Stages 3 and 4 of the sleep cycle with repair of other parts of the body. Wedderburn & Smith (1980) report that in babies there is more of both types of sleep but in adults it has been found that there is additional REM sleep following unusually emotional episodes, whereas there is more Stages 3 and 4 sleep after intense physical exercise. It is not yet clear how this is accomplished but there seem to be changes in protein synthesis and circulating hormones. The adrenal gland releases adrenaline, noradrenaline and corticosteroids in large amounts during wakefulness but only in small quantities during sleep and among other things, these hormones inhibit the formation of new protein in tissues. When asleep, the relative absence of adrenocorticosteroids, and the presence of other hormones, especially the growth hormone and testosterone promote renewal of body tissue. Of course these activities are only part of a complex chemical and enzymatic system controlling the body's renewal and restoration, which is not yet fully understood.

There are however a number of other theories about sleep. Some writers consider that the function of sleep might simply be energy conservation. The decreasing amount of sleep taken in old age might therefore be due to the decreasing metabolic rate and energy usage associated with advancing years (Canavan, 1984). Another theorist has suggested that sleep is merely an instinct — a genetic hangover from an earlier era when secluded inactivity at night alternated with daytime activity as part of a survival strategy (Meddis, 1977).

LIFESPAN: EFFECT ON SLEEPING

The component of the model called the lifespan is certainly relevant when considering sleeping. This AL is affected by age both in terms of duration and quality.

Not only do the young require more sleep than adults, as already stated, but their sleep has relatively more Stages 3 and 4 sleep in which the growth hormones are secreted, and this is not surprising in view of their rapid physical growth. They also have relatively more REM sleep which is understandable because of the vast amount of brain development and learning in the early years of life. Babies sleep for about 16 hours each day split into 6 to 8 sleep periods but gradually there are longer periods of sleep, mostly at night, and longer periods awake. By the age of 4, the average child sleeps for 11 hours each night, perhaps with an additional short day-time nap. However although babies and toddlers seem to spend quite a lot of time asleep, waking problems in young children are not uncommon. Richman (1983) found that about 20% of children in their second year waken regularly at night. The wakefulness can be related to factors within the child, or stress and tension within the family, but sometimes it is due to parental overresponsiveness to wakefulness which in fact, reinforces the pattern.

By the age of 15 years, most people have a sleep period which, on average, is of 7-8 hours' duration. Healthy adolescents and young adults usually sleep so well that little will disturb them. However as these same sound sleepers become middle-aged they may complain of insufficient or broken sleep, especially the women (Oswald, 1980).

In general, the older person, according to Adam (1980) sleeps for a shorter period than the young and it is more broken by periods of wakefulness; it also contains relatively less REM sleep. She describes an interesting study of 212 healthy people aged 65-93, carried out in the U.S.A., which found that by the age of 75, the older person (and no difference was found between males and females) spends more time in bed, though not necessarily asleep, and had more naps than younger people; and that by age 85, there was an increasing use of sedatives probably indicating more difficulty in falling asleep. It would seem that the over 85s require more rest and sleep. In this study, 92% of these healthy elderly believed that they got the right amount of sleep.

FACTORS INFLUENCING SLEEPING

Like all other ALs sleeping is influenced by a variety of factors. In keeping with the relevant component of the model, these are described under the following headings — physical, psychological, sociocultural, environmental and politicoeconomic factors.

Physical factors
Some physiological functions are closely related to sleeping. As far as circadian rhythms are concerned it appears that the 24-hourly cycle of light and dark is one to which most species synchronise their bodily rhythms. During a 24-hour period there is a cycle of many physiological functions such as heart rate, metabolic rate, respiratory rate and body temperature all tending to reach maximum values during the late afternoon and early evening, and minimum values in the early hours of the morning (Hawkins & Armstrong-Esther, 1978). Perhaps this would be expected. Most people are active during the day and asleep at night. There is evidence that these internally controlled rhythms are timed to synchronise with external cues and when the harmony is upset for example by travelling rapidly across time zones, there is desynchronisation which manifests itself as fatigue, malaise, lassitude and inability to make effective decisions — the syndrome known as jet-lag. The period varies with the individual, but it usually takes about 3 to 7 days to correct jet-lag and get body time and sleep time back in harmony (Smith & Wedderburn, 1980). It used to be thought that the same mechanism applied for shift workers but this is now questioned (see politicoeconomic factors p. 320).

Physical exercise may affect sleep. Children enjoy a great deal of exercise during their waking hours, and although overstimulation may, on occasion, prevent them from falling asleep quickly, exercise usually induces sleep and may contribute to their sleep having relatively longer periods of Stages 3 and 4 sleep when the growth hormones are secreted in large amounts. It has been shown too that after exercise, athletes have more Stages 3 and 4 sleep, and even adults taking more exercise than usual will secrete more growth hormone from the pituitary gland during the succeeding sleep period, thus facilitating maximal protein synthesis and restoration of the body cells (Oswald & Adam, 1983).

Eating certain foods and drinking certain beverages is also said to affect sleep. There is a popular belief, for example, that cheese and coffee cause disturbed sleep. Although there does not seem to be much evidence about cheese perhaps there is some justification for condemning coffee — unless it is the decaffeinated variety. Two cupfuls of coffee (300 mg caffeine) have been found to cause disturbed sleep in old people whereas a group of researchers found that a milk and cereal drink, Horlicks, led to less wakefulness when compared with nights when a placebo pill was taken (Brezinova & Oswald 1972). However Oswald & Adam subsequently concluded (1983) that although milk and proprietary food drinks, being easily digestible sources of nourishment, probably are helpful in inducing sleep their effect should not be exaggerated. The effect of a change in the pattern of food and fluid intake at bedtime is more important than the actual type of food/drink taken.

Some people consider that alcohol helps them to sleep. This belief may be true if taken in moderation especially if related to a pattern of fluid intake as a bedtime beverage but it has been shown that alcohol produces a lighter sleep pattern with more awakenings (Whitfield, 1982). There is certainly evidence of disturbed sleep, and indeed bad dreams, when there is withdrawal from alcohol dependence. When calorie intake affects weight, it has been found that the change in weight affects sleep. As obese people lose weight, they sleep less; and when patients with anorexia nervosa are regaining weight, they sleep longer and REM sleep is increased (Adam, 1980).

Snoring may affect sleep although it is the listener who is kept awake. Snoring may be indicative of a number of pathological conditions so should not be dismissed lightly but it may have no known cause or cure. Usually any mention of snoring is greeted with hilarity but in fact it can be justification for divorce in the U.S.A. (Feldstein, 1979).

Psychological factors

The individual's psychological status is linked to sleeping. Mood can be considered as a continuum with excitement at one pole and depression at the other. Transient insomnia caused by excitement has been experienced by most people and may not cause undue distress. The sleeplessness associated with depression may however be severe, and continue over a period of weeks. The depressed person can lie awake for hours dwelling on unhappy themes of hopelessness, and when sleep does come, is easily wakened, only to resume thoughts of rejection and failure, or even suicide. However the primary characteristic of sleep change in depression is early morning wakening; indeed, it is a major diagnostic feature.

Perhaps worry and anxiety rather than excitement and depression are the most common disturbers of sleep. It would seem that people who are worried or dissatisfied with their day-time lives are often worried and dissatisfied with their sleep. Almost everyone has had periods of anxiety and apprehension at some point in their lives even over such episodes as examinations or employment interviews. However Oswald (1980) considers that the individual should be 'protected from over-treatment'. After all, a certain amount of anxiety is inevitable in the process of living.

Dreams are believed by some people to have enormous psychological significance. They certainly have a strange fascination for man. At one time it was thought that the soul departed from the body during sleep in order to mingle with supernatural beings who would provide guidance about the future. The possible symbolism of dreams has also been given considerable credence and reinforced by writers such as Freud and Jung. Cohen (1979) maintains that 'the heart (and soul) of classic sleep research was to attempt to ... establish correlations between specific physiological events and dream characteristics.'

It is now known that dreaming occurs mainly during REM sleep. The researchers assure us that everyone dreams but most are not remembered. The rate of forgetting is remarkably fast. Subjects in the Sleep Research Laboratory in Edinburgh who were wakened during REM sleep recalled a dream in about 80% of cases; wakened 5 minutes after REM sleep, there was only fragmentary recall; aroused 10 minutes later, there was scarcely any recall. So anyone who wakens up recalling a vivid dream, has probably surfaced out of REM sleep. When volunteers were wakened persistently out of REM sleep over a few nights, it was found that they were anxious, tense and irritable; so reduced REM sleep would appear to be linked to mood. Dreams themselves can be frightening, some are bizarre, some are amusing; most are interesting to recount; indeed not uncommonly, dreams are the substance of art, music, drama, and literature.

Whatever the quantity or quality of sleep, the psychological effect of wakening up refreshed or unrefreshed determines a person's belief about being a good or bad sleeper.

Sociocultural factors

Sociocultural factors also influence sleeping. For example they will determine where a person sleeps and with whom. In Western cultures, it is usual to sleep in a bed which is raised up from the floor but in Japan, the bedroll on the floor is traditional; and in some nomadic, ethnic groups it is usual to sleep on the ground in the open, or in a tent or in a hammock.

In Western cultures, it is usual for a husband and wife or a couple who are co-habiting to sleep together in one bed but most other people sleep alone. However in other cultures it is not uncommon for several members of the family (or extended family) to sleep in the same 'sleeping-space' and if they do sleep singly or in couples, it may not be in a segregated personal bedroom; it could be in a room common to the entire family.

Cultural differences can also be identified with regard to what is worn for sleeping. Nomadic Eskimos, for example, wear the same clothes during the day and at night; in other cultures, nightdresses or pyjamas are worn, and for some people are a means of expressing sexuality; for other people the accepted norm is to sleep in the nude.

Some of these sociocultural characteristics related to sleeping do seem strange on first encounter but with the ease of international travel and the popularity of television-viewing, many people know much more about the effect that social and cultural characteristics have on the AL of sleeping.

Environmental factors

Sleep can be affected by a number of environmental factors. Sleep tends to come more easily in a familiar environment — a cool, quiet dark room in surroundings which are well known, with personal belongings at hand and so on. The safety of the environment is also important. A high bed, where there is difficulty getting in and out and anxiety of falling, may disturb the sleep of an elderly or disabled person; and the sleep of parents may be affected when a child changes from sleeping in a cot to sleeping in a bed. People who know they are sleep-walkers may not be able to fall asleep unless they are reassured that windows have been closed, and that objects which potentially could cause accidents have been removed from the immediate environment; indeed some sleep-walkers tie themselves to the bed so that they will wake up rather than sleep walk. People affected by unfamiliar surroundings like a hotel or hospital ward may have to reassure themselves by becoming fully conversant with the fire precautions and the siting of fire escape doors.

Environmental noise may or may not affect sleep. Again familiarity with the environment allows many people to sleep despite for example, the noise of a nearby factory or a busy thoroughfare or an aircraft flight path. Yet these same people may have difficulty falling asleep in a strange environment perhaps because of the sound of the waves on a beach or even by the excessive quietness of a rural setting. Night shift workers may have major complaints about noise when they are attempting to sleep during the day; although if habitually on night shift, many seem to learn to ignore the noise.

Room temperature may affect the ability to fall asleep and to remain asleep. The body temperature actually falls during sleep; there is a slight normal lowering between the hours of 0200 and 0600 which is not surprising because during sleep, there is minimal functioning of the various body systems. However, any further lowering of temperature usually wakens the sleeper, as indeed does any increase. Perhaps to be expected, the climate has an influence, and where there are extremes of climate, attempts are made to control and modify the indoor temperature. In hot climates bedrooms will probably have air-conditioning systems; some are sophisticated and ex-

pensive; others primitive although sometimes amazingly effective. Likewise in cold climates, insulation and central heating systems are used or some other means of providing heat and warmth. The physiological control of body temperature is less efficient in children and the elderly so it is recommended in the U.K. for example that bedroom temperatures should not fall below 18°C during the night.

It is interesting that latitude does not seem to alter sleeping. Within the Arctic Circle, the inhabitants sleep similar hours to us despite experiencing unending daylight in the summer and months of darkness during the winter. In countries where an afternoon siesta is the norm, the people sleep again at night.

The effect of space and weightlessness on sleep is still being researched. During the last two decades there have been spectacular advances in space exploration and data are being collected about the effect of this somewhat novel environment on human sleeping patterns.

Politicoeconomic factors

It may not strike one immediately that the AL of sleeping is influenced by politicoeconomic factors. However any consideration of where people sleep will usually involve housing or a shelter of some kind and certainly in Western culture, this will be related to economic status. The size of the house will influence whether family members have their own bedroom or a shared one, their own bed or a shared one. Some people, however, because of low earning power (for whatever reason), may have to cope with a living space which is grossly overcrowded and the family may have to sleep in the room in which they have lived and cooked all day; there is no choice. For others who would be considered as vagrants it may be necessary, even in a cold climate, to sleep 'rough', exposed to unfavourable weather conditions which endanger health and are certainly not conducive to satisfactory sleep. In some countries the government or voluntary agencies will make provision for such people, usually in the form of communal sleeping accommodation at low cost.

Type of work of course is closely related to politico-economic factors, and during the last few decades, there have been a number of studies about shift work and its effect on sleep. As a rule the 24-hour biological clock makes man fall asleep at night and awaken in the morning, and this reflects the individual's normal body rhythms, with their characteristic low level of arousal at night and higher level during the day. However night shift removes sleeping from the night sequence and out of harmony with body time. Much of the early research on sleep and nightshift work concluded that the body clock would gradually be reset over a period of about 7 nights, and then following a spell of night work, there would be a delayed return to normal. However results of later studies quoted in Smith & Wedderburn (1980) and covering a wide range of variables (including deep body temperature, potassium excretion, adrenalin excretion, blood pressure and reaction time) all show that experienced shift workers demonstrate a flatter than normal night shift curve of these readings on the first night, and that this is retained without much deviation over subsequent consecutive night shifts. It is replaced by a typical day curve on the first full day without night work. So the body clocks of shift workers remain set to 'real' time. Smith & Wedderburn suggest that these findings were made possible because the researchers were able to collect more data; instead of using one or two readings each night, as in the older studies, they used body-borne microchip recorders which collected continuous readings of several variables. They conclude that although shift workers get used to night work, this is because they 'become better at handling the contradiction of being biologically geared to day activity while being required to work at night, and not because they reset their body clocks!' Typically the duration of day-time sleeps after night shifts are short and often, although feeling fatigued, it is difficult to fall asleep. So a sleep debt builds up.

Long hours of work and interruptions of sleep by telephone calls also cause a sleep debt. In a study of young hospital doctors in Cambridge, U.K. and New York, and reported by Oswald & Adam (1983), it was shown that sleep loss caused them to be more easily irritated; they could not react to complexity and could only think of one thing at a time. Shift systems, long hours, interruptions of sleep, indeed any factor which causes persistent sleep loss, has implications for health workers such as doctors and nurses where impairment of performance can affect the safety of the patient as well as the worker. Some occupational groups have strict rules and regulations which limit the length of tiring duties, for example aircrew and long-distance truck drivers. The International Labour Organisation has recommendations for all occupational groups regarding working hours but they are not always implemented.

DEPENDENCE/INDEPENDENCE IN SLEEPING

Unlike some of the other ALs already discussed, each individual is independent for the actual activity of sleeping. Unlike the majority of the other ALs too, this component does not have a direct relationship with the lifespan component. Babies, although helpless for many ALs, spend most of their time sleeping; and the elderly, at the opposite end of the lifespan and sometimes dependent for other ALs, also spend more time at rest in bed or asleep than younger adults. However, while the activity itself is independent, the environmental conditions for sleep are not necessarily so. The infant is dependent on others for maintaining a suitable temperature conducive to sleep, at least by use of clothing if not by control of atmospheric

temperature. The safety of the environment is also controlled by others and there are accidents, sometimes with fatal sequelae because a baby has rolled out of a high bed when asleep, or has smothered in a pillow, or has been overlaid by a domestic pet.

Children and adolescents can also be dependent on others for sleep. If there is prolonged stress or tension in the family they may develop disturbed sleeping patterns (Richman, 1983) and when there is noise, for whatever reason, there may be difficulty in getting to sleep and periods of wakefulness.

The sleep of adults may also be dependent on others, especially in relation to disturbance by excessive noise and particularly if on shiftwork. Perhaps the major concern about dependence in adulthood, however, is related to the use of sleeping pills. A considerable number of people, especially in industrialised countries, are anxious about difficulties with falling asleep and staying asleep for what they believe to be an appropriate period, and they resort to drugs to enhance their own capacity for this AL. The widespread use and abuse of drugs has created considerable problems not only in terms of cost to the taxpayer (if there is a national health service where they are free or heavily subsidised) but also in terms of creating dependence on drugs. It is salutary that studies of people who have taken sleep medications for months or years indicate few beneficial effects in terms of either falling asleep or staying asleep (Canavan, 1984). So it would seem that long-term dependence on sleeping pills is not a satisfactory solution to a person's sleep problem, whatever its nature.

INDIVIDUALITY IN SLEEPING

Individuality is the final component of the model. From the foregoing discussion, it is evident that there are many dimensions in each component of the model which help one to describe how a particular person develops individuality in the AL of sleeping. Below is a résumé of the main points of the discussion.

Lifespan: effect on sleeping
- Length/frequency/type of sleep in infancy and childhood
- Average duration in adolescence and adulthood
- Time in bed/time asleep/wakefulness in old age

Factors influencing sleeping
- Physical   — biological clock
  - length of sleeping period
  - pre-sleep routine
  - time of going to sleep
  - movement during sleep
  - snoring

— wakening during sleep/time/cause
— time of wakening at end of sleeping period
— sex differences
— effect of exercise
— effect of food/drink

- Psychological
  — personal feelings about sleeping
  good or bad sleeper
  refreshed/unrefreshed on waking
  mood on rising
  — knowledge and attitudes
  need for sleep
  dreaming

- Sociocultural
  — sleeping space
  — type of bed/bedding
  — own/shared bed

- Environmental
  — noise/quietness
  — hot/cold atmosphere
  — standard of safety

- Politicoeconomic
  — income/type of housing
  — own/shared room
  — type of work/night duty

Dependence/independence in sleeping
- Provision of conditions conducive to sleep
- Use of sleeping pills

Sleeping: patients' problems and related nursing activities

Sleeping is such a complex activity and highly sensitive to change, so perhaps it is to be expected that when a person is ill, some problems will be encountered, even transiently, in relation to this AL. However, as refreshing sleep is considered to be therapeutic, it is important for the nurse to know about the person's usual habits in relation to sleeping so that this knowledge can be used to devise an individualised plan of nursing and everything possible can be done to induce natural sleep.

In order to individualise nursing, it is necessary to assess the activity of sleeping insofar as it is relevant to the particular person. Assessing involves observing the patient; acquiring information about the patient's sleeping habits partly by asking appropriate questions, partly

by listening to the patient and/or relatives; and using relevant material from available records such as medical records. The nurse would be seeking answers to the following questions:

- how often in 24 hours does the individual usually sleep?
- when does the individual usually sleep?
- where does the individual sleep?
- what factors influence the way the individual carries out the AL of sleeping?
- what does the individual know about sleeping?
- what is the individual's attitude to sleeping?
- how well does the individual sleep?
- has the individual any long-standing difficulties with sleeping and if so, how have these been coped with?
- what problems, if any, does the individual have at present with sleeping or seem likely to develop?

Of course the nurse does not necessarily ask these actual questions because much of the information can be acquired in the course of conversing with the patient.

The collected information can then be examined to identify any problems being experienced with the AL and these can be arranged in some order of priority. The nurse may recognise potential problems which can also be discussed with the patient. Mutual realistic short- and, where appropriate, long-term goals can then be set to prevent potential problems from becoming actual ones; to alleviate or solve the actual problems; or to help the patient cope with those which cannot be alleviated or solved.

Keeping in mind what the patient can and cannot do for himself, the nursing interventions to achieve the set goals can then be selected according to local circumstances and available resources. These interventions should be written on the nursing plan along with the date on which evaluation will be carried out, in order to discern whether or not the stated goals are achieved. Of course, other professional groups such as doctors, physiotherapists, dietitians are usually involved in the care programme and it is important to ensure that the total care of the patient is discussed and mutually agreed. On the Nursing Plan proforma suggested by Roper/Logan/Tierney (p. 352) there is a page for appropriate entries of this type in order to indicate the relationship between nursing interventions derived from medical/other prescription and nurse-initiated interventions.

However, before student nurses can begin to think in terms of individualised nursing, they require a general idea of the conditions which can be responsible for, or can change, the dependence/independence status for the AL of sleeping and which can be experienced by the person as a problem in carrying out the AL. The remainder of this section is a general discussion of the types of patients' problems related to sleeping and the relevant nursing activities. They are grouped under headings which indicate how the problems can arise:

- Change of environment and routine
- Change of dependence/independence status
- Discomforts associated with sleeping
- Altered consciousness.

CHANGE OF ENVIRONMENT AND ROUTINE

There are many reasons for a newly-admitted patient experiencing sleep problems. One major reason may be the strange environment of a hospital ward. Whatever their previous sleeping arrangements, the majority of patients in the U.K. are admitted into an open Nightingale type of ward; some into two-, four- or six-bedded bays, recesses or rooms; and only a minority have single rooms. In many instances a patient has no choice about sleeping in the presence of others.

The hospital bed. The bed itself may be very different. All patients are admitted into a single bed, yet many married couples have been used to sleeping in a double bed. The majority of hospital beds are higher than the divan type of bed used in most homes although new models can be mechanically adjusted. If the height cannot be adjusted, this can be anxiety-producing for those who are not bedfast and who need to eliminate, especially during the night; the nurse can help when she identifies these patients at the initial assessment by discussing their preference for a commode/bedpan/urinal. This information would be written in the nursing plan so that all staff would be informed. Where adjustable height beds are in use, it is important for nurses to remember to lower them before the patient goes to sleep.

Some beds are specially designed. One for example is adjustable so that the sitting position can be maintained during sleep. If it is necessary for the patient to adopt this position because of severe dyspnoea, it is often a relief to be so well supported, and although not a natural position for sleeping, the patient usually adapts reasonably well. Other special beds which may be used by patients include: air, low air loss, water, sand, fluidised sand, mud, bead, net suspension, Ko-Ro, Stryker and flotation beds. Sleeping on these types of beds is 'different' and initially there is a period of adaptation until the patient becomes gradually used to the change. The objective in using them is dispersal of body weight over a greater surface area for the prevention of pressure sores (p. 222). The patient needs to understand why such a bed is necessary and should be encouraged to talk about his reaction to it.

Most people's concept of a bed includes careful selection of a mattress and the choice can be very personal. Hospital mattresses can be sufficiently different to interfere with sleep, particularly on the first few nights.

Apart from the bed itself, hospital bedding can differ from that used at home and patients who experience such a difference may require some time for adjustment. Nowadays many people favour one single covering article for ease of bed-making such as a quilt or a downie. However some people like to feel the weight of bedclothes and therefore choose to use conventional sheets and blankets. Wherever possible, arrangements should be made to interfere as little as possible with patients' preferences and thereby provide the greatest possibility of continuance of good sleeping habits. To this end an increasing number of hospitals offer patients the choice between a quilt and conventional bedding. Waterproof protection of the mattress can make patients restless; if the restlessness is due to the patient feeling hot and perspiring the nurse can offer cooling measures as appropriate; if it is due to discomfort from wrinkling of the waterproof protection, it can either be straightened or removed.

Wearing night attire provided by the hospital is much less common than previously, but just as day clothes are personal and important to one's self-image, so are night clothes and any difference can therefore interfere with sleep. In some cases where night clothes are soiled with excreta or vomit, it is preferable for the patient to wear hospital gowns. In the interests of maintaining morale, it is important that they are attractive as well as comfortable.

Pre-sleep routine. Each patient has been socialised into a pre-sleep routine with an individualised sequence which is necessary for comfort and conducive to relaxation. Many patients continue to be capable of carrying out that routine while in hospital and they should be encouraged to do so.

Information from dependent patients, or their relatives if patients are not able to give it, will help nurses develop a nursing plan which includes pre-sleep routines along lines with which the patient is familiar.

Posture. Depending on the cause for admission to hospital, a changed posture may be necessary, and help may be required to adapt to the change. For example, in the absence of a special bed when a patient has to be nursed sitting up it may be more comfortable to use an adjustable height bed-table with a pillow on it, on which to rest with flexed arms, thus ensuring the best conditions for breathing and sleeping. Lying supine over a length of time for any reason, can cause a feeling of fullness in the abdomen; this can be due to the upper abdominal organs resting against the diaphragm, so slight raising of the head of the bed may allow the organs to slide down a little, relieving the pressure and permitting sleep. Patients with a lower limb on traction are usually nursed in a high bed with the bedclothes arranged in two sections around the elevated limb; such patients may feel more comfortable if a pillow is placed close to each side of the body on which they can rest their arms. When a solution has been found it should be written in the nursing plan so that all staff are informed of these measures for inducing sleep.

Temperature. People who have sleeping problems are often highly sensitive to the environmental temperature. Sometimes however, it is difficult for the nurse to exert any control over local conditions. For example for safety reasons, in a few high-rise hospitals, the windows on the upper floors cannot be opened, so natural ventilation is not possible. Also the heating or cooling system is often controlled centrally and not all radiators have individual heat control mechanisms. In such circumstances, an immediate solution is to make adjustments to night attire and to bedding if patients feel they are too hot or too cold; or to use cooling fans, or adequately covered hot water bottles or an electric blanket.

Noise. In the last few decades, almost everyone has had to become more tolerant to an increase in the noise level from a variety of environmental sources; the term 'noise pollution' is now used and discussed in Chapter 7 in relation to maintaining a safe environment. But even people who appear to enjoy bombardment by noise when well, can rarely tolerate it when they are ill. The night nurse's work can be pre-planned so that noisy trolleys are not needed in the ward after patients have settled for the night, and any procedures which must be performed during the night should be carried out as quietly as possible. Empty beds for possible new admissions can be near the ward entrance so that their occupation will cause as little disturbance to as few patients as possible. The same applies if the death of a patient is expected during the night.

When a patient becomes disorientated at night removal to a single room may be helpful where adequate lighting simulates daytime and lessens shadows which may be the cause of distress; staff can speak normally, as opposed to whispering which is thought to increase the patient's confusion. On the other hand, the patient may be more confused by the move, in which case re-orientation in the ward may be more practical; a short period of disturbance there being preferable for all concerned to a longer one in a sideward.

Light. Many people are very sensitive to and disturbed by even a low intensity of light for sleeping. Night lighting in the newer hospitals is well dimmed and arranged near floor level so that it is below the eye level of patients in bed. If a nurse decides to help a patient to sleep by shading a nearby light, fire safety factors should be complied with; otherwise drawing bed curtains or using a mobile screen may help to intercept the disturbing light.

Disturbance of circadian rhythm. It is useful to remember that there are a few people admitted to hospital who have been working on night duty and they may have problems with sleeping because shift work has altered their sleeping pattern. Also travellers who have passed through time zones can become ill or have an accident and may arrive in hospital before their biological sleep rhythm has been re-established. A study done by Armstrong-Esther & Hawkins (1982) tentatively suggests that elderly people, for pathophysiological reasons such as opaqueness of the eye or reduced function of the pineal gland may be substituting normal exogenous cues related to the sleep cycle for social cues. It is possible, they say, that some elderly may have lost their physical responsiveness to light and dark and come to rely more on social synchronisers. Once these are disturbed by admission to hospital, the elderly patient may have no reliable cues and goes into a state of internal desynchronisation. This state in which the body's rhythms are out of synchrony may be the cause of sleep disturbance, as well as confusion and incontinence, which indeed is often observed in the elderly after admission to hospital. Nurses should be alert to these possible variants when gathering information about a patient's sleeping habits.

CHANGE OF DEPENDENCE/INDEPENDENCE STATUS

Apart from environmental factors, people who would normally be considered 'good' sleepers, may require some assistance to sleep when in hospital. Before interfering with a person's independence in this AL however, it is important that the nurse identifies the patient's usual sleeping pattern. After all there are people whom Meddis (1977) labels nonsomniacs, some of them requiring as little as 2 hours of sleep per night, and they are not upset by wakefulness. Nevertheless, most people expect to sleep at night and three broad categories of insomnia have come to be recognised.

Sleeplessness
Inability to get to sleep. Some people report that it takes them as long as 90 minutes to get to sleep and they are likely to continue this pattern during their stay in hospital. Provided the nurse has ascertained that they are not unduly anxious about it and that it is not interfering with their health, it does not need to be treated. But should such patients remain wakeful for an even longer period, they may need help from the nurse. Among the 'delayed onset' sleepers are a group who could be termed 'worriers'; having ensured that they are physically comfortable, an opportunity to talk about the cause of the worry may leave them feeling less anxious which can encourage sleep. Whenever possible this group could be left to sleep until they awaken naturally in the morning.

Excessive wakefulness. There are those who fall asleep quickly but report that they waken frequently and stay awake for longer or shorter periods. When this information appears on the nursing assessment, the night nurse should be alerted to observing the patient frequently throughout the night in an attempt to record the sleep pattern. It is well-known that a few minutes awake during the night can seem much longer. The patient who stays awake for longer periods may fall asleep again quite naturally after voiding and having a hot drink. Being punitive to patients who state that they have had a poor night, but to the nurse appear to have been asleep, is unrealistic; if the patient feels that he has had a poor night, then the quality of sleep has not been sufficient to produce a feeling of refreshment. Sleep researchers acknowledge that the EEG does not record the 'quality' of sleep. A sympathetic understanding of these patients' problem, expressed by attending to their pre-sleep routine, can help them to relax and fall into a refreshing sleep. The nurse should attempt to identify any change in the patient's daytime activities and note if, because of lack of sleep, they are more easily fatigued. Appetite should also be observed; tired people seldom eat well.

People who suffer from depression, may be troubled by excessive wakefulness and in the long periods when they are awake are helped by having someone to whom they can talk about their problems. It is an illness which can now be treated successfully and if patients have not already sought medical help, they can be encouraged to do so.

Early morning waking. Depression can also be characterised by early morning waking, but the age group most commonly reporting early waking, as early as 0500 hours, is the elderly. If patients awaken early feeling refreshed, they can be offered a morning beverage; those in single rooms may wish to read or occupy themselves in some way; those in large wards can be encouraged to continue resting in bed to avoid disturbing the other patients. Should such patients need a rest during the day, Hayter (1984) maintains that a morning nap is more beneficial than an afternoon nap.

Restlessness

Restlessness is a feature found in many patients with insomnia. After an extensive literature survey and many observations of restlessness in patients Norris (1975) wrote:

Restlessness is a universal, discontinuous, animal behaviour evidenced by nonspecific, repetitive, unorganised, diffuse, apparently nonpurposeful motor activity that is subject to limited control.

It is not always possible to identify the cause but careful documentation of restless behaviour exhibited by many different patients will provide a data bank from which should come a better understanding of this form of interference with sleep. Nowadays, records and tape-recordings are available which teach pre-sleep relaxation, the intention being to reduce restlessness and promote sleep and some people find them effective. The use of rhythmic sound on tape recordings has also proved helpful, such as the noise of waves on a seashore, but more research would be required before making generalisations about this method of reducing restlessness and thus inducing sleep.

Although certain forms of restlessness may be nonspecific the nurse must realise that some drugs prescribed for purposes other than sleeping, are disturbers of sleep and promote restlessness. A commonly used medication in this category is the diuretic group. As well as relieving, for example, oedema they promote frequent elimination of urine, and although these drugs are normally administered in the early part of the day to preclude disturbance of sleep, their effect may persist into the night. Drugs given to relieve constipation may also cause minor abdominal discomfort and disturbed sleep, or even promote defaecation during the night unless administered at a time which will produce the desired effect during the day. Some antidepressant drugs may cause not only disturbance of sleep but actually induce wakefulness because they act in a manner similar to caffeine. When assessing a patient's sleeping pattern, it is therefore important that the nurse is aware of the effect of other currently prescribed drugs which may in fact be the cause of restlessness.

It is worth noting too, that restlessness may occur because some people admitted to hospital do not mention, initially, that they have been accustomed to taking sedatives at home. After all, in a survey of over 2000 people it was found that 15% of men and 25% of women (Whitfield, 1982) who go to see the family doctor attend because of insomnia, and any sleep difficulties will probably be exacerbated by admission to hospital.

Drug dependence

Apart from this group who have been on sedation at home there are some patients who, in spite of all general comfort measures, fail to sleep and require to have sleeping pills which are prescribed by the doctor and given by the nurse. When hypnotic drugs have been ordered to induce sleep, they should be given a few minutes before lights are turned out. If analgesics are also required to relieve pain they should be administered sufficiently early for them to take effect before the hypnotic is given thus enhancing the effect of the hypnotic. The name of the drug, and the dose and time at which it is given are recorded, and also the time at which the patient fell asleep, the time of waking, and mood on waking.

Almost paradoxically, sleeping drugs, although given to induce sleep, can have a detrimental effect on the individual's sleeping pattern. Following many experiments carried out at the Edinburgh Sleep Research Laboratory, it was found that after taking sleeping pills for several nights, the person slept badly when the pills were discontinued, indeed return to a natural sleeping pattern could take up to 6–8 weeks (Oswald & Adam 1983). It is important that the nurse should be aware of this and ensure that the patient who has had hypnotics in hospital is informed of this effect, (and also relatives) when being discharged from hospital. The patient can be reassured that independence in sleeping will return even if there are difficulties during the initial period at home.

DISCOMFORTS ASSOCIATED WITH SLEEPING

Sleeping is such a sensitive and highly individualised activity, and discomfort of any kind may interfere with a person's ability to rest and sleep.

Pain is always a deterrent and descriptions of various sorts of pain and the related nursing activities for its relief have been included in previous chapters pertaining to each AL. However one type of pain which, rightly or wrongly, is sometimes associated with sleep is cramp. The patient wakens during a sleep period complaining of intense pain in the foot or calf. The surrounding muscles are tense and rigid and when the foot is affected there is inability to move, usually the big toe. It is thought to be due to interference with the blood supply; alternate raising of the leg above the level of the bed, and letting it dangle at the side below the level of the bed helps to drain the blood from, and take fresh blood into the area giving relief. Some people find that pressing the foot on a cold surface relieves the spasm but there does not appear to be any documented evidence that this is so. It is best for the nurse to find out whether or not the patient has had cramp previously and if so, how he coped with it.

Other discomforts have been described in earlier chapters which interfere with the relevant AL and often also interfere with sleep.

All aspects of promoting comfort, rest and sleep are priority items especially with ill patients, for whom rest and sleep are essential components of therapy. Many patients are aware of the sources of their discomfort and if given the opportunity will make them known so the nurse who takes time to listen can frequently identify the cause and take steps to alleviate or remove the discomfort. There are, of course, other avenues of expression. The patient who is uncomfortable may appear pale, tense, restless; he may lie rigidly in bed; he may be perspiring profusely. The nurse must be aware of these cues so that she can minimise the effect of, or eliminate the causes, and do everything possible to increase comfort and promote optimal resting and sleeping.

Clearly sleep is a state of altered consciousness but it is a normal Activity of Living. Other altered states of consciousness are found in a range of disease conditions which must be differentiated from sleep.

ALTERED CONSCIOUSNESS

In an article discussing altered states of consciousness, Findley (1984) first of all suggests a pragmatic definition of consciousness as 'a state of wakefulness, alertness and awareness of personal identity and environmental events, that is awareness of self and surroundings'. Consciousness refers to both arousal (requiring intact functioning of the ascending reticular formation of the brain stem) and the content of consciousness (requiring the intact functioning of the cerebral hemispheres). Altered consciousness according to Findley can be considered in terms of a gradual change from a normal conscious level through impaired attention, loss of alertness, drowsiness, sleep, stupor and finally coma. Clearly drowsiness and sleep are normal phenomena whereas stupor and coma are abnormal states.

Coma

The ability to assess accurately a patient's level of consciousness is one of the responsibilities of the nurse. The Glasgow Coma Scale (Fig. 17.2) is a standardised tool which is detailed enough to detect changes in consciousness, or responsiveness as some practitioners prefer to call it. It assesses three modes of behaviour:

- eye opening
- motor response
- verbal response

and is incorporated in an observation record chart (Teasdale et al, 1975; Allan, 1984) which includes recording of other vital signs namely temperature, pulse, respiration and blood pressure. Each of the three behaviours is independently assessed.

Eye opening

Spontaneous eye opening. When the patient's eyes open on the approach of someone to his bedside, it is recorded as spontaneous. This observation will not be expected when the patient is asleep but nurses should be alert to the fact that in some brain-damaged patients the diurnal rhythm is reversed. Observation must therefore be made for any patient who can respond with spontaneous eye opening during the night and not during the day.

Eye opening to speech. If the patient's eyes do not open spontaneously he should be addressed in a normal voice by name and asked to open his eyes. If he does not do so repetition in a loud voice is used, avoiding a commanding tone because it is response to stimulation by sound which is being tested.

Eye opening to pain. Lack of response to verbal stimulation is followed by testing for response to physical stimulation, such as exerting pressure on the patient's finger nail-bed as shown in Figure 17.3.

	Eye opening *Score*		Motor response *Score*		Verbal response *Score*
high *score*		6	If command such as 'lift up your hands' is obeyed		
		5	If purposeful movement to remove painful stimulus such as pressure over eyebrow	5	If oriented to person, place and time
	4 If eyes open spontaneously to approach of nurse to bedside	4	If finger withdrawn after application of painful stimulus to it	4	If conversation confused
	3 If eyes open in response to speech	3	If painful stimulation at finger tip flexes the elbow	3	If inappropriate words are used
	2 If eyes open in response to pain at finger tip	2	If the patient's arms are flexed and finger tip stimulation results in extension of elbow	2	If only incomprehensible sounds are uttered
low *score*	1 If eyes do not open in response to pain at finger tip	1	If there is no detectable response to repeated and various stimuli	1	If no verbal response

A normal person would score 15 on the scale; the lowest possible score is 3 which is compatible with, but does not necessarily indicate, brain death. A score of 7 is used as a definition of coma.

Fig. 17.2 Glasgow coma scale

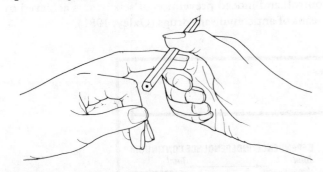

Fig. 17.3 Pressure on finger nail-bed (Teasdale, 1975)

Best motor response

Obeys commands. The patient is required to perform the specific movements requested. Should the relatives have informed the nurse (in the initial assessment phase) that the patient was deaf before the brain damage, then the request will be made by gesture or even in writing. It is preferable to ask him to raise an arm or a leg rather than asking him to squeeze the tester's fingers which can trigger off a reflex contraction; if the latter test is used, it is wise to test that the patient will also release and squeeze again several times before recording this score.

Localises pain. Pressure applied over say the eyebrows (supra-orbital ridge) should stimulate the patient to move his arm thus showing that he has located the pain and is attempting to remove the stimulus.

Withdraws from painful stimulus. Pressure as in Figure 17.3 causes withdrawal of the finger.

Flexion response. Painful stimulation at the finger tip (Fig. 17.3) flexes the elbow but the patient does not achieve a localising response when stimulus is applied at other sites.

Extension response. The patient's arms are flexed and finger tip stimulation (Fig. 17.3) produces straightening at the elbow.

No response to pain. This is scored when there is no detectable response to repeated and various stimuli.

Verbal response

Orientated. After arousal, the patient is asked who he is, where he is and what year and month it is; he is not expected to give the exact day of the month. If accurate answers are given it is recorded that he is orientated.

Confused conversation. A patient can sometimes produce language, even phrases, but if he cannot give the correct answers to questions about orientation then it is recorded that his conversation is confused.

Inappropriate words. When a patient only utters one or two words, more often in response to physical stimulation than to speech, it is recorded that he is using inappropriate words.

Incomprehensible sounds. The utterance of groans, moans or indistinct mumbling without any intelligible words is recorded on this score.

No verbal response. If prolonged and repeated stimulation does not produce phonation then the nil score is recorded.

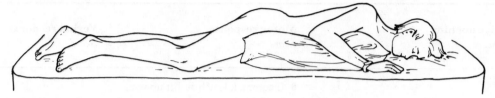

Fig. 17.4 Safest position for an unconscious patient

Use of some type of chart for factual information renders obsolete such terms as deeply unconscious, unconscious and semi-conscious; deeply comatose, comatose and semi-comatose — all terms which can mean different things to different people. The chart can be marked and kept at the bedside so that any member of the team caring for the patient can see by glancing at the chart whether or not there has been any change on any item in the scale.

The Glasgow Coma Scale provides an indication of overall brain dysfunction and can be scored out of 15. It is quick and easy to use and allows data to be documented in a logical manner. As well as assessing responsiveness level it will be necessary for members of the caring team to accept responsibility for managing several of the unresponding comatose patient's other activities of living. These are breathing, eating and drinking, eliminating, personal cleansing and dressing (prevention of pressure sores), controlling body temperature, mobilising passively and maintaining a safe environment. All procedures associated with these ALs should be carried out by the nurse in such a way that not only life is maintained but also the patient's dignity is safeguarded. The unconscious patient is usually nursed in the semiprone position illustrated in Figure 17.4.

Convulsions (fits)

A form of transient unconsciousness sometimes occurs as a feature of what is termed a convulsion. When a baby has a convulsion or seizure it often heralds a febrile illness. In other age groups, there may be a variety of causes, including cerebral anoxaemia, hypoglycaemia, disturbance of calcium balance, electrolyte imbalance, excessive hydration, the injection of certain drugs and poisons, infections which produce high temperature elevations, and a number of metabolic disorders. Convulsions are also a feature of epilepsy but nowadays, good control, and indeed prevention of seizures, is achieved by means of anticonvulsant drugs (Oxley, 1981).

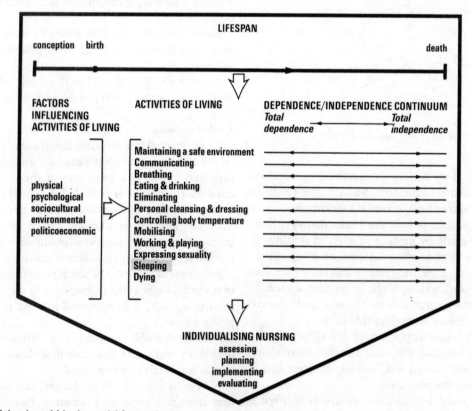

Fig. 17.5 The AL of sleeping within the model for nursing

Anaesthesia

Convulsions or seizures may occur without much warning but it is possible to alter deliberately the level of human consciousness. This occurs when a patient is given a general anaesthetic. The anaesthetised person appears to be in a state of induced unconsciousness although there is increasing evidence that appearances are misleading; the patient on the operating table may actually hear what is being said and may be 'aware' of the inability to move. These findings certainly have implications for staff in the operating suite both prior to surgery and in the recovery room. Nowadays, for many operations, light anaesthetics are used so patients recover consciousness quite quickly after surgery. Stephens & Boaler (1977) maintain that deliberately wakening patients is undesirable; they should be given time to regain consciousness at their own pace.

In circumstances where there is altered consciousness — coma, convulsions, general anaesthetic — the skill and adaptability of the nurse are of paramount importance. In these states, even when transient in nature, the person is dependent for all Activities of Living, indeed for survival.

Like sleep, as might be expected, these states of altered consciousness are characterised by changes in the electrical activity of the cerebral cortex when recorded by EEG. Every advance in the research centres provides more information about the 'how' and 'why' of altered consciousness, including sleep. Perhaps in the not too distant future, it will be possible to refute Dr Johnson's observation some decades ago:

no searcher ... can tell by what power the mind and body are thus chained down in irresistible stupefaction ... the witty and the dull, the clamerous and the silent, the busy and the idle, are all overpowered by the gentle tyrant, and all lie down in the equality of sleep.

In the second half of this chapter some of the problems and discomforts which can be experienced by patients in relation to the AL of sleeping have been described. This provides the beginning nurse with a generalised idea of these; it will be useful in assessing, planning, implementing and evaluating an individualised programme for each patient's AL of sleeping.

This chapter has been concerned with the AL of sleeping. However, as stated previously it is only for the purpose of discussion that any AL can be considered on its own; in reality the various activities are so closely related and do not have distinct boundaries. Figure 17.5 is a reminder that the AL of sleeping is related to the other ALs and also to the various components of the model for nursing.

REFERENCES

Adam K 1980 A time for rest and a time for play. Nursing Mirror 150(10) March 6:17–18
Allan D 1984 Glasgow Coma Scale. Nursing Mirror 158(23) June 13:32–34
Armstrong-Esther C, Hawkins L 1982 Day for night: circadian rhythms in the elderly. Nursing Times 78(30) July 28:1263–1265
Brezinova V, Oswald I 1972 Sleep after a bedtime beverage. British Medical Journal 2 May 20:431–433
Canavan T 1984 The psychobiology of sleep. Nursing 2(23) March:682–683
Cohen D 1979 Sleep and dreaming. Pergamon Press, Oxford
Felstein I 1979 The sufferer who doesn't suffer. Nursing Mirror 146 April 12:42–43
Findley L 1984 Altered consciousness. Nursing 2(23) March: 663–666
Hawkins L, Armstrong-Esther C 1978 Circadian rhythms and night shift working in nurses. Nursing Times Occasional Paper 74(13) May 4:49–52
Hayter J 1983 Sleep behaviours of older persons. Nursing Research 32(4) July/August:242–246
Lathlean J 1980 Relaxation using yoga. Nursing 1(20) December:882–884
Meddis R 1977 The sleep instinct. Routledge & Kegan Paul, London
Norris C 1975 Restlessness: a nursing phenomenon in search of a meaning. Nursing Outlook 23:103–107
Oswald I 1980 No peace for the worried. Nursing Times 150(11) March 13:34–35
Oswald I, Adam K 1983 Get a better night's sleep. Martin Dunitz, London
Oxley J 1981 Fitting the symptoms. Nursing Mirror Clinical Forum Supplement 12, December 9
Richman N 1983 Management of sleep problems. Maternal and Child Health 8(6) June: 227–233
Smith P, Wedderburn Z 1980 Sleep, body rhythms and night-work. Nursing 1(20) December: 889–892
Stephens D, Boaler J 1977 The nurse's role in immediate post-operative care. British Medical Journal 1:1199–1202
Teasdale G, Galbraith S, Clarke K 1975 Observation record chart. Nursing Times 71(25) June 19:972–973
Wedderburn Z, Smith P 1980 Sleep: its function and measurement. Nursing 1(20) December:852–855
Whitfield W 1982 Breaking the habit. Nursing Mirror 155(10) September 8:59–60

ADDITIONAL READING

Hearne K 1980 Insight into dreams. Nursing Mirror 150(10) March 6:20–22
Sleep and Comfort 1980 Nursing 1(20) December:851–892
Thornton P et al 1984 The sleep clinic. Nursing Times 80(11) March 14:40–43

18

Dying

The activity of dying

Dying is the final act of living. Death is what marks the end of life on earth, just as the event of birth marks its beginning. The only certain thing in all our lives is that we will die one day; but there are many uncertainties as to why, when, where and how.

It is probably these uncertainties about dying which provoke uneasy feelings when people think about the prospect of their own death and the death of those they love. Life would not be worth living if death became a preoccupation but, if the subject is ignored, how can people develop the resources needed to comfort the bereaved, bear the sorrow of grieving and face death with dignity?

THE NATURE OF DYING

Death and dying

To die suddenly from natural causes, in old age, and without loss of dignity is what most people would regard as a 'good' death. It may be sudden as occurs for example following a massive coronary or cardiovascular accident; or it may be preceded by a process of dying. Accompanying an acute terminal illness or surgery, dying may take only a few days or a few weeks. On the other hand, when there is chronic illness with a poor prognosis, the process of dying may span several months.

Some people die suddenly not from natural causes but in quite violent circumstances. In most countries of the Western world, road accidents are a major cause of death in young adults, normally a particularly healthy group; international publicity is given to serious aircraft accidents which, although rare, almost always have a high mortality rate; industrial accidents for example in mines often cause mass deaths in large numbers; and in areas of the world where natural disasters such as floods, earthquakes, and hurricanes occur with relative frequency, there may be a heavy death toll. Every country has its major tragedies when whole families or even communities can be wiped out by such events.

Sudden violent death may not be accidental, however, but deliberate. Murder is not common but the incidence is rising in most industrialised nations. Most countries are aware of the increasing violence and terrorism in the modern world and of the corresponding need to protect individuals from undesirable and preventable acts of homicide. For many obvious reasons, the relatives' grief may be complicated by feelings of lust for revenge and fear for their own personal safety, and this may precipitate yet more deaths.

Violent death on a large scale as a result of war seems to be a constant feature in modern society; and in response to apparently unwarranted aggression perhaps war is inevitable as a means of national self-defence. However, following the Second World War, the United Nations Organisation was created to provide a forum for discussion about disputes in order to preclude the waging of war. Unfortunately this option is not always accepted and the death toll among armed forces and civilians is only one feature of the horror of war. The possibility of a nuclear holocaust adds considerably to the horror with the prospect of mass annihilation or, in its aftermath, the painful process of dying from the effects of radiation.

Most people, even those with a strong religious faith about an afterlife, are afraid of death and dying. However there are some individuals who, for a variety of reasons, want to die and intentionally take their own lives by committing suicide. Self-poisoning is the most frequently used method and attempted suicide (para-suicide) is currently a common emergency in the casualty department of any busy hospital in most industrialised countries. In the U.K., suicide is more than twice as common in men than women; the rate rises as age increases; a large proportion of victims have a history of a broken home or marriage; and the risk rate is higher among professional and executive workers than among manual workers (Roberts, 1977). Until relatively recently suicide was a criminal offence in the U.K. and, although the law has now changed, there is still a stigma attached to suicide which may serve to increase the already great amount of distress and guilt suffered by the relatives.

Although not suicidal in intent, there is another group of people who, when they are dying, want to die quickly; and there are some people attending a dying person, who want to 'help' them to die quickly. 'Bringing about an easy death' is the actual meaning of the term euthanasia, although mercy killing is a phrase often used as a synonym. It is a topic which evokes strong emotions and heated debate. Those with particular religious or personal convictions argue that it is morally wrong to end life deliberately. Others consider that euthanasia is not a deliberate act of killing but merely allows death to occur for example by not treating with antibiotics a respiratory infection in an old, incapacitated person although providing care and comfort in every other way.

The subject of euthanasia has provoked lengthy debate about the 'right to die' in balance with the 'right to live'. The debate is not new. It has gone on down through the centuries but has currently re-emerged with some force because of procedures made possible by recent technological advances; although often life-saving and often appropriate to use, they do raise ethical problems. Saunders (1976) writing about some of these problems maintains:

As often happens, we discover *how* to do something and only later *when* to do it. No treatment . . . carries with it the automatic commitment to use it just because it is technically feasible.

In a number of countries, proponents of euthanasia have formed societies to discuss and propagate their beliefs, and to provide information to people who wish assistance in reducing the distress of dying. In some instances, an even more positive stance has been taken and attempts have been made to introduce legislation making voluntary euthanasia possible. As yet, however, these measures have not been successful, essentially because of public anxiety regarding potential abuse of such laws about death.

It is difficult to discuss the nature of death and dying without considering the nature of grieving and bereavement. Most adults have some experience of these emotions following the death of a relative or friend; indeed grieving and bereavement are a part of the process of living although related to the process of dying and death.

Bereavement and grieving

Although, thankfully, the dying person does not necessarily suffer great distress, those who are left behind almost inevitably suffer a deep sense of desolation at the loss of someone who is significant to them. Grief is the emotional reaction which follows and is one of the most intense emotional experiences. Murray Parkes (1972) in his book, *Bereavement* maintains that grief is 'the cost of commitment' in our lives.

It is not necessarily only husbands, wives or children who are bereaved, although one's immediate reaction is to think of these close relatives. Many others may be affected by a death, such as friends, colleagues, neighbours, co-patients, doctors and nurses. Gyulay (1975) identifies, in the case of a child's death, the 'forgotten grievers' as the father, siblings, grandparents, peers and friends, neighbours and teachers, and Copper (1982) makes the same point in relation to stillbirth although in this instance, the baby has not been known to those others as an individual with a separate identity.

It may seem surprising to include the father in this list until one remembers that in Western culture men are not expected to reveal deep emotion and so there has been the assumption that men do not feel grief so intensely as women. So intense is the emotion of grief that it affects even those sometimes wrongly assumed to be untouched by loss: the very young and the very old, the mentally ill and the mentally handicapped. 'The bereaved' are, by definition, those who suffer loss and grief in response to a death; those who were, in some important way, committed to the person who died.

Although feelings of loss and grief are almost universal responses in bereavement, many other reactions can occur. Shock, disbelief, anger, denial, shame, guilt, resentment, anxiety, fear, depression and despair are among the emotional reactions which may be experienced by the bereaved to a varying degree and at different times throughout the grieving process. However, sometimes a death brings relief to those left behind and this may be the case, for example, if the family has had to watch suffering in someone they love and bear the burden of care during a prolonged terminal illness.

Initially there is usually a short period of intense grief when the bereaved person suffers profound despair and sorrow and openly mourns. Shock and total disbelief can be experienced at this time, especially in the case of sudden death, and the experience may seem unreal. Then there is a long period of sadness. Pining for the dead person is common and often this takes the form of 'searching behaviour' involving attachment to places and objects associated with the dead person's life and their relationship.

While grieving, a sense of the persisting presence of the dead person appears to be a comforting phenomenon and illusions, hallucinations and dreams often occur. Such events seem to help to compensate for the reality of the loss, and the loneliness felt. Sometimes the bereaved person experiences intense anxieties for the future and feels totally incapable of taking decisions and coping with everyday demands.

Depression is not uncommon and, even long after the death, episodes of intense grief and despair may return. Restitution from bereavement involves adaptation to a new life as the death of a significant person inevitably alters the role and function of the bereaved; a widow is no longer a wife and a son may now be the head of the household. The old identity must be given up and a new one evolved. Usually, the new life is moulded gradually and some significant milestones include events such as returning to work, moving house and making new friends.

Bereavement can be a long and painful process.

Although it is probably true that 'time heals', a person seldom remains unaffected by a bereavement even after a long time lapse.

THE PURPOSE OF DYING

All of the Activities of Living discussed so far can be seen to have a clear purpose. Some, such as breathing, are performed for survival; others like eating and drinking not only for survival but also for comfort and enjoyment; and yet others, the ALs of communicating and expressing sexuality, have as their purpose the interaction of human beings with one another in the process of living. In the same kind of way, is it possible to discern a purpose of dying?

Many people have some kind of personal belief about the meaning of death and often this is based on the philosophy of a particular religion. Most religions have some strong belief about the fate of man's spirit and soul after death. For example Christianity purports that there is life after death; Roman Catholics, Protestants and Jews believe that death marks the beginning of an afterlife with God, some being convinced that this existence is everlasting and will hold greater joy and peace than life on earth. Within such a philosophy then, the purpose of dying is to allow progression from life on earth to the afterlife. For those who do not hold such beliefs, dying may be seen to have no purpose other than being an inevitable end to living.

The purpose of grieving is essentially to come to terms with the irreparable loss of someone who is significant in one's life. The fact that the grief is shared with family and friends provides support while emotional and other adjustments are made and the threads of everyday living are picked up again.

LIFESPAN: EFFECT ON DYING

The model of living includes the lifespan as one of its components; conception is the lifespan's starting point and death is its endpoint. However death can occur at any age and when it comes, it determines the length of an individual's lifespan. When the lifespan of groups of individuals is investigated, it is possible to detect trends in death rates within and between groups and as most countries maintain population statistics, international comparisons can be made about average age of death and life expectancy. A century ago in most industrialised countries the life expectancy was around 40 years, slightly higher for females; nowadays, it is around 70 years.

The stages of the lifespan were discussed as a component of the model in an earlier part of the book and it is useful to review the effect of death and dying in relation to the different age groups.

Prenatal period. Death can occur during early uterine existence associated with what is termed a spontaneous abortion, or the fetus may die at a late stage in pregnancy and the mother knows that the period of labour will produce only a dead baby. It is not possible to know the 'reaction' of the fetus in these circumstances, but it is possible to observe the desolation experienced by parents who, in these instances, are the most directly affected. Richardson (1980) quotes a mother describing the experience of stillbirth as 'the loneliest of losses; you are the only one who has had a relationship with the baby'. Some babies die during the process of birth or in the neonatal period or during the first 12 months of life sometimes in inexplicable, so-called 'cot deaths' (Limerick, 1984), but in industrialised countries, if infants survive the first year, they have a good life expectancy.

Childhood. In industrialised countries, deaths during childhood are rare, for example in the U.K., they account for less than 1% of all deaths and the most common cause is accidents; theoretically accidents are preventable, a topic which is discussed on page 84 in Chapter 7, Maintaining a Safe Environment. Children do become aware of death and dying at quite an early age and it is interesting to note the findings of studies which have been conducted to ascertain what young children think about death. One of the earlier studies was carried out by Nagy (Teifel, 1969) in Hungary following the Second World War. A group of 378 children aged 3–10 years from different socioeconomic backgrounds and religions, and of varying intellectual ability were asked to express death-related thoughts verbally, in drawing and in writing. Nagy categorised the findings in three stages. In Stage I (3–5 years) there was no clear distinction between living and lifeless. The dead person was 'less alive' or asleep or had gone away and would return. In Stage II (5–6 years) death was personified as a death-man or skeleton who carried away living people and there was no return. In Stage III (9–10 years) death was inevitable and permanent; it was a termination of life.

Adolescence. Although the teenager understands intellectually about the finality of life, time is a sort of insulation between the adolescent and eventual death. So the dying adolescent who is just beginning to enjoy independence and self-confidence does not want to end what has just begun, and in the confusion and distress and often anger, may feel isolated from both parents and peers.

The death of an adolescent (and of a child) is devastating especially to parents. In industrialised countries, parents do not expect to outlive their children and it is very difficult to comfort them after such a loss. Such premature death may be greatly resented. They have been cheated of time together which they had the right to expect; the dead person had so much to give and so much to live for. Hopes and faith about life are dealt a severe blow which can have a lifelong effect on the family. However many bereaved parents consider that although the loss leaves a permanent scar, it is possible to grow because of the experience and help others in similar circumstances.

Adulthood. During early adulthood, people are considered to be in the 'prime of life' and a consideration of personal death and dying is almost totally alien, at least in industrialised countries where life expectancy is high. Sudden death, therefore, perhaps as a result of a road accident, comes as a shock to the family. There has been no time to contemplate the event and no opportunity to begin the process of grieving in anticipation of death. There has been no chance to say goodbye, and often there is an aura of unreality in the immediate post-death period. For the bereaved family there may also be an untimely change in status; perhaps a young family bereft of a parent and spouse, perhaps a sudden termination of a promising career.

In later adulthood the physical and other changes associated with the male and female menopause probably serve to remind the individual of man's mortality; and an increasing incidence of disease in this age group, either personally or observed in friends and colleagues, make the possibility of death and the process of dying a reality. For a spouse who is bereaved in this age group it can mean intense loneliness despite the support of family and friends; and for the young adults of the family, it may mean the loss of a supportive parent and perhaps taking on increasing responsibility for the remaining parent.

The elderly. For the elderly there is the realisation that they are coming to the end of the lifespan and they are made aware of this by an increasing number of deaths in their peer group. The majority of elderly people are healthy and retain their independence and may die suddenly or have a very short terminal illness. For some however, if they are ill and dependent, death may be welcomed as a release from pain and discomfort; for a few, the process of dying can be a long, courageously endured struggle to cherish their dignity and self-esteem despite a frail body.

A long terminal illness may cause great difficulties for relations also. Although able to prepare themselves for the bereavement they have, in addition to their anxieties and fears, the burden of care at home, or hospital visiting, over a long period of time. For those who are bereaved by the death of an elderly person, it may mean the loss of a spouse with whom they have spent a lifetime, and for the younger generation it may mean the loss of a much-loved parent or grandparent.

Human death is never really absent from our personal lives or from the community in general; indeed there is truth in the popular philosophy that we are 'dying from the moment we are born'.

FACTORS INFLUENCING DYING

Apart from the differences associated with the various stages of the lifespan, a number of factors influence death and dying. The various factors are discussed, using the categories which appear in the model, under the headings physical, psychological, sociocultural, environmental and politicoeconomic factors.

Physical factors

In old age, it is normal for systems of the body to become less efficient and to undergo a gradual process of degeneration. Physically, the process of dying is not dissimilar except that the progressive decline is brought about by disease and the nature of the particular pathology involved determines the course and speed of the irreversible degeneration of biological functioning. It is therefore difficult to diagnose the onset of 'dying' as a physical process but it may be helpful to say it begins when medical treatment cannot halt the course of a disease, and can only alleviate the symptoms of the fatal illness. In many instances a considerable length of time may elapse between the medical diagnosis of fatal illness and the onset of rapid physical decline in the terminal stages of the illness which precede the event of death.

Dying as a physical process, is a very complicated phenomenon and it is important to appreciate that it is seldom possible for doctors to diagnose the exact time of its onset or to give a precise prognosis of when death will occur.

In contrast, it is usually possible to determine with accuracy the time at which death ultimately occurs. For most purposes it can be assumed that death has occurred when a person's pulse and respiration have ceased. But sometimes a much more elaborate diagnosis of death is required especially if there has been admission to hospital and sophisticated, artificial, 'life-support systems' are being used to maintain vital body functions. Although not spelled out in legal terms, there is medical agreement about tests ascertaining complete and irreversible brain death, requiring confirmation by at least two experienced doctors. The criteria include fixation of pupils, absence of corneal and of vestibulo-ocular reflexes; absence of response within the cranial nerve distribution to sensory stimuli; no response to bronchial stimulation when a catheter is passed into the trachea; no spontaneous breathing movement when the patient is disconnected from a mechanical ventilator (Taber, 1982). Agreed criteria for the definition of death are essential when removal of organs for transplant surgery is being considered, and they are strictly applied by a medical team quite separate from the transplant team. A recent report produced by the Health Departments of Great Britain and Northern Ireland ('Cadaveric Organs for Transplantation' 1983) provides a code of practice and deals with the various physical and ethical issues in detail. To cope with the many ethical problems surrounding the criteria, the concepts of 'clinical death' (death of the person), 'biological death' (death of the tissues) and 'brain death' (irreversible brain damage) have been introduced and recognised by a number of countries.

Most Activities of Living are affected by the physical changes which occur in the process of dying, and all cease when life ends — when the event of death occurs. After death, the body cools, the tissues and muscles lose their tone and rigor mortis (stiffening of the body) sets in after 2 or 3 hours.

There are also physical factors which are relevant in relation to bereavement. For those who are bereaved, there is usually extreme physical exhaustion. Unless the death is sudden and unexpected, there will probably have been a period of time prior to the death when it was necessary either to pay frequent visits to the hospital or to provide 24-hour care at home. Perhaps also there is a young family to be supervised in the usual Activities of Living, or full-time employment to be carried on during the dying period of the family member and immediately after, and inevitably there is accompanying physical stress.

The bereaved seem to be more susceptible to physical illness. Statistics indicate that the bereaved spouse is admitted to hospital more frequently than married persons of the same age, and that elderly bereaved are more likely to become physically ill than those in a younger age group (Madison & Viola, 1968). The elderly person is often in a precarious physical state anyway, and the stress of the death of a spouse may exacerbate physical weakness. Some writers do not hesitate to refer to the 'broken heart syndrome' and Pike (1983) quotes a reference which showed that 12% of surviving spouses die within a year of their wives' or husbands' dying, while mortality in a non-bereaved control group was only 1.2% for the same period. Frederich (1978) believes that the intensity of the trauma of grief has a direct effect on the body's physical functioning. He considers that the pituitary gland releases more adrenocorticotrophic hormones as part of the body's reaction to stress; this in turn stimulates the adrenal cortex and the release of corticosteroids; these depress the body's immune system and suppress the response to infections and neoplastic disorders. As a consequence, physical disease processes become evident and in turn these lead to further stress. Obviously there is a close link between physical and psychological factors.

Psychological factors

It is much less easy to describe psychological aspects of the dying process because no two individuals respond in the same way and because any one person's reaction to dying is influenced by his personality, personal beliefs and total life experience. Whether or not the person suspects or knows for certain that he is dying is also an important factor. It is no virtue in itself that all people should be told they are dying, or discover the fact for themselves. However, the person's understanding of his prognosis will affect his attitude, mood and behaviour. Those with experience of caring for dying people tend to agree that they usually *are* aware, without needing to be told, of their fatal prognosis. After all, the person is able to feel and see the symptoms and signs of the disease and to realise that he does not seem to be getting any better; he is able to consider the possibilites and probabilities of whether or not he will recover; and most of all, he becomes aware of the altered way in which those around him begin to behave towards him. His increasing awareness of his situation is discernible in the way his own behaviour begins to change.

For some people, awareness of impending death may be accompanied by intense fear. Fear of death has been a source of speculation in both personality theory and psychotherapeutic clinic work but in two studies done in the U.S.A. and quoted in McCarthy (1980) the amount of education and level of intelligence have no direct influence on fear of death, nor does there seem to be a significant relationship between death, anxiety and age.

Of course, the psychological changes which take place are not the same for any two individuals but it appears that there are certain kinds of reactions which commonly occur in the dying process. Some of these have been described by Kubler-Ross (1969) following her interviews in North America with dying patients.

She says that, on realising what is happening, most people pass through a phase of 'denial and isolation' in which they refuse to accept that they are dying. As denial lessens, the common reaction is one of 'anger' and the person will ask 'Why me?' ... 'What have I done to deserve this?' Sometimes attempts to cope with the situation then involve a stage of 'bargaining'. The person tries to find ways of believing that a miracle recovery will happen or that he might be given more time and he makes 'bargains' with the doctor or with God. When these fail and the imminent loss of life and loved ones becomes a reality, 'depression' is experienced and this is an almost universal feature of the dying process. There is profound regret over missed opportunities and failures of the past and an overwhelming sadness engulfs the dying person. With sensitive care the person can be helped through this by being reminded of the achievements of his life, by being shown that he is respected and loved, and reassured that he will be looked after to the end and that what is important is to cope with each day at a time, to make the most of what is left.

It does seem that dying need not be the terrible nightmare which many people fear so much. There can be serenity and composure in dying and many people die peacefully in their sleep with no apparent struggle or distress. Indeed McCarthy (1980) describes the prospect of death as representing not only 'the end of growth, pleasure, thought, consciousness, accomplishment, striving ... it constitutes a final opportunity to experience the self, maintain self-esteem, relate to others, care for loved ones' and this is echoed by a young general practitioner who himself was dying. He considered that dying 'makes life suddenly real ... it has been the greatest adventure of my life' (Cassons, 1980).

The immediate family and friends of the dying person are often under great stress, concerned about the discomforts and pain of a loved one and also about the impending loss of someone who is significant to them. When the death occurs, there is inevitably emotional upset reflecting the sense of desolation and loss. As memories flood back, those who are grieving may find it difficult to concentrate on other activities, often there is tearfulness, and there may be loss of appetite and loss of weight. These are expected symptoms of grief and are usually relatively transient; the person usually uses coping mechanisms to resume at least a semblance of normal activities of living. However there may be more prolonged psychological dysfunction related to grief.

Occasionally, the feelings of helplessness and hopelessness prove too much and the grief reaction is so intense and prolonged that the bereaved person suffers a mental breakdown which requires specialised medical treatment. This is more likely to happen to women than to men, to those of unstable personality, and to those bereaved by a sudden death, the death of a child or death as a result of suicide.

Sociocultural factors

In societies where care of the dying is still very much a family responsibility, the social customs which surround death tend to be elaborate. The various rituals and the ceremonies performed are designed to encourage the bereaved to mourn openly and to seek the sympathy and support of members of their community. Each society has its own way of treating death according to its culture.

Social customs throughout the world vary markedly. In the Middle East some funeral rituals involve prolonged and public exhibitions of grief; and in some African tribes mourners gather together to 'drown their sorrows' publicly in drinking ceremonies. Although the rituals differ, the common element is the emphasis on the importance and necessity of communal and overt mourning.

In Western societies elaborate ritual surrounding death is fast disappearing. In Victorian times, funerals were grand occasions and the whole community engaged in mourning. The family wore black and withdrew to the confines of their home, ceasing for a while to participate in any social activities and centring life around opportunities to share their sorrow and grief and show respect to the dead. Nowadays, death is almost a taboo subject and people feel they must mourn discreetly and 'get over it' quickly.

Cremation is now much more popular than burial; the cremation service is brief and there is not even a grave to remind the community of the death and allow the bereaved to maintain some kind of contact with the memory of the dead person. Of course although in Western culture the choice of cremation may seem to sever the final link, for other cultures it is the norm. The Navajo Indians for example, after elaborate mourning rituals, *must* burn the body in a special house or 'hogan'.

Many of the social customs surrounding death have their origin in religion and involve a ceremonial which ensures proper disposal of the dead body. For the Muslim there are strict religious practices. Every Muslim believes that the time of his death is predetermined and nobody can do anything to alter it. While dying, the family and friends recite parts of the Koran so that these are the last words heard. After death, perfumes are applied to the body, it is wrapped in a special cloth, then placed in a grave facing Mecca. In the Islamic view, a Muslim is not the owner of his own body; it is held in trust from God. Suicide is therefore forbidden; a post-mortem removal of organs for transplant is not allowed, and cremation is not permitted (Walker, 1982). The practice of Orthodox Jews also requires that a dying person has a fellow Jew in attendance to read scriptures and recite prayers during his last hours. There is also a special way of laying out the corpse and similarly, mutilation of the body is forbidden. The ritual purification is a reflection of the belief that death is not the final end but the beginning of an afterlife with the Almighty (Levenstein & Joseph, 1978). For the Hindu too, death is not the end. Their faith is centred on the transmigration of souls with indefinite reincarnation, and the form of the new body depends on the type of life the person has led; and the Dayak tribe of Borneo (Kastenbaum, 1981) believe the soul stays in heaven for a period of seven generations then is reborn on earth.

The beliefs held by the individual obviously affect his view of himself and of life. Someone who believes that life after death exists is less likely to fear death and more likely to see within the sorrow, an element of joy. In contrast, a person who believes that death is the end of everything may fear dying and find only despair and loss in bereavement.

Environmental factors

In urbanised, industrialised countries there has been a clear trend towards death in *institutions* rather than at home as once was the case. Now in the U.K., more than half of the deaths which occur each year take place in hospitals and the rate is even higher among the elderly population.

Roughly one in three deaths occur *at home* and, compared to patients who die in institutions, the people who die at home tend to be from a younger age group and to have a wife, daughter or daughter-in-law able to look after them in their terminal illness. Cartwright et al (1973) found from their study of *Life Before Death* that a sizeable proportion (37%) of those who died at home had been in a hospital during the preceding year; half of the group had cancer and many had problems which required a good deal of care. The majority of families concerned, when asked about this in the course of the study, expressed pleasure that their relative had died at home rather than in a hospital.

Providing care for the dying at home, although often desirable, is not always possible. Hospital care, the main alternative, is frequently considered to be undesirable as appropriate facilities are not usually available in busy general wards. Because of the difficulties inherent in both institutional and home care for the dying, a new development has emerged in the form of *hospices*: small, homely places set up to cater especially for the needs of the dying. The name of St Christopher's Hospice in London and the pioneering work of Dr Cicely Saunders are known throughout the world.

The decision of where a person should be looked after in his terminal illness depends on many factors. Consideration must be given to the individual's particular needs and to his own wishes as well as those of the family. Although a terminal illness is not usually protracted, the majority of deaths do not happen quickly.

In societies where hospitals are a scarce resource, particularly in developing countries, the decision is less complicated. Care of the dying is accepted as a family responsibility and in such circumstances the dying person is able to remain at home, to end his life in the care and company of close relatives.

For the bereaved, particularly following the death of a spouse, there is an obvious change in the immediate environment of the house; all around are constant reminders of previous routines in everyday Activities of Living which are no longer shared. The painfulness of the memories may be assuaged by packing or giving away the dead person's clothes and belongings, perhaps to family members, yet this in itself is a stressful activity. In some instances there may be an enforced change of environment, perhaps to a smaller house in a strange neighbourhood, because the death has caused a major change in economic circumstances.

Politicoeconomic factors

In Western society, the commemoration of death is often an occasion when economic distinctions are emphasised. The type of funeral, the degree of ceremony, whether or not there are commemorative plaques or headstones are activities which reflect the economic status of the individual.

The economic status of a country is reflected in the cause of death and the life expectancy of the population. The most important causes of death in industrialised countries today are heart disease, cancer and stroke. Taken together in the U.K., for example, these diseases account for two-thirds of all mortality in the late adulthood and old age stages of the lifespan, and some of these fatal diseases can be caused or aggravated by factors such as overindulgence in food or alcohol or smoking. In industrialised countries, life expectancy is around 70 years of age, slightly higher for women than for men, and mortality rates among the young are very low indeed. Even so there are social class differences and the less good mortality rates in the lower social classes are highlighted in a recent U.K. Report 'Inequalities in health' (Black, 1980). The legislature usually determines how the death is recorded, and politicoeconomic factors influence the provision made by the state for funeral costs and financial assistance to dependants.

In many developing countries, however, the picture is quite different and reflects the lower economic status; infant mortality rates are high, preventable infectious diseases claim many lives, people still die from starvation and even those who manage to remain relatively healthy have a much shorter life expectancy than in the Western world. The economic status of a country to some extent influences what can be done to prevent the circumstances which lead to avoidable early deaths but the political decisions determine how much of the national budget can be relegated for health services. Political decisions also determine how much will be spent on costly hospital life-saving procedures which reach such a small percentage of the population, and how much will be used in the community rectifying the conditions which are the cause of so many deaths. In many instances, no financial provision is made by the state for dependants and in a number of these countries, it is not yet a legal requirement to record the death.

DEPENDENCE/INDEPENDENCE IN DYING

Death is universal and inevitable, and apart perhaps from suicide, there is little personal independence about the time of death although there are some who maintain that individuals 'have turned their face to the wall' and willed themselves to die.

In the presence of general weakness and disease, the dying person is often aware that with the passing of each day, there is some slight erosion of independence in the physical aspects of ALs. However at home and in hospital, as well as in a hospice, the care providers may be sufficiently empathetic to encourage the person to continue making choices for as long as possible and remain in control of pain relief (if pain is present), in control of his quality of living, and in control of the immediate environment. Self-esteem can remain intact and even with increasing physical dependence, there can be independence of spirit. So while preserving the right to live independently to the optimum for these circumstances, the care providers have to help the dying person to balance the degree of personal dependence/independence in the Activities of Living up until the time of death.

For the family of the dying person, there will probably be varying degrees of dependence on others during the period prior to death when family, friends, neighbours and colleagues often offer to assist with, for example, family transport and shopping as well as visiting the dying person. In the period of grieving, the presence and thoughtfulness of others can be comforting and supportive although the bereaved person knows that this is a transient phase until physical and emotional strength is renewed, and the props of dependence can be withdrawn.

INDIVIDUALITY IN DYING

Each individual has personal beliefs about life, and about death and dying. The experience of death is unique to each person, and using the components of the model already discussed, it is possible to identify not only the problems related to dying but also the wishes of the individual during this terminal activity. Below is a résumé of the main points of the preceding discussion.

Lifespan: effect on dying
- Age group of dying person and family/friends

Factors influencing dying
- Physical
  - terminal illness/cause of death
  - diagnosis of death
  - physical effects on other ALs
  - physical effect on family/friends

- Psychological
  - personality and temperament
  - fears and anxieties about dying and death
  - awareness of approaching death
  - whether or not significant others know of prognosis
  - behaviour of others towards the dying person
  - effect of grieving and bereavement on family/friends

- Sociocultural
  - past life experience
  - personal beliefs about dying and death
  - religious/cultural rituals surrounding death and bereavement

- Environmental — selection of home/hospital/hospice
  — change of environment for family
- Politicoeconomic — home/family/financial circumstances
  — effect on cause of death and life expectancy
  — availability of health and support services

Dependence/independence in dying
- Status in relation to all ALs
- Suicide/other causes of death
- Status during grieving and bereavement

Dying: patients' problems and related nursing activities

The dying person and the family are faced with many problems and emotional demands of a highly complex nature. Not all dying people require, or even wish, the help of a nurse but for many people at the endpoint of the lifespan, some of their problems can at least be alleviated with skilled and sensitive nursing. Individualised nursing can only be carried out if the nurse knows about the patient's (and family's) problems, and about personal wishes (and those of the family) related to this last Activity of Living. While observing and while conversing with the patient and the family, the nurse would be seeking answers to the following questions:

- when is the individual likely to die?
- what factors influence the way the individual is dying?
- what does the individual (and family) know about the prognosis?
- what are the individual's beliefs about dying and death?
- what problems does the individual have at present or seem likely to develop?
- what effect does the dying process have on the family and how does this affect the individual?
- what effect will bereavement have on the family?

The information collected should then be examined to identify any problems being experienced in the process of dying. Potential problems should be identified and prevented when possible; and actual problems should be solved or alleviated; or the patient should be helped to cope with them. When possible, the patient and family should be involved in the process of assessment and should help to set realistic goals.

The nursing interventions (and what the patient agrees to do) to achieve the set goals should be selected according to local circumstances and available resources; these are then written on the nursing plan. In many instances, evaluation will have to be done daily because although, in the process of dying, there is often a gradual erosion of independence in all ALs, this may fluctuate from day to day, and the person who is dying should be helped to live to the optimum for that day. Cure is not the objective; comfort and well-being are of paramount importance.

Of course, a multidisciplinary team may often be involved in the care programme of a dying person and it is important that the individualised nursing plan is congruent with the team's mutually agreed objectives, so that the patient can be helped to be as comfortable as possible for as long as possible, and can die with dignity.

In order to provide individualised nursing, the nurse needs to have a background knowledge of the general conditions which can be responsible for, or can change the individual's dependence/independence status, and which can be experienced by the person as problems. The general problem areas are discussed under the following headings:

- change of environment and routine
- physical problems associated with dying
- psychological problems associated with dying
- the family's problems.

CHANGE OF ENVIRONMENT AND ROUTINE

When dying people are nursed in their own home setting, at least they are surrounded by family, friends, neighbours, and many of their personal possessions are in view or can be brought to them. The individual at least has a semblance of control over the immediate environment. Currently however, in many industrialised countries, people are transferred to hospital to die, totally removed from familiar surroundings. So following hospitalisation there comes a moment when they realise that they will not again see their own home and their worldly possessions. This very final environmental separation must be coped with as well as the other fears and anxieties and physical discomforts.

Most of the points made about change of environment earlier in the text, when discussing the preceding ALs, are augmented when the person appreciates that his own death will take place within the restricted personal living space of the hospital. Certainly initially the person is concerned that hospital routines will be unfamiliar, especially those associated with washing and toileting; that privacy will be threatened; that eating and drinking likes and dislikes may not be given much consideration, and the type of food may be alien to his taste; that ward temperature and humidity may be uncomfortable for him; that noise levels and the presence of other people will disturb periods of sleep; that if bedfast, the capacity to mobilise will be out of his control; that there will be difficulty communicating with staff and other patients who are all strangers. All of these potential problems are exacerbated if the person comes from a different cultural group, especially if there are strict religious/cultural practices associated with dying and death, some of which may not be feasible to countenance in an institutional setting.

In Western culture, because hospitals and a lot of their equipment and procedures are so geared to 'cure' — and lack of ability to cure is often seen as professional failure — it is not surprising that the prospect of dying and death in a hospital environment can create such problems for the patient and family.

It is, in fact, a sad reflection on our lack of preparation and provision for care of the dying that it was seen to be necessary to create what has become known as the hospice movement. It is undeniable that, in a hospice, there is expertise in terminal care; that there are calm, relaxed surroundings where care and concern for the wishes of the patient are paramount, and this permeates the environment. Indeed there is almost dismay that they have acquired 'an aura of élitism, an idea of excellence in practice that can neither be achieved in the home nor in general hospitals'. (Nursing Times Editorial, 1976).

It is important to the nurse to appreciate that despite the physical constraints of a hospital ward, everything possible should be done to provide an environment which will assist the patient to die peacefully and with dignity.

PHYSICAL PROBLEMS ASSOCIATED WITH DYING

Pain. Pain is probably what many people fear most about the process of dying and, although it is experienced at other times throughout life, it can be of particular distress to the dying. As long ago as 1972 Hinton was reporting that about one patient in eight suffered pain in the terminal illness and Cartwright et al in 1973 reported that in their sample, two-thirds of patients who died at home suffered from a distressing degree of pain. These findings are corroborated in more recent studies (Hockley, 1984).

For a long time it seemed to be assumed that the pain of dying could not be controlled and had to be endured.

The work of Dr Cicely Saunders and others has radically altered medical thinking about this and it is now quite clear that with prudent use of analgesic drugs, control of terminal pain can and should be achieved. The basic principle of management is that sufficiently potent analgesics are given *regularly* so that pain is not only relieved, but prevented and if pain does occur, then the dose should be increased or the drug changed.

The prescribing of drugs is of course a medical responsibility but it is one which relies on competent nursing assessment of pain (p. 40) and regular evaluation of the effectiveness of the pain control methods employed. Very often nurses do patients a disservice by being reluctant to give analgesics unless the patient's pain is obvious and debilitating, thinking that the drugs may not be effective if given too often or too early in the terminal phase. In fact, routine administration of drugs can be effective for months in the majority of cases.

In addition to pain caused by the terminal illness, the patient may suffer from other types of pain too. If he is confined to bed he may experience pain due to pressure or lack of movement. Joint pains and muscular tension can be alleviated with careful positioning, massage and the application of local heat.

Wilkes (1974) tried to find out what particular discomforts were suffered by terminally ill patients and he identified the 10 major symptoms experienced after admission to hospital as outlined in Table 18.1.

Table 18.1 Discomforts suffered by terminally ill patients

Symptom	Suffered by terminally ill patients (%)
Pain	58
Incontinence	38
Confusion	21
Dyspnoea	17
Nausea	16
Bedsores	15
Vomiting	13
Open wounds	13
Cough	5
Dysphagia	3

Wilkes 1974

More recently Hockley (1984) carried out a study in two different hospitals, interviewing patients, relatives and nursing staff and found that there were distressing physical symptoms related to mouth infections, anorexia, sleeplessness, pressure sores, as well as pain. In order to identify whether or not a patient is experiencing any of these problems, or may be likely to, the nurse needs to carry out an assessment of all ALs. Some of the nursing activities which may be implemented to alleviate these problems are mentioned below, with reference made to earlier discussion of them.

Anorexia, nausea and vomiting (pp. 171, 179, 179). It is

helpful if nurses pay special attention to the patient's food and fluid intake. Small, easily digested meals which are appetising to the individual should be offered at regular intervals. The patient should be encouraged, and helped if necessary, to clean his teeth in the hope that he will feel more comfortable and perhaps therefore more inclined to take food. Anti-emetic drugs may be prescribed to relieve persistent nausea; a nasogastric tube may be passed to prevent constant retching.

Difficulty in swallowing. Dysphagia makes eating and drinking very uncomfortable. A local anaesthetic in gel form given before food, or food given in semi-solid form, may help to ease the patient's difficulty.

Dehydration (p. 173). Frequent small drinks of the patient's choice should be made available and help may be needed if the patient is weak or unable to sit up. The nurse may find that it is fear of incontinence which causes the patient to reduce fluid intake. Adequate hydration is by far the best method of preventing a 'dirty' mouth.

Incontinence (p. 195). The dying person can be extremely distressed by incontinence and it is necessary for the nurse to approach this problem with sympathy and tact. Despite its hazards, catheterisation may be the best way to deal with urinary incontinence in these circumstances.

Constipation (p. 194). Undernutrition may contribute to constipation as well as lack of exercise and inadequate fluid intake and the patient suffers considerable discomfort. Treatment by laxatives may be necessary if faecal impaction becomes a potential problem.

Pressure sores (p. 222). General debility, reduced movement, reduced food intake and lack of vitamin C, and impaired sensation may cause pressure sores to develop more readily in the dying person. Regular turning to relieve prolonged pressure on any one part may be carried out, but if this is too disturbing, bed appliances alone should be used. Although prevention of pressure sores is important, it is more important to allow the dying person as much comfort and peace as possible in the absolutely final stages of life. Dying patients often seem to become very sensitive to pressure, such as from bedclothes, and great patience and skill may be needed to help the patient to remain comfortable in bed.

Difficulty in breathing (p. 150). The patient and the visitors can be very distressed by dyspnoea. Chemotherapy is often used to ease it but administration of oxygen is seldom helpful because use of the mask often merely increases the feeling of suffocation. Ventilating the room, placing the bed near a window even if only for the psychological effect, and being with the patient may ease the sense of panic and fear. The very noisy breathing known as the 'death rattle' can be subdued with drugs which dry up the excessive secretions in the respiratory tract.

Unpleasant odour. Unless the nurses are meticulous in carrying out nursing activities related to such conditions as incontinence or discharging wounds, an unpleasant smell can result and it is distressing to all concerned. Hormones or other drugs can be used to reduce the smell from a fungating lesion, such as may occur in advanced cancer of the breast. Good ventilation of the room and discreet use of aerosol sprays can be helpful and the patients will appreciate any attempt to minimise what for them is also a distressing problem.

Nursing activities aimed to promote physical comfort for the dying are not substantially different from those applicable to problems of ALs described earlier. However greater skill and patience are often demanded of the nurse because 'minor' discomforts can assume major proportions as the patient's independence and strength diminish. Encouragement can be given for the patient to participate in his care if he so wishes and nursing routines must be flexible to allow attention to be given at times when the patient feels able to cope with disturbance and when pain control is at its optimum.

PSYCHOLOGICAL PROBLEMS ASSOCIATED WITH DYING

Each dying patient and those close to him will react to the approaching death in a very individual way. The psychological and emotional reactions will vary as will the nature of the problems experienced. There will be differences too according to whether the dying person is cared for at home or in hospital; and whether either or both parties are aware of the prognosis and the likely course of the terminal illness.

Fear and anxiety. Almost universally, dying people experience fear and anxiety in the process of dying. These are reactions to any illness but are particularly intense in terminal illness because there is no prospect of recovery. There are so many things about which the dying person may feel apprehensive and afraid: fear of death, fear of pain, fear of the process of dying, fear of loss of control and dignity, and fear of being alone or of being rejected are just some of them.

The knowledge that death will mean parting from family and friends obviously is a source of great sadness to the dying person and often there is considerable anxiety about their future and about how they will cope with their bereavement. The onset of depression, described earlier as a common feature of the dying process, is sometimes mistaken as a physical symptom but most probably is more often caused by the dying person's feelings of sadness, fear and regret.

In gaining strength and courage to face death without fear many people find their religious beliefs an invaluable resource. For some patients who die in hospital the chaplain becomes an important source of comfort and companionship. The hospital chaplain (or any other representative of any faith) who is a welcome visitor for the patient should be made to feel welcome in the ward by the nursing staff. He is, after all, a member of the multiprofessional health care team with a special role and function. With his religious knowledge and ability to give spiritual guidance, the chaplain has a particular contribution to make to the care of the dying patient. Often he becomes the person in whom the patient confides innermost fears and anxieties; sometimes the chaplain helps the dying patient to understand the significance of death and to accept it with dignity and without fear.

Loneliness. According to Kastenbaum (1981) one of the greatest concerns among people who are dying is that they will be left alone. People who die in hospital sometimes can experience an overwhelming sense of loneliness; although they are not 'alone', they are without close companionship. The contact which the nurse has with the patient who is dying is frequent and, if allowed, can become the basis of a trusting relationship which will prevent loneliness and isolation. There is probably no patient who is more in need of tender loving care than the patient who is nearing death. McNulty (1974) makes this point well when she says: 'We are sometimes so overwhelmed by the broader issues raised by our technical ability to maintain a semblance of life and defer the moment of death, that we are in danger of losing sight of that precious, human personal touch that is our role to give.'

Forming a supportive relationship with a dying patient is not easy and often nurses seem to avoid getting involved at all. Sometimes this is because they do not understand that reactions such as anger and depression are 'normal' in the process of dying. Often it is because they are afraid of being faced with the question 'Am I dying?' In fact, this question is not often asked but, if it is, it means the patient wants to talk about his fears and uncertainties. It is important for nurses to remember that dying patients usually *are* aware of their prognosis. Even though the patient has not been told explicitly there are many subtle ways in which the information may be transmitted to him by doctors and nurses. Sometimes both the patient and family choose not to admit openly that they know the prognosis; in other cases the knowledge is frankly shared. Whether or not dying patients should be told of their prognosis is a complex and delicate question.

There are good reasons on practical, psychological and spiritual grounds for adopting a policy in favour of telling the truth. But equally there may be reasons on occasions for withholding this information in the best interests of the patient. In practice, the decision should not be difficult if dying patients are given time and opportunity, with someone they can talk to and trust, to explore their fears and suspicions and to indicate what they want (and don't want) to know. What is important is for the nurse to be sensitive to the patient's own awareness of his situation and to know what he has been told by his doctor and relatives.

This of course means that the nurse must assess the patient's situation and the most important source of information is the patient. The nurse will learn what she needs to know by listening carefully, observing astutely and communicating effectively. Once she knows what the patient feels and understands about the situation, she can gain confidence to form a close relationship and show the patient that she is willing to listen. A dying patient, feeling lonely and afraid, will gain comfort from companionship and closeness. Spending time with him, talking or sharing in his silence, and taking care over physical needs can restore tranquillity to an existence which in so many ways is in turmoil. Showing sympathy and compassion are important aspects of nursing a dying patient and essential if the nurse is to help with the many psychological problems which may arise in the dying process.

THE FAMILY'S PROBLEMS

The patient's family too may feel afraid and anxious. They find it hard to watch if their loved one is suffering and find it difficult to understand the fluctuating moods, and sometimes unpredictable reactions to their visits. They may fear their own ability to cope with the event of death, to control their emotions and to face the future alone.

If the person is being looked after in hospital, the family may feel cut off and unable to find ways of expressing their love and concern; and in the publicity of an open ward they may find that maintaining their close relationship becomes difficult. In caring for a dying person at home the family faces other stresses arising from the total involvement of that situation. Their ability to cope emotionally may be eroded by the exhaustion of providing for all the needs of the dying person in the last stages of illness.

The positive value of establishing a supportive and humane relationship with the relatives of a dying patient is emphasised by McNulty (1974) when she says:

Nurses have a lot to answer for in their apparent insensitivity to the needs of relatives . . . I think that we are sometimes afraid to stop for fear we might not be able to answer the questions asked; afraid because we cannot give the so much wanted good news; afraid because we might have to say 'I don't know'. If only we could realise that just by stopping for a moment and sharing our presence, we may have to some degree lightened the family's burden.

Being accessible is the essential point. The relatives should be encouraged to see the nurse or doctor in charge, and at visiting times, nurses must be available and able to make such arrangements. Yet Bond (1982) in a series of articles called 'Relatively Speaking' found that despite a great deal of literature about the need for communication, nurses still do not seem to make themselves available. Practical advice about when and how often to visit can be helpful to the family, and allowing close relatives to help in the care of the patient, for example by helping him to wash or have a meal, may be greatly appreciated as this gives a purpose to visits and provides the opportunity for affection and concern to be expressed.

It is often the nurse who has to break the news of the actual event of death to the patient's next-of-kin and this is a task which must be done as sensitively and compassionately as possible. The nurse can do little to ease the relative's distress; what is important is that she is prepared for the fact that reactions cannot be predicted. The relative may appear totally inconsolable or almost unconcerned; sometimes anger is directed at the nurse or doctor. Whatever the reaction the nurse must remain calm and kind. Requests to see the body should be allowed as this can be important in confirming the reality and allowing the saying of a final farewell.

Dealing kindly with the practicalities will be appreciated. It is important that the next-of-kin understands what is written on the death certificate given by the doctor and knows that this has to be taken within a certain time to the office of the Registrar of Births, Deaths and Marriages in the district in which the hospital is situated (not the district of the deceased person's home). The Registrar provides the certificate which authorises an undertaker to arrange the funeral. Usually the nurse also returns the deceased person's effects to the next-of-kin and this should be done sympathetically, making sure that the person has some means of transport home. The way in which nurses deal with the family at this final contact with the hospital is very important. Kindness and practical help will be remembered with gratitude whereas lack of this may well contribute to a lingering bad memory of the patient's time in hospital.

Following the death, there are many problems which may face the bereaved as they attempt to accept and cope with the loss. There are emotional problems of grief, the difficulties of social adjustment and sometimes there are economic strains too, if the deceased person was the family breadwinner.

The early stage of acute grief is particularly distressing and sometimes involves feelings of self-criticism and guilt, the person wondering if the death could have been prevented. Acute reactive depression and even suicidal thoughts may occur. Sometimes the problem is that the grief reaction may be delayed, particularly if the bereaved had much to do with the practicalities of the funeral or if the death was very sudden or totally unexpected in the illness. Then they may wonder why they do not feel shocked and sad, only later having to cope with these intense feelings. Some people find it distressing to mourn openly and find the funeral traumatic; others may be worried by the intensity of their emotions when alone and

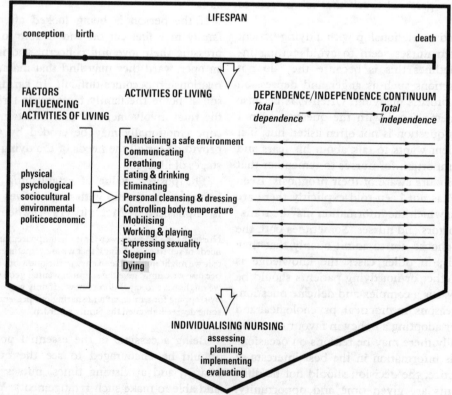

Fig. 18.1 The AL of dying within the model for nursing

wonder if they might be on the verge of a complete mental breakdown. Most people appear to be surprised by just how long their feelings of loss and sadness last and begin to wonder if they will ever readjust and resume a normal life again. Bereavement is probably the most devastating experience which is faced in life and it disrupts every Activity of Living.

The most helpful contribution the nurse can make is to help the bereaved persons to face up to and work through the emotional difficulties. This means that they must be given time: time to grieve, time to talk, to reminisce, to express openly fears and worries and to begin to plan a new future. The community nurse is in an ideal position to assess the needs and problems of a bereaved person. An elderly man now on his own could be helped to cope with the domestic tasks previously done by his wife. A mother left to bring up young children might be given help to consider what to tell the children and how to support them in their grief.

In fact helping bereaved people is a communal responsibility; a basic human concern which can be shared by both professionals and the public. Bereavement is not an illness but a life event with which most people need the help of others. Giving help to the bereaved needs to begin before the death if this is possible, so that grief can be anticipated and preparations made for readjustment.

Grief cannot be cured, but it can be shared. Showing compassion to the bereaved will be a reminder that, despite their loss, they are not entirely alone and that there is some reason to renew their sources of faith and hope, and have the courage to begin again.

Caring for the dying and bereaved is an important aspect of nursing. The emphasis of all nursing is on helping people to cope with the Activities of Living; dealing with death is no different. Caring for the dying is concerned with life before death and helping the bereaved is about life after death.

In the first chapter of this book the role of the nurse in caring for the dying was mentioned when Virginia Henderson's famous definition of the function of nursing was discussed. She wrote: 'Nursing is primarily assisting the individual (sick or well) in the performance of those activities contributing to health, or its recovery (*or to a peaceful death*) that he would perform unaided if he had the necessary strength, will or knowledge ...'

Nursing is concerned with helping people, both in living and in dying.

In the second half of this chapter some of the problems and discomforts which can be experienced by patients in relation to the AL of dying have been described. This provides the beginning nurse with a generalised idea of these; it will be useful in assessing, planning, implementing and evaluating an individualised programme for each patient's AL of dying.

This chapter has been concerned with the AL of dying. However, as stated previously it is only for the purpose of discussion that any AL can be considered on its own; in reality the various activities are so closely related and do not have distinct boundaries. Figure 18.1 is a reminder that the AL of dying is related to the other ALs and also to the various components of the model for nursing.

REFERENCES

Black D 1980 Working group on inequalities in health, HMSO, London
Bond S 1982 Communicating with families of cancer patients. Nursing Times 78 (24) June 16: 1027–1029
Capper E 1982 Stillbirth. Nursing 34 February: 1490
Cartwright A et al 1973 Life before death. Routledge & Kegan Paul, London
Cassons J 1980 Dying — the greatest adventure of my life. Christian Medical Fellowship, London
Editorial 1976 The hospice movement. Nursing Times 72 (26) July 1: 3
Frederich J 1976 Grief as a disease process. Omega 7: 297–306
Gyulay J A 1975 The forgotten grievers. American Journal of Nursing 75 (9) September: 1476–1479
Health Departments of GB and N Ireland 1983 Cadaveric organs for transplantation. DHSS, London
Hockley J 1984 Complaints from terminally ill. Nursing Mirror 158 (12) March 21: 12
Kubler-Ross E 1969 On death and dying. Macmillan, New York
Kastenbaum R 1981 Death, society and human experience. Mosby, St Louis
Levenstein R, Joseph B 1978 Jewish teaching concerning death. Nursing Times Occasional Paper 74 (9) March 23: 35–36
Limerick S 1984 Sudden infant death. Nursing Times 80 (10) March 7: 28–29
McCarthy J 1980 Death, anxiety and loss of the self. Gardner Press, New York
McNulty B 1974 The nurse's contribution in terminal care. Nursing Mirror 139 (15) October 10: 59–61
Madison D, Viola A 1968 The health of widows in the year following bereavement. Journal of Psychosomatic Research 12: 297
Murray Parkes C 1972 Bereavement: studies of grief in adult life. Penguin, Harmondworth
Nagy M 1969 The child's theories concerning death. In: Teifal (ed) The meaning of death. McGraw Hill, New York
Pike C 1983 The broken heart syndrome and the elderly patient. Nursing Times 79 (19) March 2: 50–53
Richardson R 1980 Losses: talking about bereavement. Open Books, Somerset
Roberts L 1977 Suicide. Nursing Mirror 144 (2) January 13: 68–69
Saunders C 1976 Problems of euthanasia. Nursing Times 72 (26) July 1: 4–9
Taber S 1982 The role of the transplant co-ordinator. Nursing Times 78 (23) June 9: 973–978
Walker C 1982 Attitudes to death and bereavement among cultural minority groups. Nursing Times 78 (50) December 15: 2106–2109
Wilkes E 1974 Relatives, professional care and the dying patient. Nursing Mirror 139 (15) October 10: 53–56

ADDITIONAL READING

Clinical Forum 10 Bereavement. Nursing Mirror 157 (19) November 9: i–xvi
Sofaer B 1983 Pain relief — the core of nursing practice. Nursing Times 79 (47) November 23: 38–42
Williams J 1980 Appetite in the terminally ill patient. Nursing Times 76 (20) May 15: 875–876

Documentation of Nursing

19

Using the model in practice

We firmly believe that to be useful, a model for nursing has to be applicable in the real world of nursing — that is in everyday practice. In order to begin to evaluate the usefulness of our model in practice we initiated a small project in which nurses in nine different practice settings tried out the model with one patient. Data from assessment of all nine patients were recorded on the Patient Assessment Form in the format in which it was first published in *The Elements of Nursing* (1980); it reflects our model for nursing. For the three other phases of the process of nursing the nurses designed their own documents and these were presented in the publication arising from the project — *Using a Model for Nursing* (1983a). On the basis of the contributors' presentations and suggestions, we designed and presented in that book a more comprehensive document which not only reflects our model for nursing, but also incorporates all four phases of the process of nursing. The document is made up of four pages (A4 size), headed as follows:

- Patient Assessment Form: Biographical and health data
- Patient Assessment Form: Assessment of ALs
- Nursing Plan: Related to ALs
- Nursing Plan: Derived from medical/other prescription

Before proceeding to comment further on this document and various issues related to documentation, a brief reminder of our model for nursing might be helpful; it is based on a model of living which describes individuality in living, and the equivalent component in the model for nursing is 'individualising nursing'. The five components of the model for nursing are:

- 12 Activities of Living
- lifespan

347

- dependence/independence continuum
- factors influencing the ALs
- individualising nursing

In the model for nursing (Fig. 19.1) the first four components lead into the fifth, individualising nursing, and the process of nursing — assessing, planning, implementing and evaluating — is used to achieve this objective.

The four phases of the process of nursing will be discussed in turn, together with information about the re-

- collecting information from/about patients
- reviewing the collected information
- identifying the patient's problems
- identifying priority among problems

Patient Asssessment Form
The most comprehensive patient assessment is carried out as soon as possible after the patient's admission/referral, and in more or less detail at that time, according to circumstances. As already mentioned we divided our

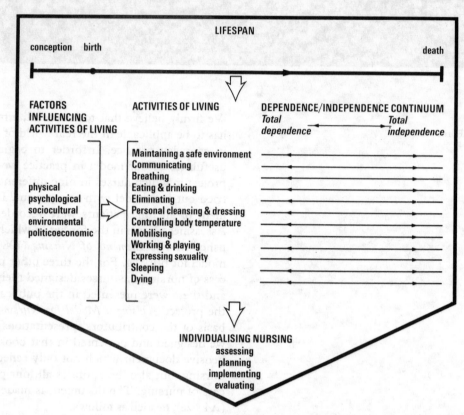

Fig. 19.1 Model for nursing

cording of collected information on the simple documents which we designed. In the context of the model for nursing, this chapter focuses on documentation, because in practice it is a crucial part of implementing the process. It is from what is recorded on nursing documents that beginning nurses will develop much of their understanding of the process, and what is involved in individualising nursing. Assessing is the first phase of the process, and its documentation will now be discussed.

ASSESSING

The assessing phase of the process of nursing was described on pages 72 to 76, but here, in case there is doubt about what assessment includes, it will be helpful to remind readers of our use of the word. It includes:

Patient Assessment Form into two pages on which to document two different kinds of assessment data. Here further guidance will be given about the use of page one, Figure 19.2 for documentation of biographical and health data.

Biographical and health data. The type of biographical and health data to be collected at the initial assessment was discussed on pages 73 to 74. Here a few more points will be made about specific entries on Figure 19.2, page one.

At 'Type of accommodation' there is an item 'including mode of entry if relevant'. This may seem strange to beginning nurses but it was included on the advice of community nurses who need to know how to gain entry when, for example, the patient is alone and cannot get to the door.

The information collected at 'Significant others' puts

Patient Assessment Form : Biographical and health data

Date of admission   Date of assessment   Nurse's signature

Surname   Forenames

Male ☐   Age ☐   Prefers to be addressed as

Female ☐   Date of birth _____
              Single/Married/Widowed/Other

Address of usual residence

Type of accommodation
(incl. mode of entry
if relevant)

Family/Others at this residence

Next of kin   Name   Address

                   Relationship   Tel. no.

Significant others
(incl. relatives/dependents
visitors/helpers
neighbours)

Support services

Occupation

Religious beliefs and relevant practices

Recent significant life crises

Patient's perception of current health status

Family's perception of patient's health status

Reason for admission/referral

Medical information (e.g. diagnosis, past history, allergies)

GP Address Tel. no.   Consultant Address Tel. no.

Plans for discharge

Fig. 19.2

Page one   *Roper, Logan, Tierney*   ©Longman Group Limited 1985

Patient Assessment Form: Assessment of ALs

Date

Activity of living AL	Usual routines: what can/cannot be done independently previous coping mechanisms	Patient's problems: actual / potential (p)
Reminder of the 12 ALs Maintaining a safe environment Communicating Breathing Eating and drinking Eliminating Personal cleansing and dressing Controlling body temperature Mobilising Working and playing Expressing sexuality Sleeping Dying		

Fig. 19.2

Page two

Roper, Logan, Tierney   © Longman Group Limited 1985

Nursing Plan: Related to ALs

Goals	Nursing interventions related to ALs	Evaluation

Roper, Logan, Tierney

Nursing Plan: Derived from medical/other prescription

Nursing interventions derived from medical/other prescription	Goals	Evaluation

Other Notes

Fig. 19.2

Roper, Logan, Tierney

©Longman Group Limited 1985

the patient in the context of his family and friends and as the nurses on the different shifts read this item and use it in conversation with individual patients, it helps them to feel that the nurses know each one of them as a person and not just as a patient. On the other hand discussion of this item with the patient may reveal that all significant others live at some distance: or as may be the case with elderly patients, information can reveal their social isolation, and in both instances nurses would know that talking with these patients would be an important part of their nursing care.

There is an item 'Medical information (e.g. diagnosis, past history, allergies)': this would include the medical diagnosis as well as any other pertinent medical information relevant to the patient's nursing and it may well be taken from the patient's case-notes. The past history would include any previous hospital admissions. And it is important that staff know of any allergies early in the patient's stay. Other information which could be recorded here might be, in the case of midwifery, when a woman has had a previous baby or babies, the midwife needs to have some details about the pregnancies, deliveries and postnatal care. Any medicine which the patient is taking can also be recorded here.

The information collected at 'Support services' will probably be useful when planning the patient's discharge. It is important for nurses to know the sorts of services which a patient has had before admission and may require after discharge. These can include for example, home helps, meals-on-wheels, attendance at day hospital, district nurse visits, voluntary visitors in the case of patients who are socially isolated, and a laundry service for those who are incontinent. Information about support services is almost always required by nurses in the community.

Activities of Living data. In our second book *Learning to Use the Process of Nursing* (1981) there are examples of the completed Assessment of Activities of Living part of the Patient Assessment Form. This is the original version of the form; it has a ruled space for each AL. The updated version is illustrated in Figure 19.2. The second page is designed for recording data from assessment of the ALs. The main portion of the page is blank so that the nurse can use the space to best advantage for the particular patient. On the left there is a prompt list of the 12 ALs and reference to these is essential in translating our model into practice. The information can be collected by observing, interviewing and measuring. However, information may not need to be collected about all the ALs nor in any particular order and guidance about this is given later, but here the AL framework is set in the context of the other components of the model for nursing.

While collecting information about the patient's ALs the nurse will necessarily take account of the stage on the lifespan, one of the components of the model. There is a reminder to consider the patient's 'Previous routines' and

it is necessary to remember that these will have been fashioned by physical, psychological, sociocultural, environmental and politicoeconomic factors — another component of the model; they are discussed in each of the AL chapters (7 to 18). The nurse is reminded of the dependence/independence continuum of the model by the heading 'what can/cannot be done independently'. And there is a prompt 'previous coping mechanisms' for the nurse to remember that if there are problems or discomforts with any of the ALs, enquiry should be made about how these have been coped with. On page 72 we gave our interpretation of what 'assessment' includes, and this is the reason for the column (on the right of the Patient Assessment Form) headed 'Patient's problems' and there is a reminder that they can be actual or potential.

To return to the blank space on the assessment form (page two, Fig. 19.2): absence of a ruled space for each of the 12 ALs allows documentation of assessment data about the most *problematic* ALs first. To give a few examples, in some cases of acutely ill or injured patients the AL of breathing might take priority and be assessed first: this will be essential when a patient is admitted because of haemoptysis. Data from assessing a patient who has a severe nose bleed will be recorded first, at the entry for the AL of breathing. Should the bleeding be from the stomach (haematemesis) assessment of the AL of eating and drinking would take priority. Bleeding from the rectum would give priority to the AL of eliminating; and haemorrhage from the vagina would give priority to assessing the AL of expressing sexuality. These are examples of circumstances in which the patient's problems are readily apparent and documented in order of priority, an advantage of designing that part of the assessment form as a blank space.

In less acute circumstances however, the blank space can be used to document information about the ALs in the order which seems most appropriate for each patient. Often the actual and potential problems and their priority will be apparent only after reviewing the data collected, in stark contrast to the problems mentioned in the previous paragraph.

On the other hand, patients may have their own priority, for example a person who is both obese and a heavy smoker may opt for tackling one of the problems before the other. And we repeat that in the majority of instances information about the ALs need not be collected in any specific order and indeed in the case of short stay patients, or at subsequent 'assessments' of longer term patients, information about all the ALs may not be necessary.

However, some information about ALs which are not problematic will be useful, and in some cases, essential throughout the patient's stay. This does not need to be re-written on the Nursing Plan, but nevertheless, since it is about the patient's individuality in living, nurses need this information if they are to facilitate the maintaining of independence; to interfere as little as possible with previous habits of living, and to interact with the patient as a person. For example, the entry at personal cleansing and dressing may state 'baths independently each morning' alerting the nurse to make sure that a bathroom is available; the entry at mobilising may say 'exercises for 10 minutes each morning' and it may be desirable to provide privacy and avoid interfering with this healthy habit. The entry at working and playing can provide a relevant topic of conversation manifesting the nurse's interest in the patient as a person thereby alleviating some of the negative feelings which can be the experience of being a patient. However for those ALs which are presenting a problem the information is likely to change as the nursing intervention is achieving/not achieving the set goals by the set date.

Here it is pertinent to clarify an important point about using our model; choosing the relevant AL at which to document assessment data. In most instances it is self-evident but there is some information which does not always appear to link specifically to one AL; examples are pain, haemorrhage and pressure sores. These examples were brought to our notice by the contributors to *Using a Model for Nursing* (1983a). Although 'Body structure and function' required for each AL is not a 'component' of the model, it is necessary for users of the model to know which of these are required for each AL because it indicates at which AL to document assessment data about the examples given above — pain, haemorrhage and pressure sores.

The nervous system is necessary for awareness of pain, and in our model, the nervous system is part of the body structure and function required for the AL of communicating, so assessment data about pain (which is not specifically related to any of the other ALs) should be documented at the AL of communicating. Examples of such pain would be headache, angina at rest, and abdominal pain not related to eating and drinking, or eliminating. However, pain which mainly interferes with a particular AL should be documented at that AL; for example pain in the lower limbs interferes mainly with mobilising so should be documented there.

Some guidance about the documentation of assessment data related to haemorrhage has already been given in the context of priorities in assessing ALs, and some particular types of haemorrhage related to specific ALs were mentioned there. But when the bleeding is from vessels unrelated to a particular AL, then the effects of the loss of blood will manifest in the cardiopulmonary system, which, in our model for nursing, is part of the body structure and function required for the AL of breathing. Consequently information about this sort of haemorrhage and its assessment will be documented at the AL of breathing.

Similarly the skin was discussed as one of the body structures and functions required for the AL of personal cleansing and dressing. And the subject of pressure sores was included in the discussion of this AL (Ch. 12). Consequently the assessment data about any potential or actual problem of pressure sores will be documented at the AL of personal cleansing and dressing.

There need not be hard and fast rules about where to document particular data but obviously it is helpful if nurses who work together and are using this model adopt a similar classification and, in the main, it becomes self-evident as familiarity with the model is acquired.

Summarising this section — assessment of ALs is not complete until the collected data have been reviewed, and the patient's actual and potential problems with particular ALs have been identified, then arranged in order of priority if this is relevant.

PLANNING

Planning was discussed on pages 76 to 77: it is the second phase of the process of nursing and it cannot be carried out until information from the initial assessment is available. As a reminder, it starts with setting short- and/or long-term goals for each identified actual and potential problem. The goal-setting part of planning should, whenever possible, be written in terms amenable to observing, interviewing, measuring and testing where appropriate to facilitate evaluation at a later date as specified on the Nursing Plan. The nursing interventions to achieve the set goals by the set time are then selected. To document the planning phase of the process of nursing we designed the Nursing Plan (Fig. 19.2, pages three and four).

Nursing Plan

The Nursing Plan should not only inform the nurses of the particular nursing interventions which have to be implemented during the spell of duty, but should contain all the planned nursing interventions; for example, some interventions may only be carried out weekly but could have nursing implications in the intervening period. We designed the Nursing Plan so that information about nursing interventions related to ALs could be documented separately from those derived from medical prescription.

Nursing Plan related to ALs. The Nursing Plan on page three of our document (Fig. 19.2) is related to the ALs and it forms the right side of the double fold. This positioning is deliberate so that the problems, both actual and potential, identified at the initial assessment, do not need to be written again. In the case of an emergency admission they will be listed in order of priority, otherwise they need to be numbered in priority. Opposite the problems the goals can be written, together with the 'Nursing interventions related to ALs' and there is a column in which to record the result of 'Evaluation'. If the goal is written in terms so that the nurse can observe, interview, measure or test to discover its achievement/non-achievement, then beside the date in the evaluation column it may only be necessary to write 'Goal achieved' and the nurse's signature (Roper, Logan & Tierney, 1983b).

The Nursing Plan may have nursing interventions at an AL even although there is not a specific problem stated. An example is the patient does not have a problem with mobilising but there is a nursing intervention at that AL — 'encourage patient to do foot exercises 2 hourly'. The goal is prevention of deep vein thrombosis manifested by no change in the circumference of the calf of the leg, no increase in the temperature of the skin over the calf, and no pain in the calf. Another example is the patient who does not have a problem with the AL of eating and drinking but there is a nursing intervention at that AL — 'encourage patient to eat adequate protein and vitamin C'. The goal is to prevent pressure sores by having adequately nourished tissues over the pressure areas.

The Nursing Plan is just that — a *plan* which tells nurses what to do and when. Extra information should only be written on it when a goal has been achieved; when the nursing intervention has to be changed to achieve the already set goal; when for any reason the goal has to be modified; when the date for evaluation is changed (delayed) to allow more time for the nursing intervention to achieve the set goal; or if the patient develops another problem. Before discussing where day-to-day information about the patient should be recorded we will finish this section by discussing page four of our Nursing Plan (Fig. 19.2).

Nursing Plan derived from medical/other prescription. The documents we have discussed so far cater for the nurse-initiated nursing interventions related to ALs but clearly there are nursing interventions which are derived directly from medical prescription (Fig. 19.2, page four). Already most hospitals and local authorities have a method of documenting prescribed drugs such as: name of drug, dose, time of administration, route by which it has to be given, together with the nurse's signature. There are also many charts in use for recording prescribed measurements such as fluid intake and output; blood pressure; temperature, pulse and respiration. They are filled in by nurses who, as well as doctors, use information from these documents. However, these do not cater for other nursing interventions which also derive from medical or other prescription and contributors to the third book *Using a Model for Nursing* (1983a) experienced difficulty with this. Reflecting on their uncertainty about where to document nursing interventions from such prescriptions as lumbar puncture and so on, we decided to add page four (Fig. 19.2) to our Nursing Plan, thereby documenting the medically derived nursing interventions separately.

At the bottom of this part of the Nursing Plan is a space for 'Other Notes'. The information which could be recorded here might be about the time and place of clinic appointments; arrangements for transport to and from these clinics; and particulars about the loan of equipment, such as a walking frame for the patient to use at home. These examples alert the nurse to the fact that planning is necessary for the patient's discharge. However, there is no constraint on the type of relevant information which nurses may find necessary to record in this space.

IMPLEMENTING

While introducing documentation for the process of nursing, many hospitals have designed an assessment form and a 'care plan' or a nursing plan as we prefer to call it. We also recommend the use of a document separate from our four-page Patient Assessment Form and Nursing Plan for recording the individualised nursing resulting from use of the other two documents. This is the Patient's Nursing Notes, the use of which will now be discussed.

Patient's Nursing Notes

The Patient's Nursing Notes must be used in conjunction with the Patient Assessment Form and the Nursing Plan but unlike them, it does not have a particular design because it is a 'daily report' on the individual patient. On it should be written for each shift when relevant: additional assessment data; all planned nursing interventions which have been carried out; any additional evaluation data, together with any other pertinent information, for instance, the patient feeling transient nausea during an intervention. Or perhaps the patient did not eat supper, which in the absence of nausea and/or vomiting does not constitute a problem, but the nurses on the next shift need to be aware of this to alert them to monitor the patient's appetite.

If the additional assessment data on the Patient's Nursing Notes reveal a new problem, it will be added to the Nursing Plan where it will have a goal, a nursing intervention and a date for evaluation. If the entry in the Nursing Notes is 'dressing changed, wound now infected' then this new problem of infection will be added to the Nursing Plan at the AL of personal cleansing and dressing. Should the additional evaluation data on the Nursing Notes show that the set goal has been achieved, this will be recorded on the Nursing Plan and the nursing intervention will be cancelled. If the Nursing Notes reveal that the goal has only been partially achieved by the set date, a decision will have to be made about delaying the date for evaluation. Should the notes say that the problem is unchanged, extra assessment data will be collected and a decision made about changing the nursing intervention to achieve the already set goal. If the Nursing Notes reveal that the problem has become worse, extra assessment information will guide the decision about the nursing intervention and perhaps restating the goal on the Nursing Plan.

The Patient's Nursing Notes, the Patient Assessment Form and the Nursing Plan should be a permanent part of nursing documentation. Writing on them should not be erased and they should be filed with other records on the patient's discharge or transfer. Because of an increasingly litigation-conscious public, most hospitals now recognise the legal status of nursing documents and are filing them so that there is a permanent record after a patient's discharge from the health service. Well-designed, well-written records which are concise and precise will be of inestimable value to a defence lawyer providing evidence in a court of law in relation to a litigant's claim (Roper, Logan & Tierney, 1983b).

However the accuracy of nursing records is up for criticism. Castledine (1982) states '... there have already been at least two legal cases in this country this year which have questioned the quality and content of nursing records — and progress notes in particular.' It is obvious that the content of nursing records must be improved.

EVALUATING

The relatedness of evaluating to the other three phases of the process of nursing cannot be overemphasised. In the foregoing discussion of the *implementing* phase we wrote about collecting evaluation data. Evaluation could be said to start whenever a goal is set and that is the first activity in the *planning* phase. To set the goal there must be an identified problem and that is the last activity in the *assessing* phase. Goal-setting then, is an integral part of evaluating. We advocated patient participation in goal-setting and this is no less true for evaluating (Roper, Logan & Tierney, 1983c).

The close relationship between goal-setting in the planning phase of the process of nursing, and the evaluating phase has already been referred to in this chapter. Here it is important to point out that the evaluating phase is the only one which does not have a separate document. The quality of evaluating is entirely dependent on the quality of the written goals which, it cannot be too strongly stressed, should be in terms so that the nurse can observe, interview, measure or test to discover their achievement/non-achievement. Ongoing evaluation data should be written on the Patient's Nursing Notes; and on the set date for 'evaluation', information will be written in the appropriate column of the Nursing Plan.

In most cases there should be a combination of the nurse's objective evaluation and the patient's subjective evaluation, and these may not correlate. For example, the nurse may observe that a patient looks less flushed and appears to be less restless which could indicate less pain; however the patient may say that the pain has not lessened. Of course in this instance the patient's subjective evaluation will override the nurse's objective evaluation because 'pain is what the patient says it is' (p. 133). If a dehydrated patient has to drink from a glass a measured amount of fluid in each 2 hours, there will be 2 hourly evaluation (by observation) of whether the prescribed amount has been taken; if not, the remaining fluid will be measured, thus providing objective data that the goal has only been partially achieved. Should the goal include 'clean moist mouth' and 'lack of thirst', inspection of the patient's mouth followed by a descriptive observation would be objective information, and the patient's response to enquiry about being thirsty would be subjective information.

In the general discussion about assessing (p. 72) and evaluating (p. 78), data collecting instruments were mentioned. These include the Norton scale, (p. 226) for identifying patients at risk of developing pressure sores; and a painometer (p. 41).

Elsewhere in this book (p. 327) there is discussion of the Glasgow coma scale. Use of these types of instrument is becoming increasingly common in health care. When used in assessing they give an objective measure thereby permitting goals to be stated specifically, and evaluation will reveal whether or not there has been change in the desired direction.

Before change can be quantitatively evaluated, measurement is required. However the development of measuring scales is still in its infancy in nursing. Scales could be formulated by practising nurses when they recognise entities which are measurable; but of course the scales should then be subjected to systematic trials with a representative sample to establish reliability and validity.

DOCUMENTATION

Increased paperwork is one of the most common negative criticisms about using the process of nursing in practice (Roper, Logan & Tierney, 1983b). But to be fair the 'process' paperwork has to be compared with previous paperwork which is mostly in the form of nursing orders and daily reports in the Kardex and in books such as the 'TPR book'; and lists of patients requiring medicines, injections, wound dressings and so on. And even if there *is* more paperwork the important questions are: is it helpful for patients, nurses and nursing, and is it manageable within the constraints of time and staffing levels?

Answering these questions briefly, and taking patients first, most of the contributors to *Using a Model for Nursing* (1983a) mentioned that the patient had found the 'try-out' of the model helpful. It is difficult to determine factually whether or not using the process is of benefit to patients. As yet, criteria for measuring quality of nursing are underdeveloped.

However Miller (1984) found little difference in the result of nursing carried out by task-allocation, and by using the process of nursing in the short-term; but in the long-term, patients in the 'process' ward were less dependent, less incontinent and happier. There is sufficient anecdotal evidence that the majority of patients welcome the increased interest which nurses take in them, particularly during the initial assessment. Set against this is a minority of patients who may feel that their privacy is threatened by the more comprehensive nursing assessment.

Next, is it helpful to nurses? All those in the small project were positive about trying out our model for nursing with one patient and said that the different paperwork was worthwhile. Substantiating this, there is considerable anecdotal evidence, some of it published in nursing journals, that nurses, particularly students, find using the process of nursing in practice helpful.

With regard to whether or not practical use of the process of nursing is helpful to nursing, it would only be fair to say that there are some nurses who are against it. In an article entitled 'Is there a danger of "processing" patients?' (Roper, Logan & Tierney, 1983c) we discussed the concern that because the nursing process is so heavily weighted on the scientific method, it seems to belittle the intuitive, artistic side of nursing. We argued that this does not have to be the case.

Here however we make our stance clear: we believe that the nursing documents will be the means of achieving *continuity of nursing* and not *continuity of nurses*; the latter less feasible because of the increasing use of part-time workers, and decreasing weekly working hours. Furthermore we believe that analysis of accumulated available nursing data, documented in process format, could refine nurses' concept of nursing and keep it congruent with reality.

To make documentation of nursing manageable within the constraints of time and staffing levels, the search is for comprehensive but simple documents (reflecting a model for nursing) on which to record the four phases of the process precisely and concisely.

In this chapter we have given guidance about using our simple Patient Assessment Form and Nursing Plan and we have discussed use of the Patient's Nursing Notes. But all of the book contributes to the thinking which will guide the nurse in using these simple documents, and familiarity with our model for nursing is a pre-requisite to using the documents.

However we have no doubt about the complexity of documenting nursing because the process of nursing involves a complex network of activities, their relatedness compounding this complexity. Furthermore the unique individuality of each patient requires nurses to acquire the necessary skills to be adaptable and imaginative in coping with this. And it is the patient's individuality in living which is the basis for individualising nursing.

REFERENCES

Castledine G 1982 The patient's progress. Nursing Mirror 155 (16) October 20: 41

Miller A F 1984 Nursing Process and patient care. Nursing Times Occasional Paper 80 (13) June 27: 56–58

Roper N, Logan W, Tierney A 1980 The elements of nursing. Churchill Livingstone, Edinburgh

Roper N, Logan W, Tierney A 1981 Learning to use the process of nursing. Churchill Livingstone, Edinburgh

Roper N, Logan W, Tierney A (eds) 1983a Using a model for nursing. Churchill Livingstone, Edinburgh

Roper N, Logan W, Tierney A 1983b Endless paperwork? Nursing Mirror 156 (25) June 22: 34–35

Roper N, Logan W, Tierney A 1983c Is there a danger of 'processing' patients? Nursing Mirror 156 (22) June 1: 32–33

ADDITIONAL READING

Roper N, Logan W, Tierney A 1983 A model for nursing. Nursing Times 79 (9) March 2: 24–27

Roper N, Logan W, Tierney A 1983 A nursing model. Nursing Mirror 156 (21) May 25: 17–19

Roper N, Logan W, Tierney A 1983 Problems or needs? Nursing Mirror 156 (23) June 8: 43–44

Roper N, Logan W, Tierney A 1983 Identifying the goals. Nursing Mirror 156 (24) June 15: 22–23

Roper N, Logan W, Tierney A 1983 Unity with diversity. Nursing Mirror 156 (26) June 29: 35

Appendices

Appendix 1

WORLD HEALTH ORGANIZATION (WHO)

International health organisations

International co-operation on health matters began in 1851 with the 1st International Sanitary Conference, held in Paris. It was mainly concerned with the many controversies over quarantine regulations in the Mediterranean ports. Epidemic diseases such as cholera and yellow fever were rife in Europe but at that time the cause was still unknown; pathogenic microorganisms were only beginning to be isolated in the 1880s.

During the next hundred years, other International Sanitary Conferences were held. Gradually, in step with the rapid progress in technological and medical knowledge, the scope of international co-operation was broadened to deal with topics related to health such as nutrition and housing, and with the creation of research centres to study disease.

The activities associated with international health were halted during the Second World War but when it ended, the United Nations Organization approved the establishment in 1946 of the World Health Organization, the first worldwide body of its kind.

The structure of WHO

The headquarters of WHO is in Geneva, Switzerland, but in keeping with its policy of decentralisation of control, it has six Regional Offices in:

Alexandria:	E. Mediterranean region
Brazzaville:	African region
Copenhagen:	European region
Manila:	W. Pacific region
New Delhi:	S.E. Asia region
Washington:	Region for the Americas.

The staff of the secretariats are highly qualified experts from many disciplines, including nursing, along with the necessary support staff.

The role of WHO

According to its constitution, WHO's main role is to encourage and assist the governments in its 160 member countries to fulfil their responsibilities for the health of the people. Among other things, its functions are:

- to promote the development and improvement of health services
- to collate and disseminate information on all matters pertaining to the public health
- to further research and the application of recent advances in health care

The activities of WHO

WHO's objective is defined in its constitution as: 'the attainment by all peoples of the highest possible level of health.' To achieve this broad objective, the constitution mentions activities such as:

- stimulating the eradication of epidemic, endemic and other diseases
- promoting the prevention of accidental injuries
- providing safe water supplies
- improving nutrition, housing, sanitation, recreation, working conditions and other aspects of environmental hygiene
- promoting maternal and child health; family health
- improving mental health
- promoting co-operation among scientific and professional groups contributing to the advancement of health
- maintaining epidemiological and statistical services
- promoting international standards for food, biological and pharmaceutical products
- assisting and developing informed public opinion on health matters
- educating and training appropriate health personnel

The publications of WHO

WHO has a wide range of publications associated with its activities. Technical publications deal with the results of scientific work supported or promoted by WHO, such as the recommendations of expert groups who investigate a specific topic, and information from member countries about, for example, health statistics or health legislation. Official publications include decisions of the Executive Board and the World Health Assembly, its policy-making body. In addition, there is *World Health*, an illustrated magazine for the general public highlighting some of the striking aspects of public health work; the *WHO Chronicle*, available every 2 months for the medical and public health professions and providing information about the principal health activities undertaken in the various countries; and *World Health Forum*, a quarterly for policy-makers, health planners, administrators, health educators and public health workers of all kinds for international exchange of health information.

WHO's response to changing needs

The profound changes which have occurred in the world since WHO was founded have inevitably affected the methods used by the organisation in dealing with health problems. For example, from many world-scale attacks on epidemic diseases, the emphasis is now shifting to issues such as the poverty-malnutrition-infection syndrome; community organisation at village level as a prerequisite for rural health development; the risks to mothers and children of unplanned fertility; and the maldistribution of health resources.

For these types of problems, relationships with ministries of health are not enough; there must be co-operation with other ministries and agencies whose activities are closely related to the maintenance of health. The emphasis is therefore altering. Instead of mounting a WHO project in a country as was the case in the early years, the accent is on technical co-operation with a national programme planned by the country itself. In essence it is a change from what was termed a well-intentioned, international paternalism to an era of international collaboration; from a donor/recipient relationship to democratic co-operation. At the annual meeting of the World Health Assembly in Geneva, Dr H. Mahler the Director-General maintained that the shift to technical co-operation was far from complete and emphasised that one of the main objectives of the 1984–85 budget (US $520 million) was to build up each country's capacity to work out and carry out a national strategy for 'health for all by the year 2000' and strengthen the health infrastructure. The emphasis on primary health care as a means of achieving 'health for all by the year 2000' has been a central theme in WHO's activities since the WHO/UNICEF Conference in Alma Ata 1978, when 142 member states agreed to adopt this approach to the promotion of health.

The methods of achieving its objectives have changed but the basic principles of WHO's constitution remain valid, one of which is often quoted:

… the enjoyment of the highest attainable standard of health is one of the fundamental rights of every human being without distinction of race, religion, political belief, economic or social condition.

Appendix 2

THE INTERNATIONAL COUNCIL OF NURSES

The International Council of Nurses was founded in 1899 and is the oldest international professional organisation in the health care field. It is an independent, non-governmental federation of national nurses' associations from 95 countries (June 1984) for example in the U.K. it is the Royal College of Nursing, and in the U.S.A. the American Nurses Association. Through them ICN represents almost a million nurses around the world. The ICN is supported by annual dues from member associations based on a stipulated fee for each nurse in membership. In recent years all member associations paid the full per capita fee but the governing body, the CNR, agreed that from 1984, the fee would be graduated according to the World Bank Atlas GNP population and growth rate for the country in which the member Association is situated. In this way, some member associations pay 50% of the fee, some 75% and others 100% of the stipulated fee. Only one association from each country can be in membership with ICN.

Objectives

- to promote the development of strong national nurses' associations
- to assist national nurses' associations to improve the standards of nursing and the competence of nurses
- to assist national nurses' associations to improve the status of nurses within their countries
- to serve as the authoritative voice for nurses and nursing internationally

Policy statements

The activities of ICN reflect the interest of its international membership and policy statements have been devised on topics such as nursing practice, nursing education, planning and policy-making, nursing research, legislation, and economic and general welfare of nurses.

Broader issues are also included, such as statements on the role of the nurse in relation to family planning, to safeguarding the environment, to smoking, to the care of detainees and prisoners, to refugees and displaced persons, and to nuclear war.

Publications

A bi-monthly journal, the *International Nursing Review*, is published by ICN with articles and information on topical issues around the world. There are also several professional publications dealing with, for example, ethical considerations in nursing and the socioeconomic welfare of nurses.

Fellowships

The ICM/3M Nursing Fellowship programme awards fellowships annually for further study in nursing to three international winners selected by ICN from a list of national nominees submitted by member associations.

The Florence Nightingale International Foundation

This endowed trust, administered by ICN, was established to maintain a permanent memorial to Florence Nightingale. The monies can be used for any educational purpose related to the nursing profession in any part of the world.

Structure

CNR and Congress

The governing body of the ICN is the Council of National Representatives (CNR) which is composed of the presidents of the 95 member associations. The CNR meets every 2 years to determine policy matters and each of the 95 countries has one vote in the decision-making process. Every fourth year the CNR is held in conjunction with a Congress, which is open to nurses throughout the world.

Board of Directors

At the quadrennial Congress, the CNR elects the 15-member Board of Directors: a President, 3 Vice-Presidents, 7 area representatives (Africa, Eastern Mediterranean, Europe, North America, South and Central America, Southeast Asia and Western Pacific) and 4 members-at-large. The Board meets at least once a year. It takes decisions between meetings of the CNR, appoints committees, considers issues of topical interest and recommends action to the CNR.

Executive Staff

The programme of ICN is carried out by the staff of ICN. As well as visiting member associations and giving guidance when appropriate regarding their development, ICN staff deal with requests for assistance from non-member countries, giving advice on matters related to nursing and nurses, and assisting them in the formation/conduct of their national associations.

ICN headquarters is situated in Geneva and is favourably placed to permit maximum co-operation and collaboration with many other international organisations centred in Switzerland, such as the World Health Organization, the International Labour Office and the League of Red Cross Societies.

ICN is also in contact with the work of the United Nations by means of its relationship with the United Nations Educational, Scientific, and Cultural Organization (UNESCO) and the United Nations International Children's Fund (UNICEF), and is on the Consultative Register of the Economic and Social Council (ECOSOC).

The ICN programme covers a number of issues but currently there is a major emphasis on two areas — the contribution of nursing to primary health care (PHC) as defined by WHO/UNICEF at the Alma Ata Conference in 1978; and the socioeconomic welfare of nurses.

ICN was represented at the WHO/UNICEF Conference on Primary Health Care and made a Statement about nursing's contribution to PHC. A year later at the CNR in Kenya, a workshop was held to pool ideas from member associations and develop a strategy which would provide guidelines for action, and the resulting document was circulated to all associations by January 1980. Reports on action were made at the ICN Congress in 1981 and subsequently workshops have been held in some of the seven ICN areas to provide opportunities for collaboration and exchange of ideas on a regional basis. In every country, nurses are key members of the health team and have enormous potential to promote health, and prevent disease as well as to care for those who are sick.

PHC is concerned with nursing; socioeconomic welfare is concerned with nurses. Although all of ICN's national associations need to be concerned about the welfare of their members, the problems can be very different depending on the size and degree of influence of the association, its financial and other resources, the national legislation of the country, and a host of other factors. ICN assists associations through the provision of advice and expertise, and the sharing of information and experience. At international level, ICN works closely with other organisations especially the International Labour Organization (ILO) in promoting the status of nurses. In June 1977, the International Labour Conference adopted a Convention and Recommendation on the Conditions of Life and Work of Nursing Personnel. ICN and its member associations contributed to the content and lobbied for the adoption of these international standards.

Members

The most important people in any organisation are the members and ICN gives nurses the opportunity to be represented internationally in matters affecting their profession and, by so doing, their personal future.

The ICN is organised and functions unrestricted by considerations of nationality, race, creed, colour, politics, sex and social status.

Appendix 3

THE EEC* NURSING DIRECTIVES

The European Economic Community Nursing Directives were signed by the Council of Ministers of the EEC on 27 June 1977 and were implemented in June 1979. They refer only to nurses responsible for general care although since then Midwifery Directives have also been signed (January 1980). More recently factual information has been collected from member states about the availability, or otherwise, of specific educational programmes leading to a qualification in the nursing care of the mentally ill and a report, collating this material, was produced in 1983. In 1984 the nursing profession in countries of the EEC were consulted about the possibility of freedom of movement for psychiatric nurses. Similar information is also being gathered about programmes for the nursing of sick children, and it is expected that a similar exercise will be conducted in the near future related to nursing of people who are mentally handicapped.

In EEC terminology, a directive is a declaration which has binding force as to the result to be achieved but which leaves to the signatory national authorities, the form and method of implementation.

Historical outline

The idea of European federal union is not new. Since the time of the Roman Empire, there have been plans for corporate action, which have met with varying degrees of success. However, the idea was given new impetus in 1946 when Winston Churchill said in his famous speech at the University of Zurich: 'we must create a sort of united states of Europe'. Various countries in western Europe took up the challenge, and after many discussions the Treaty of Rome was signed in 1957 by 'the Six' — Belgium, France, Germany, Italy, Luxembourg, The

Netherlands — and the European Economic Community was created.

One of the EEC's aims was to achieve greater unity between member countries, and one means of achieving this was to have free movement of personnel. For professional groups, free movement involves common agreement about minimum standards of education. To give advice about nursing, the EEC, in 1971, recognised the Permanent Committee of Nurses in liaison with the EEC (PCN). This committee included representatives from the national nurses' associations in most western European countries and from the International Council of Nurses (ICN) and, in the course of its deliberations, it collected much data about nursing in member states.

Around this time several activities were in progress in the United Kingdom. The Royal College of Nursing (RCN) set up a Standing Committee on the EEC and also sent a representative to a similar committee set up by the British Medical Association. The U.K. became a member of the Community in 1973 (along with Denmark and Eire to create 'the Nine'); in 1975 the EEC Medical Directives were signed; and in 1977 the Nursing Directives were signed.

Main points in the EEC nursing directives

1. Mutual Recognition

One of the main issues is the mutual recognition of qualifications. Nationals of a member state who have a nursing qualification given by a member state are able to practise in any other member state by:

a. being 'established' in another member state (this usually means living or working there)
   or
b. 'providing services' while temporarily visiting a member state.

---

*In some documents there is a trend to refer to the European Community, i.e. EC.

365

This applies to individuals holding a qualification recognised by a 'competent authority' and in the U.K. the competent authority is the U.K. Central Council for Nursing, Midwifery and Health Visiting. In the U.K. the rights of nurses who have had their names entered on the appropriate register prior to the date of implementation, and have qualifications which meet EEC regulations, are treated as if they were obtained on or after the implementation date. For pre-1979 programmes which do not meet EEC requirements, the nurse must provide evidence of 3 years' practice as a registered nurse in her own country.

2. Education Qualifications
Any agreement about mutual recognition of qualifications inevitably involves agreement about minimum standards in the educational preparation of holders of the qualification. The Directives therefore stipulate that the minimum period for the basic programme of the general nurse is 46 00 hours *or* 3 years and should consist of two parts:

A. Theoretical instruction
   a. nursing:
      nature and ethics of the profession
      general principles of health and nursing
      nursing principles in relation to:
      ● general and specialist medicine
      ● general and specialist surgery
      ● child care and paediatrics
      ● maternity care
      ● mental health and psychiatry
      ● care of the old and geriatrics
   b. basic sciences:
      anatomy and physiology
      pathology
      bacteriology, virology, parasitology, biophysics,
      biochemistry and radiology
      dietetics
      hygiene: preventive medicine
                    health education
      pharmacology
   c. social sciences:
      sociology
      psychology
      principles of administration
      principles of teaching
      social and health legislation
      legal aspects of nursing
B. Clinical instruction
   nursing in relation to:
   ● general and specialist medicine
   ● general and specialist surgery
   ● child care and paediatrics
   ● maternity care
   ● mental health and psychiatry

● care of the old and geriatrics
● home nursing

The number of hours of theoretical and clinical instruction must amount to no less than one-third and one-half respectively of the total hours of instruction given in the complete programme; the remainder of the period being apportioned according to the needs of the educational programmes approved by the competent authorities in the member states.

3. Quality of care
It is understandable that in any member state there might be concern about the quality of care given by incoming nurses as a consequence of the EEC Nursing Directives. To overcome this, machinery for monitoring quality has been set up — the Advisory Committee on Training in Nursing — and its task is: 'to help to ensure a comparably high standard of training of the various categories of nursing personnel throughout the Community'. This is achieved by discussion and consultation, by exchange of information about content and methods of teaching, and by reviewing developments in nursing practice and in the medical and social sciences.

4. Discipline
Another subject closely allied to the maintenance of standards is the provision of machinery to deal with disciplinary matters. In the U.K. as far as the Nursing (and Midwifery) Directives are concerned, the conduct of a nurse from another EEC country is subject to discipline by the U.K. Central Council for Nursing, Midwifery and Health Visiting as if she or he were a U.K. registered nurse and a U.K. national. Provision is made within the directives for the competent authority in each country to inform member states when 'knowledge of a serious matter' comes to their attention if this impinges on professional recognition.

5. Language
Article 15.3 of the Directive, concerned with mutual recognition, places a duty on member states to: 'see to it that, where appropriate, the persons concerned acquire, in their interests and that of their patients, the linguistic knowledge necessary for the exercise of their profession in the host member state'. In all countries of 'the Ten it has been agreed that the responsibility lies with the employing authority to ascertain language competence.'*

6. Implementation
When the Medical Directives were signed, the Committee of Senior Officials on Public Health was created with the task of identifying any difficulties which might

*Greece joined the EEC in 1980

arise from the implementation of the Directives. When the Nursing Directives were signed, the terms of reference of the Committee of Senior Officials were extended to collect all relevant information on the conditions under which nursing care is given by nurses responsible for general care in member states; and this committee is now concerned on an intercountry basis with the implementation of directives related to all professional groups.

SUGGESTED READING

Allan P. 1984 Making the European connection. Nursing Times 80(18) May 2:19–20

Official Journal of the European Communities 1977 Legislation 20: L176. HMSO, London

Quinn S. 1978 Nursing — the EEC dimension. Nursing Times Occasional Paper 74(1) January 5:1–4

Standing Committee of Nurses of the EEC (PCN) 1983 Outline of the conditions of service of first level nurses in the countries of the European Communities. Royal College of Nursing, London

Appendix 4

SYSTÈME INTERNATIONAL (SI) UNITS

In the White Paper Command 4880, 1972, the U.K. Government announced its intention to change over to metrication in 1975. At an international convention in 1960, the General Conference of Weights and Measures had agreed to promulgate an International System of Units, frequently described as SI or Système International. This is merely the name for the current version of the metric system, first introduced in France at the end of the 18th century.

In any system of measurement, the magnitude of some physical quantities must be arbitrarily selected and declared to have unit value. These magnitudes form a set of standards and are called *basic units*. All other units are *derived units*.

Basic units

The SI has seven basic units and nurses will commonly be using four of these:

Name of SI Unit	Symbol for SI Unit	Quantity
metre	m	length
kilogram	kg	mass
second	s	time
mole	mol	amount of substance

Derived units

Derived units are obtained by appropriate combinations of basic units:

  unit area results when unit length is multiplied by unit length
  unit density results when unit weight (mass) is divided by unit volume

Some derived units have special names and symbols and will be encountered in relation to dietetics and laboratory reports:

Name of SI Unit	Symbol for SI Unit	Quantity
joule	J	work, energy, quantiy of heat
pascal	Pa	pressure
newton	N	force

Decimal multiples and submultiples

The metric system uses multiples of 10 to express number.

Multiples and submultiples of the basic unit are expressed as decimals and the following prefixes are used:

Multiples and sub-multiples of units

Multiplication factor		Prefix	Symbol
1 000 000 000 000	10^{12}	tera	T
1 000 000 000	10^9	giga	G
1 000 000	10^6	mega	M
1 000	10^3	kilo	k
100	10^2	hecto	h
10	10^1	deca	da
0.1	10^{-1}	deci	d
0.01	10^{-3}	centi	c
0.001	10^{-3}	milli	m
0.000 001	10^{-6}	micro	μ
0.000 000 001	10^{-9}	nano	n
0.000 000 000 001	10^{-12}	pico	p
0.000 000 000 000 001	10^{-15}	femto	f
0.000 000 000 000 000 001	10^{-18}	atto	a

The most widely used prefixes are kilo, mili and micro (μ):

$$0.000\,001\,g = 10 - {}^6g = 1\,\mu g$$

Rules for using units

a. The symbol for a unit is unaltered in the plural and should not be followed by a full stop except at the end of the sentence:

> 5 cm *not* 5cm. or 5 cms.

b. The decimal sign between digits is indicated by a full stop in typing. No commas are used to divide large numbers into groups of three, but a half-space (whole space in typing) is left after every third digit. If the numerical value of the number is less than 1 unit, a zero should precede the decimal sign:

> 0.123 456 *not* .123,456

c. The SI symbol for 'day' (i.e. 24 hours) is 'd', but urine and faecal excretions of substances should preferably be expressed as 'per 24 hours':

> g/24 h

d. 'Squared' and 'cubed' are expressed as numerical powers and not by abbreviation:

> square centimetre is cm^2 *not* sq cm.

Commonly used measurements

a. Temperature is expressed as degrees Celsius (°C) and the standard thermometer is graded 32–42°C.

> 1° Celsius = 1°Centigrade

b. The calorie is replaced by the joule:

> 1 calorie = 4.2 J
> 1 Calorie (dietetic use) = 4.2 kilojoules = 4.2 kJ

The previous 1000 Calorie reducing diet is expressed (approximately) as a 4000 kJ diet.

1 g of fat provides	38 kJ
1 g of protein provides	17 kJ
1 g of carbohydrate provides	16 kJ

c. Equivalent concentration mEq/1 is commonly used for reporting results of monovalent electrolyte measurements (sodium, potassium, chloride and bicarbonate). It is not part of the SI system and should be replaced by molar concentration — in these examples mmol/1.

For these four measurements, the numerical value will not change.

d. The SI unit of pressure is the pascal (Pa). Blood gas measurements should be given in the SI unit kPa instead of mmHg.

> 1 mmHg = 133.32 Pa
> 1 kPa = 7.5006 mmHg

Column measurement will be *retained* in clinical practice *as at present*.

> blood pressure (in mmHg)
> cerebrospinal fluid (in mmH_2O)
> central venous pressure (in cmH_2O)

SUGGESTED READING

Department of Trade and Industry 1972 Metrication. HMSO, London
Have you gone SI, nurse? 1973 Nursing Mirror, 136 (1): 18; (2): 14; (3): 42; (4): 33; (5): 29
SI: the international system of units. 1973 HMSO, London

Appendix 5

PUBLICATIONS BY ROPER, LOGAN & TIERNEY

Articles

Roper N, Logan W, Tierney A 1983 A model for nursing. Nursing Times 79 (9) March 2: 24–27

Roper N, Logan W, Tierney A 1983 Nursing process
1. A nursing model. Nursing Mirror 156 (21) May 25: 17–19
2. Is there a danger of 'processing' patients? Nursing Mirror 156 (22) June 1: 32–33
3. Problems or needs? Nursing Mirror 156 (23) June 8: 43–44
4. Identifying the goals. Nursing Mirror 156 (24) June 15: 22–23
5. Endless paperwork? Nursing Mirror 156 (25) June 22: 34–35
6. Unity — with diversity. Nursing Mirror 156 (26) June 29: 35

Books

Roper N, Logan W, Tierney A 1980 The elements of nursing. Churchill Livingstone, Edinburgh

Roper N, Logan W, Tierney A 1981 Learning to use the process of nursing. Churchill Livingstone, Edinburgh

Roper N, Logan W, Tierney A (eds) 1983 Using a model for nursing. Churchill Livingstone, Edinburgh

Index